U.S. Department of
Homeland Security

United States
Coast Guard

Commandant
United States Coast Guard

2100 2ND ST SW STOP 7902
Washington DC 20593-7902
Staff Symbol: CG-11
Phone: (202) 475-5173
Fax: (202) 475-5909

COMDTINST M6000.1E
APR 29 2011

COMMANDANT INSTRUCTION M6000.1E

I0297058

Subj: COAST GUARD MEDICAL MANUAL

1. PURPOSE. This Manual establishes policies, procedures, and health care standards for all active duty and reserve Coast Guard members and other Service Members assigned to duty with the Coast Guard.

2. ACTION. All Coast Guard unit commanders, commanding officers, officers-in-charge, deputy/assistant commanders, and chief of headquarters staff elements shall comply with the provisions of this Notice, Instruction, or Manual. Internet release is authorized.

3. DIRECTIVES AFFECTED. The Coast Guard Medical Manual, COMDTINST M6000.1D, is cancelled.

4. MAJOR CHANGES. Major changes to this Manual include: updated guidance on the Periodic Health Assessment and incorporation of modernization initiatives, more specifically the Health, Safety, and Work-Life Service Center.

5. PROCEDURES. No paper distribution will be made of this Manual. Official distribution will be via the Coast Guard Directives System (CGDS) DVD. An electronic version will be located on the following Information and Technology CG-612 web sites Intranet: http://cgweb.comdt.uscg.mil/CGDirectives/Welcome.htm, Internet: http://www.uscg.mil/directives/, and CGPortal: http://cgportal.uscg.mil/delivery/Satellite/CG612.

6. ENVIRONMENTAL ASPECT AND IMPACT CONSIDERATIONS. Environmental considerations were examined in the development of this Manual and have been determined not to be applicable.

DISTRIBUTION – SDL No. 158

	a	b	c	d	e	f	g	h	i	j	k	l	m	n	o	p	q	r	s	t	u	v	w	x	y	z
A	1	1	1	1	1	1	1	1	1	1		1	1	1	1	1		1		1						
B	1	1	1	1	1	1	1	1	1	1	1	1	1	1		1	1	1	1	1	1	1	1	1	1	
C	1	1	1	1	1	1	1	1	1		1	1	1	1	1	1	1	1	1	1	1	1	1	1	1	1
D	1	1	1	1			1	1			1	1		1	1	1		1			1					
E	1	1		1	1		1	1										1								
F																	1	1	1							
G			1	1	1																					
H																										

COMDTINST M6000.1E

7. **PRIVACY COMPLIANCE.** When completed, the numerous forms identified in this Manual contain Sensitive Personally Identifiable Information (SPII). The Privacy Act of 1974, 5 U.S.C. 552a mandates that agencies establish administrative, technical, and physical safeguards to ensure the integrity of records maintained on individuals. The Privacy Act also requires the protection against any anticipated threats which could result in substantial harm, embarrassment or compromise to an individual. In order to maintain the public's trust and prevent privacy breaches, the Coast Guard has a duty to safeguard all types of Personally Identifiable Information (PII) in its possession. Unintended disclosure or compromise of an individual's PII constitutes a Privacy Incident and must be reported in accordance with COMDTINST 5260.5 (series), Privacy Incident Response, Notification and Reporting Procedures for Personally Identifiable Information.

8. **RECORDS MANAGEMENT.** All data/documents created for Coast Guard use and delivered to, or falling under the legal control of the Coast Guard are Federal records. Ensure that all records created as a result of processes prescribed in this directive are maintained and disposed of in accordance with the Coast Guard Information and Life Cycle Management Manual, COMDTINST M5212.12 (series).

9. **FORMS/REPORTS.** The forms referenced in this Manual are available in USCG Electronic Forms on the Standard Workstation or on the Internet: http://www.uscg.mil/forms/, CG Central at http://cgcentral.uscg.mil/, and Intranet at http://cgweb2.comdt.uscg.mil/CGFORMS/Welcome.htm.

                                                Mark J. Tedesco /s/
                                                Director of Health, Safety, and Work-Life

RECORD OF CHANGES			
CHANGE NUMBER	DATE OF CHANGE	DATE ENTERED	BY WHOM ENTERED

This page intentionally left blank.

Medical Manual
Table of Contents

CHAPTER 1

ORGANIZATION AND PERSONNEL

Section A. Organization.

1. Mission of the CG Health Services Program 1
2. Director of Health, Safety, and Work-Life 1
3. Health, Safety, and Work-Life Service Center (HSWL SC) 3
4. Responsibilities of Commands with Health Care Facilities 5
5. Governance 5

Section B. Personnel.

1. Chief of the Clinical Staff 1
2. Collateral Duty Command Surgeons 1
3. Regional Manager (RM) 1
4. Regional Practice Director (RPD) 3
5. Regional Practice Senior Medical Executives (SME) 3
6. Regional Practice Senior Dental Executive (SDE) 5
7. Regional Practice Senior Independent Duty Health Services Technician (SIDHS) 6
8. Regional Pharmacy Executive (RPE) 6
9. Senior Health Services Officer (SHSO) 6
10. General Duties of Medical Officers 7
11. Duties of Flight Surgeons 13
12. General Duties of Dental Officers 15
13. General Duties of Pharmacy Officers 17
14. HSWL SC Pharmacy Officers 18
15. Environmental Health Officers 19
16. Clinic Administrators 21
17. Physician Assistants (PA) and Nurse Practitioners (NP) 23
18. Contract Health Care Providers 25
19. TRICARE Management Activity-Aurora (TMA) Liaison Officer 25
20. Health Services Technicians 26
21. Health Services Technicians - with a Dental Qualification Code (13) 28
22. Independent Duty Health Services Technicians (IDHS) 29
23. CG Beneficiary Representatives at Uniformed Services Medical Treatment Facilities (USMTF) 33
24. CG Representative at the Department of Defense Medical Examination Review Board (DODMERB) 35
25. Health Benefits Advisors (HBA) 36
26. Dental Hygienists 38
27. Red Cross Volunteers 39

28. Volunteers...39

Section C. CG Health Services Officer Training Matrix.

1. Introduction..1

Tables.

Table 1-C-1 CG Medical Officer Matrix..1
Table 1-C-2 CG Dental Officer Matrix..2
Table 1-C-3 CG Leadership Courses Matrix...3
Table 1-C-4 CG Chemical, Biological, Radiological, Nuclear, and Explosive
(CBRNE) Courses Matirx...4
Table 1-C-5 CG Disaster Training Matrix...5

CHAPTER 2

HEALTH CARE AND FACILITIES

Section A. Health Care for Active Duty Personnel.

1. Care at Uniformed Services Medical Treatment Facilities...................................1
2. Emergency Care..3
3. Dental Care and Treatment 6
4. Consent to and Refusal of Treatment..11
5. Elective Surgery for Pre-Existing Defects 13
6. Elective Health Care 13
7. Other Health Insurance (OHI) 14
8. Procedures for Obtaining Non-Emergent Health Care from Nonfederal Sources.............15
9. Obtaining Vasectomies and Tubal Ligations from Nonfederal Providers.........17
10. Care at Department of Veterans Affairs (DVA) Medical Facilities 17
11. HIPAA and the Uses and Disclosures of Health Information of Active Duty
Personnel..18

Section B. Health Care for Reserve Personnel.

1. Eligibility for Emergency Treatment at any DOD, CG or Civilian Medical Facility..........1
2. Care at Uniformed Services Medical Treatment Facilities..................................1
3. Non-Emergent Care at Other Than CG or DOD Facilities..................................3

Section C. Health Care for Retired Personnel.

1. Care at Uniformed Services Medical Treatment Facilities..................................1
2. Care under TRICARE Standard and Extra (formerly CHAMPUS)....................1
3. Care at Veterans Administration Medical Facilities...1

Section D. Health Care for Dependents.

1. Care at Uniformed Services Medical Treatment Facilities 1
2. Referral for Civilian Medical Care (DD-2161) 1
3. Rights of Minors to Health Care Services 2

Section E. Care for Preadoptive Children and Wards of the Court.

1. General 1
2. Secretary's Designation 1

Section F. Health Care for Other Persons.

1. Members of the Auxiliary 1
2. Temporary Members of the Reserve 1
3. Members of Foreign Military Services 2
4. Federal Employees 3
5. Seamen 3
6. Non-Federally Employed Civilians Aboard CG Vessels 3
7. Civilians Physical Exams prior to Entry to the CG 4

Section G. Medical Regulating.

1. Transfer of Patients at CG Expense 1
2. Travel Via Ambulance of Patients to Obtain Care 1
3. Aeromedical Evacuation of Patients 1

Section H. Defense Enrollment Eligibility Reporting System (DEERS) in CG Health Care Facilities.

1. Defense Enrollment Eligibility Reporting System 1
2. Responsibilities 1
3. Performing DEERS Checks 1
4. Eligibility/Enrollment Questions, Fraud and Abuse 2
5. Denial of Non-emergency Health Care Benefits for Individuals Not Enrolled in Defense Enrollment Eligibility Reporting System (DEERS) 3
6. DEERS Eligibility Overrides 3

Section I. Health Care Facility Definitions.

1. CG Facilities 1
2. Department of Defense Medical Facilities 2
3. Uniformed Services Military Treatment Facilities (USMTFs) 2

Section J. Policies and Procedures Required at CG Health Care Facilities.

1. Administrative Policies and Procedures 1
2. Operational Policies and Procedures 1
3. Patient Rights..2
4. Health Care Provider Identification 3

Section K. General Standards of Care.

1. Standard of care 1
2. Diagnosis and therapy..1
3. Bases for Diagnoses..1
4. Treatment 1
5. Time Line for Treatment..1
6. Correct-site Surgery Policy..2
7. Patients role..2
8. Documentation...2

CHAPTER 3

PHYSICAL STANDARDS AND EXAMINATION

Section A. Administrative Procedures

1. Applicability of Physical Standards...1
2. Prescribing of Physical Standards..1
3. Purpose of Physical Standards..1
4. Application of Physical Standards..1
5. Interpretation of Physical Standards...2
6. Definitions of Terms Used in this Chapter 2
7. Required Physical Examinations and Their Time Limitations 3
8. Waiver of Physical Standards 10
9. Substitution of Physical Examinations 12

Section B. Medical Examination (DD-2808) and Medical History (DD-2807-1)

1. Report of Medical Examination DD-2808..1
2. Report of Medical History DD-2807-1 1
3. Findings and Recommendations of Report of Medical Examination (DD-2808) 1
4. Correction of Defects Prior to Overseas Transfer or Sea Duty Deployment........................5
5. Objection to Assumption of Fitness for Duty at Separation 5
6. Separation Not Appropriate by Reason of Physical Disability 6
7. Procedures for Physical Defects Found Prior to Separation 6

Figure 3-B-1 7
Figure 3-B-2 8

Section C. Medical Examination Techniques and Lab Testing Standards

1. Scope 1
2. Speech Impediment 1
3. Head, Face, Neck, and Scalp (Item 17 of DD-2808) 1
4. Nose, Sinuses, Mouth, and Throat (Item 19, 20 of DD-2808) 2
5. Ears (General) and Drums (Item 21, 22 of DD-2808) 2
6. Eyes (General), Ophthalmoscopic, and Pupils (Item 23, 24, 25 of DD-2808) ..3
7. Ocular Mobility (Item 26 of DD-2808) 5
8. Heart and Vascular System (Item 27 of DD-2808) 5
9. Lungs and Chest (Item 28 of DD-2808) 9
10. Anus and Rectum (Item 30 of DD-2808) 11
11. Abdomen and Viscera (Item 31 of DD-2808) 11
12. Genitourinary System (Item 32 of DD-2808) 11
13. Extremities (Item 33, 34, 35 of DD-2808) 12
14. Spine and Other Musculoskeletal (Item 36 of DD-2808) 14
15. Identifying Body Marks, Scars, and Tattoos (Item 37 of DD-2808) 15
16. Neurologic (Item 39 of DD-2808) 16
17. Psychiatric (Item 40 of DD-2808) 17
18. Endocrine System 18
19. Dental (Item 43 of DD-2808) 18
20. Laboratory Findings 19
Figure 3-C-1 25
21. Height, Weight and Body Build 26
22. Distant Visual Acuity and Other Eye Tests 26
23. Audiometer 33
24. Psychological and Psychomotor 33
Figure 3-C-2 34
Figure 3-C-3 37
Figure 3-C-4 38

Section D. Medical Standards for Appointment, Enlistment and Induction in the Armed Forces

1. Scope 1
2. Medical Standards 1
3. Policy 2
4. Responsibilities of Commandant (CG-11) 2
5. Height 3
6. Weight 3
7. Head 3
8. Eyes 3
9. Vision 7
10. Ears 8

11.	Hearing	8
12.	Nose, Sinuses, Mouth and Larynx	9
13.	Dental	10
14.	Neck	11
15.	Lungs, Chest Wall, Pleura, and Mediastinum	11
16.	Heart	13
17.	Abdominal Organs and Gastrointestinal System	16
18.	Female Genitalia	19
19.	Male Genitalia	20
20.	Urinary System	21
21.	Spine and Sacroiliac Joints	22
22.	Upper Extremities	23
23.	Lower Extremities	25
24.	Miscellaneous Conditions of the Extremities	27
25.	Vascular System	28
26.	Skin and Cellular Tissues	29
27.	Blood and Blood-Forming Tissues	31
28.	Systemic	31
29.	Endocrine and Metabolic	34
30.	Neurologic	35
31.	Learning, Psychiatric, and Behavioral	37
32.	Tumors and Malignancies	40
33.	Miscellaneous	40
Figure 3-D-1 Evaluation for Risk OF Head Injury Sequelae		42
Figure 3-D-2 Classification and Comparative nomenclature of Cervical Smears		43

Section E. Physical Standards for Programs Leading to Commission

1.	Appointment as Cadet, USCG Academy	1
2.	Commissioning of Cadets	2
3.	Enrollment as an Officer Candidate	2
4.	Commissioning of Officer Candidates	3
5.	Coast Guard Direct Commission Program	4
6.	Direct Commission in the CG Reserve	4
7.	Direct Commission of Licensed Officers of U. S. Merchant Marine	4
8.	Appointment to Warrant Grade	4

Section F. Physical Standards Applicable to All Personnel (Regular and Reserve) For: Reenlistment; Enlistment of Prior Service USCG Personnel; Retention; Overseas Duty; and Sea Duty

1.	General Instructions	1
2.	Use of List of Disqualifying Conditions and Defects	1
3.	Head and Neck	2
4.	Esophagus, Nose, Pharynx, Larynx, and Trachea	2

5.	Eyes	2
6.	Ears and Hearing	5
7.	Lungs and Chest Wall	5
8.	Heart and Vascular System	7
9.	Abdomen and Gastrointestinal System	9
10.	Endocrine and Metabolic Conditions (Diseases)	11
11.	Genitourinary System	12
12.	Extremities	14
13.	Spine, Scapulae, Ribs, and Sacroiliac Joints	17
14.	Skin and Cellular Tissues	18
15.	Neurological Disorders	19
16.	Psychiatric Disorders. (See section 5-B concerning disposition)	20
17.	Dental	21
18.	Blood and Blood-Forming Tissue Diseases	21
19.	Systemic Diseases, General Defects, and Miscellaneous Conditions	22
20.	Tumors and Malignant Diseases	23
21.	Sexually Transmitted Diseases	23
22.	Human Immunodeficiency Virus (HIV)	23
23.	Transplant recipient	24

Section G. Physical Standards for Aviation

1.	Classification of Aviation Personnel	1
2.	General Instructions for Aviation Examinations	1
3.	Restrictions Until Physically Qualified	4
4.	Standards for Class 1	4
5.	Candidates for Flight Training	7
6.	Requirements for Class 2 Aircrew	10
7.	Requirements for Class 2 Medical Personnel	10
8.	Requirements for Class 2 Technical Observers	11
9.	Requirements for Class 2 Air Traffic Controllers	11
10.	Requirements for Landing Signal Officer (LSO)	11
11.	Refractive Surgery	12
12.	Contact Lenses	13

<u>Section H. Physical Examinations and Standards for Diving Duty</u>

| 1. | Examinations | 1 |
| 2. | Standards | 2 |

CHAPTER 4

HEALTH RECORDS AND FORMS

Section A. Health Records.

1. Purpose and Background 1
2. Contents of the Health Record 1
3. Custody of Health Records 4
4. Opening Health Records 6
5. Checking out the Health Record 7
6. Terminating Health Records 10
7. Creating an Additional Volume 13
8. Lost, Damaged, or Destroyed Health Records 13
9. Accuracy and Completeness Check 14

Section B. Health Record Forms.

FORM	TITLE	
1. CG-3443	Health Record Cover	1
2. CG-5266	Drug Sensitivity Sticker	2
3. DD-2766	Adult Preventive and Chronic Care Flowsheet Form	2
4. SF-513	Consultation Sheet	3
5. SF-507	Medical Record	4
6. DD-2795	Pre-Deployment Health Assessment	4
7. DD-2796	Post-Deployment Health Assessment	4
8. DD-2900	Post-Deployment Health Re-Assessment	4
9. CG-6020	Medical Recommendation for Flying	5
10. DD-2808	Report of Medical Examination	5
11. DD-2807-1	Report of Medical History	11
12. CG-5447	History and Report of OMSEP Examination	15
13. CG-5447A	Periodic History and Report of OMSEP Examination	18
14. CG-5684	Medical Board Report Cover Sheet	19
15. SF-600	Chronological Record of Medical Care	19
16. SF-558	Emergency Care and Treatment	22
17. CG-5214	Emergency Medical Treatment Report	23
18. SF-519	Radiographic Reports	25
19. Laboratory Reports		26
20. DD-771	Eyewear Prescription	26
21. SF-602	Syphilis Record	28
22. OF-522	Authorization for Anesthesia, Operations, etc.	28
23. DD-1141	Record of Occupational Exposure to Ionizing Radiation	28
24. Audiogram Results		30
25. DD-2215	Reference Audiogram	30

26. DD-2216	Hearing Conservation Data	30
27. CG-4057	Chronological Record of Service	30
28. DD-2870	Authorization for Disclosure of Medical or Dental Information	31
29. DD-2871	Request to Restrict Medical or Dental Information	31
30. PHS-731	International Certificate of Vaccination	31
31. SF-515	Tissue Examination	32
32. DD-877	Request for Medical/Dental Records or Information	32
33. CG-6100	Modified Screening For: Overseas Assignment and/or Sea Duty Health Screening	33
34. CG-6201	Bloodborne Pathogens Exposure Guidelines	33
35. CG-6202	Examination Protocol for Exposure to: CHROMIUM COMPOUNDS	33
36. CG-6203	Examination Protocol for Exposure to: ASBESTOS	33
37. CG-6204	Examination Protocol for Exposure to: BENZENE	33
38. CG-6205	Examination Protocol for Exposure to: NOISE	33
39. CG-6206	Examination Protocol for Exposure to: HAZARDOUS WASTE	33
40. CG-6207	Examination Protocol for Exposure to: LEAD	33
41. CG-6208	Examination Protocol for Exposure to: RESPIRATOR WEAR	33
42. CG-6209	Examination Protocol for Exposure to: PESTICIDES	34
43. CG-6210	Examination Protocol for Exposure to: RESPIRATORY SENSITIZERS	34
44. CG-6211	Examination Protocol for Exposure to: BLOODBORNE PATHOGENS	34
45. CG-6212	Examination Protocol for Exposure to: TUBERCULOSIS	34
46. CG-6213	Examination Protocol for Exposure to: SOLVENTS	34
47. CG-6214	Examination Protocol for Exposure to: RADIATION	34
48. CG-6215	How to Calculate a Significant Threshold Shift	34

Section C. Dental Records Forms.

FORM   TITLE

1. CG-3443-2   Dental Record Cover 1
2. NAVMED 6600/3   Dental Health Questionnaire 2
3. SF-603   Dental Record 2
4. SF-603-A   Dental Continuation 14
5. SF-513   Consultation Sheet 14
6. Lost Dental Records 14
7. Special Dental Records Entries 14
8. Dental Examination Requirements 14
9. Recording of Dental Treatments on Chronological Record of Care, SF-600 15

Section D. Dental Records Forms.

1. Purpose and Background 1
2. Contents of Clinical Records 2
3. Extraneous Attachments 3

    4. Opening Clinical Records 3
    5. Terminating Clinical Records 4
    6. Custody of Clinical Records 4
    7. Safekeeping of Clinical Records...4
    8. Transfer of Clinical Records 4
    9. Lost Damaged or Destroyed Clinical Records..5

Section E. Employee Medical Folders.

    1. Purpose and Background 1
    2. Custody of Employee Medical Folders (EMF's)..1
    3. Contents of the Employee Medical Folders 2
    4. Accountability of Disclosures...3
    5. Opening Employee Medical Folder 3
    6. Terminating Employee Medical Folders 3
    7. Transferring to Other Government Agencies 4
    8. Lost, Damaged, or Destroyed Employee Medical Folders 4
    9. Employee Medical Folder, SF-66 D 4

Section F. Inpatient Medical Records.

    1. Purpose and Background 1
    2. Maintenance and Storage..2
    3. Disposition of IMRs..3
    4. Inpatient Medical Record Forms and Required Entries...4

Section G. Mental Health Records.

    1. Active duty..1
    2. Non-active duty...1
    3. Psychiatric Evaluation Format 1
    4. Custody of Mental Health Records...1

CHAPTER 5

DEATHS AND PSYCHIATRIC CONDITIONS

Section A. Deaths.

    1. General..1
    2. Duties of health services department 1
    3. Determining Cause of Death...1

4. Death Certificates for Deaths Occurring Away From Command or in Foreign Ports 1
5. Relations with Civilian Authorities 2
6. Reporting Deaths to Civilian Authorities 2
7. Death Forms for Civilian Agencies and Individuals 2
8. Identification of Remains 2

Section B. Psychiatric Conditions.

1. General 1
2. Personality Disorders 1
3. Adjustment Disorders 2
4. Organic Mental Disorders 2
5. Psychoactive Substance Use Disorders 3
6. Schizophrenia 3
7. Psychotic Disorders Not Elsewhere Classified 4
8. Delusional (Paranoid) Disorder 4
9. Neurotic Disorders 4
10. Mood Disorders 4
11. Anxiety Disorders (or Anxiety and Phobic Neuroses) 5
12. Somatoform Disorders 5
13. Dissociative Disorders (or Hysterical Neuroses, Dissociative Type) 5
14. Sexual Disorders 6
15. Sexual Dysfunctions 6
16. Factitious Disorders 7
17. Disorders of Impulse Control Not Elsewhere Classified 7
18. Disorders Usually First Evident in Infancy, Childhood, or Adolescence 7
19. Psychological Factors Affecting Physical Condition 9
20. V Codes for Conditions Not Attributable to a Mental Disorder that are a Focus of Attention or Treatment 9
21. Additional Codes 10

Section C. Command directed Mental Health Evaluation of Coast Guard Service members.

1. Active Duty Mental Health Evaluation Protection 1
2. Emergency Evaluations 1
3. Non-emergent Mental Health Evaluation 1
4. Service Member's Rights 2
5. Things Not To Do 2
6. Evaluations NOT covered 3
7. Memorandum Requesting a Mental Health Evaluation 3

CHAPTER 6

MEDICAL READINESS/DEPLOYMENT HEALTH

Section A. Overview.

1. Purpose..1
2. Responsibilities..1
3. Individual Medical Readiness..1
4. Standard Definitions and Scoring..1
5. Medically Ready..3
6. Deployment Definitions...3

Section B. Expeditionary Deployment.

1. Electronic Deployment Health Assessment (EDHA)..1
2. Responsibility and timeline for the EDHA..1
3. EDHA Overview..1
4. EDHA Healthcare Provider Review Process..1
5. Pre-Deployment Requirements..2
6. Deployment..3
7. Post-Deployment..3
8. DD-2900, Post-Deployment Health Reassessment via the EDHA (see above)....4
9. Compliance Program..4

Section C. Routine Deployment.

1. Pre Deployment Requirements..1
2. Deployment..1
3. Post-Deployment..1
4. Additional References..2

CHAPTER 7

PREVENTIVE MEDICINE

Section A. General.

1. Scope..1
2. Responsibilities..1

Section B. Communicable Disease Control.

1. General 1
2. Disease Outbreak 1
3. Medical Event Reporting 1
4. Figure 7-B-1 Medical Event Reporting Chart Within 24 Hours 3
5. Figure 7-B-2 Medical Event Reporting Chart Within 7 Days 4
6. Sexually Transmitted Infection (STI) Program 5
7. STI Treatment 7
8. STI Drug Prophylaxis 7
9. STI Immunizations 7
10. STI Reporting 7

Section C. Immunizations and Allergy Immunotherapy (AIT)

1. General 1
2. Unit Responsibilities 1
3. Equipment and Certification Requirement 1
4. Immunization Site Responsibilities 1
5. Immunization on Reporting for Active Duty for Training 4
6. Specific Vaccination Information 4

CHAPTER 8

FISCAL AND SUPPLY MANAGEMENT

Section A. Resource Management.

1. Unit's Commanding Officers Responsibility 1
2. Health, Safety, and Work-Life Service Center (HSWL SC) 2
3. CG Headquarters 2

Section B. General Property Management and Accountability.

1. Basic Policies 1
2. Physical Property Classifications 1
3. Property Responsibility and Accountability 1
4. Expending Property Unnecessarily 1
5. Stock Levels, Reorder Points, and Stock Limits 1
6. Transferring and Loaning Property 3

Section C. Custody, Issues, and Disposition.

1. Transferring Custody 1
2. Storerooms 1

3. Issuing Material 1
4. Inspecting Storerooms 1
5. Disposing of Property 2

Section D. Health Services Supply System.

1. Health Services Control Point..1
2. Responsibility for General Stores Items 1
3. Supply Support Assistance 1
4. Authorized Allowances...2
5. Supply Sources..2
6. Health Care Equipment...3
7. Emergency Procurement...4
8. Factors for Replacing Equipment 4

Section E. Eyeglasses and Ophthalmic Services.

1. General..1
2. Personnel Authorized Refractions 1
3. Procuring and Issuing Standard Prescription Eyewear 1
4. Aviation Prescription Lenses 3
5. Contact Lenses..3

6. Sunglasses for Polar Operations 4
7. Safety Glasses...4

CHAPTER 9

HEALTH SERVICES TECHNICIANS ASSIGNED TO INDEPENDENT DUTY

Section A. Independent Duty Afloat.

1. Introduction..1
2. Mission and Responsibilities 1
3. Providing Health Care Afloat 5
4. Training...13
5. Supply and Logistics...17
6. Health Services Department Administration 23
7. Combat Operations 26
8. Environmental Health 27

Section B. Independent Duty Ashore at Sectors, Sector Field Offices, Air Stations, and Small Boat Stations.

1. Introduction 1
2. Mission and Responsibilities 1
3. Chain Of Command 2
4. Operation of the Health Services Division 2
5. Providing Health Care 5
6. Training 9
7. Supply and Logistics 11
8. Health Services Department Administration 17
9. Search and Rescue (SAR) Operations 20
10. Environmental Health 20

Section C. Independent Duty in Support of Deployable Specialized Forces (DSF)

1. Introduction 1
2. Mission and Responsibilities 1
3. Chain Of Command 2
4. Operation of the Health Services Division 2
5. Providing Health Care 5
6. Training 10
7. Supply and Logistics 12
8. Health Services Department Administration 18
9. Tactical Operations 21
10. Environmental Health 21

Section D. Quality Improvement Compliance Program (QICP)

1. Background 1
2. Purpose 1
3. Overview 1
4. Program Elements 1
5. Collaborative Program 2
6. Monitoring the QICP 2
7. Assistance Program 2
8. Responsibility 2
9. QI Compliance Checklist 3
10. Compliance Certification Standards 3
11. Post Survey 4

Section E. Independent Duty Management of TRICARE

1. Introduction 1
2. Discussion 1
3. Access to Care 1

4. Access to Care Standards 1
5. Enrollment 2
6. Resources 2

CHAPTER 10

PHARMACY OPERATIONS AND DRUG CONTROL

Section A. Pharmacy Administration.

1. Responsibilities 1
2. Prescribers 4
3. Prescriptions 6
4. Prescribing in the Medical Record 8
5. Signatures 11
6. Dispensing 11
7. Labeling 16
8. Drug Stock 17
9. Credit Return Program (Reverse Distribution Program) 19
10. Pharmacy and Therapeutics Committee 20
11. Figure 10-A-1 Clinic Non-Prescription Medication Program 22

Section B. Controlled Substances.

1. General 1
2. Custody and Controlled Substance Audits 1
3. Drug Enforcement Administration (DEA) Registration 4
4. Reporting Theft or Loss 4
5. Procuring, Storing, Transferring, and Disposing of Controlled Substances 5
6. Prescribing Practices 7

Section C. Forms and Records.

1. General 1
2. Prescription Forms 1
3. Quality Control Forms 2
4. Controlled Drug Forms 2
5. Forms Availability 5

Section D. Drug Dispensing Without a Medical Officer.

1. General 1
2. Child-Resistant Containers 1
3. Controlled Substances 1
4. Formulary 1

5. Non-prescription Medication Program 2

CHAPTER 11

HEALTH CARE PROCUREMENT

Section A. Contracting For Health Care Services.

1. General 1
2. Type of Services 1
3. Eligibility For Contract Health Care Services 2
4. Approval to Contract for Services 2
5. Funding 3
6. Pre-contract Award Actions 4
7. Award Evaluation Factors 6
8. Post-Contract Award Actions 6

Section B. Health Care Services Invoice Review and Auditing.

1. General 1
2. Invoices Subject to Review and Audit 1
3. Review and Audit Procedures 1
4. Report of Potential Third Party Liability (RCN 6000-2) 2

Section C. Claims Processing.

1. General 1
2. Certification 1
3. Administrative Screen 1
4. Technical Screen 2
5. Appropriateness Review 3
6. Peer Review 4
7. Guidelines for Initial Appropriateness and Peer Reviews 5

CHAPTER 12

OCCUPATIONAL MEDICAL SURVEILLANCE AND EVALUATION PROGRAM (OMSEP)

Section A. General Requirements.

1. Description 1
2. Enrollment 1
3. Reporting Requirements 3

4. Medical Removal Protection..4
5. Roles and Responsibilities 4

Section B. Administrative Procedures.

1. General 1
2. Examination Types 1
3. Use of OMSEP Forms 5
4. Medical Removal Standards 6
5. Reporting of Examination Results 6

Section C. Medical Examination Protocols.

1. General 1
2. Asbestos, CG-6203 1
3. Benzene, CG-6204 4
4. Chromium Compounds, CG-6202 6
5. Hazardous Waste, CG-6206 8
6. Lead, CG-6207 10
7. Noise, CG-6205 and CG-6215 12
8. Pesticides, CG-6209 17
9. Respirator Wear, CG-6208 19
10. Respiratory Sensitizers, CG-6210 21
11. Solvents, CG-6213 23
12. Tuberculosis, CG-6212 26
13. Bloodborne Pathogens, CG-6211 27
14. Radiation (Ionizing/Non-ionizing), CG-6214 32

CHAPTER 13

QUALITY IMPROVEMENT

Section A. Quality Improvement Program.

1. Mission..1
2. Background 1
3. Internal Quality Assurance Reviews...1
4. External Quality Improvement Reviews...1
5. Goals 2
6. Operational Health Readiness Program (OHRP)..2
7. Objectives 2
8. Definitions...3
9. Responsibilities 4
10. Confidentiality Statement 7

11. QIP Review and Evaluation 7

Section B. Credentials Maintenance and Review.

    1. Background 1
    2. Definitions 1
    3. Pre-selection Credentials Review 2
    4. Provider Credentials File (PCF) 3
    5. Documentation 4
    6. Verification 5
    7. Contract Provider Credentials Review 6
    8. Reverification 6
    9. National Practitioner Data Bank (NPDB) 7
    10. National Provider Identifiers Type 1 (NPI) 7

Section C. Clinical Privileges.

    1. Purpose 1
    2. Background 1
    3. Definitions 1
    4. Applicability and Scope 3
    5. Clinical Privileges 4

Section D. Operational Health Readiness Program.

    1. Background 1
    2. Purpose 1
    3. Overview 1
    4. OHRP Compliance Process 2

Section E. Quality Improvement Implementation Guide (QIIG).

    1. Background 1
    2. Responsibilities 1

Section F. National Provider Identifiers.

    1. National Provider Identifiers (NPI) Type 1 1
    2. Clinic National Provider Identifiers (NPI) Type 2 1

Section G. Health Insurance Portability and Accountability Act (HIPAA).

    1. Background 1
    2. HIPAA Privacy/Security Officials (P/SO) 1
    3. HIPAA Training Requirements 4

4. Handling HIPAA Complaints and Mitigation 7
5. Unintentional Disclosures of Protected Health Information 9
6. Protected Health Information and the Coast Guard Messaging System 10
7. Other CG Members Who Utilize Protected Health Information 10
8. Electronic Transmission of Protected Health Information 11

Section H. Quality Improvement Studies.

1. Background 1
2. Responsibilities 1
3. Definitions 1
4. General information 2
5. QIS Focus 2
6. QIS Process 2
7. QIS Report Form 2
8. Frequency of Quality Improvement Studies 2
9. Completing the QIS Report Form 2
10. Follow-up Reporting 5
11. Integration 5
12. Filing 5

Section I. Peer Review Program.

1. Background 1
2. Characteristics of a Peer Review Program 1
3. Responsibilities 1
4. Process 2
5. Definitions 2

Section J. Infection and Exposure Control Program.

1. Introduction 1
2. Policy 2
3. Standard Precautions 2
4. Precautions for Invasive Procedures 5
5. Precautions for Medical Laboratories 6
6. Handling Biopsy Specimens 6
7. Using and Caring for Sharp Instruments and Needles 7
8. Infection Control Procedures for Minor Surgery Areas and Dental Operatories 8
9. Sterilizing and Disinfecting 14
10. Clinic Attire 19
11. Storage and Laundering of Clinic Attire, PPE and Linen 19
12. Cleaning and Decontaminating Blood or Other Body Fluid Spills 20
13. Infectious Waste 20
14. Managing Exposures (Bloodborne Pathogen Exposure Control) 21

  15. Training Personnel for Occupational Exposure 26

Section K. Patient Safety and Risk Management Program.

  1. Purpose 1
  2. Informed Consent 1
  3. Adverse Event Monitoring and Reporting 4
  4. Patient Safety Training 8

Section L. Training and Professional Development.

  1. Definitions 1
  2. Unit Health Services Training Plan (In-Service Training) 1
  3. Emergency Medical Training Requirements 3
  4. Health Services Technician "A" School 4
  5. Health Services Technician "C" Schools 4
  6. Continuing Education Programs 5
  7. Long-Term Training Programs 6

Section M. Patient Affairs Program.

  1. Patient Sensitivity 1
  2. Patient Advisory Committee (PAC) 1
  3. Patient Satisfaction Assessment 2
  4. Patient Grievance Protocol 2
  5. Congressional Inquiries 3
  6. Patient Bill of Rights and Responsibilities 3

CHAPTER 14

MEDICAL INFORMATION SYSTEM (MIS) PROGRAM

Section A. Medical Information Systems (MIS) Plan.

  1. Purpose 1
  2. Background 1
  3. Privacy rights 2
  4. Applicability and Scope 4
  5. Objectives 5
  6. Definitions 5
  7. Organizational Responsibilities 6

Section B. Medical Information System.

  1. Background 1

2. Systems 1

Section C. Medical Readiness Reporting System (MRRS).

1. Description 1
2. Recorded tests 1
3. Questions Related to MRRS 1
4. Access Instructions 1

Section D. Medical Information Implementation Guide (MIIG)

1. Background 1
2. Responsibilities 1

CHAPTER 1

ORGANIZATION AND PERSONNEL

Section A. Organization.

1. Mission of the CG Health Services Program 1
2. Director of Health, Safety, and Work-Life 1
3. Health, Safety, and Work-Life Service Center (HSWL SC) 3
4. Responsibilities of Commands with Health Care Facilities 5
5. Governance 5

Section B. Personnel.

1. Chief of the Clinical Staff 1
2. Collateral Duty Command Surgeons 1
3. Regional Manager (RM) 1
4. Regional Practice Director (RPD) 3
5. Regional Practice Senior Medical Executives (SME) 3
6. Regional Practice Senior Dental Executive (SDE) 5
7. Regional Practice Senior Independent Duty Health Services Technician (SIDHS) 6
8. Regional Pharmacy Executive (RPE) 6
9. Senior Health Services Officer (SHSO) 6
10. General Duties of Medical Officers 7
11. Duties of Flight Surgeons 13
12. General Duties of Dental Officers 15
13. General Duties of Pharmacy Officers 17
14. HSWL SC Pharmacy Officers 18
15. Environmental Health Officers 19
16. Clinic Administrators 21
17. Physician Assistants (PA) and Nurse Practitioners (NP) 23
18. Contract Health Care Providers 25
19. TRICARE Management Activity-Aurora (TMA) Liaison Officer 25
20. Health Services Technicians 26
21. Health Services Technicians - with a Dental Qualification Code (13) 28
22. Independent Duty Health Services Technicians (IDHS) 29
23. CG Beneficiary Representatives at Uniformed Services Medical Treatment Facilities (USMTF) 33
24. CG Representative at the Department of Defense Medical Examination Review Board (DODMERB) 35
25. Health Benefits Advisors (HBA) 36
26. Dental Hygienists 38
27. Red Cross Volunteers 39
28. Volunteers 39

COMDTINST M6000.1E

Section C. CG Health Services Officer Training Matrix.

   1. Introduction 1

Tables.

   Table 1-C-1 CG Medical Officer Matrix..1
   Table 1-C-2 CG Dental Officer Matrix..2
   Table 1-C-3 CG Leadership Courses Matrix..3
   Table 1-C-4 CG Chemical, Biological, Radiological, Nuclear, and Explosive (CBRNE) Courses Matirx..4
   Table 1-C-5 CG Disaster Training Matrix..5

COMDTINST M6000.1E

Section A. Organization.

1. Mission of the CG Health Services Program 1
2. Director of Health, Safety, and Work-Life 1
3. Health, Safety, and Work-Life Service Center (HSWL SC) 3
4. Responsibilities of Commands with Health Care Facilities 5
5. Governance 5

This page intentionally left blank.

COMDTINST M6000.1E

CHAPTER ONE – ORGANIZATION AND PERSONNEL

Section A. Organization.

1. Mission of the CG Health Services Program. The mission of the CG Health Services Program is to provide health care to active duty and reserve members in support of CG missions, to ensure the medical and dental readiness of all CG members to maintain ability for world-wide deployment and to ensure the availability of quality, cost-effective health care for all eligible beneficiaries.

2. Director of Health, Safety and Work-Life (CG-11).

    a. Mission. The mission of the Director of Health, Safety and Work-Life is to:

        (1) Serve as advisor to the CG Commandant.

        (2) Develop the CG's overall health care program.

        (3) Develop the CG's overall safety program.

        (4) Develop the CG's overall work-life program.

        (5) Administer a comprehensive automated Medical Information System.

    b. Duties and Responsibilities. Under the general direction and supervision of the Commandant, Vice Commandant, the Chief of Staff, and DCMS, the Director of Health, Safety and Work-Life shall assume the following duties and responsibilities:

        (1) Serve as Program Director (PD) for Work-Life Office (CG-111), the Health Services Office (CG-112), and the Safety and Environmental Health Office (CG-113).

        (2) Act as advisor to the CG Commandant in providing counsel and advice on:

            (a) Health care issues affecting operational readiness and quality of life in the CG.

            (b) Interdepartmental and inter-service agreements for health care of CG personnel.

            (c) The significance of legislative matters affecting the CG Health Services, Work-life and Safety and Environmental Health Programs.

            (d) Important developments in the Department of Defense (DoD) and the Department of Health and Human Services which affect the

CG Health Services, Work-life and Safety and Environmental Health Programs.

(3) Ensure availability of a comprehensive, high quality health care program and determine the priority and capacity for delivery of services to all eligible beneficiary groups.

(4) Plan, develop, and administer a comprehensive program for the prevention of illness and injury of CG personnel and dependents, to reduce losses and protect the environment in CG working facilities and living spaces by establishing and maintaining adequate safety and environmental health standards for aircraft, vessel, shore facilities, and motor vehicles providing information and encouragement to beneficiaries for personal wellness programs and providing healthy and pleasing meals at CG dining facilities.

(5) Liaison with TRICARE Management Activity (TMA), including the appropriation of funds, on behalf of the CG as provided in the Dependents Medical Care Act and regulations pursuant thereto.

(6) Monitor and protect the health of personnel attached to the CG through the Occupational Medical Surveillance and Evaluation Program (OMSEP).

(7) Direct the administration of funds in those appropriations or allotment fund codes under the control of the Director of Health, Safety and Work-Life, including furnishing total budget estimates and apportionment or allotment recommendations to the Chief of Staff.

(8) Advise responsible offices concerning establishing physical standards for military duty and special operational programs.

(9) Procure and recommend assignments to the Commander, Personnel Service Center (PSC), and review the performance of Public Health Service (PHS) personnel detailed to the CG.

(10) Provide professional health care guidance to all health services personnel.

(11) Maintain liaison with the PHS, the Department of Veterans Affairs (DVA), the DoD, and other Federal agencies and serve on interservice boards and committees as appointed.

(12) Set policy and guidelines for the subsistence program.

(13) Provide technical advice to operating program managers.

(14) Set policy and guidelines for health care quality assurance; and act as the Governing Body for CG health care.

(15) Set policy and guidelines for the Substance Abuse Program.

(16) Serve as a member of the Human Resources Coordinating Council.

(17) Administer the CG Emergency Response System.

(18) Oversee the detailed PHS personnel. The responsibility of the PHS for providing physicians, dentists, and other allied health personnel support to the CG is set forth in 42 USC, 253. These personnel are provided on a reimbursable basis and are subject to CG regulations and the Uniform Code of Military Justice (UCMJ).

(19) Set policy and guidelines for the enforcement of the Health Insurance Portability and Accountability Act (HIPAA) at CG health care facilities.

3. Health, Safety, and Work-Life Service Center (HSWL SC).

   a. Mission. The mission of HSWL SC is to:

      (1) Ensure/coordinate access to and/or delivery of Health, Safety, and Work-Life (HSWL) services to CG members and employees.

      (2) Implement Commandant (CG-11) program policies as set forth in applicable guidance.

      (3) Assess and respond to identified program needs of CG units and prioritize the delivery of available resources.

      (4) Work under the direction of CG Directorate COMDT (CG-11), and collaboratively with DoD, and TRICARE contract entities in ensuring/coordinating access to and/or delivery of cohesive HSWL services to eligible and authorized beneficiaries.

      (5) Ensure the integration of readiness data, delivery/coordination of direct care, and provide oversight and advice to all field units for all HSWL programs.

   b. Functions and Responsibilities. Under the direction and supervision of the Director, Health, Safety, Work-Life Commandant (CG-11), the Commanding Officer of Health, Safety and Work-Life SC shall:

      (1) Serve as the CG Military Treatment Facility (MTF) Commander, providing counsel and advice on:

         (a) Interagency and inter-service agreements for health care of CG personnel.

(b) The significance of legislative matters affecting the CG health care delivery program.

(c) Important developments in the DoD which affect the CG health care program.

(2) Designate Regional Practices within each District area of responsibility (AOR), the National Capital Area (NCA), the CG Academy, Training Center (TRACEN) Cape May and the Puerto Rico AOR.

(3) Administer a comprehensive health care program for all active duty (AD) and select reserve (SELRES) beneficiaries.

(4) Develop health services mobilization requirements and support documents.

(5) Review and act on requests for contract health care services.

(6) Act as contracting officer's technical representative (COTR) in reviewing health care contract proposals.

(7) Administer the health care quality improvement program.

(8) Administer Safety and Environmental Health Programs.

(9) Administer the Substance Abuse and Treatment Prevention Program in accordance with Personnel Manual, COMDTINST M1000.6 (series) and The Coast Guard Promotion Manual, COMDTINST M6200.1 (series).

(10) Develop and implement pharmaceutical support services.

(11) Supervise the laboratory certification process.

(12) Be responsible for providing funding for direct health care expenditures.

(13) Be responsible for the general oversight of health care budgets.

(14) Be responsible for the oversight of general clinic policy to include setting standards for clinic operations and prioritizing of clinic functions IAW Commandant (CG-11) policies.

(15) Designate clinics as catchment area patient management sites.

(16) Maintain liaison with the PHS, the DVA, the DoD, and other Federal agencies within the area of responsibility.

(17) Ensure compliance with Health Insurance Portability and Accountability Act (HIPAA) requirements.

(18) Be responsible for implementing a comprehensive Medical Information System.

(19) Be responsible for assigning Designated Medical Officer Advisors (DMOA) to all independent duty Health Service Technicians (HS's) and for oversight of the DMOA program.

(20) Review and validate all area health care proposals submitted to meet current and out year mission planning requirements (this includes proposed personnel billet restructuring, facility renovation/construction proposals, and electronic resource proposals subject to programmatic approval.)

(21) Ensure each CG unit is assigned to a CG clinic or sick bay for the purposes of operational medical readiness and health service support. Ensure every clinic/sickbay is aware of their responsibility for the units within their designated area of responsibility (AOR).

(22) Coordinate with unit Commanding Officers to detail health services personnel (Officer and Enlisted, CG, and USPHS) for special assignments including meeting short-term staffing needs.

4. <u>Responsibilities of Commands with Health Care Facilities</u>. Unit Commanding Officers shall be responsible for:

   a. Maintenance, repair and general support of clinic facilities.

   b. Working with HSWL SC in fostering quality, productivity and operating efficiencies.

   c. Support the utilization of assigned health services personnel for maintaining operational medical readiness health service support to CG personnel within the designated clinic/sickbay AOR. This includes medical and dental readiness support and regional Flight Surgeon on-call responsibilities.

5. <u>Governance</u>. An Executive Leadership Council will make policy recommendations to CG-11. The Council shall be chaired by CG-11(d) and consist of CG-11, CG-11 Office Chiefs, CG-1123, the CO of HSWL SC, the HSWL SC deputy, the HSWL SC Chief of Clinical Staff, and the HS Rating Force Master Chief. The Board shall meet at least quarterly and at the discretion of the Chair.

This page intentionally left blank

Section B. Personnel.

1. Chief of the Clinical Staff 1
2. Collateral Duty Command Surgeons 1
3. Regional Manager (RM) 1
4. Regional Practice Director (RPD) 3
5. Regional Practice Senior Medical Executives (SME) 3
6. Regional Practice Senior Dental Executive (SDE) 5
7. Regional Practice Senior Independent Duty Health Services Technician (SIDHS) 6
8. Regional Pharmacy Executive (RPE) 6
9. Senior Health Services Officer (SHSO) 6
10. General Duties of Medical Officers 7
11. Duties of Flight Surgeons 13
12. General Duties of Dental Officers 15
13. General Duties of Pharmacy Officers 17
14. HSWL SC Pharmacy Officers 18
15. Environmental Health Officers 19
16. Clinic Administrators 21
17. Physician Assistants (PA) and Nurse Practitioners (NP) 23
18. Contract Health Care Providers 25
19. TRICARE Management Activity-Aurora (TMA) Liaison Officer 25
20. Health Services Technicians 26
21. Health Services Technicians - with a Dental Qualification Code (13) 28
22. Independent Duty Health Services Technicians (IDHS) 29
23. CG Beneficiary Representatives at Uniformed Services Medical Treatment Facilities (USMTF) 33
24. CG Representative at the Department of Defense Medical Examination Review Board (DODMERB) 35
25. Health Benefits Advisors (HBA) 36
26. Dental Hygienists 38
27. Red Cross Volunteers 39
28. Volunteers 39

This page intentionally left blank.

B. Personnel. This section describes the primary duties and responsibilities of personnel assigned to provide health service support within the CG direct care system. The primary missions of the CG direct care system are to provide/coordinate health care for active duty (AD) and selected reserve (SELRES) members in support of CG missions and ensuring the medical and dental readiness of CG members for world-wide deployment.

1. Chief of the Clinical Staff. Under the general direction of the HSWL Commanding Officer, serve as the Senior Clinical and Public Health Service (PHS) advisor to HSWL SC, providing counsel and advice as delineated in Health, Safety, and Work-Life Support Activity Organization Manual, HSWLSUPACTINST M5401.1 (series).

2. Collateral Duty Command Surgeons. HSWL SC shall assign in writing, on a collateral duty basis, to LANTAREA and PACAREA and each District Commander, a Medical Officer to serve as the Command Surgeon to manage District-level flight surgeon coverage, providing counsel, advice, and other duties as delineated in Health, Safety, and Work-Life Support Activity Organization Manual, HSWLSUPACTINST M5401.1 (series).

3. Regional Manager (RM). CG Officer with health care administration training and experience. Will report to HSWL SC via Chief, Medical Administration Division. The RM will:

    a. Maintain liaison with HSWL and Commanders of units in their AOR

    b. Provide oversight and supervision of medical administrative functions of all clinics, sickbays and Work-Life staffs in the HSWL Regional Practice AOR

    c. Ensure that all health and work-life related services under the purview of the FO are carried out in accordance with current policy, regulations and standard of practice in the following areas:

        (1) Family Advocacy
        (2) Employee Assistance Program
        (3) Dependent Care
        (4) Sexual Assault
        (5) Suicide Prevention
        (6) Health promotion
        (7) Transition and Relocation
        (8) Personal Financial Competency Program
        (9) Adoption Reimbursement
        (10) Child and Elder Care
        (11) Services to Family Members with Special Needs
        (12) Crisis Intervention

(13) Addiction Prevention

(14) Substance Abuse Prevention

(15) Critical Incident Stress Management

(16) Leading and participating in the interview and hiring process for new W-L Office employees in collaboration with Commandant (CG-111) Program managers.

(17) Advising HSWL SC staff of sensitive urgent Work-Life related issues.

d. Regularly evaluate metrics for financial, clinical, workload, staffing and other data to ensure compliance with benchmarks, regulations, and external accreditation requirements.

e. Ensure Timely access to health care and work-life services.

f. Monitor active duty primary care enrollment in the HSWL RP AOR.

g. Optimize resource utilization, including, but not limited to, AFC-57 funding, and capital within the HSWL RP AOR.

h. Oversee the administrative and personnel functions for the HSWL RP organization. Examples include, but are not limited to:

(1) TAD activity

(2) Track OERs, EERS, COERs and EARS and routing up rating chains.

(3) Designating staff property custodians.

(4) Random Urinalysis (N/A for OPCON units).

(5) Weight Program (N/A for OPCON units).

(6) Awards (N/A for OPCON units).

(7) Coordinate with SHSO for Leave reports.

(8) UCMJ (N/A for OPCON units).

i. Ensure timely access to health care service providers and oversee referrals to non-Federal health care service providers ("white space" activities).

j. Oversee non-Federal medical and dental preauthorization processing for designated units.

k. Participate in and conduct meetings with leadership in HSWL initiatives and partnerships with federal (DOD, VA, etc), state and local delivery systems as authorized by HSWL and in accordance with policies promulgated by COMDT (CG-11).

l. Partner with SME and SIDHS to ensure that DMOA and DSMO duties are carried out IAW established policy.

m. Provide health benefits support and direction to designated units through health benefits advisors, clinics with TRICARE Service Centers and other resources.

n. Monitor performance of contracted personnel.

o. Coordinate Quality Improvement program activities delineated in policy including but not limited to Pharmacy and Therapeutics meetings and Quality Improvement Focus Group meetings.

p. Oversee the HSWL informational marketing throughout the AOR, making information and training concerning HSWL services available to all eligible users.

q. Ensure HSWL staff participates in on-going required professional training and maintains all appropriate certifications/licensures as required by policy.

r. Ensure appropriate procedures are in place to protect any personally identifiable information (PII) used or collected, for all users of RP services.

s. Collaborate and coordinate with Program Managers (CG-11) and HSWL SC staff with respect to program oversight, operational health readiness and quality assurance site visits.

t. Perform other duties as directed by the HSWL SC Commanding Officer.

4. <u>Regional Practice Director (RPD)</u>. The large, mission specific RP at the CG accession points, CG Academy and TRACEN Cape May will have a USPHS Officer as Director in lieu of RM and be supported in the performance of their duties by a Clinic Administrator.

5. <u>Regional Practice Senior Medical Executive (SME)</u>. In addition to the primary duties of a Medical Officer (MO), SME is responsible for the provision of the services delivered by or supervised by all Medical Officers in the FO, and duties include supervision of all Medical Officers and OER/COER rating/endorsement. The SME will perform or delegate the following duties:

   a. <u>Ensuring medical readiness compliance</u>. Directly and through the DMOA, DSMO and HSs assigned ensure medical readiness compliance at all units in AOR.

   b. <u>Prescribed regulations</u>. Performing those duties as prescribed in United States Coast Guard Regulations, COMDTINST M5000.3 (series).

   c. <u>Advise Commanding Officer</u>. Advising the Commanding Officer of any deleterious environmental health factors.

   d. <u>Supervising any assigned PAs and NPs</u>. Supervising any assigned PAs and NPs including, on a monthly basis, random review for approximately five percent of the PA's/NP's charts for adequacy and appropriateness of treatment rendered. May designate, in writing, supervisory responsibility of assigned mid-level provider(s) to other active duty physicians within the command.

e. Pharmacy duties. In the absence of a Pharmacy Officer, maintaining antidotes for narcotics and poisons and ensuring only properly trained personnel are assigned to the pharmacy.

f. Commanding Officer's representative. Acting as the Commanding Officer's representative on local emergency planning boards, and during emergencies or disasters furnishing advice to the Commanding Officer, formulating plans, and helping civilian authorities meet health care needs using the guidance and policy outlined in Alignment With The National Incident Management System and National Response Plan COMDTINST 16000.27 (series) on the Incident Command System in the CG.

g. Managing the quality of health care services provided.

h. Quality improvement technical supervisor. Acting as quality improvement technical supervisor for all contracted health services.

i. Use of personnel. Ensuring efficient and effective use of all assigned MOs and civilian consultants.

j. Overseeing the HS training program. Overseeing the HS training program outlined above to include ensuring, through training and experience, that Health Services Technicians are prepared for independent duty assignments. This includes the development of and effective supervision of training through assigned DSMOs and DMOAs.

k. Recommending the DSMO. Recommending to the command a DSMO for each HS who provides medical treatment to patients and overseeing this responsibility for other MOs in the chain-of-command.

l. Convening medical boards. Convening medical boards as appropriate in accordance with Chapter 3, Physical Disability Evaluation System, COMDTINST M1850.2 (series).

m. Quality ancillary services. Ensuring that all ancillary service areas (e.g., laboratory, radiology, etc.) maintain adequate policy, certification, radiation safety, and procedures manuals.

n. Professional oversight. In conjunction with the HSWL SC, providing professional oversight and establishing qualifications standards and privileging for assigned personnel, including contract, reserve, auxiliary and student providers.

o. Assigning the duties of MO and HS personnel. Assigning the duties of MO and HS personnel and ensuring position and billet descriptions are accurate and that credentials and privileging requirements are met. For HS personnel, this should occur in coordination with the Clinic Administrator.

p. Provide the range of services for each beneficiary group as directed by COMDT (CG-11).

q. Maintaining liaison. Maintaining liaison with counterparts in nearby (75 miles) Military Treatment Facility (MTF), Uniformed Services Treatment Facility (USTF), Veterans Administration (VA) and private sector facilities.

r. Preparing performance appraisals for assigned staff.

s. Reviewing and ensuring accuracy of CG MIS data. Reviewing and ensuring accuracy of Composite Health Care System (CHCS), Medical Readiness Reporting System (MRRS), CG Business Intelligence (CGBI), and other statistical and informational reports.

t. Quality Improvement Program. Ensuring active participation and compliance with the Quality Improvement Program.

u. Infection control procedures. Ensuring strict adherence to current infection control procedures and standards.

v. Keeping the Senior Health Services Officer informed.

w. Other duties assigned by the Commanding Officer and Senior Health Services Officer.

6. Regional Practice Senior Dental Executive (SDE). In addition to the primary duties of a Dental Officer (DO), SDE is responsible for the provision of the services delivered by or supervised by all Dental Officers in the RP, and duties include supervision of USPHS Dental Officers and COER rating/endorsement. The SDE will perform or delegate the following duties:

   a. Ensuring dental readiness.

   b. Preventive dentistry and dental health education program. Conduct and organize preventive dentistry and dental health education programs for all eligible beneficiaries.

   c. Prescribed regulations. Performing those duties as prescribed in United States Coast Guard Regulations 1992, COMDTINST M5000.3 (series).

   d. Training. Preparing, through training and experience, health services technicians for independent duty assignments.

   e. Administration. Overseeing the preparation of reports, updating the dental clinic policy and procedures manual, and maintaining records connected with assigned duties.

   f. Supervising. Overseeing the overall working condition, cleanliness and infection control of the dental clinic, which includes sterilization procedures, dental supply, equipment, publications maintenance, and the establishment of a preventive maintenance program for dental equipment and supplies.

   g. Dental supplies. Maintaining custody, security, and records of the dispensing of dental supplies, including all controlled substances and poisons under the cognizance of the dental branch.

   h. Prescriptions. Issuing prescriptions for, and supervising the dispensing of controlled substances, used in the dental branch.

i. Oversceing personnel. In conjunction with the HSWL SC, providing professional oversight and establishing qualification standards and privileging for assigned personnel, including contract, reserve and student providers.

j. Managing the quality of dental care services provided.

k. Assigning personnel. Ensuring position and billet descriptions are accurate and that credentials and privileging requirements are met.

l. Determining the priority and range of services for each beneficiary group. Within general CG and unit guidelines, determining the priority and range of services for each beneficiary group.

m. Maintaining liaison. Maintaining liaison with counterparts in USMTF, USTF, VA and private sector facilities.

n. Preparing performance appraisals for assigned staff.

o. Statistical and informational reports. Reviewing and ensuring accuracy of Dental Common Access System (DENCAS), Composite Health Care System (CHCS), and CG Business Intelligence (CGBI) and other statistical and informational reports.

p. Training. Ensuring that appropriate training is conducted on a regularly scheduled basis.

q. Quality Improvement Program. Ensuring active participation and compliance with the Quality Improvement Program.

r. Ensuring strict adherence to current infection control procedures and standards.

s. Keeping the Senior Health Services Officer informed.

t. Other duties assigned by the Senior Health Services Officer.

7. Regional Practice Senior Independent Duty Health Services Technician (SIDHS). The SIDHS is responsible for administrative oversight/mentoring of all IDHSs in their respective AOR.

8. Regional Pharmacy Executive (RPE). In addition to services delivered at the location assigned, the RPE is responsible for the provision of the pharmacist delivered services and oversight of all pharmacy services provided by non-pharmacists for an assigned AOR.

9. Senior Health Services Officer (SHSO). The SHSO is a senior health care provider, in charge of day-to-day operations of a local medical/dental practice site. The SHSO is designated by HSWL SC with Commandant (CG-112) input.

    a. Advisor to the Commanding Officer. Act as an advisor to the Commanding Officer regarding all health related matters.

    b. Daily routine. Under the unit Executive Officer, carry out the plan of the day as it pertains to the Health Services Division.

c. <u>Administrative functions</u>. Responsible for the oversight of the administrative, as well clinical functions of the clinic, and the supervision of the Clinic Administrator (CA).

d. <u>Support role</u>. Ensure that the clinic performs supporting clinic duties for units designated by the HSWL SC in their area of responsibility IAW this Instruction, cognizant HSWL SC Instructions, their SOP, and other pertinent directives. These duties include but are not limited to the following:

   (1) Ensure that health care delivery is provided in a timely manner to units for which a clinic is designated as their Primary Care Manager (PCM).

   (2) Assist with the timely completion of Medical Boards.

   (3) Be responsible for the allocation of resources (personnel, funds, space, and equipment) within the division.

   (4) When directed by the command, represent the division at staff meetings and ensure timely dissemination of the information to division personnel.

   (5) Prepare performance appraisals as appropriate and ensure that performance evaluations for all health services personnel are prepared and submitted in accordance with current directives.

   (6) Review all division reports.

   (7) Be responsible for the division training program, including rotation of personnel assignments for training and familiarization, in the health care delivery system.

   (8) Oversee clinic policies, procedures and protocols for compliance with this Manual, HSWL SC Instructions, Standard Operating Procedure (SOP), HIPAA and other pertinent directives.

   (9) Participate in health care initiatives with local/regional DoD delivery systems, under Headquarters and HSWL SC guidance.

   (10) Ensure strict compliance to current infection control procedures and standards.

   (11) Serve as chair of the Patient Advisory Committee.

   (12) Perform other duties as directed by the HSWL Commanding Officer.

10. <u>Duties of Medical Officers (MO)</u>. The principal mission of MOs is to support the operational missions of the CG. MOs include Physicians, Physician Assistants (PA), and Nurse Practitioners (NPs) who are members of the CG or PHS detailed to the CG. MOs are required to have appropriate certification or licensure while assigned to the CG. Physicians must have an unrestricted state license to practice medicine. See 1-B-11 for nurse practitioner and physician assistant credential requirements. Civilian medical practitioners (under contract to the CG or GS employees) assigned to a medical treatment facility are considered MOs to the limits defined by the language of their contract and/or job description. Civilian

medical practitioners who have a contract with the CG to see patients in their private offices are not considered MOs for the purpose of this Manual.

a. <u>Primary duties and responsibilities</u>. The primary duties and responsibilities of the CG MO, in support of CG missions as authorized by applicable laws and regulations are:

(1) To provide health care for all CG AD and SELRES. This will be accomplished, in part, by:

   (a) Treatment of sick and injured personnel.

   (b) Prevention and control of disease.

   (c) Making the appropriate referrals IAW existing policy and regulation.

   (d) Promotion of healthy lifestyle choices.

   (e) Giving advice on such matters as hygiene, sanitation, and safety.

   (f) Recommend one of the following duty status of active duty/reserve personnel (and CG civil service employees, if applicable):

   (1) Fit for Full Duty (FFD). The member is able to perform the essential duties of the member's office, grade, rank, or rating. This includes the physical ability to perform world wide assignment. (The exception to this is if a member is HIV positive; refer to Coast Guard Human Immunodeficiency Virus (HIV) Program, COMDTINST 6230.9 (series) for details)

   (2) Fit for Limited Duty (FLD). The interim status of a member who is temporarily unable to perform all of the duties of the member's office, grade, rank, or rating. This includes the physical ability to perform world wide assignment. A member placed in this temporary status will have duty limitations specified, such as: no prolonged standing, lifting, climbing; or unfit for sea or flying duty.

   (3) Not Fit for Duty (NFD). The member is unable to perform the essential duties of the member's office, grade, rank, or rating. (If needed specific instructions should be given (i.e. confined to rack, sick in quarters or sick at home).

   (g) Ensuring that the member is notified of results of all Papanicolaou (PAP) smears, mammograms, biopsies, pregnancy tests, and all tests that are abnormal or whose results indicate a need to initiate or change treatment and/or duty status.

   (h) Ensure the medical and dental fitness/readiness for unrestricted worldwide duty of active duty and reserve personnel.

   (i) Ensure all appropriate documentation is completed in appropriate Medical Information Systems (MIS). Medical Readiness Reporting System (MRRS), Composite Health Care System (CHCS) (including proper utilization and completion of Current Procedural Terminology (CPT) and International Classification of Diseases (ICD) codes in CHCS) and Dental Common Access System (DENCAS), as applicable (see Chapter 14 for information about CG MIS).

(j) Ensure that all HSs under their responsibility are properly trained in the clinical and emergency medicine aspects of the HS rate and proactively participate in the HS training program in order to prepare the HS for Independent Duty. This is primarily accomplished through the function as Designated Medical Officer Advisor (DMOA) and Designated Supervising Medical Officer (DSMO) to the HSs so assigned (see below for further description). Every HS performing duties in a CG clinic or sickbay shall be assigned a DSMO or a DMOA as appropriate. The DSMO and DMOA will function as the signature authority for clinical practical factors/qualifications for HSs assigned. The duties include:

   (1) Ensuring that HSs who participate in Emergency Medical Technician (EMT) operations maintain their certification, knowledge and health services skills in EMT operations.

   (2) Provide health services refresher training on clinical and emergency procedures.

   (3) Preparing HS for independent duty assignments through training, daily clinical supervision, feedback, and experience.

(k) Thoroughly understand all operational missions of the unit and other CG units within the clinic/sickbay AOR and the human factors involved in performing them.

(l) Maintain an active interest and participate in the local unit's safety program, assist the safety officers in planning, implementing, and coordinating the unit safety program, and advise the command on safety issues.

(m) Be thoroughly familiar with the types of personal protective and survival equipment carried at the unit. Be familiar with the CG Rescue and Survival System Manual, COMDTINST M10470.10 (series).

(n) Actively participate in the unit and clinic training programs to ensure that personnel are capable of coping with the hazards of mission performance by presenting lectures and demonstrations which include, but are not limited to:

   (1) Fatigue.

   (2) Emergency medicine.

   (3) Stress.

(4) Drug and alcohol use and abuse.

(o) Participate in a program of continuing education and training in operational medicine including training with other branches of the Armed Forces. This is accomplished primarily through attendance at annual training offered through various DoD sources. (See chapter 1C of this Manual for further guidance).

(p) Participate in all required initial and annual training in the privacy and security requirements mandated by Health Insurance Portability and Accountability Act (HIPAA).

(q) Serve as the medical member in physical disability evaluation cases.

(r) Advise local commands on health status of personnel, the physical fitness of personnel, immunization/medical readiness standards, nutritional adequacy/weight control, food handling and preparation, heating, ventilation and air conditioning, housing, insect, pest and rodent control, water supply and waste disposal, and safety.

b. Amplifying policy/guidance for MO's. Amplifying policy/guidance for the appropriate performance of the CG MOs duties will include:

(1) Designated Supervising Medical Officer (DSMO). MOs assigned as a "Designated Supervising Medical Officer" (DSMO) will assume clinical responsibility for the treatment provided by each HS in their clinic for whom they are responsible. Additionally, the DSMO is responsible for ensuring the completion of clinical practical factors/qualifications for each HS that is supervised and is the signature authority for signing off on these qualifications. Assignment as a DSMO shall be made in writing and signed by the DSMO's Commanding Officer. Clinical supervision and accountability is defined as follows:

(a) During normal clinic hours, HS consultation with the DSMO as determined by that MO and review 100 percent of all patient encounters seen only by the HS. (Ideally these reviews would include the patient's presentation to the MO.) The DSMO shall countersign all records reviewed.

(b) Outside normal clinic hours, direct or telephone consultations may be coordinated with the DSMO or duty MO. The following working day, a review of 100 percent of all visits seen only by the HS will be done by the DSMO or duty MO. The DSMO or duty MO shall countersign all records reviewed.

(c) The DSMO shall use the variety of clinical presentations of illness and injury to provide ongoing clinical training to the HSs that provide care under their oversight. It is imperative that MOs use every available teaching opportunity to ensure that HSs are trained to provide care as an Independent Duty HS.

(2) Designated Medical Officer Advisor (DMOA). HSs on independent duty (IDHSs) shall have a DMOA identified. The DMOA shall provide professional advice and consultation to the IDHS and shall ensure that the IDHS maintains his/her clinical competency. The DMOA, along with the XO of the IDHS's unit, is responsible for ensuring the medical and dental readiness compliance through the supervised IDHS. The DMOA is responsible for ensuring the completion of clinical practical factors/ qualifications for each IDHS that is supervised and is the signature authority for signing off on these qualifications. The DMOA and the IDHS shall fill out the IDHS Operational Integration Form, in Chapter 9, Section D. The Health, Safety, and Work-Life Service Center (HSWL SC) shall apportion units with IDHSs to units with MOs attached. HSWL SC will make such assignments in writing, addressed to the Senior Health Services Officer (SHSO) of the clinic providing support. Upon the SHSO's assignment of a DMOA to an IDHS, the assignment letter will be forwarded to the DMOA. A copy of this assignment letter shall be forwarded, by the clinic administrator, to the IDHS' unit (CO/XO), the HSWL SC, and Commandant (CG-1121). Assignment letters shall be addressed to the specific individuals involved, and new letters shall be issued following a change of DMOA or IDHS. The HSWL SC shall make assignment changes as necessary and forward such information to Commandant (CG-1121). The DMOA shall be thoroughly familiar with the duties and responsibilities of the IDHS as outlined in this section and in Chapter 9 of this Manual. Professional advice and consultation, in this instance, is defined as follows:

(a) Telephone, radio, or e-mail/electronic consultation regarding specific cases as necessary between the HS and the DMOA. This does not preclude consultation between the HS and another CG MO, an MO of the Army, Navy, Air Force, USPHS, or a physician under contract to the CG whose contract provides for such consultations.

(b) Visit with assigned HS. The DMOA shall have all assigned HSs report to the clinic for a personal visit. Travel will be funded by HSWL SC. This visit should be scheduled as soon as the HS completes IDHS school. This visit will normally be scheduled for a period of at least two weeks as this will allow the time required for the DMOA to complete the IDHS Operational Integration Form, CG-6000-4. This visit is an excellent opportunity for a more junior corpsman at the clinic to gain experience as an IDHS by providing backfill at the IDHS's unit.

(c) Schedule regular visits with assigned IDHS's (once a quarter) when practical, or at minimum, regular telephone calls.

(d) Treatment record review: All patient encounters shall be entered by the IDHS into the electronic health record and countersigned by the DMOA. The DMOA is encouraged to provide input to the unit CO or

XO regarding the professional performance of the IDHS. Additional information can be found in QIIG 46.

(e) Review of HSWL SC quality improvement site survey reports for the independent duty site. The DMOA and IDHS shall review the HSWL SC quality improvement site reports for the site. They shall collaborate on the required written plan of corrective actions which must be submitted to the HSWL SC following the site survey. The DMOA should also consult with the unit CO regarding the findings of the survey report. HSWL SC shall ensure that the reports are made available for review by the DMOA and the IDHS.

(f) Special situations. Additional responsibilities for DMOAs assigned to support Maritime Safety and Security Teams (MSST) and Enhanced Maritime Safety and Security Teams (EMSST) are described in the Tactical Medical Manual, COMDTINST M16601.16 (series). Overall, they shall include the active involvement, oversight of medical training, and mission assistance incumbent on developing a special operations/tactical medical operations program for the assigned units. It is anticipated that MSST DMOAs will have responsibility for providing medical control duties for the supported unit. DMOAs assigned to MSSTs shall be physicians and will be expected to attend additional training for tactical medical knowledge and experience.

(3) Physical Examinations and Periodic Health Assessments (PHA). MOs shall conduct physical examinations in accordance with Section 3-C of this Manual. MOs shall conduct PHA in accordance with Coast Guard Periodic Health Assessment (PHA), COMDTINST M6150.3 (series). Cases involving disability evaluation shall be guided by the Physical Disability Evaluation System, COMDTINST M1850.2 (series), the Department of Veterans Affairs Publication, Physician's Guide for Disability Evaluation Examinations.

(4) Reports to Command. Report injuries or deaths of personnel, damage, destruction, or loss of health services department property, and any other important occurrence, to the local command for entry into appropriate log. Report any suspected child/spouse abuse to the local command and local law enforcement/child protective agency in accordance with the Coast Guard Family Advocacy Program, COMDTINST 1750.7 (series), and other local, state, or Federal law. Report patients in serious or critical condition to the local command with the information needed to notify the next of kin.

(5) Educational Measures. Conduct health education programs, including disseminating information about preventing disease and other subjects pertaining to hygiene and sanitation regarding sexually transmitted infections (STIs) and advise them of:

(a) Sexually Transmitted Infections (STI). Conduct or supervise the instruction of personnel regarding sexually transmitted infections and advise them of the associated dangers.

(b) First Aid Instruction. Conduct or supervise a program which will ensure knowledge and ability in first aid.

(c) Occupational Medical Surveillance and Evaluation Program (OMSEP). Conduct or supervise a program to indoctrinate personnel in the various aspects of occupational health and the OMSEP.

(d) Human Immunodeficiency Virus (HIV). Conduct or supervise the instruction of personnel regarding HIV and advise them of the associated dangers. Refer to CG HIV Program, COMDTINST M6230.9 (series) for further information.

(e) Wellness. Conduct or supervise a program to emphasize the importance of life-styles in maintaining health.

(f) Human Services. Conduct or supervise the instruction of Health Services personnel to ensure they are aware of all the services available to maintain a state of well being for personnel.

(g) Cooperation with other agencies. Cooperate with Federal, state, and local agencies for preventing disease, reporting communicable diseases, and collecting vital statistics.

(6) MOs may also provide health care for other eligible beneficiaries as authorized by applicable laws and regulations as resources allow.

(7) SME or MOs co-located at Child Care Development Centers (CDC) and Family Child Care Homes (FCC), are responsible for serving on the Special Needs Resource Team (SNRT) to help determine if a dependent child with special needs can be accommodated in CG CDC/FCC programs. Specific roles and responsibilities as a SNRT member include:

(a) Reviewing medical documentation on each child,

(b) Recommending program modifications/adaptations,

(c) Making recommendations for training that address specific issues of children with special needs,

(d) Providing training (if requested) for CDC staff and FCC providers. Additionally, SME/MO are responsible for providing medical guidance regarding specific infectious disease exposure risks at CDC and FCC.

11. <u>Duties of Flight Surgeons (FS)</u>. In addition to fulfilling the general duties of an MO (and SHSO/SME, if applicable), FS assigned to duties involving flight operation (DIFOPS) billets must provide a significant degree of operational oversight and interaction within the Air Station community in order to ensure the

highest level of health and safety well-being within the unit. FS shall maintain current aircrew qualifications and minimums, including flight time, as stipulated in the Coast Guard Air Operations Manual, COMDTINST M3710.1 (series). All FS shall have the responsibility of participating in a regional Flight Surgeon on-call program. FSs shall support this regional on-call system to the fullest extent possible. Additionally, provisions of a comprehensive Aeromedical Program will require significant attention to the non-clinical operational duties described below that will involve a significant amount of the FS's duty time:

a. Expert in the Aviation Medicine Manual. Be a subject matter expert in the Coast Guard Aviation Medicine Manual, COMDTINST M6410.3 (series).

b. Know the unit. Thoroughly understand all operational missions of the aviation unit and participate as a frequent flight crew member during routine training missions and on operational missions such as MEDEVACS and SAR, as appropriate. Must meet the requirements as set forth in the Coast Guard Air Operations Manual, COMDTINST M3710.1 (series) and the Coast Guard Aviation Medicine Manual, COMDTINST M6410.3 (series).

c. Be familiar with the operational missions of other CG units in the local area.

d. Know the aircraft. Obtain a significant understanding of the flight characteristics of all aircraft assigned to the unit and be thoroughly familiar with the human factors involved in pilot and crew member interaction with the aircraft.

e. Air Operations Manual. Be familiar with the CG Air Operations Manual, COMDTINST M3710.1 (series), with specific emphasis on Chapter 6, Rescue and Survival Equipment, Chapter 7, Flight Safety, and the sections of Chapter 3 (Flight Rules) dealing with protective clothing and flotation equipment.

f. Aviation personnel are fit for flight duty. Ensure that aviation personnel are physically and psychologically fit for flight duty and attempt to learn any unusual circumstances which might adversely affect their flight proficiency; this includes getting acquainted with each pilot and crew member.

g. Recommendations to the CO. Make recommendations to the CO concerning the health status of aviation personnel. In particular, only a FS, Aviation Medical Officer (AMO) or Aeromedical PA (APA) shall issue "up" chits, except as noted in the Coast Guard Aviation Medicine Manual, COMDTINST M6410.3 (series).

h. Air Station flight safety program. Maintain an active interest in the Air Station flight safety program by assisting the Flight Safety Officer in planning, implementing, and coordinating the station flight safety program, and advising the command on the aeromedical aspects of flight safety.

i. Aircraft Mishap Analysis Boards. When so assigned by Commandant (CG-11), participate as the medical member of Aircraft Mishap Analysis Boards and be responsible for completing the MO's report in accordance with Chapter 2 of Safety and Environmental Health Manual, COMDTINST M5100.47 (series).

j. Personal protective and survival equipment. Be thoroughly familiar with the types and uses of personal protective and survival equipment carried on aircraft at the unit. The Flight Surgeon shall be familiar with the CG Rescue and Survival Systems Manual, COMDTINST M10470.10 (series).

k. Aviation training program. Actively participate in the unit aviation physiology training program to ensure that aviation personnel are capable of coping with the hazards of flight by presenting lectures and demonstrations which include, but are not limited to:

   (1) Fatigue.

   (2) Medication and nutritional supplement use in aviation personnel.

   (3) Emergency medicine.

   (4) Survival.

   (5) Disorientation.

   (6) Night vision.

   (7) Reduced barometric pressure.

   (8) Crash injury avoidance.

   (9) Stress.

   (10) Drug and alcohol use and abuse.

l. MEDEVAC. Advise the command on MEDEVAC operations and participate in the Regional Flight Surgeon on-call program as outlined in the CG Aviation Medicine Manual, COMDTINST M6410.3 (series) (details under development).

m. Refresher training. Ensure that Emergency Medical Technicians (EMT) who participate in aviation operations maintain their knowledge and skills in aeromedical physiology, and provide refresher training lectures and demonstrations to EMT and health services technicians on emergency medical procedures. FSs may authorize, in writing, EMTs to perform ACLS skills only if properly trained and have demonstrated proficiency.

n. Continuing education. Participate in a program of continuing education and training in aviation and operational medicine. This shall include familiarity with information published for and training with FSs in other branches of the Armed Forces (see chapter 1C of this Manual and the CG Aviation Medicine Manual, COMDTINST M6410.3 (series) for further guidance).

12. General Duties of Dental Officers (DO). The principal duty of a DO is to support the CG operational mission by determining and maintaining each member's dental fitness for unrestricted duty on a worldwide basis. CG DOs are assigned to perform duties as general DO. Exceptions will be authorized in writing by Commander, Personnel Service Center (PSC).

   a. General Responsibilities. CG DOs must stay informed in all fields of general and military dentistry and be responsible for:

(1) Ensuring the fitness for unrestricted duty of active duty personnel on a worldwide basis and ensure all appropriate documentation is completed in appropriate Medical Information Systems (MIS). This includes Medical Readiness Reporting System (MRRS), Dental Common Access System (DENCAS) and Composite Health Care System (CHCS).

(2) Providing dental care for all eligible beneficiaries as authorized by applicable laws and regulations including the TRICARE dental plan and Active Duty Dental Plan.

(3) Preventing and controlling dental disease (this includes performing dental prophylaxis).

(4) Promoting dental health.

(5) Referring eligible beneficiaries for dental treatment per HSWL SC SOP, and the Active Duty Dental Plan.

(6) Prioritizing the delivery of dental care to meet CG unit operational readiness requirements.

(7) Ensuring that patients with periodontal disease have the opportunity to receive follow-up care.

(8) Ensuring that results of all biopsies are received and reviewed by a dentist to ensure that the appropriate action is taken.

(9) Ensuring that when dental externs are assigned to the clinic that a protocol is developed detailing lodging and subsistence arrangements, types of procedures allowed, available population to be treated, and supervising DO responsibilities. See Student Externship Programs (SEP), COMDTINST 6400.1 (series), for amplifying information. The protocol must be signed by the local command and provided to all participating dental schools.

(10) Ensuring that procedures for handling medical emergencies within the dental clinic are clearly written and emergency drills are practiced periodically.

(11) Participate in all required initial and annual training in the privacy and security requirements mandated by HIPAA.

(12) Actively utilize and be thoroughly familiar with required applications and modules of appropriate Medical Information Systems (MIS).

b. <u>Dental examinations</u>. DOs shall conduct the dental examination portion of physical examinations in accordance with Chapter 3 of this Manual. Dental examinations shall be conducted as soon as practical on personnel who report for duty so as to determine the need for dental treatment and to verify their dental records. Annual Type 2 dental examinations shall be conducted on all active duty and reserve personnel collocated with dental examiners (e.g, CG DOs, DoD DOs, or civilian contract dentists).

c. Care of Mass Casualties. DOs shall be qualified to perform first aid procedures in order to treat or assist in treating mass casualties.

d. State Licensure. While assigned with the CG, DOs are required to have an unrestricted state license to practice dentistry.

e. Continuing Education. Participate in a program of continuing training in operational medicine/dentistry including familiarity with information published for other branches of the Armed Forces.

13. General Duties of Pharmacy Officers. While assigned with the CG, Pharmacy Officers are required to have an unrestricted state license to practice pharmacy. Pharmacy Officers shall ensure that medications are acquired, stored, compounded, and dispensed according to applicable Federal laws in their primary and collateral duty clinics. This includes the direct supervision and management of the following:

    a. Dispensing and labeling of all drugs, chemicals, and pharmaceutical products.

    b. Information and guidance regarding collateral duty oversight of clinics, satellite clinics and sickbays is provided in QIIG 45.

    c. Patient-oriented pharmaceutical services. Patient-oriented pharmaceutical services include monitoring for appropriate drug therapy, allergies, therapeutic duplication, and medication interactions. Significant patient interactions should be documented on the Chronological Record of Medical Care, SF-600.

    d. Providing verbal and written patient medication counseling when appropriate.

    e. Collateral Duties. Carry out collateral duties as further outlined in Chapter 10 of this Manual.

    f. Supplies. Maintaining routinely stocked pharmaceuticals and vaccines at levels consistent with anticipated usage between regularly scheduled procurements of pharmacy supplies.

    g. Security measures. Ensuring that security measures are instituted to prevent unauthorized entrance into the pharmacy or misappropriation of pharmacy stock.

    h. Controlled substance. Receiving, safeguarding, and issuing all controlled substances as the designated custodian of controlled substances.

    i. Quality control. Ensuring adequate quality control of all pharmaceuticals locally compounded.

    j. References. Maintaining current drug information references and a reference library of pertinent textbooks and professional journals.

    k. Pharmacy and Therapeutics Committee. Serving as subject matter expert and implementing the decisions of the Pharmacy and Therapeutics Committee and serving as Secretary of that committee.

    l. Monthly inspections. Inspecting monthly all clinic stocks of drugs and biologicals.

m. Formulary. Developing and maintaining a formulary for local use by Medical and Dental Officers.

n. Drug information. Informing the clinical staff of new drug information, policy changes, or other pertinent data on drugs.

o. Continuing education. Participate in a program of continuing education in pharmacy or related fields.

p. Monthly inspections of emergency drug supplies. Maintaining, updating, and documenting monthly inspections of emergency drug supplies.

q. Technical advice. Providing technical advice concerning pharmaceutical matters.

r. Immunization requirements. Providing technical guidance and advice to the medical staff on current immunization requirements.

s. Resource for designated therapeutic categories. Serving as a resource for designated therapeutic categories of medications as they relate to the CG Health Services Allowance Lists, DoD Basic Core formulary, HS Drug Formulary and other drug lists.

t. Continuing education. Participate in a program of continuing training in operational medicine/pharmacy including familiarity with information published for other branches of the Armed Forces.

u. HIPAA and MIS. Participate in all required initial and annual training in the privacy and security requirements mandated by HIPAA and actively utilize and be thoroughly familiar with required applications and modules of appropriate Medical Information Systems (MIS).

14. Health, Safety, and Work-Life Service Center (HSWL SC) Pharmacy Officer(s). Under the general direction and supervision of the Chief, Operational Medicine Branch, HSWL SC, the HSWL SC Pharmacy Officer shall:

    a. Quality improvement program. Plan, develop and implement, within the resources available, a HSWL SC-wide pharmacy quality improvement program to:

        (1) Review and evaluate the delivery of pharmaceutical services in support of mission operations, implement established policies pertaining to pharmaceutical services, and recommend appropriate changes.

        (2) Monitor pharmacy operations, via quality improvement site visits, financial monitoring, and other workload indicators to ensure optimum utilization of personnel and financial resources.

    b. Plan and administer the acquisition and distribution of pharmaceuticals.

        (1) Review, analyze, and recommend the most efficient and cost effective means for providing pharmaceutical services throughout the Area, including the financial resources to be allocated to each operating facility under HSWL SC oversight.

(2) Monitor the procurement of controlled substances by CG units within the Area.

(3) Provide to HSWL SC a system for the random monitoring of drugs procured from nonfederal sources.

c. Consultant. Serve as pharmaceutical consultant on pharmacology, pharmacy, and drug utilization and provide technical pharmacy expertise, assistance and advice to the COMDT (CG-11) and command elements within the Area.

d. Provide guidance and advice. Regarding the evaluation, training, and justification for pharmacy personnel to meet operational needs of units within the Area.

e. Provide liaison. Provide liaison or representation to regional Federal and professional pharmacy groups and committees.

f. Collateral duty assignments. Administer and monitor the collateral duty assignments of pharmacy officers in their respective Area.

g. MIS Project Review Board (PRB). Provide guidance, advice, and technical support as needed as subject matter expert in matters pertaining to the MIS Project Review Board (PRB).

15. Environmental Health Officers. Environmental Health Officers are responsible for recognition, evaluation, and control of biological, chemical, physical, and ergonomic factors or stresses arising from the environment which may cause sickness, impaired health and well-being, or significant discomfort and inefficiency, property damage, or which could adversely affect the CG's industrial hygiene, pest management, radiological health, and sanitation. Specific responsibilities can include:

a. Environmental health program. Planning, budgeting, implementing and directing an environmental health program to support commands within their geographic area of jurisdiction.

b. Health audits. Conducting environmental health audits of CG facilities and operations in order to detect health hazards and noncompliance with applicable safety and environmental health laws, regulations, standards, and procedures. Facilities and operations include:

(1) Work environments.

(2) Storage, handling, treatment, and disposal of hazardous materials and hazardous waste.

(3) Storage, handling, treatment, and disposal of infectious medical waste.

(4) Food preparation, service, and storage operations.

(5) Solid wastes storage, handling, treatment, and disposal.

(6) Pest management operations.

(7) Potable water treatment, storage, and distribution systems.

(8) Waste water collection, treatment, and disposal system.

(9) Housing facilities.

(10) Ionizing radiation sources.

(11) Non-ionizing radiation sources.

(12) Recreational facilities.

(13) Health care facilities.

(14) Child care facilities.

(15) Laundry and dry-cleaning operations.

(16) Barber shop operations.

c. <u>Technical assistance</u>. Providing technical assistance to units to abate deficiencies identified by the Environmental Health Officer during the audit.

d. <u>Hazard abatement</u>. Monitoring ongoing hazard abatement actions to ensure that identified hazards are being eliminated promptly.

e. <u>Training</u>. Providing environmental health training to commands within their jurisdiction.

f. <u>Technical assistance</u>. Providing technical assistance to units on request to identify and abate health risks.

g. <u>Plans and specifications</u>. Reviewing engineering plans and specifications for new facilities and modifications to existing facilities to ensure conformance with environmental health standards and practices.

h. <u>Technical advisor</u>. Serving as technical advisor to commands within their jurisdiction.

i. <u>Health risk assessment</u>. Initiating and conducting special health risk assessment studies.

j. <u>Liaison</u>. Maintaining liaison with Federal, state, and local government agencies concerning environmental health for commands within their jurisdiction.

k. <u>Medical monitoring data</u>. In consultation with a Medical Officer, advise commands when medical monitoring data indicates the possibility of occupationally-induced or aggravated disease and investigating possible causes so that corrective measures can be initiated.

l. <u>Occupational Medical Surveillance and Evaluation Program (OMSEP)</u>. Providing consultation, advice, and training on the OMSEP to CG commands within their area of jurisdiction.

m. <u>Enrolling personnel in the OMSEP</u>. Enrolling personnel in the OMSEP when they meet the criteria of occupational exposure as defined in paragraph 12-A-2 of this Manual.

n. Disenrolling personnel from the OMSEP. Disenrolling personnel from the OMSEP when they do not meet the criteria of occupational exposure as defined in paragraph 12-B-4 of this Manual.

o. Reports. Environmental Health Officers shall submit reports to the HSWL SC about environmental health conditions observed during their surveys.

p. Duty Limitations. Environmental Health Officers shall carry out all management functions required to operate the safety and environmental health program within their AOR. They may be required to perform only those technical duties for which they are trained. They may represent the health services division at various staff meetings in matters relating to the management and budgetary aspects of their assignment. They will be primarily responsible for special studies as in the case of monitoring chemical spill response and enforcement personnel. They will be responsible to the HSWL SC for proper implementation of the safety and environmental health program.

16. Clinic Administrators (CA). Officers, Chief Warrant Officers (experience indicator 19), or senior enlisted personnel assigned under the direction of the SHSO to manage and administer health care facilities. The CA will not be required to, nor attempt to, perform clinical duties for which he/she is not qualified. The general duties and responsibilities of the CA will be:

a. Medical/dental readiness. Ensure the medical/dental readiness of all AD and SELRES personnel within their AOR and ensure that, as appropriate, all documentation is completed in appropriate Medical Information Systems (Medical Readiness Reporting System (MRRS), Dental Common Access System (DENCAS), CG Business Intelligence (CGBI) and Composite Health Care System (CHCS)).

b. Plan, supervise, and coordinate general administration of the health services facility. Prepare and submit annual business plan to the RP. Provide administrative oversight to contract providers and IDHS's within their AOR.

c. Budgets. Prepare, submit, manage, and exercise fiduciary control and accountability over the clinic's AFC-30 and AFC-57 funds.

d. Acquisition of supplies and equipment. Provide fiscal oversight over the acquisition of equipment and supplies.

e. Maintain a planned program of equipment maintenance and replacement.

f. Security. Provide physical security of health services division supplies and pharmaceuticals.

g. Liaison. Maintain liaison with other local agencies (military and civilian) in all health care related matters.

h. Resources. Provide resources to assist Medical and Dental Officers in emergency care of the sick and injured when necessary.

i. Develop disaster preparedness plan. Develop disaster and pandemic influenza force health protection preparedness plans. Refer to Coast Guard Pandemic Influenza Force Health Protection Policy, COMDTINST M6220.12.

j. Heavy weather bill. Prepare the heavy weather bill as it relates to the health services division.

k. Cost reduction and enhancement. Seek opportunities for cost reduction and enhancement to patient care through billet conversions, resource sharing, contracting, etc.

l. Advisor to the SHSO. Serve as an advisor to the SHSO on all administrative matters.

m. Supervision of enlisted personnel. Oversee, with the SHSO, the supervision of enlisted personnel assigned to the health services division for the adequate performance of all non-clinical HS performance factors/qualifications (the DSMO is required to sign for clinical qualifications).

n. Correspondence, reports, and records. Ensure that correspondence, reports, and records comply with appropriate instructions. Consult Information and Life Cycle Management Manual COMDTINST M5212.12 (series) and the Correspondence Manual, COMDTINST M5216.4 (series) for further guidance.

o. Maintain an adequate health services division reference library.

p. Mentoring. Train subordinates, conduct classes, instruct enlisted personnel in their duties, and supervise their study of regulatory and professional publications and courses for advancement in rating.

q. Continuing education. CAs must participate in a continuing education program in Health Care Administration. A link in CG Central will be provided. Verification will be during the HSWL SC quality improvement surveys.

r. Assist beneficiaries with health benefits information.

s. Appearance and conduct. Enforce standards of appearance and conduct of health services personnel.

t. Medical Information Systems (MIS). Ensure that accurate, appropriate data is submitted to all automated MIS. Ensure staff is appropriately trained for applicable MIS access.

u. Coding. Ensure proper coding of medical procedures is being conducted.

v. HS clinical assignments. Oversee clinical rotation of assigned HSs.

w. Implement Policies. Implement clinic policies, procedures, and protocols, to ensure compliance with United States Coast Guard Regulations 1992, COMDTINST M5000.3 (series), the Medical Manual, COMDTINST M6000.1 (series), HSWL SC INST/SOP, and other pertinent directives.

x. Compliance with regulations. Ensure compliance with all applicable Federal, state, and local statutes, together with the Medical, Dental and Pharmacy Officers.

y. Work-life issue. Oversee and promote work-life programs pertaining to health care.

z. Patient Advisory Committee. Serve as assistant chair for the Patient Advisory Committee.

aa. Personnel evaluations. Ensure that enlisted personnel evaluations for members assigned to the health services division are prepared and submitted in accordance with the Personnel Manual, COMDTINST M1000.6 (series).

bb. Nonfederal (NONFED) health care, contracts, and Blanket Purchase Agreement (BPA). Provide administrative oversight in the areas of NONFED health care, contracts, and BPAs.

cc. Health care invoices. Ensure that health care invoices are processed in accordance with HSWL SC INST/SOP.

dd. Physical examinations and PHAs. Ensure that local physical examinations and PHAs comply with current standards. Function as the reviewing/approving authority for all non-aviation/non-diving physical exams.

ee. Environmental sanitation program. Promote and administer the unit's environmental sanitation program (in the absence of an Environmental Health Officer).

ff. Occupational Medical Surveillance and Evaluation Program (OMSEP). Collaborate with the unit's OMSEP coordinators to provide needed medical support.

gg. Health Insurance Portability and Accountability Act (HIPAA) local Privacy/Security Official. Serve as the HIPAA local Privacy/Security Official or delegate these responsibilities in writing.

hh. Radiation safety. Ensure compliance with radiation safety requirements (periodic radiation equipment inspections and personal dosimetry) per Safety and Environmental Health Manual, COMDTINST M5100.47 (series).

ii. Health Risk Assessments (HRA) Administrator. Serve as the HRA administrator for the PHA.

jj. Medical Event Report Coordinator. Serve as the medical event report coordinator to ensure the timely submission of reports and ensure adherence with applicable instructions, (i.e., Coast Guard Human Immunodeficiency Virus (HIV) Program, COMDTINST M6230.9 (series)).

17. Physician Assistants (PA) and Nurse Practitioners (NP).

    a. General Responsibilities. PA and NP responsibilities as general MOs are defined in Section 1-B-1. The further duties of PA designated Aeromedical Physician Assistants are detailed in the Coast Guard Aviation Medicine

Manual, COMDTINST M6410.3 (series). Under the supervision of the Senior Medical Executive (SME) they are subject to the duty limitations listed below. In lieu of state licensing, PAs are required to maintain certification from the National Commission on Certification of Physician Assistants (NCCPA) and local clinical privileging. Since NP are commissioned in the PHS, an active, unrestricted state license as NP and certification shall be from either the American Academy of Nurse Practitioners or American Nurses Credentialing Center, and local clinical privileging as an NP is required for clinical practice with the CG.

b. Duty Limitations.

(1) Senior Medical Executive (SME) of units with mid-level providers (PAs or NPs) assigned shall assign clinical duties and responsibilities to each provider and shall be accountable for the actions of those providers.

  (a) To determine the extent of oversight required, SMEs shall be guided by this section, the provider's clinical training, and previous experience, by personal observation, and Chapter 13-C, Clinical Privileges.

  (b) The SME may delegate supervisory responsibility to another staff physician. A copy of this delegation shall be filed in the non-certified provider's Professional Credentials File (PCF).

  (c) Physicians responsible for supervising mid-level providers shall perform and document reviews of at least five percent of the mid-level provider's charts each calendar month for accuracy of diagnosis and appropriateness of treatment rendered. This will be determined on the charting, previous experience and personal observation of the performance of the mid-level provider by the designated supervising MO.

c. Not Certified. PAs who are not certified by the National Commission on Certification of Physician Assistants (NCCPA), recent graduates who have not taken or passed the NCCPA examination, and NPs who do not have an active, unrestricted RN license and who have not taken or passed a specialty board examination offered by the American Academy of Nurse Practitioners or the American Nurses Credentialing Center, shall practice in CG facilities only under the following conditions:

(1) All health record entries shall be co-signed by a licensed physician by the end of the next working day.

(2) When a supervisory physician is not present at the unit, non-certified mid-level providers shall be restricted to providing medical care, except for emergencies, to active duty members only.

(3) Non-certified mid-level providers may stand clinic watches providing a standby licensed physician is available via telephone to discuss any questions or concerns.

(4) With the exception of operational emergencies, non certified mid-level providers are not eligible for independent TAD assignments at locations where a supervisory physician is not present.

(5) Nothing in this section limits PA or NP access to any available source of information or advice during an emergency.

(6) Policy regarding supervision, duties and responsibilities of mid-level providers is further amplified in the Health Services Quality Improvement Implementation Guide (QIIG) Eight.

18. <u>Contract Health Care Providers</u>. All contract health care providers shall meet the credential requirements for certification, licensure and malpractice insurance set forth in Chapter 13 Section B of this Manual.

19. <u>TRICARE Management Activity-Aurora (TMA) Liaison Officer</u>.

   a. <u>Responsibilities</u>. The CG TMA liaison officer maintains liaison between TRICARE and Commandant (CG-11) on matters of policy, operations, and program administration. This function will not involve the responsibility for formulating department policies. Departmental policies will continue to be developed by members of the liaison group for the Uniformed Services Health Benefits Program.

   b. <u>Duties</u>. Specific duties include, but are not limited to the following:

      (1) Coordinate and assist, as necessary, in preparing and submitting uniform workload data for use in budgetary programming at departmental level.

      (2) Ensure timely notification to Commandant (CG-11) concerning changes in TRICARE operational or administrative procedures.

      (3) Identify gaps in the TRICARE information program and recommend solutions.

      (4) Represent CG viewpoints on matters relating to TRICARE operational and administrative procedures.

      (5) Assist in developing future TRICARE information programs.

      (6) Keep the CG informed of problem areas relating to service beneficiaries and service health care facilities, where appropriate, and recommend changes which will benefit the TRICARE operation.

      (7) Monitor purchases of high-cost equipment for use by TRICARE beneficiaries and make recommendations concerning future purchases as opposed to rental.

   c. <u>Duties within TMA Liaison Division</u>.

      (1) Investigate and respond to Presidential, Congressional, and beneficiary inquiries and complaints. Investigate and respond to inquiries concerning eligibility.

      (2) Make public presentations concerning program benefits to various groups.

(3) Prepare special studies relating to program activities.

(4) Serve as liaison representative for United States Public Health Service (USPHS), Department Veterans Affairs (DVA), and National Oceanic & Atmospheric Association (NOAA).

(5) Other Duties. Participate in contract performance appraisal visits to the fiscal administrators. This function involves a comprehensive review and evaluation of the operations of the civilian agencies which, under contract, administer the program within each region.

20. Health Services Technicians (HS).

   a. Rating Structure. The rating structure for health services technicians is contained in Group VIII, Enlisted Performance Qualifications Manual, COMDTINST M1414.8 (series). One of the primary goals of the HS rate is to have all HSs capable and trained as Independent Duty HSs.

   b. General Duties of HS.

   (1) The primary purpose of a HS is to provide supportive services to Medical and Dental Officers and provide primary health care in the absence of such officers.

   (2) In particular, HS are responsible for all administrative aspects of health care and health record maintenance for both their command and subordinate commands without HS attached. Geographically separate subordinate commands will retain responsibility for security (i.e. physical custody) of health records. In addition to the military duties common to all enlisted personnel, HS perform health services department functions, such as:

   (a) Respond to calls for emergency medical assistance or evacuations (MEDEVACs).

   (b) Maintain appointments and appointment records utilizing the appropriate CHCS module.

   (c) Ensure that all appropriate documentation is completed in appropriate MRRS, DENCAS, and CHCS to assist in the tracking of operational medical and dental readiness.

   (d) Maintain a Health Services Log. Each unit with health services personnel shall maintain a Health Services Log. This log is used to document the daily operations of the clinic or sickbay. At a minimum it is used to record all individuals reporting to sick call or for treatment, inspections and inventories conducted, and the results of potable water test.

   1. Sickbays and clinics shall submit the Health Services Log to the CO for review, approval, and signature on a schedule to be determined by the CO.

2. The patient listing portion of the Health Services Log can be produced by CHCS. At a minimum it must contain the name of patient, date of visit, Division or Department, members unit OPFAC (for active duty CG only), and branch of service.

(e) Maintain a Binnacle List: The Binnacle List can be produced by CHCS. At a minimum it must be sorted by OPFAC and Department/Division and include patient name, duty status, date of onset, and date of expiration of duty status. The Binnacle List shall be distributed to local command(s) as determined by the health care facility command.

(f) Perform OMSEP duties.

(g) Render first aid.

(h) Perform tentative diagnosis and emergency treatment. (In doing so, appropriate drugs, oral or injectable, may be administered as required in emergency situations to prevent or treat shock or extreme pain. In all other incidents where injection of controlled substances is required, permission must be obtained from a physician prior to administration. In either case, the local command shall be notified immediately and entries shall be made in the patient's health record).

(i) Provide nursing care where trained.

(j) Provide definitive treatment.

(k) Provide prophylactic treatments.

(l) Instruct crew members in first aid and oral hygiene.

(m) Prepare materials (including sterile instruments) and medications for use.

(n) Maintain military readiness of the health services division by complying with the appropriate Health Services Allowance List.

(o) Perform administrative procedures in health care matters, maintain health and dental records current in all aspects.

(p) Adhere to regulations, instructions, and control of precious metals, controlled substances, and poisons.

(q) Exercise responsibility for all equipment and stores placed in their charge, and exercise personal supervision over their condition, safekeeping, and economic expenditure.

(r) Maintain cleanliness of all health services spaces.

(s) Provide services as a health benefits advisor.

(t) Assist in the processing of nonfederal health care requests and invoices.

(u) Maintain the security and confidentiality of all medical and dental records and databases and any other protected health information and actively utilize and be thoroughly familiar with required applications and modules of appropriate Medical Information Systems (MIS).

(3) Each HS who provides medical treatment to patients at a CG clinic staffed by one or more MO shall have an MO from that facility assigned in writing as his/her Designated Supervising Medical Officer (DSMO). The DSMO shall assume responsibility for all clinical treatment provided by the HS. Each independent duty HS, and HSs assigned to sickbays without an MO, shall have an MO assigned in writing as his/her "Designated Medical Officer Advisor" (DMOA) to provide professional advice and consultation when needed. Refer to 1-B-11.b(2) for further details concerning DSMO/DMOA. Health Services Technicians assigned to units without an MO shall provide only "first response" emergency care to non-active duty personnel.

(a) Care shall be taken during medical examinations which involve chest, genital, and rectal areas to afford maximum privacy and minimum exposure of the patient. A chaperone of the same gender as the patient may be requested by the patient during examination or treatment. HS are authorized to conduct examinations to include: auscultation, palpation, percussion, and visual inspection as indicated by the medical complaint. However, HS shall not perform:

1. Routine digital examinations of the prostate.

2. Routine examinations through instrumentation of the urethra.

3. Routine gynecological examinations.

Such routine examinations shall be referred to an MO. In situations where no MO is readily available and such examination is necessary to provide emergency care, the HS is authorized to do so. If the HS and patient are of different gender, a chaperone of the same gender as the patient shall accompany the patient during the examination or treatment.

(b) Participate in a course of continuing education, either clinical or administrative, through correspondence courses, resident courses, etc, including all required initial and annual training in the privacy and security requirements mandated by HIPAA.

21. <u>HS – with a Dental qualification code (13)</u>.

a. <u>Primary responsibility</u>. The primary responsibility of Dental Technicians is to provide chairside assistance to DOs.

b. <u>Additional duties include</u>.

(1) Cleansing, sterilization, maintenance, and preparation of dental instruments.

(2) Cleansing, disinfecting, and maintenance of dental equipment and dental operatories.

(3) Preparing of dental materials.

(4) Assessing, referral, and treatment (under direct supervision of a DO) of common dental conditions. Charting dental conditions.

(5) Maintaining dental records.

(6) Exposure and development of dental radiographs.

(7) Providing oral hygiene instruction, taking impressions, and fabricating study models.

(8) Performance of emergency intervention as necessary.

(9) Maintain the security and confidentiality of all dental records, databases, and other protected health information and actively utilize and be thoroughly familiar with required applications and modules of appropriate Medical Information Systems (MIS).

(10) Ensure that all appropriate documentation is completed in appropriate Medical Information Systems, (Medical Readiness Reporting System (MRRS), Dental Common Access System (DENCAS), and Composite Health Care System (CHCS) to assist in the tracking of operational medical and dental readiness.

22. <u>Independent Duty Health Services Technicians (IDHS)</u>. Formerly referred to as IDTs, the IDHSs will follow the guidance in Chapter 9 of this Manual. The identification or term Independent Duty Health Services Technician, used in any form, only identifies those Health Services Technicians that have successfully completed one of the three recognized Independent Duty Training courses, i.e. the CG's Independent Duty Health Services Technician, USN Independent Duty Corpsman, or USAF Independent Duty Medical Technician courses.

   a. <u>General Duties</u>.

      (1) HS on independent duty perform the administrative duties and, to the extent for which qualified, the clinical duties prescribed for MOs of vessels and stations. (See United States Coast Guard Regulations 1992, COMDTINST M5000.3 (series) and Section 1-B of this Manual.). They shall not attempt, nor be required to provide, health care for which they are not professionally qualified. They shall provide care only for AD personnel; however they may provide care to non-active duty patients on an emergency basis. The filling of prescriptions for other than AD personnel shall be strictly limited to emergency situations and to authorized stock on hand under the allowance list for the unit. They may, under the guidance set in Chapter 10 of this Manual, establish non-prescription medication programs for eligible beneficiaries.

      (2) Under certain circumstances, HS assigned to Deployable Specialized Forces (DSF) may be detailed to perform combatant duties, which are not

prohibited by the Geneva Conventions. However, under routine situations, in accordance with Paragraph 7-5-4, United States Coast Guard Regulations 1992, COMDTINST M5000.3 (series).

(3) In accordance with the Personnel Manual, COMDTINST M1000.6 (series), CO are authorized to use HS for general duties except noted below:

    (a) HS shall not be used for duties that require bearing arms (except for the limited purposes allowed by Shipboard Regulations Manual, COMDTINST 5000.7 (series) and the Geneva Convention for their own defense or protection of the wounded and sick in their charge) even though the bearing of arms may be purely ceremonial.

    (b) HS shall not be used for combat duties that are unrelated to health care or administration.

b. <u>Specific Duties (see Chapter 9)</u>. Use the Health Services Log to document and keep track of your specific duties such as those listed below.

    (1) <u>Sanitation of the Command</u>. Make daily inspections to ensure that appropriate sanitation practices are maintained. Maintain a log that includes heat stress monitoring, potable water testing and pest control.

    (2) <u>Health of Personnel</u>. The IDHS's will assist the command in ensuring the medical and dental readiness for the personnel in their AOR by providing monthly Medical and Dental Readiness reports to the command, through CGBI, scheduling the crew for required readiness exams and procedures as needed, and informing the command when a given crew member or department fails to cooperate with the IDHS's efforts to comply with readiness requirements. The IDHS shall also maintain a tickler system to include all return appointments requested by physicians or dentists from outside referrals requested by the command.

    (3) <u>Care of Sick and Injured</u>. Hold daily sick call. Diagnose and treat patients within capabilities. When indicated, refer cases to facilities where Medical or Dental Officers are available or, if this is not practical, obtain help and advice by radio or other expeditious means.

    (4) <u>Procurement, Storage, and Custody of Property</u>. All parts of the Health Services Allowance List Afloat, COMDTINST M6700.6 (series), and Health Service Allowance List Ashore, COMDTINST M6700.5 (series) contain information needed for ordering and procuring supplies. The HSAL also contains procedures for storage and custody of property.

    (5) <u>Reports</u>. Prepare and submit reports required by this Manual and other directives, specifically inpatient hospitalization and medical event reporting.

    (6) <u>Health Records</u>. Maintain health records as required by Chapter 4 of this Manual. Ensure that all treatment records and/or consults from outside referrals are obtained and placed in the health record. In addition, ensure

that each patient is notified of all physical exams, consultations, and diagnostic tests (e.g., pap smears, mammograms, biopsies, x-rays, etc.) performed at any facility prior to filing in the health record. Maintain the security and confidentiality of all medical/dental records, databases and any other protected health information.

- (7) Training. Prepare and carry out a program for training non-medical personnel in first and self-aid, personal hygiene, sexually transmitted infection prevention, medical aspects of CBR warfare, cardiopulmonary resuscitation, etc, as part of the unit's regular training program.
- (8) Other Duties as assigned by the CO.

c. Reporting Procedures.

- (1) Policy. Upon reporting for independent duty, the HS shall consult with the local command to determine their policies regarding health care and the administration of the health services department.
- (2) Inventory. Obtain the unit Health Services Allowance List and inspect the inventory of all health services department equipment, supplies, and publications. Initiate action for repair, survey, or replenishment of equipment, supplies, and publications. Verify inventory records and check logs of controlled substances. Report any discrepancies to the local command without delay. Amplification of requirements and procedures is contained in Chapters 8 and 10 of this Manual.
- (3) Health Records. Check health records against the personnel roster. Any missing records should be accounted for or requested from previous duty stations. If records cannot be accounted for within one month's time, open a new health record. Check health records for completeness, and if not current, obtain and enter all missing information to the fullest extent possible. (See Chapter 4 of this Manual for further instructions pertaining to health records).
- (4) Operational Medical Readiness. Ascertain the state of operational medical readiness of the health services department and advise the local command. Operational readiness refers to the immediate ability to meet all health care demands within the unit's capabilities.

d. Responsibilities. The CO is responsible for the health and readiness of the command. The health services department is charged with advising the CO of conditions existing that may be detrimental to the health of personnel and for making appropriate recommendations for correcting such conditions. Meticulous attention to all details and aspects of preventing disease must be a continuing program. It is imperative that shipboard and station sanitation and preventive health practices be reviewed constantly in order that any disease promoting situation may be discovered immediately and promptly eradicated.

e. Routines. Many of the items listed in the daily, weekly, monthly and yearly requirements can be documented in the Health Services Log.

(1) Daily Routines.
   (a) Sickcall. Hold sickcall daily at a time prescribed by the Commanding Officer.
   (b) Binnacle List. Prepare the unit binnacle list and submit it to the CO.
   (c) Inspections. The following shall be inspected daily:
      1. Living spaces.
      2. Heads and washrooms.
      3. Fresh provisions received (particularly milk and ice cream).
      4. Scullery in operation.
      5. Drinking fountains.
      6. Garbage disposals.
      7. Sewage disposals.
      8. Coffee messes.
      9. Water supplies.
      10. Industrial activities. (See Chapter 7 of this Manual and the Food Service Sanitation Manual, COMDTINST 6240.4 (series)).
   (d) Testing of Water. Perform water tests for chlorine/bromine content daily outside of CONUS and at all units that make or chlorinate/brominate their own water and record the results in the Health Services Log. Consult the Water Supply and Wastewater Disposal Manual, COMDTINST M6240.5 (series).
   (e) Cleaning. Health services department spaces shall be cleaned daily and all used instruments cleaned and stored until sterilization can be accomplished.
(2) Weekly Routines.
   (a) Inspections. Conduct sanitation inspection of the ship or station with emphasis on food service, living spaces, sanitary spaces, specifically including food handlers, refrigerators, chill boxes, galley spaces, and pantries. Submit a written report to the CO and make an appropriate entry in the health services log.
   (b) Training. Conduct training in some aspect of health care or treatment unless required more frequently by the CO or other directive.
   (c) Field Day.
   (d) Resuscitators. Inspect and test resuscitators to ensure proper functioning. Record results in the health services log.
(3) Monthly Routines.

(a) Reports. Submit all required health services monthly reports, outlined by Chapter 9 of this Manual and other appropriate directives.

(b) Inspection of Battle Dressing Station Supplies. Inspect battle dressing station supplies to ensure adequate and full inventory. Check sterile supplies and re-sterilize every six months. Replace expired or deteriorated supplies and materials. Enter an appropriate entry in the health services log indicating that the inspection was conducted and the action taken.

(c) First Aid Kits. Inspect hinges and hasps to ensure that they are free from rust, corrosion, or excessive paint.

(d) Poison Antidote Locker. Inspect poison antidote locker for proper equipment and medications as per allowance list.

(4) Quarterly Routines.

(a) Inventory of Controlled Substances. The Controlled Substances Inventory Board shall conduct an inventory, as required by Chapter 10 of this Manual, and submit a written report of the findings to the CO.

(b) Reports. Submit all required health services reports as outlined in Chapter 6 of this Manual and other appropriate directives.

(c) Inventory. Conduct a sight inventory of all health services consumable supplies/equipment as required by Chapter 8 of this Manual and the Health Services Allowance List.

(d) First Aid Kits. Inspect the contents to ensure adequate and full inventory. Replace expired and deteriorated supplies and materials. Make an appropriate entry in the health services log.

23. CG Beneficiary Representatives at Uniformed Services Medical Treatment Facilities (USMTF).

   a. Duties. Ensure CG active duty personnel and the commands of those personnel are provided the following:

   (1) CG authorities are provided prompt and current information concerning the status of CG personnel being treated.

   (2) CG personnel being treated receive necessary command administrative support.

   (3) The USMTF use the patient's CG health record and that entries are made in it or on forms that are filed in it.

   (4) The necessary health records and forms either accompany the patient or are forwarded to the command having custody of the health record.

   b. Responsibilities. The representative is responsible for the following:

   (1) Notification of Patient Status. It is essential that the representative keep cognizant command levels advised of the status of CG patients admitted for inpatient treatment. Notify commands, by the most expedient means

possible, within 24 hours of admission or discharge of members of their command.

(2) <u>Health Record Entries</u>. The representative is responsible for ensuring that all information concerning inpatient hospitalization, (e.g., admissions, operative summaries, discharge summaries) which is required to be entered in the health record, is furnished to the command which maintains the patient's health record. The representative shall also make the USMTF aware that all entries or forms associated with outpatient medical and dental activity must be entered in the patient's CG health record.

(3) <u>Copies of Forms</u>. The USMTF is responsible for completing and furnishing at least one copy of the following forms to the representative. The representative is responsible for preparing any additional copies needed.

(a) Inpatient hospitalizations:

1. Medical Record, SF-507 (or other discharge summary form).

2. Operative summary if surgery was done.

(b) Physical examinations/Periodic Health Assessments:

1. Report of Medical Examination, DD-2808.

2. Report of Medical History, DD-2807-1

3. ANY specialty reports obtained pursuant to the physical examination.

(c) Medical Evaluation Boards (MEB):

1. Medical Board Report Cover Sheet, CG-5684 for IMB/DMB.

2. Current Report of Medical Examination, DD-2808 for IMB.

3. Current Report of Medical History, DD-2807-1 for IMB.

4. Current Medical Record, SF-507 for IMB/DMB.

5. ANY specialty reports obtained pursuant to the physical examination for IMB/DMB.

6. Evaluee's Statement Regarding the Findings of the Medical Board, CG-4920 signed by the patient for IMB/DMB.

7. The command endorsement, Line of Duty/Misconduct Statement (if any), and members rebuttal (if any) should normally be done at/by the command for IMB/DMB.

(4) <u>Liaison and Assistance</u>. The representative shall:

(a) Maintain liaison between the CG units in the area and the USMTF as follows:

1. Clinical services to obtain timely appointments for CG personnel.

2. Pharmacy to facilitate drug exchange with CG units.

3. Biomedical repair to help originate and maintain agreements for repair and maintenance of local CG medical equipment.

(b) Whenever possible, personally meet with each hospitalized CG AD and SELRES member and meet or phone the immediate family of the member, offering them assistance.

(c) In appropriate cases, channel other CG and DoD resources such as Mutual Assistance, Family Programs, Red Cross, etc. to assist hospitalized members and their dependents.

(5) <u>Assignment and Duties</u>. HS assigned to a USMTF as CG Beneficiary Representatives are attached to the HSWL SC which will exercise military control over them. The representative is expected to comply with the rules and orders of the USMTF to which assigned, and is subject to the orders of the hospital commander. However, it is expected that any duties assigned will be consistent with the purpose noted in subparagraph 13a. above.

24. <u>CG Representative at the Department of Defense Medical Examination Review Board (DODMERB)</u>.

   a. <u>General</u>. DODMERB is located at the USAF Academy, CO and is a joint agency of the military departments responsible for scheduling, reviewing, and certifying service academy and ROTC scholarship applicant medical examinations, and other programs assigned by the Office of the Assistant Secretary of Defense, Health Affairs.

   b. <u>Responsibilities</u>.

   (1) As a member of DODMERB, the CG:

      (a) Establishes entrance standards for the CG Academy.

      (b) Makes its health care facilities available for completing entrance physical examinations for all service academies.

   (2) As a member of DODMERB, the CG liaison:

      (a) Is assigned as an examination evaluator/administrator.

      (b) Participates in implementing plans and organizational procedures for board actions.

   c. <u>Duties</u>.

   (1) Maintain a current list of examining centers which includes dates and examination quotas.

   (2) Schedule examinations for the applicants.

   (3) Notify applicants and program managers of scheduled examinations.

   (4) Review and apply medical standards.

(5) Notify applicants and program managers of the status and qualifications of applicants.

(6) Provide copies of medical examinations and medical information to the various programs on applicants until they are no longer eligible.

(7) Provide copies of medical examinations and medical information to eligible applicants as requested.

25. Health Benefits Advisors (HBA).

   a. Responsibilities. Individuals designated as Health Benefits Advisors (HBAs) at CGMTFs are responsible for advising and assisting beneficiaries concerning their health benefits. This individual shall:

   (1) Keep current on the multiple health and dental care programs and options available to AD, SELRES, retirees and their family members such as: TRICARE, Uniformed Services Family Health Benefits Program (USFHBP), Retiree Dental Program, TRICARE Dental program, etc.

   (2) Advise all beneficiaries on matters pertaining to healthcare benefits, including.

   (a) Obtaining Non-availability Statements and using the local appeal system for Non-availability Statements.

   (b) Obtaining prior authorization for specialty care under TRICARE prime.

   (c) Educating Prime enrollees on access standards for Acute, Routine and Specialty healthcare.

   (3) Advise TRICARE beneficiaries on the relationship between TRICARE, DVA programs, Social Security, Medicare, insurance provided through employment, and the effect of employment and private insurance on benefits available under TRICARE. Emphasize the following:

   (a) Availability of TRICARE and explain financial implications of using non-participating providers.

   (b) Provide beneficiaries the names and addresses of participating providers of the specific services the beneficiary requires.

   (c) Caution beneficiaries to verify that the provider participates in TRICARE at the time of service and if they are accepting new patients.

   (4) Coordinate TRICARE problem cases with the HSWL SC and TRICARE contractors.

   (5) Assist all beneficiaries in properly completing TRICARE enrollment and claim forms.

   (6) Serve as a single point of contact for all health benefits programs available to active duty and retired members and their dependents.

(7) Provide information and assistance based upon personal, written, or telephone inquiries concerning healthcare benefits.

(8) Keep beneficiaries informed of changes within the various programs, e.g., legislative changes affecting benefits available or other policy/procedures impacting upon the usage of civilian medical care. Provides for an ongoing program of lecture services, informational seminars, and group counseling to various beneficiary groups, service clubs, retirement briefings, etc.

(9) Maintain liaison with local providers and encourages them to increase their acceptance of the TRICARE program.

(10) Maintain liaison with the HSWL SC and unit collateral duty HBAs in local area.

b. Training.

(1) Individuals designated as HBAs must be trained in TRICARE benefits, exclusions, claims preparation, processing, cost-sharing formulas, eligibility criteria, and alternatives to TRICARE.

(2) Training Schedule.

(a) Requests for attendance at the TRICARE course should be submitted via the Chain of Command to the CG TRICARE Liaison Officer at TMA-Aurora.

(b) TRICARE course registration form is available at http://www.tricare.osd.mil/. This form may be submitted electronically or by mail.

(3) TMA-Aurora Liaison Staff Seminars. The Liaison Office at TMA-Aurora provides seminars for large beneficiary groups, e.g., recruiter, career counselor, etc. Arrangements for seminars should be made directly with the CG Liaison.

(4) Funding. Training requests for the TRICARE course will be funded by the cognizant unit.

c. Sources of Reference Materials. HBAs shall acquire and become familiar with specific reference materials on Federal and nonfederal health programs. Specifically, as TRICARE policies change, the HBA shall maintain an updated reference library through distribution channels as outlined below:

(1) TRICARE Information: www.tricare.osd.mil.

(2) TRICARE Publications: www.tricare.osd.mil/smart

(3) Beneficiaries can check their own claim status and eligibility at www.mytricare.com

(4) TRICARE Claim Forms (DD-2642, 04/2003) Now available at http:// www.tricare.osd.mil or by contacting:

NAVY PUBLICATIONS AND FORMS CENTER
5801 TABOR AVE
PHILADELPHIA, PA 19120-5013
U/I: PD

(5) Referral for Civilian Medical Care (DD-2161). May be printed locally by accessing CG Standard Workstation III, USCG Adobe Forms or by contacting:

NAVY PUBLICATIONS AND FORMS CENTER
5801 TABOR AVE
PHILADELPHIA, PA 19120-5013
U/I: PD

(6) Fiscal Intermediary Distribution by Region. Fiscal Intermediary Newsletter.

(7) Local Community. Local Publication - Social Services Directory.

26. <u>Dental Hygienists</u>. Dental hygienists are licensed graduates of American Dental Association accredited schools of dental hygiene. Whether contract or active duty providers, they are authorized to treat beneficiaries in CG dental clinics under the oversight of a DO. Restrictions on the degree of required oversight and the scope of services vary from state to state.

　a. <u>Scope of practice</u>. In the interests of standardization, quality improvement, and risk management, Dental Hygienists in CG health care facilities shall, in most circumstances, treat patients only when a DO is present for duty at the command. At the discretion of the SDE, and in the interest of expediency, this guideline may be overridden if each of the following conditions is met on each patient:

　　(1) Only active duty members are treated.

　　(2) An MO is present in the building.

　　(3) Patients' Periodontal Screening and Recording (PSR) scores are 10 or less.

　　(4) The licenses of the SDE and Dental Hygienist are not jeopardized by this action.

　b. <u>Patient criteria</u>. In every case, patients must receive a Type 2 examination by a DO no more than six months prior to treatment by a Dental Hygienist.

　c. <u>Patient review</u>. The SDE, or a staff DO designated by the SDE, shall conduct an intra-oral review of no fewer than 5% of the Dental Hygienist's patients for completeness of plaque/deposit removal and damage to hard/soft tissues. The responsible DO shall document these reviews in the patients' dental records.

　d. <u>State laws</u>. The scope of the Dental Hygienist's services shall be governed by either the state in which the license is held or the state in which the clinic is located, whichever is more restrictive, and shall be itemized in the clinic's SOP.

e. Injections. In some cases the state license may contain an addendum certificate which "privileges" the Dental Hygienist to administer injections of local anesthesia under the direct oversight of a licensed dentist. This practice is not authorized in Coast Guard clinics.

27. Red Cross Volunteers. Red Cross Volunteers are people who have completed a formal training program offered by a Red Cross Chapter and have a certificate of successful completion. Red Cross training is a screening and educational tool that enables individuals with an interest in helping others to function as supervised medical assistants in the clinic.

    a. Responsibilities. Red Cross Volunteers are responsible for scheduling their time in the clinic with clinic staff, accepting supervision, and carrying out activities mutually agreed upon by themselves and the clinic. These duties must fall within the scope of duties for which Red Cross training has prepared the volunteer. Duties may include: patient transport via gurney or wheelchair within the clinic, assessing and properly recording temperature, respiratory rate, heart rate, and blood pressure, acting as a chaperone during exams or treatment, assisting in specialty areas, i.e., laboratory (with appropriate additional training and supervision), answering telephones, filing and other clerical duties, cleaning and wrapping instruments.

    b. Supervision. Supervision of Red Cross volunteers is the responsibility of the CA and may be delegated.

    c. Orientation. Each volunteer must have an initial orientation to the clinic documented. Orientation shall include at least the following topics:

        (1) Fire Safety.

        (2) Emergency procedures (bomb threats, mass casualty, power outages, hurricanes/tornadoes).

        (3) Standard precautions and infection control.

        (4) Proper handling of telephone emergency calls.

        (5) Phone etiquette, paging, proper message taking.

        (6) Patient Bill of Rights and Responsibilities, to include confidentiality, and chaperone duties in accordance with Chapter 2-J-3-b of this Manual.

        (7) Privacy Act and HIPAA.

28. Volunteers.

    a. Volunteer Health Care Workers (HCW). Volunteer health care workers (HCW) who are not privileged providers with the PHS, DOD or CG Auxiliary (AUX) shall work under the supervision of clinic staff, as determined by the

SHSO. (Note: All volunteers, except PHS, DOD, CG AUX, or Red Cross volunteers which are covered elsewhere in this chapter, are required to sign a gratuitous service agreement. These volunteers may provide support services that include but are not limited to: patient transport via gurney or wheelchair within the clinic, assessing and recording vital signs, acting as a chaperone during examination or treatment, clerical duties such as answering telephone or filing, cleaning and wrapping instruments, etc. Non-privileged health care providers with special skill sets (e.g. RN, EMT, Paramedic, Dental Hygienist) may work up to the level of their license/certification at the discretion of and supervision by the SHSO. Verification of the capabilities of the provider is the responsibility of the SHSO. Written documentation that the member has received/understood instructions concerning items listed in 1-B-21-g.(1) through (7), must be signed by the CA and counter signed by the SHSO.

b. CG non-rate volunteers. CG non-rate (active/reserve) who wish to learn more about the HS rating by participating in clinical activities prior to applying/attending HS "A" school are considered volunteers and must follow the same guidelines set forth in Chapter 1-B-21-b. and g. of this Manual. Additionally, written documentation that the member has received/understood instructions concerning items listed in 1-B-21-g.(1) through (7), must be signed by the CA and counter signed by the SHSO. Additional requirements include:

   (1) Priority should be given to the non-rate (active/reserve) that are on the HS "A" school list. Other non-rate (active/reserve) personnel will be considered by the CA on a case-by-case basis.

   (2) All non-rates (active/reserve) must obtain written approval by their department supervisor prior to being assigned to the health services division.

   (3) The non-rate (active/reserve) must be supervised at all times within the clinic by a senior HS1/HS2 and may not provide independent patient care.

   (4) The non-rate (active/reserve) will not to be utilized as part of the HS clinical duty rotation schedule and must work during normal clinical hours Monday-Friday while assigned to the clinic. This clinical participation will not preclude non-clinical duties or assignments.

   (5) Non-rates (active/reserve) aboard cutters must be directly supervised by the ship's IDHS and follow the same guidelines in Chapter 1-B-21-b. and g. Written documentation as stated in 1-B-21-g. must be signed by the XO and IDHS.

c. TAD "non-medical personnel". TAD "non-medical personnel" who are assigned to medical will follow the same guidelines in Chapter 1-21-g., and will not be utilized in the delivery of patient care.

d. Health care providers up to fourteen (14) days. Health care providers who are members of the PHS or DOD and volunteer to work in CG clinics for up to fourteen (14) days per year will not be required to apply to Commandant (CG-11) for clinical privileges.

    (1) Volunteer providers in this category will submit a copy of a current active state license, copy of current clinical privileges and a current CPR card to the local clinic when they report in. They will also complete a request for clinical privileges appropriate to their category and submit to the SHSO. Volunteer providers can also submit a Credentials Transfer Brief in lieu of their license and CPR card.

    (2) For all categories of volunteer health care providers, only one active, unrestricted license from a state or U.S. Territory is required. Volunteers are authorized to work in any CG clinic in any state or territory even if they are not licensed in that jurisdiction.

    (3) The SHSO will evaluate the clinical privileges requested and by signing the request will authorize the provider to perform those health care services.

e. <u>Health care providers who volunteer more than fourteen (14) days</u>. Health care providers who are members of the PHS or DOD and volunteer to work in CG clinics for more than fourteen (14) days per year will be required to apply for clinical privileges from Commandant (CG-11) as described in Chapter 13-B and C of this Manual.

f. <u>Auxiliary</u>. Volunteer health care providers who are members of the CG Auxiliary, will be required to apply for clinical privileges from Commandant (CG-11), IAW with protocols described in the Medical Manual, COMDTINST M6000.1(series), Chapter-13-B and C and are required to satisfy the same standards for credentialing and privileging that are required for active duty health care providers in the CG. Volunteer providers will work under the direct or indirect supervision of CG clinic providers IAW COMDTINST 6010.2B.

g. <u>Initial orientation</u>. Each volunteer must have an initial orientation to clinic standard operating procedures which must be documented and must include at the minimum:

    (1) Fire safety.

    (2) Emergency procedures (e.g., bomb threats, mass casualty, power outages, and hurricanes/tornadoes).

    (3) Standard precautions and infection control.

    (4) Proper management of telephone calls, emergency calls.

    (5) Telephone etiquette, paging, taking messages.

    (6) Patient sensitivity and confidentiality.

    (7) Privacy Act and HIPAA

This page intentionally left blank

COMDT INST M6000.1E

Section C. CG Health Services Officer Training Matrix

1. Introduction…………………………………………………………………....1
Table 1-C-1 CG Medical Officer Matrix………………………………………………1
Table 1-C-2 CG Dental Officer Matrix……………………………………………….. 2
Table 1-C-3 CG Leadership Courses Matrix………………………………………….3
Table 1-C-4 CG Chemical, Biological, Radiological, Nuclear, and
             Explosive (CBRNE) Courses Matrix……………………………….4
Table 1-C-5 CG Disaster Training Matrix……………………………………………...5

This page intentionally left blank.

C. CG Health Services Officer Training Matrix.

1. Introduction. Emerging national and military strategies in support of wartime, humanitarian assistance, homeland security/defense and disaster response contingencies are the driving forces behind the training requirements to provide initial and sustainment training for all CG Health Services personnel. Training for Health Services enlisted personnel is contained in Chapter 9 of this Manual and in the Cutter Training and Qualification Manual, COMDTINST 3502.4 (series). Officers serving in the CG Health Services system may require training in a variety of specific subject areas. Some of this training is necessary for all officers in the CG Health Services system and some is specific based on the type of duty position to which the officer is currently assigned and/or the specific professional category of the officer. The following information provides a matrix showing required and recommended training for officers in the CG Health Services system. Unless otherwise specified, required training should be completed within the first three years of the tour requiring that training.

2. CG Medical Officer Training Matrix.

Name of course	Description	Duration	Funding source	Notes	Target audience
Operational & Primary Care Medical Training	Annual operational medicine and primary care training for all CG MOs	1 week	AFC-56 (central)	See annual solicitation letter sent from Commandant (CG-1121)	Required at least every 3 years for CG primary care providers
Operational Aviation Medical Training	Annual refresher aviation and operational medicine training for CG FS, AMOs and APAs	4 days	AFC-56 (central)	See annual solicitation letter sent from Commandant (CG-1121)	Required at least every 3 years for CG aviation medicine providers

Table 1-C-1

CG Medical Officer Training Matrix (con't)

Name of course	Description	Duration	Funding source	Notes	Target audience
Flight Surgeon/ Aeromedical Physician Assistant Training	Required training to provide care in aviation medicine	7 weeks	AFC-56 (central)	Apply through Commandant (CG-1121); Army or AF course followed by a 1 week CG transition course at ATC Mobile	Required for any MO in order to provide aviation medicine care
Physician Assistant Training	Operational medicine and primary care training for CG Pas	5 days	AFC-56 (central)	See annual solicitation letter sent from Commandant (CG-1121)	Required at least every 3 years for CG mid-level providers

Table 1-C-1 (cont.)

3. <u>CG Dental Officer Training Matrix</u>.

Name of course	Description	Duration	Funding source	Notes	Target audience
Dental Officer Training	Refresher and upgrade training for CG Dental Officers	5 days	AFC-56 (central)	Apply through Dental Program Manager at Commandant (CG-1122)	Required every other year for CG Dental Officers

Table 1-C-2

4. <u>CG Leadership Courses Matrix</u>.

Name of course	Description	Duration	Funding source	Notes	Target audience
Joint Operations Medical Manager's Course	Training in medical support for expeditionary operations	5 days	AFC-56 (limited – central funding) or local funding	DOD course, apply through Commandant (CG-1121)	Highly recommended for clinic SMEs, Commandant (CG-1121) and HSWL SC MOs
Homeland Security Medical Executive Course	Training in the federal, state and local responses to domestic mass casualty/care situations	5 days	AFC-56 (limited – central funding) or local funding	DOD course, apply through Commandant (CG-1121)	Highly recommended for clinic SMEs, SHSOs, Commandant (CG-1121), and HSWL SC MOs
CG Senior Leadership Principles and Skills (SLPS) Course	Standard CG course for developing leadership and negotiation skills	5 days	AFC-56 (central)	Commandant (CG-112) will contact target audience	Required for all SHSOs within 3 years of assignment; recommended for all SMEs/ SDEs
Direct Commission Officer School	Training to prepare recently commissioned officers of the CG	4 weeks	AFC-56 (central)	Commandant (CG-112) will contact target audience	Required for all new PHS Officers detailed to CG billets
Officer Basic Course	Recommended PHS training	2 weeks	Local funding	Commandant (CG-112) will contact target audience or arrange through local channels	Recommended for all PHS officers

Table 1-C-3

5. **CG Chemical, Biological, Radiological, Nuclear, and Explosive (CBRNE) Courses Matrix.**

Name of course	Description	Duration	Funding source	Notes	Target audience
CBRNE Emergency Preparedness and Response Course	On-line training for all health care providers in the CG	N/A	Web-based	Provided for the CG by the AF; see Commandant (CG-112) website for further details	MOs take Clinician Course. DOs, Pharmacists and all other PHS categories take Operator/ Responder Course. Required within 12 months of assignment
Medical Management of Chemical and Biological Casualties	Medical principles relating to chemical and biological weapons attacks	6 days	AFC-56 (central)	Army course- apply through Commandant (CG-1121)	Required for MOs within 3 years of assignment. Optional for all DOs, Pharmacy Officers, and EHOs
Combat Casualty Care Course	Combat casualty care training is provided in austere environment and in mass casualty situations	9 days	AFC-56 (central)	Army course- apply through Commandant (CG-1121)	Required for MOs within 3 years of assignment. Recommended for all DOs. Officers who have previously taken this course through DOD are not required to attend
OFRD Response Modules – Core	Required PHS training	N/A	Web-based	Apply through PHS OFRD website	Required for all PHS officers
OFRD Response Modules - Clinical	Recommended PHS training	N/A	Web-based	Apply through PHS OFRD website	Recommended for all appropriate PHS officers

Table 1-C-4

CG CBRNE Courses Matrix (con't)

Name of course	Description	Duration	Funding source	Notes	Target audience
Advanced Cardiac Life Support- Basic Provider	Advanced life support training for adverse cardiac events	2-3 days			All MOs in clinical billets are required to maintain current ACLS certification as a condition of employment
Basic Life Support for Healthcare Providers	CPR training required for all CG Healthcare Providers	4-8 hours	Local training	Local funding	Required maintenance of certification for all CG Health Care providers

Table 1-C-4 (cont.)

6. <u>CG Disaster Training Matrix</u>.

Name of course	Description	Duration	Funding source	Notes	Target audience
Incident Command System 100	Basic orientation to the Incident Command System	N/A	Web-based	Web training is through FEMA's website; check Commandant (CG-1121) website for further info	Required for all MOs, DOs, Pharmacy, Med Admin and Environmental Health Officers
Incident Command System 200	Second-level orientation to the Incident Command System	N/A	Web-based	Web training is through FEMA's website; check Commandant (CG-1121) website for further info	Required for all MOs, DOs, Pharmacy, Med Admin and Environmental Health Officers

Table 1-C-5

CG Disaster Training Matrix (con't)

Name of course	Description	Duration	Funding source	Notes	Target audience
Incident Command System 300	Advanced orientation to the Incident Command System	2-3 days	Local funding; Local TAD	Check on Commandant (CG-1121) website for further info	Required for SME, SHSO and HQ and HSWL SC MOs
Incident Command System 700	Introduction to the National Incident Management System	N/A	Web-based	Web training is through FEMA's website; check Commandant (CG-1121) website for further info	Required for all MOs, DOs, Pharmacy, Med Admin and Environmental Health Officers
Incident Command System 800	Introduction to the National Response Framework	N/A	Web-based	Web training is through FEMA's website; check Commandant (CG-1121) website for further info	Required for all MOs, DOs, Pharmacy, Med Admin and Environmental Health Officers
Advanced Disaster Life Support	Orientation for advanced medical response in disasters	2 days	Local funding	Check Commandant (CG-1121) website for further info	Recommended

Table 1-C-5 (cont.)

CHAPTER 2
HEALTH CARE AND FACILITIES

Section A. Health Care for Active Duty Personnel.

1. Care at Uniformed Services Medical Treatment Facilities 1
2. Emergency Care 3
3. Dental Care and Treatment 6
4. Consent to and Refusal of Treatment 11
5. Elective Surgery for Pre-Existing Defects 13
6. Elective Health Care 13
7. Other Health Insurance (OHI) 14
8. Procedures for Obtaining Non-Emergent Health Care from Nonfederal Sources 15
9. Obtaining Vasectomies and Tubal Ligations from Nonfederal Providers 17
10. Care at Department of Veterans Affairs (DVA) Medical Facilities 17
11. HIPAA and the Uses and Disclosures of Health Information of Active Duty Personnel 18

Section B. Health Care for Reserve Personnel.

1. Eligibility for Emergency Treatment at any DOD, CG or Civilian Medical Facility 1
2. Care at Uniformed Services Medical Treatment Facilities 1
3. Non-Emergent Care at Other Than CG or DOD Facilities 3

Section C. Health Care for Retired Personnel.

1. Care at Uniformed Services Medical Treatment Facilities 1
2. Care under TRICARE Standard and Extra (formerly CHAMPUS) 1
3. Care at Veterans Administration Medical Facilities 1

Section D. Health Care for Dependents.

1. Care at Uniformed Services Medical Treatment Facilities 1
2. Referral for Civilian Medical Care (DD-2161) 1
3. Rights of Minors to Health Care Services 2

Section E. Care for Preadoptive Children and Wards of the Court.

1. General 1
2. Secretary's Designation 1

Section F. Health Care for Other Persons.

1. Members of the Auxiliary 1
2. Temporary Members of the Reserve 1
3. Members of Foreign Military Services 2
4. Federal Employees 3

COMDTINST M6000.1E

 5. Seamen 3
 6. Non-Federally Employed Civilians Aboard CG Vessels......................................3
 7. Civilians Physical Exams prior to Entry to the CG 4

Section G. Medical Regulating.

 1. Transfer of Patients at CG Expense 1
 2. Travel Via Ambulance of Patients to Obtain Care 1
 3. Aeromedical Evacuation of Patients 1

Section H. Defense Enrollment Eligibility Reporting System (DEERS) in CG Health Care Facilities.

 1. Defense Enrollment Eligibility Reporting System 1
 2. Responsibilities 1
 3. Performing DEERS Checks 1
 4. Eligibility/Enrollment Questions, Fraud and Abuse 2
 5. Denial of Non-emergency Health Care Benefits for Individuals Not Enrolled in Defense Enrollment Eligibility Reporting System (DEERS) 3
 6. DEERS Eligibility Overrides 3

Section I. Health Care Facility Definitions.

 1. CG Facilities 1
 2. Department of Defense Medical Facilities 2
 3. Uniformed Services Military Treatment Facilities (USMTFs).............................2

Section J. Policies and Procedures Required at CG Health Care Facilities.

 1. Administrative Policies and Procedures 1
 2. Operational Policies and Procedures 1
 3. Patient Rights 2
 4. Health Care Provider Identification 3

Section K. General Standards of Care.

 1. Standard of care 1
 2. Diagnosis and therapy 1
 3. Bases for Diagnoses 1
 4. Treatment 1
 5. Time Line for Treatment...1
 6. Correct-site Surgery Policy 2
 7. Patients role..2
 8. Documentation 2

Section A. Health Care for Active Duty Personnel

1. Care at Uniformed Services Medical Treatment Facilities (USMTF). 1
2. Emergency Care. 3
3. Dental Care and Treatment. 6
4. Consent to and Refusal of Treatment. 11
5. Elective Surgery for Pre-Existing Defects. 13
6. Elective Health Care. 13
7. Other Health Insurance (OHI). 14
8. Procedures for Obtaining Non-Emergent Health Care from Nonfederal Sources. 15
9. Obtaining Vasectomies and Tubal Ligations from Nonfederal Providers. 17
10. Care at Department of Veterans Affairs (DVA) Medical Facilities. 17
11. HIPAA and the Uses and Disclosures of Health Information of Active Duty Personnel. ..18

This page intentionally left blank.

CHAPTER TWO – HEALTH CARE AND FACILITIES

Section A. Health Care for Active Duty Personnel.

1. Care at Uniformed Services Medical Treatment Facilities (USMTF).

    a. Authority for Health Care. Title 10 USC, 1074(a) provides that under joint regulations to be prescribed by the Secretary of Defense and the Secretary of Homeland Security, a member of a uniformed service who is on active duty is entitled to health care in any facility of any uniformed service. Members of the reserve components who are on active duty (including active duty for training) for periods prescribed for more than 30 days are entitled to the same health care in any facility of the uniformed services as that provided for active duty members of the regular services.

    b. Use of Own Service Medical Treatment Facilities. Under ordinary circumstances, members shall be enrolled in Active Duty TRICARE Prime, assigned a Primary Care Manager (PCM) and receive health care at that organization to which the member is assigned. However, Commanding Officers may request assignment to another USMTF through HSWL SC. Members away from their duty station or on duty where there is no USMTF of their own service may receive care at the nearest USMTF.

    c. Medical readiness. The CO/OIC of the unit is responsible for ensuring the medical and dental readiness of their unit. All CG members are required to be medically ready for deployment. All Individual Medical Readiness (IMR) requirements that are delineated in CG periodic Health Assessment, COMDTINST M6150.3 are required to be met by CG AD and SELRES members (to include Direct Commission Officers). For the purposes of fulfilling medical/dental readiness data entry requirements, all AD and SELRES personnel (via their assigned unit) will be assigned to a CG clinic or sick bay based on the district or sector of their unit location. The following web page lists the units and their assigned CG Clinic responsible for entering their MRRS entries http://www.uscg.mil/hq/cg1/cg112/docs/pdf/Clinic%20List%20For%20Web.pdf (Exceptions may be granted on a case-by-case basis, in writing, by the HSWL SC). CO/OIC of units with a CG clinic or sickbay shall support the medical readiness data entry requirements of those units assigned to their clinic/sickbay by ensuring the appropriate entries are made in MRRS. When an individual goes to a civilian or military physician for immunizations or exams, the information shall be sent to the supporting clinic or sickbay for entry into MRRS. Determination of units assigned to a clinic or sickbay may also be found by reviewing the spreadsheet on CG-Central: Medical Community >Medical Policy>Clinic Responsibility Unit Report.

d. Dental Readiness. When an individual goes to a non Active Duty Dental Plan dentist or DoD dentist for an exam or treatment, the DD-2813 shall be filled out and sent via fax to the supporting clinic or sickbay for entry into DENCAS.

e. <u>Use of Other Services Medical Treatment Facilities and/or Civilian Facilities</u>. The closest USMTF having the appropriate capabilities shall be used for non-emergency health care. Health care in civilian medical facilities for non-emergent conditions is not authorized without prior approval from HSWL SC. All health care received at other treatment facilities (military/civilian) shall be recorded in the CG health record.

f. <u>Definitions</u>.

   (1) Uniformed Services are the Army, Navy, Air Force, Marine Corps, CG, Commissioned Corps of the Public Health Service, and the Commissioned Corps of the National Oceanic and Atmospheric Administration.

   (2) Active Duty means full-time duty in a Uniformed Service of the United States, to include full-time training duty; annual training duty, and attendance, while in the service, at a school designated as a service school by law or by the Secretary of the Uniformed Service concerned.

   (3) Protected Health Information (PHI). Some of the purposes for which the PHI may be used or disclosed relate to the execution of a member's military mission. These include disclosures needed when determining the member's fitness for duty, determining the member's fitness to perform any particular mission, and to report on casualties. The PHI that is released to a command authority is on a "need to know" basis. Appropriate military command authorities include all commanders who exercise authority over an individual who is a member of the Armed Forces, or other person designated by such a Commander to receive PHI in order to carry out an activity under the authority of the Commander. They can only be provided information that is necessary to assess the active duty member's ability to carry out a specific duty.

   (4) Health Care means outpatient and inpatient professional care and treatment, nursing care, diagnostic tests and procedures, physical examinations, immunizations, prophylactic treatment, medicines, biologicals, other similar medical services, and ambulance service. Prostheses, hearing aids, spectacles, orthopedic footwear, and similar adjuncts to health care may be furnished only where such adjuncts are medically indicated.

g. <u>Application for Care</u>. Members of the CG on active duty may be provided health care by a USMTF when requested by appropriate CG authority, a Public Health Service Medical Officer detailed to the CG, or by the member by presenting a Geneva Convention Identification Card.

h. Subsistence Charges. All active duty members of the uniformed services are required to pay subsistence in a USMTF at a rate prescribed by the Department of Defense.

i. Loss of Entitlement. A member of the CG who is separated from active duty for any reason other than retirement, is not eligible for health care at a USMTF by reason of that previous service unless otherwise noted on the Certificate of Release or Discharge from Active Duty form DD-214.

2. Emergency Care.

   a. Definition of Emergency Condition.

      (1) An emergency medical condition exists when the patient's condition is such that, in a Medical Officer's opinion, failure to provide treatment or hospitalization would result in undue suffering or endanger life or limb.

      (2) In an emergency, the patient's safety and welfare, as well as that of the personnel around the patient, must be protected. When a USMTF cannot render immediate care, other local medical facilities, Federal or civilian, may be used. The decision to admit the patient to any of these facilities shall be made by the command with regard for only the health and welfare of the patient and the other personnel of the command.

   b. Responsibilities.

      (1) Patient.

         (a) The patient is responsible for notifying the civilian or military physician or dentist that he or she is in one of the following:

            1. Active Duty CG.
            2. CG Reserve on active duty or active duty for training.
            3. CG Reserve in an inactive duty training drill or appropriate duty status.

         (b) It is also the responsibility of the patient or someone acting in the patient's behalf to request that the physician or dentist notify the member's command or the closest CG organization and PCM that he or she is undergoing emergency treatment at a civilian or military medical facility.

         (c) The patient shall provide, to their PCM, all information needed to verify the course of treatment received and authorize release of all records associated with the episode of care.

(2) <u>Commanding Officer</u>. When notified that a member of the CG is hospitalized, in either a civilian hospital or MTF, transferred to another facility, or discharged from an inpatient status, the unit CO or designated representative shall notify HQ and HSWL SC via e-mail within 24 hours. The e-mail address is HQS-DG-HSWL Inpatient Hospitalization. No other individuals shall be included or copied on this e-mail. This e-mail will only be viewed by command designated individuals at HSWL SC and HQ on a need to know basis. If you cannot access this e-mail site contact the HSWL SC or Commandant (CG-1121) for assistance. Use the following format when sending the e-mail, including the statement at the end of the e-mail.

SUBJ: INPATIENT HOSPITALIZATION – (Initial, update or Final)
1. RATE/RANK, FIRST NAME LAST NAME, EMPLID, USCG/USCGR.
2. UNIT
3. DATE AND FACILITY WHERE MEMBER ADMITTED.
4. DIAGNOSIS (use plain language i.e., appendicitis)
5. ESTIMATED DURATION
6. POC RATE/RANK NAME, PHONE # AND E-MAIL ADDRESS

This communication and its attachments are confidential to the Coast Guard Health Care Program and to the intended recipient(s). Information contained in this communication may be subject to the provisions of the Privacy Act of 1974 and Health Insurance Portability and Accountability Act. If you have received this email in error, please advise the sender immediately and delete the entire message together with all attachments. All unintended recipients are hereby notified that any use, distribution, copying or any other action regarding this email is strictly prohibited.

(3) <u>Chain of command notification</u>. COs shall utilize a separate e-mail to notify other personnel on a need to know basis. The information contained in this e-mail shall only be the minimum necessary to accomplish the intended goal. Information sent shall be considered PHI and the guidelines provided in (1.e. (3)) of this section shall be followed. Use the following format when sending the e-mail to include the statement at the end of the e-mail.

SUBJ: INPATIENT HOSPITALIZATION
1. RATE/RANK, FIRST NAME LAST NAME, EMPLID, USCG/USCGR
2. UNIT
3. DATE AND FACILITY WHERE MEMBER ADMITTED
4. ESTIMATED DURATION
5. POC RATE/RANK NAME, PHONE # AND E-MAIL ADDRESS

This communication and its attachments are confidential to the Coast Guard Health Care Program and to the intended recipient(s). Information contained in this communication may be subject to the provisions of the Privacy Act of 1974 and Health Insurance Portability and Accountability Act. If you have received this email in error, please advise the sender immediately and delete the entire message together with all attachments. All unintended recipients are hereby notified that any use, distribution, copying or any other action regarding this email is strictly prohibited.

- (4) <u>CO, Health, Safety, and Work-Life Service Center (HSWL SC)</u>. When notified that a member of the CG is hospitalized, HSWL SC shall:

    (a) Assure the confidentiality of inpatient E-mails.

    (b) Be responsible for coordinating additional inpatient care at a civilian medical facility prior to transferring the patient to a USMTF. Nothing in the above should be construed as precluding the necessary care for the patient concerned. HSWL SC shall notify the member's unit of any transfer action.

    (c) Assist in ascertaining all necessary background information about the case, whether the patient should be moved, and the location of the nearest USMTF which can accept the case. Patients shall be transferred in accordance with the provisions of Medical Regulating to and Within the Continental U.S., COMDTINST M6320.8 (series).

- (5) <u>COs with Reservists</u>.

    (a) A Reservist needing emergency treatment while on orders and engaged in active duty training shall be taken to the nearest appropriate medical facility. If outpatient follow-up treatment is required, (i.e., office visits, tests, etc.) such treatment must be preauthorized by HSWL SC after issuance of a Notice of Eligibility by the local command.

    (b) The CO of the reserve member shall comply with Chapter 6 of the Reserve Policy Manual, COMDTINST M1001.28 (series) in notifying the Commander, HSWL SC and the local command when a Reservist engaged in active duty training is admitted to a civilian hospital or USMTF, and subsequent follow-up.

- (6) <u>Government Responsibility</u>. Non-adherence to these notification directives cannot limit the Government's liability to pay bills for emergency medical and dental treatment to authorized CG beneficiaries. However, if prior approval is not obtained for NON-EMERGENT treatment in nonfederal facilities, the member receiving the care will be liable for payment.

c. <u>Emergency Care Outside the Continental United States</u>. CG active duty personnel outside the continental limits of the United States are entitled to health care at USMTFs, where available. If such facilities are not available, emergency health care may be obtained at CG expense without prior authorization.

d. <u>Absentees or Deserters</u>. Charges incurred by CG personnel for civilian health care when absent without authority or in desertion is the sole responsibility of the individual. However, charges for civilian health care after actual or constructive return of the individual to CG or military control may be paid from

CG funds. Refer questions on payment of health care in regards to constructive return to HSWL SC.

   e. Appellant Leave. CG personnel in appellant leave status shall obtain health care and enroll in TRICARE Prime at the nearest USMTF to their appellant leave address (residence). CG personnel on appellant leave are not eligible for TRICARE Prime Remote because they lack a permanent assignment to a TPR location. CG personnel may transfer their enrollment to another USMTF at the direction of HSWL SC.

3. Dental Care and Treatment.

   a. Extent of Dental Services.

      (1) Active duty CG personnel are entitled to emergency, routine, and accessory dental treatment at all USMTFs. Dental care from Active Duty Dental Plan participating dentists is authorized only as prescribed in Chapter 11 of this Manual.

      (2) Reserve CG personnel ordered to active duty with their consent for less than thirty days are eligible for emergency dental treatment only, and are also subject to the following modifications:

         (a) Reserve personnel are responsible for all dental diseases and conditions in existence prior to the initiation of or call to active duty. They must be in a class 1 or 2 dental status. (See Chapter 4 Section C.3.c.)

         (b) Reserve personnel shall not be eligible for routine or accessory dental treatment, which cannot be completed prior to termination of or release from active duty status.

         (c) Reserve personnel are responsible for maintaining their dental fitness for duty while on inactive status or during periods of active duty less than 30 days.

         (d) CG Reserve personnel ordered to active duty for 30 days or more are eligible for emergency, routine, and accessory dental treatment at all USMTFs, and are also subject to the modifications listed above.

         (e) Reservists who are not on extended active duty are required to obtain an annual dental exam to facilitate readiness. These exams can be obtained from a Coast Guard clinic, Reserve Health Readiness Program, or the reservist's civilian dentist. Payment for civilian dental examinations is covered by the reservist's own dental insurance. In the event the member does not have dental insurance, the HSWL SC will provide payment for the annual dental exam only.

(f) All dental visits shall be entered in DENCAS whether the care is received at a CG health care facility or other treatment facility. Active Duty and Reserve members are responsible for ensuring that dental care recorded at a facility other than a CG health care facility is recorded in DENCAS. The Active Duty Dental Plan will ensure DENCAS entry for the exam visits.

b. Definitions of Types of Dental Treatment.

(1) Emergency Dental Treatment. Emergency dental treatment includes those procedures directed toward the immediate relief of pain, uncontrolled bleeding, orofacial trauma and/or swelling, the removal of oral infection which endangers the health of the patient, and repair of prosthetic appliances where the lack of such repair would cause the patient physical suffering.

(2) Routine Dental Treatment. Routine dental treatment reflects those procedures listed as, required primary core privileges, on the Request for Clinical Privileges – Dentist, CG-5575B, (which includes but is not limited to: examinations, radiographs, diagnosis and treatment planning, amalgam and resin restorations, prophylaxis, scaling and root planing, surgical periodontal procedures, cast and ceramic restorations, removable partial and complete dentures, extractions, non-surgical root canal therapy, vital and non-vital bleaching, mouthguards, sealants, and removable and fixed retainers).

(3) Accessory Dental Treatment. Accessory dental treatment reflects those procedures listed as, supplemental privileges, on Request for Clinical Privileges – Dentist, CG-5575B which includes but is not limited to: implant restorations, limited orthodontics (Invisalign® is not authorized except at the member's expense), molar uprighting, guided tissue regeneration, free soft tissue and connective tissue grafts, mucogingival surgery, and surgical root canal therapy.

(a) Implant restorations placed by CG Dental Officers (DOs) shall be performed by one of the following:

1. Those DOs specifically privileged to do so by DOD facilities.

2. Those DOs who have received implant training as part of a residency program.

3. Those DOs who have had extensive training and experience restoring implants may be privileged to restore implants on an individual basis.

(b) Implant maintenance is the responsibility of all DOs. Each DO shall be familiar with the techniques and armamentarium of implant maintenance, as well as diagnosis of successful and unsuccessful implants.

    (c) Requests for implants from non-Federal providers for active duty members shall be submitted for review and approval to the Active Duty Dental Plan prior to initiation of treatment. Factors to be considered include:

        1. Oral hygiene.

        2. Treatment alternatives.

        3. Feasibility and expectations for long-term success.

        4. Length of service and anticipated rotation date.

c. <u>Dental Care of Recruits</u>. Only emergency dental treatment should be provided to those recruits who are to be separated from the Service prior to completing recruit training. It is important that recruits in this category do not have teeth extracted in preparation for prosthetic treatment and then be separated from the Service prior to the time prosthetic appliances are provided.

d. <u>Emergency Dental Treatment in Nonfederal and Non-contract Facilities</u>.

    (1) If an Active Duty Dental Plan (ADDP) dentist is not available, emergency dental treatment required for the immediate relief of pain or infection may be obtained by active duty CG personnel from any available dentist. Once the emergency has been alleviated, all follow-up treatment must be from a USMTF or ADDP dentist unless preauthorized by ADDP.

e. <u>Criteria To Be Followed When Requesting Orthodontic/Orthognathic Surgical Care</u>.

    (1) Orthodontic/orthognathic surgical treatment can affect release from active duty, rotation dates, and fitness for duty. Therefore, written authorization to commence all orthodontic/orthognathic surgical treatment (whether elective or not, and whether provided by Federal or Nonfederal practitioners) must be requested from Commander (PSC-epm) for enlisted and (PSC-opm) for officers via HSWL SC prior to its initiation. Command endorsement must include a copy of Administrative Remarks, CG-3307 documentation described in article 2-A-3.e.(4)(a) below. Request for nonfederal care from HSWL SC must follow the established guidelines:

        (a) DTF completes the attached DTF Orthodontic Referral and UCCI DTF Referral Request form which may be found at: https://secure.ucci.com/non-ldap/forms/addp/forms/referral-form.pdf.

(b) DTF forwards completed forms to TRICARE Management Activity Dental Service Point of Contact (DSPOC) via fax at 703-681-9090.

(c) The DSPOC will review the 2 forms submitted by the DTF and either approve or disapprove the referral or request additional info. The DSPOC will notify the DTF Point of Contact of the decision.

(d) If approved, the DSPOC will scan and securely e-mail the approved DTF Referral Request to UCCI. The UCCI Dental Care Finder will then initiate the scheduling of the appointment.

(e) If disapproved, the DTF may appeal through their respective Dental Chain of Command.

(2) Submit a memo from the member requesting Orthodontic treatment detailing the end of enlistment and rotation dates, treatment plan from Orthodontist detailing reason for and length of treatment, and Service Record Administrative Remarks, CG-3307 documenting command approval for treatment.

(3) Preexisting conditions are the member's responsibility.

(4) Treatment not required to maintain the member's fitness for duty is elective in nature and is not authorized for payment by the CG. If the member's condition does not impair job function, the treatment shall be considered elective.

(5) Elective care may be obtained, if available, from an MTF or nonfederal provider. Any payments may be the responsibility of the member. In addition, the member is financially responsible for any care arising from complications that require additional treatment. Because complications could lead to subsequent action by the Physical Disability Evaluation System (PDES), and to protect the interests of both the service member and the CG, the member's command is responsible for Service Record Administrative Remarks, CG-3307 documentation detailing:

(a) Command approval and the personnel action to be taken by the command regarding the granting of absence.

(b) That the service member was instructed regarding the provisions contained herein and other applicable directives.

(c) That the service member must obtain copies of all treatment records from the provider for inclusion into the CG dental record, including (e.g. initial evaluation, treatment plan, progress notes, and follow-up care).

(d) Member must be evaluated by a Dental Officer and given a duty status prior to returning to work.

(6) If elective treatment is approved, PDES processing shall be suspended pending the outcome of the elective treatment. Aviation personnel, divers and cadets are required to have a waiver request approved by PSC (opm or epm). In addition, members whose duties preclude regular visits to an orthodontist (e.g., icebreakers crews, isolated LORAN duty, etc.) fall under this category.

(7) If the condition is service-related, the CG shall be responsible to acquire care sufficient to return the member to a fit for full duty status (e.g., that which existed at the time of the member's entry to the service), but not necessarily to ideal conditions not impacting on performance of duties. If treatment is not available at a local MTF, use of ADDP provider(s) may be authorized.

(8) If orofacial pain is the only symptom causing the member to be not fit for full duty, then it must be treated. Treatment may include, but is not limited to physical therapy, stabilization splints, stress management, and medications. Since orthodontic treatment is of long duration, it is not an appropriate method to relieve acute pain.

(9) All treatment must be completed, inactivated, or terminated prior to transfer or release from active duty. Personnel who are being transferred or released from active duty, and who request inactivation of orthodontic appliances, shall sign an entry in the Dental Record / Continuation, SF-603/603-A, stating their intention to seek orthodontic therapy at their own expense.

(10) Orthodontic treatment utilizing a series of clear removable aligners such as Invisalign® does not require written authorization. These aligners are removable so treatment is inactivated when appliances are no longer used.

f. <u>Third Molar Extraction Criteria</u>.

(1) The management of third molars is complicated by the age of CG personnel and the seagoing and isolated nature of CG service. A growing body of evidence suggests that prophylactic removal of all pathology-free non-erupted third molars results in unnecessary morbidity and cost. Nevertheless, there are several conditions associated with third molars, which warrant prompt intervention.

(2) Criteria for extraction of third molars include:

(a) Symptomology.

(b) Associated pathology includes follicular cyst development, external or internal resorption of third molar, recurrent episodes of pericoronitis or single episode of pericoronitis that was unresponsive to treatment, caries in second or third molar not amenable to restorative measures, and third molar contributing to periodontal disease.

(c) Communication with oral cavity, including being able to be probed.

4. <u>Consent to and Refusal of Treatment</u>.

   a. <u>Regulatory Restrictions</u>. United States Coast Guard Regulations, COMDTINST M5000.3 (series), state in Section 8-2-1 that:

      (1) "Persons in the Coast Guard shall not refuse to submit to necessary and proper medical or dental treatments to render them fit for duty, or refuse to submit to a necessary and proper operation not endangering life."

      (2) "Persons in the Coast Guard shall permit such action to be taken to immunize them against disease as is prescribed by competent authority."

   b. <u>Policy Concerning Refusal of Treatment</u>.

      (1) Policy.

         (a) It is the Commandant's policy that compulsion is not permissible at any time to require CG personnel to submit to various types of medical or dental treatment, diagnostic procedures, or examinations.

         (b) Surgery will not be performed on persons over their protest if they are mentally competent.

         (c) Individuals who refuse to submit to measures considered by competent Medical or Dental Officers to be necessary to render them fit for duty may be processed for separation from the CG in accordance with applicable regulations unless granted a medical or administrative exemption as per Immunizations and Chemoprophylaxis, COMDTINST 6230.4 (series). Individuals may be subjected to disciplinary action for refusal of necessary treatment or surgery if the refusal is determined to be unreasonable. Refusal of medical care by vegetative or comatose individuals in accordance with a Living Will shall not be considered unreasonable.

         (d) Refusal of mandatory immunizations will be processed for separation from the Coast Guard unless granted a medical or administrative exemption as per Immunizations and Chemoprophylaxis, COMDTINST 6230.4 (series).

      (2) Non-Emergent Operations on Minors. A minor who enlists or otherwise enters active duty with parental or guardian consent is considered emancipated during the term of enlistment. There is therefore, no legal requirement that the consent of any person, other than the minor, be obtained prior to instituting surgical procedures.

(3) Refusal of Emergency or Lifesaving Treatment or Emergency Diagnostic Procedures. The refusal of recommended emergency or lifesaving treatment or emergency diagnostic procedure required to prevent increased level of impairment or threat to life is ordinarily determined to be unreasonable. However, refusal of medical care by vegetative or comatose patients under the authorization of a Living Will is not considered unreasonable. A medical board shall be convened in accordance with the Physical Disability Evaluation System, COMDTINST M1850.2 (series) for unreasonable refusal of emergency or lifesaving treatment or emergency diagnostic procedures.

(4) Refusal of Non-Emergent Treatment. If a member of the CG refuses non-emergent medical, surgical, dental, or diagnostic procedures that are required to maintain a fit for full duty status, a determination of reasonable basis for this refusal is required. A medical board shall be convened in accordance with Physical Disability Evaluation System, COMDTINST M1850.2 (series).

c. <u>Advance Directives (Living Wills)</u>.

(1) Federal law enacted in 1993 requires hospitals to ask about advance directives at the time of admission and provide patients with information to create advance directives. Advance directives, commonly known as living wills, express a person's wishes regarding certain aspects of treatment and care, including but not restricted to CPR, mechanical life support measures, etc., which may arise in the course of hospitalization.

(2) CG health care facilities are not required to provide such information under the law. Clinics may elect to provide standardized information to patients on request. Information given out shall conform to the implementing laws of the state in which the clinic is located. Clinics providing such information shall notify patients of its availability either by posted notice or via patient handout materials.

(3) Clinic staff members usually do not have the required training and experience to advise patients on the legal issues concerning creation of advance directives. Patients shall be referred to the appropriate source of legal support, e.g., command or district Legal Officers.

(4) Clinic staff members, where allowed by state law, may serve as witnesses to advance directive signatures.

(5) Advance directive documents shall be held by the member and/or the member's next of kin. Advance directive documents shall not be filed in the member's health record since health records are not universally available 24 hours a day, seven days a week, for reference by a treating hospital.

5. Elective Surgery for Pre-Existing Defects.

   a. General. Elective surgery for defects that existed prior to entrance (EPTE) have often resulted in long periods of convalescence with subsequent periods of limited duty, outpatient care, and observation which render the Government liable for benefits by reason of aggravation of these defects.

   b. Criteria. The following conditions must be met before attempting surgical correction of an EPTE defect.

      (1) The procedure being considered is an accepted one, carries a minimal risk to life, and is not likely to result in complications.

      (2) There should be a reasonable certainty that the procedure will correct the defect and restore the member to full duty within a reasonable time (three months) without residual disability. If the defect does not meet the above conditions and the member is, in fact, unfit to perform the duties of grade or rate, action shall be taken to separate the member from the Service.

   c. Discussion. Whether elective medical/dental care should be undertaken in any particular case is a command decision which should be decided using the above guidelines. In questionable cases, the member may be referred to a Medical Evaluation Board (MEB) for final decision prior to undertaking elective treatment for an EPTE defect.

6. Elective Health Care.

   a. Definition. Medical/Dental treatment not required to maintain the member's fitness for duty is elective in nature and is not authorized for payment by the CG. If the member's condition does not interfere with their ability to perform duty, the treatment shall be considered elective.

      (1) Elective care may be obtained, if available, from USMTFs. In accordance with the Health Affairs (HA) Policy 05-020 "Policy for Cosmetic Surgery" expenses incurred in obtaining elective care or follow-up care at USMTFs may be the responsibility of the member.

      (2) If obtained from nonfederal providers, payment is the member's responsibility. In addition, the member is financially responsible for any care arising from complications that require additional treatment, even if it is non-elective.

      (3) Because complications could lead to subsequent action by the Physical Disability Evaluation System (PDES), and to protect the interests of both the service member and the CG, the member's health record must contain a SF-600 entry detailing:

         (a) Command approval and the personnel action taken regarding the granting of absence.

(b) That the service member was counseled regarding the provisions contained herein and other applicable directives. Counseling will be provided at the local CG primary care facility, or if there is no nearby CG primary care facility, then HSWL SC will provide counseling via phone. A SF-600 will be faxed to HSWL SC for appropriate entries, then faxed or mailed back to the unit for incorporation into the member's health record.

(c) That the service member must obtain copies of all treatment records from the provider for inclusion into the CG health record, including initial evaluation, treatment plan, progress notes, and follow-up care.

(d) Members must be evaluated by a Medical Officer and given a duty status prior to returning to work.

(4) Members shall understand that once they have received an elective treatment or procedure, they may be adversely affected for present or future assignments or specialized duty .

(5) Liposuction and paniculectomy are elective procedures that are allowed if the member otherwise is compliant with weight and body fat standards. Bariatric surgery including gastric banding and/or bypass is not authorized.

7. Other Health Insurance (OHI).

   a. General. In some situations a member may desire to utilize their spouses' health insurance (OHI) to obtain health care outside of the Military Health Care System. Whether elective health care or all other areas of health care, this decision has an impact on the command and possibly on a member's access to the Physical Disability Evaluation System (PDES).

   b. Criteria. The following conditions must be met before utilizing a spouse's health insurance or OHI:

   (1) ALL payments are the member's responsibility. In addition, the member is financially responsible for any care arising from complications that require additional treatment, even if it is non-elective.

   (2) Because complications could lead to a loss of access to the Physical Disability Evaluation System (PDES), and to protect the interests of both the service member and the Coast Guard, the member's CG health record must contain a SF-600 entry detailing:

   (a) Command approval and the personnel action to be taken by the command regarding the granting of absence. That the service member was instructed regarding the provisions contained herein and other applicable directives. Counseling will be provided at the local CG primary care facility, or if there is no nearby CG primary care facility, then HSWL SC will provide counseling via phone. An SF-600 will be faxed to HSWL SC for appropriate entries, then faxed or mailed back to the unit for incorporation into the member's health record.

    (b) That the service member must obtain copies of all treatment records from the provider for inclusion into the CG health record, including initial evaluation, treatment plan, progress notes, and follow-up care.

8. Procedures for Obtaining Non-Emergent Health Care from Nonfederal Sources.

   a. Nonfederal sources for active duty. Nonfederal sources for active duty care are intended to supplement and not substitute for care that is available through the federal system. USMTF's or DVA facilities, if located within a 40 mile radius of the member's unit (except a 30 mile radius for maternity care), shall be used first for non-emergent, non-elective health care before nonfederal sources are used. Each case must be evaluated for:

      (1) Appropriateness of care.

      (2) Urgency of treatment.

      (3) Time and cost factors associated with obtaining such care from a USMTF.

      (4) The member's anticipated length of stay at the given station.

      (5) Operational need of the unit for the member.

      (6) Before active duty personnel are treated in a nonfederal medical facility for non-emergent conditions, prior approval from HSWL SC must be obtained. Non-elective conditions are those which, without repair or treatment, would render the member unfit for duty.

   b. HSWL SC. HSWL SC may approve requests for nonfederal health care (both medical and dental) and may delegate, in writing, limited authority to Clinic Administrators.

   c. Requests for nonfederal health care beyond a Clinic Administrator's authority. Requests for nonfederal health care beyond a Clinic Administrator's authority will be submitted by following HSWL SC policy. Telephone authorization will not be provided without a hard copy of the request. At a minimum, the following information must be provided, as applicable:

      (1) Name, grade/rate, social security number.

      (2) Anticipated rotation date and expiration of enlistment.

      (3) Whether care will be completed before transfer or separation.

      (4) Diagnosis reported by International Classification of Diseases, (current edition) Revision, Clinical Modification (ICD-9-CM) code number and a brief explanation.

      (5) History of patient's condition.

(6) Total amount of local and/or HSWL SC approved nonfederal expenditures to date for this condition.

(7) The necessity of treatment to maintain fitness to perform duty.

(8) Treatment plan: length, type of therapy/treatment, and estimated cost (cost estimates must include total scope of care not just primary provider or hospital costs).

(9) Name of facility where treatment will be done.

(10) Attending physician's prognosis with and without treatment, including likelihood of medical board action.

(11) Name of nearest USMTF capable of providing care:

   (a) Distance to facility (miles).

   (b) Earliest appointment available (not available is unacceptable).

   (c) Travel/per diem cost.

   (d) Estimated total lost time.

   (e) Other factors for consideration, e.g., travel time, road conditions, operational impact, etc.

(12) Indicate date of original submission and reason for resubmission, if previous requests were submitted for this procedure.

d. <u>If approval is granted</u>. If approval is granted, HSWL SC will provide the requester with an authorization number. This authorization number must be noted on all invoices submitted. Invoices will be submitted to HSWL SC. If approval is denied, HSWL SC will outline the appropriate appeals process to follow in their denial transmittal.

e. <u>Personnel transferred prior to completing the approved care</u>. When personnel are transferred prior to completing the approved care, the request is canceled. Personnel are required to submit another request after reporting for their new assignment.

f. <u>Authorization of funds</u>. Amounts authorized shall not be exceeded without further authorization from HSWL SC which requires additional justification.

g. <u>Inpatient hospitalization</u>. Inpatient hospitalization in nonfederal facilities shall be monitored closely by HSWL SC. Normally, an inpatient stay will not exceed seven days duration without consideration of movement to a USMTF. Cases suspected to extend past the seven-day limit shall not be placed in a civilian facility, but shall be initially referred to a USMTF. When notified that a member of the CG is hospitalized, transferred to another facility, or discharged from inpatient status, the unit CO shall notify Commandant (CG-112) and HSWL SC via e-mail as noted in 2.c.(2) of this section.

 h. <u>Penalties for non-approved care</u>. If prior approval is not obtained for non-emergent treatment in nonfederal facilities, the member receiving the care will be liable for payment.

 i. <u>Emergency treatment</u>. EMERGENCY health care does not require prior approval.

9. <u>Obtaining Vasectomies and Tubal Ligations from Nonfederal Providers</u>.

 a. <u>Preauthorization is required</u>. Submit all requests for vasectomies and tubal ligations by nonfederal providers to HSWL SC following the guidelines for requesting above. Request must show the provider of care decided on the procedure based upon applicable local and state guidelines.

 b. <u>Counseled and consent</u>. Request must contain evidence that the patient has been counseled by a physician and has given informed consent to the procedure.

 c. <u>SF-600</u>. The request must contain evidence that the patient has completed an SF-600 entry acknowledging that the CG will not pay for reversal of this procedure in a non-federal facility. The request must contain current information concerning the availability of the requested procedure from federal sources.

 d. <u>Tubal Ligations</u>. Request for a tubal ligation to be performed at the time of delivery should be submitted with the request for nonfederal maternity care.

 e. <u>Sick leave</u>. Sick leave may be granted for procedures.

10. <u>Care at Department of Veterans Affairs (DVA) Medical Facilities</u>. From time-to-time, acute medical, surgical, or psychiatric facilities are required for CG personnel when transportation to the nearest USMTF will place the individual's health or welfare in jeopardy. To preclude this and other similar situations, and to provide the best possible medical care for all active duty members, a support agreement between the CG and the DVA was completed in 1979 and remains in effect. FIGURE 2-A-1 is a copy of the medical service agreement.

 a. <u>Department of Veterans Affairs (DVA) care</u>. DVA care must be requested by the member's Commanding Officer. The agreement is limited to active duty CG personnel and does not include dependents.

 b. <u>Local contact with DVA</u>. Area Commanders and Commanding Officers should establish local contact with DVA facilities to determine mission and facility capabilities and patient admission procedures.

 c. <u>Billing procedures</u>. Forward all bills received from DVA facilities to the service member's unit for certification prior to forwarding to HSWL SC for payment.

 d. <u>MTF versus DVA</u>. When a USMTF and a DVA facility are co-located, the USMTF shall be used unless it cannot provide the required services.

11. <u>HIPAA and the Uses and Disclosures of Health Information of Active Duty Personnel.</u>

    a. <u>HIPAA</u>. The Health Insurance Portability and Accountability Act (HIPAA) contains a series of regulations, developed by the Department of Health and Human Services, and enacted into law, which are designed to provide patients with access to their medical records and provide more control over how their personal health information is used and disclosed. The rule also contains a "<u>military exception</u>" which allows health care entities, under certain circumstances, to disclose protected health information of military members without prior approval.

    b. <u>Intended uses or disclosures</u>. The CG is subject to HIPAA regulations in its role as a health care program for active duty military personnel. Accordingly, the CG has published the required Federal Register notice detailing five intended uses or disclosures of personal medical information.

        (1) The first intended use and disclosure is "to determine the member's fitness for duty, including but not limited to the member's compliance with standards and all other activities carried out under the authority of Weight /Physical Fitness Standards for Coast Guard Military Personnel, COMDTINST M1020.8 (series) for the health and well-being of CG military personnel; the Physical Disability Evaluation System, COMDTINST M1850.2 (series), and similar requirements pertaining to fitness for duty."

        (2) The second is "to determine the member's fitness to perform any particular mission, assignment, order, or duty, including any actions required as a precondition in the performance of such a mission, assignment, order, or duty."

        (3) The third is "to carry out activities under the authority of the Medical Manual, COMDTINST M6000.1 (series), Chapter 12 (Occupational Medical Surveillance & Evaluation Program)."

        (4) The fourth is "to report on casualties in any military operation or activity according to applicable CG Regulations or procedures."

        (5) The final use is "to carry out any other activity necessary to the proper execution of the mission of the Armed Forces."

        <u>Note: The CG's role as a first responder and MEDEVAC provider is not considered part of the health care program. Therefore, those activities are not subject to HIPAA limitations.</u>

    c. <u>First disclosure</u>. The first disclosure listed is designed to protect the Physical Disability Evaluation System (PDES) procedures for review of medical information. While health care professionals are permitted to continue disclosing medical information to the PDES without obtaining authorization from the member, 45 CFR 164.502b1 now requires that only the "minimum necessary to accomplish the intended purpose of the [request]" may be disclosed. More specifically, while in the past, health care professionals may have routinely disclosed a member's entire medical record to the PDES process, HIPAA regulations now require that they release the minimum necessary to the medical board (which may be the entire medical record) and the medical board may release only the information related to the injury or condition which prompted the convening of a medical board.

d. <u>Second disclosure</u>. The second disclosure listed is designed to protect a CO's ability to access necessary medical information about crewmembers. COs need this ability because they are responsible under the United States Coast Guard Regulations 1992, COMDTINST M5000.3 (series), for the well-being of the personnel in the command. This includes a CO's responsibilities to "excuse from duty any person in the command who is unable to perform because of illness or disability," "see that proper provision is made and that comforts are provided for the sick and disabled in the command" and "safeguard the health of all personnel by careful supervision of the sanitation of the unit by preventing unnecessary exposure to disease or unhealthy conditions afloat or ashore." The only constraint on a CO's access to a military member's private health information is the language of 45 CFR 164.502(b)(1). This section of the HIPAA regulations requires medical professionals to limit disclosures to the "minimum necessary to accomplish the intended purpose of the request."

e. <u>COs and Health Care Providers (HCP)</u>. In an effort to balance the CO's legitimate need for medical information with the HCP's duty to protect that information, the following guidance is offered:

  (1) COs shall, at a minimum, be entitled to a fully completed Status Profile Form, CG-5460A. Where the visible condition of the patient and the information contained in the "Duty Status" block of form CG-5460A do not provide sufficient information about a crewmember's abilities, the CO may request, and an HCP may provide, amplifying information directly related to the condition or injury specified on the form. Unrelated prior injuries or treatment and pre-existing health conditions need not be disclosed; however, medical conditions that directly aggravate the member's current condition or prognosis for recovery may be disclosed. In addition, a CO is entitled to inquire about any medication prescribed by a HCP, including any known side effects which may affect fitness for duty.

  (2) Military commanders will be required to identify their designated representatives in writing and the medical provider will have to establish procedures to validate the identity of the person making the request. If a service member presents for health care to a HCP and their supervisor, who is not their CO or CO's designee, calls to find out the member's diagnosis or their duty status, they should not be told without the service member's authorization. A Fitness for Duty chit given directly to the member who then takes it to his/her supervisor themselves is not considered disclosure of medical information.

(3) A HCP may also disclose protected health information as required by law. This includes court orders, subpoenas or summons (issued by a court, government Inspector General, or other authorized administrative body), authorized investigative demand (e.g., CGIS), or other statute or regulatory demand. The disclosure should be limited in scope to the purpose for which the information is sought.

(4) In addition, a HCP may disclose protected health information for administrative or judicial proceedings in relation to courts-martial procedures (any order from a military judge in connection with any process under the Uniform Code of Military Justice).

FIGURE 2-A-1   COMDTINST M6000.1D

IGA VI01(134A)S-79039

MEDICAL SERVICE AGREEMENT
BETWEEN THE
U. S. COAST GUARD
DEPARTMENT OF TRANSPORTATION
AND THE
VETERANS ADMINISTRATION

This agreement provides for medical services to be furnished the U.S. Coast Guard, Department of Transportation (hereinafter referred to as "CG") by the Veterans Administration (hereinafter referred to as "VA") and establishes the terms and conditions under which the services are to be furnished to active duty personnel.

I. BACKGROUND.

In February 1973, arrangements were established whereby CG active duty personnel utilized the VA hospital facilities for medical services. This agreement provides for the continuation of these services.

II. MEDICAL SERVICES TO BE FURNISHED BY THE VA.

A. Hospital care, medical services and emergency dental treatment may be provided to the extent that such care, services, or treatment are available at the VA medical facility from which requested.

B. To preclude the possibility of denying or delaying the care and treatment of an eligible veteran, VA medical services will be furnished only to the extent that there will be no reduction in the service to the veteran.

III. REFERRAL PROCEDURES.

VA medical services will be provided CG active duty personnel upon receipt of an authorization document from the responsible official at the CG facility. The authorization document will include the billing address for services to be rendered. Telephone authorizations will be accepted in emergencies pending receipt of a written authorization.

IV. REIMBURSEMENT.

A. The CG will reimburse the VA for the services performed at the current appropriate rates periodically approved by the Office of Management and Budget (OMB), except that if a CG beneficiary requires transfer to a non-VA facility, reimbursement shall be at the actual rates charged.

B. The VA medical center providing the medical services will prepare Standard Form 1081, Voucher and Schedule of Withdrawals and Credits, covering the services. The executed form will be submitted to the CG at the address shown on the authorization request.

Chapter 2. A. Page 21

V. TRANSPORTATION.

The CG will provide all necessary transportation and medical attendants, when applicable, for personnel scheduled for VA medical treatment. Travel costs to and from the VA medical facility will not be paid by the VA.

VI. LIABILITY.

Protection of the individuals furnishing services covered by this agreement will be that which is provided under 28 USC 1346(b), and by 38 USC 4116.

VII. GENERAL PROVISIONS.

A. Amendments or Cancellations:

This agreement or any of its specific provisions may be revised or amended only by the signature approval of the parties signatory to the agreement or by their respective official successors. Cancellation may be made upon 30 days written notice of either party, or their successors, to the other.

B. Effective Date:

This agreement, amendments to or cancellation thereof, shall become effective upon the date when the Chief, Office of Health Services, CG, and the Director, Supply Service, Department of Medicine and Surgery, VA, both have signed acceptance thereof.

C. Authority:

Authority for this agreement is the Economy Act of June 30, 1932, as amended (31 USC 686).

D. Previous Agreements:

This agreement supersedes previous medical service support arrangements.

ACCEPTED: ACCEPTED:

VETERANS ADMINISTRATION   DEPARTMENT OF TRANSPORTATION
                                         U. S. COAST GUARD

By: _Clyde C. Cook_   By: _Harry Allen_
    CLYDE C. COOK   HARRY ALLEN
    Director, Supply Service   Rear Admiral, U. S. Public Health Service
                                             Chief, Office of Health Services
                                             U. S. Coast Guard

Date: _Sept 24, 1979_   Date: _____

Section B. Health Care for Reserve Personnel.

    1. Eligibility for Emergency Treatment at any DOD, CG or Civilian Medical Facility..........1
    2. Care at Uniformed Services Medical Treatment Facilities..1
    3. Non-Emergent Care at Other Than CG or DOD Facilities..3

This page intentionally left blank.

COMDTINST M6000.1E

B. Health Care for Reserve Personnel.

1. Eligibility for Emergency Treatment at any DOD, CG or Civilian Medical Facility.

    a. Reserve personnel on extended active duty or temporary active duty (i.e. Active Duty Special Work (ADSW)).

    b. Reserve personnel who become ill, injured, or contract a disease in the line of duty while on active duty for training or inactive duty for training, including authorized travel to or from such duty. See Reserve Policy Manual, COMDTINST M1001.28 (series) for further details.

2. Care at Uniformed Services Medical Treatment Facilities.

    a. Authority for Reserve Personnel. Information concerning Reserve incapacitation benefits and reporting procedures is contained in the Reserve Policy Manual, COMDTINST M1001.28 (series). Additional information concerning Reserve mobilization TRICARE benefits is available at http://www.tricare.osd.mil.

    b. Application for Care. A member of the CG Reserve may be admitted to USMTFs upon written authorization from an appropriate CG authority (e.g., CO's letter, Notice of Eligibility, or appropriately endorsed orders).

    c. Definitions. The following definitions apply throughout this section:

        (1) Active duty means full-time duty in a Uniformed Service of the United States. It includes duty on the active list, full-time training duty, annual training duty and attendance, while in the service, at a school designated as a service school by law or by the Secretary of the Uniformed Service concerned.

        (2) Active Duty for Training is defined as full-time duty in a uniformed service of the United States for training purposes.

        (3) Inactive Duty Training.

            (a) Duty prescribed for reservists by the Secretary concerned with 37 USC 206 or any other provision of law.

            (b) Special additional duties authorized for reservists by an authority designated by the Secretary concerned and performed by them on voluntary basis in connection with the prescribed training or maintenance activities of the units to which they are assigned. Disability. A temporary or permanent physical impairment resulting in an inability to perform full military duties or normal civilian pursuits.

        (4) Employed. Reservists are employed on duty during the actual performance of duty, while engaged in authorized travel to or from active duty for training, and while on authorized leave or liberty.

(5) Line of Duty. An injury, illness, or disease shall be deemed to have been incurred in line of duty, if a reservist at the time of debilitating incident is performing active duty or active duty for training, or is on authorized leave or liberty, provided the disability is not the result of misconduct. While health officials may make an interim line of duty determination in order to provide timely care, the determination of whether an injury/illness was sustained or aggravated in the line of duty is a unit leadership responsibility. The provisions of Chapter 5, "Line of Duty and Misconduct", Administrative Investigations Manual, COMDTINST M5830.1 (series) apply. Continued entitlement to health care requires this level of documentation.

d. Injury Incurred in Line of Duty. A member of the CG Reserve who is ordered to active duty or to active duty for training, or to perform inactive duty training, for any period of time, and is disabled in line of duty from injury while so employed is entitled to the same hospital benefits as provided by law or required in the case of a member of the regular CG. For the purpose of these benefits, a member who is not in a pay status is treated as though receiving the pay and allowances to which entitled if serving on active duty.

e. Disease Incurred in Line of Duty While on Active Duty. A member of the CG Reserve who is ordered to active duty for training for a period of more than 30 days, and is disabled while so employed, is entitled to the hospital benefits as are provided by law or regulation in the case of a member of the regular CG. An exception is that a member of the CG Reserve ordered to perform involuntary active duty for training under the provision of 10 USC 270 is only eligible for the limited medical benefits described below, following termination of the training duty period.

f. Illness or Disease Contracted in Line of Duty in Peacetime. A member of the CG Reserve who, in time of peace, becomes ill or contracts a disease in line of duty while on active duty for training or performing inactive duty training is entitled to receive medical, hospital, and other treatment appropriate for that illness or disease. The treatment shall be continued until the disability resulting from the illness or disease cannot be materially improved by further treatment. Such a member is also entitled to necessary transportation and subsistence incident to treatment and return home upon discharge from treatment. The nature and duration of health care and related benefits for these reservists is detailed in the Reserve Policy Manual, COMDTINST M1001.28 (series), Chapter 6, "Reserve Incapacitation System".

g. Injury or Illness En Route to or from Active Duty. A member of the CG Reserve is authorized medical care for an injury or illness incurred while en route to or from active duty, active duty for training, or inactive duty for training provided the injury or disease did not result from the member's misconduct or gross negligence.

h. Injury, Illness or Disease Not in Line of Duty. A member of the CG Reserve is not entitled to medical care for an injury, illness, or disease not incurred in the line of duty.

i. Pregnancy. Personnel Manual, COMDTINST M1000.6 (series), Chapter 9, contains guidance regarding pregnancy and reserve members.

j. Periodic examinations. CG Reserve personnel are eligible to receive annual dental Type-II exams and comprehensive physical examinations for training, accession, retirement, RELAD, Medical Evaluation Boards and confinement at CG MTFs. Annual Periodic Health Assessments may be authorized by HSWL SC to be performed by CG MTFs.

3. Non-Emergent Care at Other Than CG or DOD Facilities. Any non-emergent nonfederal health care must be authorized in advance by HSWL SC.

This page intentionally left blank.

Section C. Health Care for Retired Personnel

1. Care at Uniformed Services Medical Treatment Facilities..........................2
2. Care Under TRICARE Standard and Extra (formerly CHAMPUS). 2
3. Care at Veterans Administration Medical Facilities..................................2

C. **Health Care for Retired Personnel.**

1. **Care at Uniformed Services Medical Treatment Facilities.** As set forth in 10 USC, 1074(b), retired members of the uniformed services, as specified in that Act, are entitled to required medical and dental care and adjuncts thereto to the same extent as provided for active duty members in medical facilities of the uniformed services. However, access to care is subject to mission requirements, the availability of space and facilities, and the capabilities of the medical staff as determined by the HSWL SC. Patients enrolled in TRICARE Prime Options are not eligible for non-emergent care in CG clinics. These patients shall be referred to their TRICARE primary care manager (PCM). The PCM is responsible for appropriate care and referral of such patients.

2. **Care Under TRICARE Standard and Extra.** Subject to the cost sharing provisions set forth in 10 USC, 1086, retired members who are not qualified for benefits under Title I of the Social Security Amendments of 1965 (Medicare) are entitled to receive inpatient and outpatient care from civilian sources.

3. **Care at Veterans Administration Medical Facilities.**

    a. **Eligibility for DVA Hospitalization.** CG military personnel are eligible for hospitalization in DVA facilities after separation from active duty or while in retirement under one of the following circumstances:

    (1) For injuries or diseases incurred or aggravated while on active duty during any war, the Korean conflict period 27 June 1950 through 31 January 1955 or the Vietnam conflict period (5 August 1964 through 7 March 1975).

    (2) For service-connected or nonservice-connected disabilities, if receiving disability compensation from the DVA, or if entitled to receive disability compensation from the DVA, but has elected to receive retirement pay from the CG instead of compensation from the DVA.

    b. **Medical Care Benefits.** Eligible veterans may receive hospitalization, outpatient medical care, outpatient dental care, prosthetic appliances, etc., from the VA.

COMDTINST M6000.1E

Section D. Health Care for Dependents

1. Care at Uniformed Services Medical Treatment Facilities..1
2. Referral for Civilian Medical Care (DD-2161) 1
3. Rights of Minors to Health Care Services 2

This page intentionally left blank.

COMDTINST M6000.1E

D. Health Care for Dependents.

1. Care at Uniformed Services Medical Treatment Facilities.

    a. Authority for Health Care. Title 10 USC, 1076 provides basic authority for medical and dental care for:

        (1) Dependents of active duty members and dependents of members who died while serving on active duty.

        (2) Dependents of retired members and the dependents of members who died while in a retired status.

    b. Availability of Care.

        (1) Medical and dental care for dependents in Uniformed Services Medical Treatment Facilities is subject to the availability of space and facilities and the capabilities of the medical and dental staff. With the approval of HSWL SC, the Senior Health Services Officer (SHSO) is responsible for determining the availability of space and capability of the medical and dental staffs in CG clinics. These determinations are conclusive. Patients found enrolled in TRICARE Prime are not eligible for non-emergent care in CG clinics. These patients shall be referred to their TRICARE primary care manager (PCM). The PCM is responsible for appropriate care and referral of such patients.

        (2) Dependents entitled to medical and dental care under this section shall not be denied equal opportunity for that care because the facility concerned is that of a uniformed service other than that of the sponsor.

        (3) Types of Care Authorized. Subject to the provisions set forth in 10 USC, 1079 and 1086, dependents who are not qualified for benefits under Title 1 of the Social Security amendments of 1965 (Medicare) are entitled to receive inpatient and outpatient care from civilian sources. Refer to HSWL SC for details and instructions.

        (4) All non-active duty beneficiaries seeking care in CG health care facilities are required to furnish Other Health Insurance (OHI) information to the clinic. Pursuant to Title 10 USC, Sec 1095; EO 9397, beneficiaries are required to complete the Third Party Collection Program Record of Other Health Insurance, DD Form 2569. Failure to provide complete and accurate information may result in disqualification for health care services from facilities of the Uniformed Services.

2. Referral for Civilian Medical Care, DD-2161. This form shall be used to refer non-Active duty patients from CG facilities to nonfederal facilities, either for supplemental health care or when the patient is disengaged for care. The Referral for Civilian Medical Care, DD-2161 will also be used to disengage non-CG active duty patients from CG facilities when the scope of care is beyond

the ability of the CG to provide such care. The CG facility shall contact the parent service to ensure the active duty patient has the proper direction on where to obtain necessary care. A signed Referral for Civilian Medical Care, DD-2161 disengaging the patient will accompany the patient when they depart the CG facility and a copy shall be kept on file. The Referral for Civilian Medical Care, DD-2161 is used when referring patients for supplemental health care.

3. <u>Rights of Minors to Health Care Services</u>. Where not in conflict with applicable Federal law or regulation, CG MTFs shall follow State law defining the rights of minors to health care services and counseling in substance abuse, contraception, sexually transmitted infection prevention and treatment, and pregnancy. Any protection with regard to confidentiality of care or records afforded by applicable law or regulation will be extended to minors seeking care or counseling for these services or conditions in CG MTFs.

COMDTINST M6000.1E

Section E. Care for Preadoptive Children and Wards of the Court

1. General…………………………………………………………………....1
2. Secretary's Designation……………..……………………………………….1

This page intentionally left blank.

E. Care for Preadoptive Children and Wards of the Court.

1. General.

    a. A child placed in a sponsor's home as part of a pre-adoption procedure, or by court-ordered guardianship, is not eligible for care under the Uniformed Services Health Benefits Program unless specific authority has been granted. Such authority may come from the final adoption decree, a court-ordered legal custody determination (for a period of at least 12 consecutive months), or through a Secretary's Designation authorization for limited health care in a USMTF.

    b. Eligibility for TRICARE benefits. The Uniformed Services Family Health Benefits Plan (USFHBP), or the TRICARE Dental Plan is established upon the issuance of a uniformed services dependent ID card and Defense Eligibility Enrollment Reporting System (DEERS) enrollment. Authorization for these health care programs, or for direct care (USMTF use), will be reflected on the ID card and through DEERS.

    c. Prospective dependents must meet the following eligibility rules: be unmarried; have not attained the age of 21 (or 23 if a full-time student); be dependent on the sponsor for over one-half of their support; or be incapable of self-support due to mental or physical incapacity and were otherwise eligible when incapacity occurred.

    d. If legal custody or placement is for 12 months or more, a Uniformed Services dependent ID care, DEERS enrollment, and health care eligibility may be authorized. Personnel are encouraged to contact their servicing personnel office for assistance.

2. Secretary's Designation. The following procedures apply in situations where a pre-adoptive or court ordered guardianship or placement is for less than 12 consecutive months.

    a. Children under a prospective parent or guardians care may use a USMTF by acquiring authority from the Secretary of the Uniformed Service to which the USMTF belongs. This authority is normally called a Secretary's Designation. For example, requests for care in a U. S. Navy facility must be authorized by the Secretary of the Navy or their designee. The same holds true for U. S. Army and U. S. Air Force facilities. When seeking care from a Department of Defense (DoD) MTF, contact that facility's Patient Affairs or Health Benefits Advisor staff for assistance.

    b. In cases involving CG facilities, authority has been delegated to the Commandant by the Secretary of Homeland Security to authorize treatment of pre-adoptive children and wards of the court. Letter requests must be forwarded to Commandant (CG-112) and include the following information:

(1) Member's name, grade/rate, Emplid, and duty assignment or retired status if applicable.

(2) Address of residence.

(3) Name and age of the proposed adoptive child or court-ordered ward.

(4) A copy of the court order, legal decree, or other applicable instrument issued by a court or adoption agency which indicates the child has been placed in the house for adoption or with the intent to adopt, or the court order granting guardianship of the ward to the service member and any amounts of income to which the ward is entitled.

c. Upon approval, the respective Uniformed Service will issue a letter of authority for care in one or more of their USMTFs located in the United States. This letter is the only authority for care (since designees are not DEERS-eligible) and must be presented (or on file) when seeking authorized care. These letters have expiration dates and may require the sponsor to request to reissue. When registering the patient in CHCS use the DEERS override code *10 DEERS enrollment exception* to allow the patient to be registered and to receive care.

d. When there is a need for medical care outside the United States the sponsor should contact the nearest USMTF requesting humanitarian consideration. The Service Secretaries have limited authority for designation of beneficiaries outside the United States.

COMDTINST M6000.1E

Section F. Health Care for Other Persons.

1. Members of the Auxiliary 1
2. Temporary Members of the Reserve 1
3. Members of Foreign Military Services 2
4. Federal Employees 3
5. Seamen 3
6. Non-Federally Employed Civilians Aboard CG Vessels 3
7. Civilians Physical Exams prior to Entry to the CG 4

This page intentionally left blank.

COMDTINST M6000.1E

F. Health Care for Other Persons.

1. Members of the CG Auxiliary.

    a. Authority for Care of CG Auxiliary Members. Basic authority for health care for members of the CG Auxiliary injured while performing CG duty is contained in 14 USC 832. Section 5.59 of Chapter 1, Title 33, CFR, states: "When any member of the CG Auxiliary is physically injured or dies as a result of physical injury incurred while performing patrol duty or any other specific duty to which he has been assigned, such member or his beneficiary shall be entitled to the same benefits as are now or as may hereafter be provided for temporary members of the CG Reserve who suffer physical injury incurred in the line of duty. Members of the CG Auxiliary who contract sickness or disease while performing patrol duty or any other specific duty to which they have been assigned shall be entitled to the same hospital treatment as is afforded members of the regular CG." Claims for CG Auxiliary healthcare shall be submitted to:

    DEPARTMENT OF LABOR
    ATTN OFFICE OF WORKERS' COMPENSATION PROGRAM
    1240 E 9th ST RM 851
    CLEVELAND OH 44199-2001

    All doctor reports /findings should be submitted to:

    DEPARTMENT OF LABOR
    ATTN DFEC CENTRAL MAILROOM
    PO BOX 8300
    LONDON, KY 40742-8300

    b. Compensation under Federal Employee's Compensation Act (FECA) Program. See the Detail of Appropriated Fund Civilian Employees, COMDTINST M12300.7 (series).

2. Temporary Members of the CG Reserve.

    a. Composition of the CG Reserve. The CG Reserve is a component part of the United States Coast Guard and consists of two classes of reservists: Regular and Temporary. Temporary members of the CG Reserve may be enrolled for duty under such conditions as the Commandant prescribes, including but not limited to part-time and intermittent active duty with or without pay, and without regard to age. Members of the CG Auxiliary, officers and members of the crew of any motorboat or yacht placed at the disposal of the CG, and persons (including government employees without pay other than compensation of their civilian positions) who by reason of their special training and experience are deemed by the Commandant qualified for such duty. The Commandant is authorized to define the powers and duties of temporary reserves, and to confer upon them,

COMDTINST M6000.1E

appropriate to their qualifications and experience, the same grades and ratings as are provided for regular members of the Reserve.

    b. <u>Authority for Care of Temporary CG Reservists</u>. 14 U.S.C. 707(2002) contains authority for health care and/or compensation of temporary reserves under conditions set forth therein.

    c. <u>Care at CG Expense</u>. 14 U.S.C. 707(d) states: "A temporary member of the Reserve, who incurs a physical disability or contracts sickness or disease while performing a duty to which the member has been assigned by competent authority, is entitled to the same hospital treatment afforded a member of the Regular CG."

    d. <u>Compensation under Federal Employee Compensation Act (FECA) Program</u>. See Detail of Appropriated Fund Civilian Employee, COMDTINST M12300.7 (series).

3. <u>Members of Foreign Military Services</u>.

    a. <u>General</u>. Members and dependents of foreign services assigned or attached to a CG unit for duty or training (such as Canadian Exchange Officers) or who are on active duty with a foreign military unit within the United States (such as the crew of a vessel being taken over at the CG Yard under the Military Assistance Program) are eligible for health care at DOD MTF's provided by US Code: Title 10, Section 2559. As there are several categories of foreign service members for whom medical care benefits vary, both for themselves and their dependents, if any doubt exists as to eligibility for health care and the authorized sources from which it can be obtained, contact Commandant (CG-112) for advice.

    b. <u>Care at Uniformed Services Medical Treatment Facilities</u>. Members of foreign military services and their dependents who are eligible, therefore, shall be provided inpatient health care at DOD MTFs upon request of the member's Commanding Officer or consular official, or by application of the member or dependent upon presentation of proper identification.

4. Without an existing reimbursement agreement, the CG is only authorized to provide emergency medical services to foreign nationals. Personnel reviewing requests from foreign governments or foreign citizens to attend the CG Academy, a CG training course, or serve on CG units, must ensure individuals are covered by a reimbursable agreement or purchase private health insurance.

5. <u>Federal Employees</u>.

    a. <u>Benefits Under Federal Employees Compensation Act (FECA) Program</u>. All Federal Employees assigned to CG vessels, e.g., National Marine Fishery Service (NMFS), Drug Enforcement Agents, etc., are civilian employees of the United States Government, and as such, are entitled to health care and compensation under FECA. See Detail of Appropriated Fund Civilian Employee, COMDTINST M12300.7 (series).

b. Care Aboard Ship and Outside CONUS. Federal Employees may be given medical care while serving with the CG in a locality where civilian health care is not obtainable, such as onboard a CG vessel or outside the United States. Outpatient and inpatient care may be provided at Navy medical facilities outside CONUS, if reasonably accessible and appropriate nonfederal medical facilities are not available.

6. Merchant Marine Seamen. Sick and disabled seamen may receive emergency health care aboard Coast Guard vessels.

7. Non Federally Employed Civilians Aboard CG Vessels.

a. Authority for Care. There is no statute which either prohibits or authorizes the CG to provide health care to civilians while aboard CG vessels. There is no objection to furnishing emergency health care, but routine care should not be furnished. When these civilians are aboard CG vessels for relatively lengthy periods, the Commanding Officer must determine what treatment is to be given.

b. Responsibility. Commanding Officers of vessels deployed for extended periods shall ensure that Non-Federally employed civilians who are carried aboard CG vessels under their cognizance are physically capable of withstanding the trip contemplated and that they are free from medical conditions which could cause an interruption of the vessel's mission. Non-Federally employed civilians must furnish such evidence from a physician at no expense to the CG or Federal Government.

8. Civilians Physical Exams Prior to Entry to the CG. Certain CG programs offer specific, guaranteed training schools to civilian applicants provided they can pass the required physical exam in advance of entry into the CG. Commandant (CG-11) has specifically authorized pre-entry physical exams for prospective Coast Guard members (including but not limited to) Student Naval Aviator (SNA) Candidates through the Blue 21 program as well as for pre-identified candidates for guaranteed AET "A" school upon graduation from TRACEN Cape May.

a. Responsibility.

(1) Recruiting command personnel will identify potential candidates and coordinate with the Medical Administration Officer at CG clinics that are capable of performing SNA Candidate, Class 1 and Class 2 aviation or other physical examinations to the standards identified in Chapter 3 of this Manual. Recruiters should allow a minimum of two weeks lead time in order to arrange these PEs. All potential candidates must already have completed a MEPS PE and meet basic CG accession standards.

(2) CG clinics will perform aviation PEs (SNA candidate, Class 1 and Class 2) on potential candidates identified by local recruiters. Efforts should be made to perform the PE on a single day, if possible, in order to minimize travel expenses for the potential candidate. These programs are important to the manning needs of CG Aviation, but performing these exams does not take precedence over care of active duty and reserve CG personnel.

b. Reimbursement. HSWL SC has a process to reimburse sources for expenses that are incurred in carrying out these PEs. (The clinic completes the referral for the specific service using the DD-2161 and indicating to send itemized claim back to the clinic. Upon receipt of itemized claim, the Clinic Administrator validates it and attaches a copy of the original DD-2161 before sending to HSWL SC for processing & payment). Authorization for reimbursement includes expenses for aviation PEs that the clinic would normally incur through tests done in the civilian community (e.g. X-rays, Cycloplegic eye exams, etc). Potential candidates having disqualifying conditions are noted to have such on the PE, but no further evaluation, diagnostic or treatment is authorized (except in emergencies).

c. Routing. Once completed, the original PE is sent to the requesting CG Recruiter for further processing. This is a different procedure than aviation candidate PEs on current CG members.

Section G. Medical Regulating

1. Transfer of Patients at CG Expense 1
2. Travel Via Ambulance of Patients to Obtain Care 1
3. Aeromedical Evacuation of Patients 1

COMDTINST M6000.1E

This page intentionally left blank.

COMDTINST M6000.1E

G. Medical Regulating.

1. Transfer of Patients at CG Expense.

    a. Details for the transfer of CG personnel to, from, or between hospitals and the responsibility for the expenses involved are contained in Chapter 4 of the CG Personnel Manual, COMDTINST M1000.6 (series).

    b. Information and requirements for the transfer of patients to, from, or between medical facilities is contained in Medical Regulating to and Within the Continental U.S., COMDTINST M6320.8 (series).

2. Travel Via Ambulance of Patients to Obtain Care.

    a. Active Duty Personnel. The CG is responsible for providing ambulance service (Government or civilian), for active duty members when medically necessary. Bills related to ambulance service provided to active duty personnel, shall be processed as outlined in Chapter 11 of this Manual.

    b. Retired and Dependent Personnel. Retired personnel and dependents are not provided ambulance service for initial admission, except that a Government ambulance may be used in an emergency situation as determined by the cognizant medical authority. If an ambulance is ordered by a military hospital, TRICARE Standard cannot pay for it; the military hospital must pay. TRICARE Standard cost-shares ambulances only when medically necessary; that is, the patient's condition does not allow use of regular, private transportation or taxis, "medicabs" or "ambicabs." When ambulance transportation is needed, the medical condition must be a covered TRICARE Standard benefit. Should either the provider or patient have additional questions regarding this issue, check with HSWL SC, HBA or TRICARE Service Center.

3. Aeromedical Evacuation of Patients.

    a. When the condition of the patient requires aeromedical evacuation, the transfer shall be arranged in accordance with Medical Regulating to and Within the Continental U.S. (Joint Pub), COMDTINST M6320.8 (series). If there is no USMTF in the area, a message prepared in accordance with the above instruction shall be forwarded to HSWL SC.

    b. There may be instances where civilian health care must be obtained in foreign countries. TRICARE Overseas coordinates health care of beneficiaries located in remote locations where there are no United States health care facilities through a contract with International SOS (ISOS). This contract includes coordination of urgent and emergency health care for all active duty TAD, deployed or traveling in remote locations not supported by a U.S. Medical Treatment Facility. If urgent or emergent health care is required, the medical representative should contact the ISOS at www.internationalsos.com. ISOS will require the patient's name and SSN to verify eligibility through DEERS. ISOS will coordinate health care for the patient with a local treatment facility, assist with transportation needs, and guarantee payment to the local facility on behalf of the U.S. Government. If emergency air evacuation is required and military airlift is not available, ISOS will coordinate the air evacuation with the ISOS Regional Office closest to the unit's homeport.

COMDTINST M6000.1E

Section H. Defense Enrollment Eligibility Reporting System (DEERS) in CG Health Care Facilities.

1. Defense Enrollment Eligibility Reporting System 1
2. Responsibilities 1
3. Performing DEERS Checks 1
4. Eligibility/Enrollment Questions, Fraud and Abuse 2
5. Denial of Non-emergency Health Care Benefits for Individuals Not Enrolled in Defense Enrollment Eligibility Reporting System (DEERS) 3
6. DEERS Eligibility Overrides 3

This page intentionally left blank.

H. Defense Enrollment Eligibility Reporting System (DEERS) in CG Health Care Facilities.

1. Defense Enrollment Eligibility Reporting System. This Section provides guidance for CG health care facilities on the use of the Defense Enrollment Eligibility Reporting System (DEERS) to verify patient eligibility to receive care. DEERS was established in 1979 by the Department of Defense to comply with a Congressional mandate. The two initial objectives of DEERS were to collect and provide demographic and socio-graphic data on the beneficiary population entitled to DOD health benefits, and to reduce the fraud and misuse of those benefits. The original scope of DEERS has since been broadened to include the maintenance and verification of eligibility status for all uniformed services beneficiaries. Worldwide implementation of DEERS and its registration were completed in 1985.

2. Responsibilities.

   a. Commandant (CG-1123). Commandant (CG-1123) provides overall functional management of the CG DEERS program for health services facilities. In this role, Commandant (CG-1123) provides guidance to field activities, represents the CG to the DEERS Central Systems Program Office (DCSPO), and on the DEERS Central Systems Project Officers Committees.

   b. Health, Safety, and Work-Life Service Center (HSWL SC). HSWL SC shall appoint an MLC DEERS medical project officer and alternate, who shall ensure that facilities in their respective areas participate in and comply with DEERS program requirements.

3. Performing DEERS Checks.

   a. Whom to check. All beneficiaries of the military health care system are subject to DEERS eligibility verification, with the following exceptions:

      (1) CG cadets, officer candidates, and recruits while undergoing training.

      (2) Active duty personnel receiving dental care at a military facility.

      (3) Secretarial Designees, including pre-adoptive children and wards of the Court, ARE NOT ELIGIBLE for care under the TRICARE programs. They are also not enrolled in DEERS. Verification of the eligibility of Secretarial Designees for care in a military facility is accomplished through the individual's actual letter of designation. Refer to Section 2-E for further information.

   b. When to check. CG health services facilities should verify the eligibility of all beneficiaries prior to providing health care. The following minimum eligibility checks shall be made:

      (1) 100% of all outpatient visits including visits for medical, dental, pharmacy and ancillary services.

c. <u>How to check</u>. DEERS checks for patient registration and eligibility can be done in a number of ways. The following are the most common ways to verify eligibility:

   (1) DEERS eligibility is automatically verified in CHCS upon entering patient demographics.

   (2) Use of Servicing Personnel Office (SPO)/Admin RAPIDS Terminals. Personnel in health care facilities are discouraged from performing DEERS checks using the RAPIDS terminal that may be available in their unit's Administration Office or SPO. Using this resource places an unnecessary burden on the SPO/Admin personnel, and using these terminals does not indicate that the required medical checks are being accomplished.

4. <u>Eligibility/Enrollment Questions, Fraud and Abuse</u>.

   a. <u>Eligibility/Enrollment Questions</u>. Beneficiaries of the military health care system, including active duty and retired personnel, their dependents, and survivors must provide positive proof of eligibility before being provided health care. Eligibility is determined by presenting a valid ID Card and verifying enrollment and eligibility in DEERS.

   (1) If an individual presents an ID card that is no longer valid (expired), the individual should be refused routine care and the ID card confiscated.

   (2) If the individual has a valid ID card, but is not enrolled in DEERS, they should be refused routine care, and referred to their sponsor and/or service ID card activity to be enrolled in DEERS. Following enrollment into DEERS, the patient may prove temporary eligibility (pending their enrollment showing up in the DEERS computer) by presenting a certified copy of Application for Uniformed Services Identification Card DD Form 1172 from the ID card activity. Upon presenting of this DEERS enrollment verification, the individual should be considered as fully eligible, and treatment provided.

   * Emergency care should be rendered to any individual in need.*

   b. <u>Fraud and Abuse</u>. If, in the process of verifying eligibility through DEERS, clinic personnel have reason to believe the person requesting care is doing so even though that person is no longer eligible (e.g. a divorced spouse with a valid ID card, but DEERS shows NOT ELIGIBLE), care should be refused, and the details of the situation should be reported to the appropriate personnel activity and investigation office. Clinic personnel reporting suspected fraud should document as much information about the individual as possible (name, former sponsor's name, SSN, service and status, as well as the individual's current address and telephone number if known). Do not attempt to confiscate the ID card or in any way restrict the individual. Recovery of invalid or no-longer-appropriate ID cards is the responsibility of the parent service's investigation/law enforcement personnel. Reports of possible fraud should be reported to the command of the clinic and to the Defense Manpower Data

Center Support Office (DMDC) in Monterey, CA at (800) 361-2508 Monday – Friday 0600 – 1600 PST.

5. Denial of Nonemergency Health Care Benefits for Individuals Not Enrolled in Defense Enrollment Eligibility Reporting System (DEERS).

   a. Policy.

      (1) All CONUS USMTFs will deny nonemergency health care to dependent beneficiaries not enrolled in DEERS. The DOD considers USMTFs located in Alaska, Hawaii, and Puerto Rico as being in CONUS. Patients presenting for care are required to have a valid ID card in their possession and meet DEERS enrollment requirements.

      (2) This policy affects only the delivery of nonemergency health care. Under no circumstances are CG health services personnel to deny emergency medical care or attention because a patient is not enrolled in DEERS.

      (3) Health services personnel in CG health care facilities are to conduct the minimum eligibility checks for their facility as set annually by Commandant (CG-1121). Whenever possible, prospective checking should be accomplished soon enough to allow for notifying the patient and correcting enrollment problems before a scheduled appointment.

      (4) Patients with valid ID cards, but not enrolled in DEERS, presenting for nonemergency medical care at CGMTFs will be denied care and instructed to seek proper enrollment through their cognizant personnel office.

      (5) Patients, who present for nonemergency treatment without a valid ID card and are in the DEERS data base, will not be provided health care without first providing a statement, signed by a verifying personnel officer indicating that they are eligible and providing a reason why a valid ID card is not in their possession. A copy of this statement will be maintained in the clinical record until the individual's eligibility is determined.

      (6) If the beneficiary presenting with or without an ID card is suspected of fraud, refer the case to the legal branch for appropriate investigation.

      (7) Denial of health care benefits represents a serious application of new and complex regulations. Under no circumstances will a person be denied care by the clerk performing the initial eligibility check. The decision to deny care will be made only by Clinic Administrator or by a responsible person so designated in writing by the command.

6. DEERS Eligibility Overrides. The below listed situations will override DEERS data which indicates that a patient is not enrolled or eligible. Unless otherwise stated, all situations assume that the beneficiary possesses a valid ID card:

   a. Dependents Recently Becoming Eligible for Benefits. Patients who have become eligible for benefits within the previous 120 days may be treated upon presentation of a valid ID card. In the case of children under age 10, the parent's

ID card may be used. Examples of patients expected to fall under this provision are: spouses recently married to sponsors, newly eligible step children, family members of sponsors recently entering active duty status for a period over 30 days, parents/parents-in-law, or divorced spouses (not remarried) recently determined to be eligible. After 120 days, these beneficiaries will no longer be considered recent.

b. <u>DD-1172</u>. Application for Uniformed Services Identification Card form. The patient presents an original or a copy of the DD-1172 used for DEERS enrollment and possesses a valid ID card over 120 days old, but is not enrolled in DEERS. This copy of the DD-1172 should be certified to be a True Copy by the ID Card issuing authority which prepared it. It should also contain a telephone number where the certifying individual can be contacted for verification. The person conducting the DEERS check shall contact the issuing personnel office to verify enrollment.

c. <u>Sponsors Entering Active Duty Status for a Period of Greater than 30 days</u>. If the sponsor is a reservist or guardsman recently ordered to active duty for a period of greater than 30 days, a copy of the active duty orders may be accepted as proof of eligibility for up to 120 days after the beginning of the active duty period. Additional information concerning Reserve mobilization TRICARE benefits is available at http://www.tricare.mil.

d. <u>Newborns</u>. Newborns born into Active Duty Service Member (ADSM) families or retiree families where one parent/family member is enrolled in TRICARE Prime are deemed enrolled in Prime for sixty (60) days and no Non-Availability Statement (NAS) is required for such newborns. The TRICARE Regional Director (RD) of each TRICARE Regional Office (TRO) and Deputy Director of each TRICARE Area Office (TAO) are granted the authority to extend the deemed period up to 120 days, on a case-by-case or regional basis.

e. <u>Ineligible due to ID Card Expiration</u>. When the data base shows a patient to be ineligible due to ID card expiration, care may be rendered as long as the patient has a new ID card issued within the previous 120 days.

f. <u>Sponsor's Duty Station is Outside the 50 United States with an FPO or APO address</u>. Dependents whose sponsors are assigned outside the 50 United States or to a duty station with an APO or FPO address will not be denied care as long the sponsor is enrolled in DEERS.

g. <u>Survivors</u>. In a small percentage of cases, deceased sponsors may not be enrolled in DEERS. This situation will be evidenced when the MTF does an eligibility check on the surviving beneficiary and does not find the sponsor enrolled or the survivor appears as the sponsor. In either of these situations, if the survivor has a valid ID card, he/she should be treated and referred to the local personnel support activity to correct the DEERS data base. In some situations, surviving beneficiaries who are receiving Survivor Benefit Plan (SBP) annuities will be listed in DEERS as sponsor and will be found under their own social security number. These are eligible beneficiaries and should be treated.

h. <u>Foreign Military Personnel</u>. Foreign military personnel assigned via the personnel exchange program are eligible through public law or other current directives, though not enrolled in DEERS they will be treated upon presentation of a valid ID card.

This page intentionally left blank.

Section I. Health Care Facility Definitions.

1. CG Facilities 1
2. Department of Defense Medical Facilities 2
3. Uniformed Services Military Treatment Facilities (USMTFs)..2

This page intentionally left blank.

I. Health Care Facility Definitions.

1. CG Health Care Facilities.

    a. Clinic. A CG owned or leased health care facility primarily intended to provide outpatient medical service for ambulatory patients. A clinic must perform certain non-therapeutic activities related to the health of the personnel which are necessary to support the operational mission of the unit, such as periodic health assessments (PHA), physical examinations, immunizations, medical administration, and preventive medical and sanitary measures. A clinic staff consists of at least one permanently assigned physician (Medical Officer), a Clinic Administrator, and Health Services Technicians. The staff may include Dentists, Nurses, Pharmacists, Physician Assistants and other specialists as required. A clinic may be equipped with beds for observation of patients awaiting transfer to a hospital, and for overnight care of patients who do not require complete hospital services (e.g., isolation of patients with communicable diseases). A clinic must participate in the CG's external accreditation program with the Accreditation Association for Ambulatory Health Care (AAAHC) and participate in all aspects of the CG's Quality Improvement Program as outlined in the Chapter 13 of this Manual. A clinic serves as the "parent" DMIS TRICARE enrollment site

    b. Satellite Clinic. A health care facility which is under the operational control (OPCON) of a CG clinic, but is located off-site from the clinic. It is an intermediate size medical care facility (ashore) intended to provide outpatient medical care for active duty personnel. A satellite clinic will perform activities related to the health of the personnel which are necessary to support the operational missions of all units within AOR, such as physical examinations, immunizations, medical administration, and preventive medical and sanitary measures. A satellite clinic will normally be staffed with one Medical Officer and three or more health service technicians. A satellite clinic serves as the "child" DMIS TRICARE enrollment site to the "parent" CG clinic.

    c. Dental Clinic. A facility at a CG unit for the dental care and treatment of AD personnel. Dental clinics are staffed with one or more Dental Officers and HS.

    d. Sick Bay. A small medical treatment facility (afloat or ashore) normally staffed only by Health Services Technicians for the care and treatment of AD personnel. Civilian health care providers contracted to provide in-house services at these facilities, like any facility, may provide care only within the scope of their contracts. The fact that these civilian health care providers are on board will not change the status of the medical facility.

    e. Regional Practice. Regionally located multi-site unit responsible for delivering Health, Safety, and Work-Life services programs within an AOR, thus functioning as a Group Practice. The HSWL SC acts as technical authority and

COMDTINST M6000.1E

oversees all service delivery. A CG 0-4 Regional Manager serves as the administrator of the Group Practice and Work-Life Supervisor. The Executive Staff is comprised of USPHS dental, medical and pharmacy officers serving with the CG and a CG E-7, E-8 or E-9 IDHS.

f. Resource Sharing Facility. Is a Department of Defense (DoD) or Veterans Affairs (VA) operated medical facility that provides health care to CG and DoD beneficiaries using CG or PHS Medical Officers through a resource sharing agreement.

2. Department of Defense Medical Facilities.

   a. Nomenclature and Definitions. There are three types of DoD fixed medical treatment facilities: medical centers, hospitals, and clinics. The nomenclature and definitions applicable to the classification of these facilities, as set forth below, are used by the Army, Navy, Air Force, and Marine Corps.

      (1) Medical Center. A medical center is a large hospital which has been designed, staffed and equipped to provide health care for authorized personnel, including a wide range of specialized and consultative support for all medical facilities within the geographic area of responsibility and post graduate education in the health professions.

      (2) Hospital. A medical treatment facility capable of providing definitive inpatient care. It is staffed and equipped to provide diagnostic and therapeutic services in the field of general medicine and surgery, preventive medicine services, and has the supporting facilities to perform its assigned mission and functions. A hospital may, in addition, discharge the functions of a clinic.

      (3) Clinic. A medical treatment facility primarily intended and appropriately staffed and equipped to provide emergency treatment and outpatient services. A clinic is also intended to perform certain non-therapeutic activities related to the health of the personnel served, such as PHAs, physical examinations and preventive medicine services necessary to support a primary military mission. A clinic may be equipped with beds for observation of patients awaiting transfer to a hospital, and for care of cases which cannot be cared for on an outpatient status, but which do not require hospitalization.

   b. Primary Mission. The primary mission of DoD medical facilities is to provide adequate medical care for members of the Uniformed Services on AD.

3. Uniformed Services Military Treatment Facilities (USMTFs).

   a. Former USPHS hospitals. Public Law 97-99 (1981) authorized several former USPHS hospitals (sometimes called Jackson Amendment facilities) to provide health care to active duty and retired members and their dependents. The law was modified in 1991 and the USMTF program was mandated to implement a managed care delivery and reimbursement model in order to continue as part of the Military Health System (MHS). This managed care plan went into effect on October 1, 1993 and is called the Uniformed Services Family Health Benefit Plan (USFHBP).

b. USFHBP. USFHBP is a health maintenance organization-type of plan exclusively for the dependents of active duty, retirees and their dependents. Where available, the USFHBP serves a defined population, through voluntary enrollment, and offers a comprehensive benefit package. The capacity at USFHBP sites varies and is limited. Beneficiaries enroll in the USFHBP during a yearly open season, and may disenroll after one year. Enrollment is confirmed by each USFHBP site. Those not accepted during the open season may be enrolled as openings occur on a first come-first served basis. USFHBP enrollees are not authorized to use the TRICARE Program or the direct care system (DoD and CG health care/dental facilities included) while enrolled in the USFHBP.

c. Not enrolled in the USFHBP. Dependents and retirees who do not enroll in the USFHBP or who are denied enrollment because the USFHBP is at capacity can only be treated at USMTFs on a space-available and fee-for-service basis. All USMTFs are required to be TRICARE preferred providers.

d. USFHBP is not for active duty personnel. Active duty personnel are not eligible to enroll in the USFHBP, however, they can still be treated at USMTFs under one of the following conditions:

   (1) For emergency care.

   (2) When referred by a military treatment facility.

   (3) When authorized by HSWL SC for non-emergent care.

e. No bills. When active duty care is rendered, the USMTFs are not authorized to bill or collect payment from active duty members, they must bill the CG instead.

This page intentionally left blank.

Section J. Policies and Procedures Required at CG Health Care Facilities

1. Administrative Policies andProcedures 1
2. Operational Policies and Procedures 1
3. Patient Rights..2
4. Health Care Provider Identification..3

This page intentionally left blank.

J. Policies and Procedures Required at CG Health Care Facilities.

1. Administrative Policies and Procedures. All facilities shall develop and maintain the following written administrative policies and procedures which shall be reviewed annually and updated as needed.

    a. Standard Operating Procedure. Standard Operating Procedure (SOP) defining objectives and policies for the facility.

    b. Organizational Chart. Organizational chart of the Regional Practice components in the District.

    c. Clinic Protocols. Clinic protocols, posted in the respective department, for pharmacy, medical laboratory, and medical and dental radiology.

    d. Notices if Pregnant. Notices posted in pharmacy and radiology advising female patients to notify department personnel if they are or might be pregnant or breast feeding (pharmacy only).

    e. After-hours Emergency Care. Written guidelines advising patients how to obtain after-hours emergency medical and dental advice or care. These must be readily available and widely publicized within the command and the local eligible beneficiary community.

    f. Quality Improvement Program. Quality Improvement (QI) program guidelines including assignment of a QI coordinator and QI focus group members in writing. The QI focus group shall meet at least quarterly and maintain written minutes.

    g. Patient Advisory Committee. Guidelines for a patient advisory committee (PAC) comprised of representatives of the health care facility and each major, identifiable, patient interest group. The PAC shall meet periodically and maintain written minutes.

    h. Authorized to Deny Care. Persons authorized to deny care shall be so designated in writing by the command.

    i. Time clocks. All clinics shall maintain a functioning time clock and all contract employees shall clock in and out of work every work day. Clinic administrators shall verify time cards at every pay period.

2. Operational Policies and Procedures. Facilities shall also develop and maintain the following written operational policies and procedures. These require annual review and signature by all health services personnel:

    a. Emergency Situation Bill. Emergency Situation Bill including Health Services Division response to fire, earthquake, bomb threat, heavy weather, etc.

b. Emergency Response Protocols. Health Services Emergency Response Protocols for suicide attempt/threat, rape/sexual assault, family violence and medical emergencies in the dental clinic.

c. Protocol for Managing After-hours Emergencies. Clinics at accession points and at Coast Guard units with on-base family housing shall maintain a 24-hour live watch schedule.

3. Patient Rights. Health care shall be delivered in a manner that protects the rights, privacy and dignity of the patient. Sensitivity to patient needs and concerns will always be a priority.

    a. Patient Bill of Rights and Responsibilities poster. Clinics shall post the Patient Bill of Rights and Responsibilities poster in clear view in all patient waiting and urgent care areas. Copies are available from Commandant (CG-1121).

    b. Chaperones. Chaperones shall provide comfort and support to patients during exams or treatment. All patients shall be informed of the availability of chaperones.

        (1) Chaperones are defined as persons who attend patients during medical exams or treatment. Chaperones shall be of the same gender as the patient being examined. Any nursing staff member, HS or volunteer may serve as a chaperone as part of their duties. The Senior Health Services Officer (SHSO) shall ensure that chaperones have appropriate preparation to include familiarization with the procedure and basic HIPAA policy training to enable them to carry out their duties properly. Although a patient's request for a family member or friend to be present during examination may be honored, that person is not a substitute for a chaperone.

        (2) Patients who request the presence of a chaperone shall have their request honored unless, in the opinion of the Medical Officer, the risk to the chaperone outweighs the benefit to the patient (e.g., during x-ray exposures).

        (3) Female patients undergoing breast examination or genital/rectal examination or treatment must have a chaperone present during the examination. Male patients may have a chaperone present at the patient's request.

        (4) If a provider thinks a chaperone is necessary, and the patient refuses to permit the services of a chaperone, the provider must consider whether to perform the examination or treatment or to refer the patient to another source of care.

        (5) Clinics shall have a written policy for reporting any episode of alleged misconduct during medical/dental examinations to the unit CO. Unit COs shall investigate such complaints in accordance with regulations.

c. Responsibility of the patient chaperone policy. The SHSO shall enforce the patient chaperone policy and ensure chaperones are qualified to perform their duties.

d. Allegations of misconduct. The SHSO shall ensure that allegations of misconduct are forwarded to the command in a timely manner.

e. Educational materials. Clinics shall ensure that patient educational materials concerning gender-neutral health issues (dental health, cardiovascular risk factors, colorectal cancer) and gender-related health issues (PAP smears, cervical cancer, breast disease, testicular and prostate cancer, etc.) are readily available.

4. Health Care Provider Identification.

   a. Patients right to know their physician. In accordance with the Patient Bill of Rights and Responsibilities, all patients have the right to know the identity and the professional qualifications of any person providing medical or dental care. The recent addition of Nurse Practitioners and commissioned Physician Assistants to our health care staffs has increased the chances of misidentification. Accordingly, health care providers shall introduce themselves and state their professional qualifications (level of provider) at each patient encounter.

   b. Health care name tags. The standard CG name tag does not reflect any information concerning the professional qualifications of the health care provider. Additionally, the standard CG name tag is often not visible to patients with poor eyesight, or it may be hidden by the provider's smock or lab coat. In lieu of the standard CG name tag, all health care providers, civilian and military, shall wear a specific health care provider identification tag on their outer smock or lab coat when engaged in direct patient care in CG clinics. The health care provider identification tag shall be worn above the right breast pocket (or equivalent). The following criteria shall be used by local commands and clinics in manufacturing the health care provider identification tags:

      (1) Size. The identification tag shall be 1" high by 3" wide.

      (2) Materials. Standard plastic name tag blanks which may be purchased locally or from Government sources.

      (3) Color. Standard CG blue or black with white lettering.

      (4) Contents. The identification tag shall contain the following information:

         (a) The rank, first initial and last name shall be centered on the identification name tag and placed on the top line.

(b) One of the following professional titles, or any other commonly recognized professional name, centered below the name line. Abbreviations shall not be used.

1. Physician
2. Dentist
3. Physician Assistant
4. Nurse Practitioner
5. Pharmacist
6. Physical Therapist
7. Optometrist
8. Registered Nurse
9. Health Services Technician

COMDTINST M6000.1E

Section K. General Standards of Care.

1. Standard of care 1
2. Diagnosis and therapy 1
3. Bases for Diagnoses 1
4. Treatment 1
5. Time Line for Treatment 1
6. Correct-site Surgery Policy 2
7. Patients role 2
8. Documentation 2

This page intentionally left blank.

COMDTINST M6000.1E

K. General Standards of Care.

1. Standard of care. Patients at CG clinics and sickbays shall be treated in accordance with the following general standards of care:

2. Diagnosis and therapy. Diagnosis and therapy shall be performed by a provider with appropriate credentials.

3. Basis for Diagnoses. Diagnoses shall be based upon clinical findings and appropriate tests and procedures.

4. Treatment. Treatment shall be consistent with the working diagnosis, and shall be based upon a current treatment plan. Treatment shall be provided using currently accepted clinical techniques.

5. Time Line for Treatment. Treatment shall be rendered in a timely manner. Providers should use their professional judgment in accounting for the specific needs of patients and military readiness obligations while attempting to meet the following goals for timeliness:

    a. Sick call. If provided, the patient should be triaged immediately and be seen based on urgency of the condition. The patient should be advised of the wait time to be seen and offered a later appointment if the condition does not warrant immediate attention.

    b. Urgent Care (medical). The wait time should not exceed twenty-four (24) hours. The condition must be addressed, not necessarily resolved, within this time frame.

    c. Routine Visit (medical). The wait time should not exceed 1 week (seven (7) days).

    d. Specialty Care (medical). To be determined by the Primary Care Manager (PCM) making the referral based on the nature of the care required and the acuteness of the injury, condition, or illness, but should not exceed a wait time of 4 weeks (twenty-eight (28) days) to obtain the necessary care.

    e. Well Visit. The wait time should not exceed 4 weeks. (Check TRICARE access Standards)

    f. Urgent Care (dental). The wait time should not exceed 1 day. The condition must be addressed, not necessarily resolved, within this time frame.

    g. Routine Visit (dental). The wait time should not exceed 4 weeks.

    h. Scheduled Appointment (medical or dental). The wait time should not exceed 30 minutes of appointed time. This may sometimes be delayed by the need to address prior scheduled patients, emergency care, or unforeseen military obligations.

    i. Pharmacy. Prescription available within 30 minutes.

6. Correct-site Surgery Policy. The purpose of the "Correct Site Surgery Policy" is to ensure that a comprehensive approach is in place to prevent the occurrence of a

wrong site surgery/procedure. All patients having a surgical/operative procedure shall have the surgical/operative site, confirmed by the healthcare team before any procedure is performed. Marking the correct site on radiographs and touching the correct surgical site are two examples of confirmation. Confirmation is not limited to the above examples.

    a. <u>Verify</u>. Verify that the patient and record match. (i.e. that you are performing surgery on the correct person).

    b. <u>Checklist</u>. A checklist will be used for every surgical/operative encounter to document verification of the surgical site.

        (1) Review radiograph(s) for surgical/operative site.

        (2) Review medical/dental record to verify surgical site indicated for treatment.

        (3) Review actual surgical site in presence of healthcare team.

        (4) Review informed consent.

        (5) Confirm surgical site with patient.

    c. <u>Incomplete checklist</u>. An incomplete checklist will result in postponement of the surgical/operative encounter until the documentation is completed. Any site discrepancy noted during the verification process will result in an immediate halt to the surgical encounter until the discrepancy can be resolved by members of the healthcare team.

7. <u>Patients role</u>. Patients shall participate in deciding among treatment alternatives available to them.

8. <u>Documentation</u>. All diagnosis and treatment shall be appropriately documented, including subjective complaints, pertinent positive and negative history, objective findings, clinical assessment, and plan for treatment, prescriptions, post-treatment instructions, and disposition of patient. Unusual circumstances, including complications of treatment shall be fully documented.

COMDTINST M6000.1E

CHAPTER 3

PHYSICAL STANDARDS AND EXAMINATION

Section A. Administrative Procedures

1. Applicability of Physical Standards..1
2. Prescribing of Physical Standards...1
3. Purpose of Physical Standards..1
4. Application of Physical Standards..1
5. Interpretation of Physical Standards...2
6. Definitions of Terms Used in this Chapter...2
7. Required Physical Examinations and Their Time Limitations........................3
8. Waiver of Physical Standards...10
9. Substitution of Physical Examinations...12

Section B. Medical Examination (DD-2808) and Medical History (DD-2807-1)

1. Report of Medical Examination DD-2808..1
2. Report of Medical History DD-2807-1...1
3. Findings and Recommendations of Report of Medical Examination (DD-2808).....1
4. Correction of Defects Prior to Overseas Transfer or Sea Duty Deployment...........5
5. Objection to Assumption of Fitness for Duty at Separation.............................5
6. Separation Not Appropriate by Reason of Physical Disability.........................6
7. Procedures for Physical Defects Found Prior to Separation............................6
Figure 3-B-1..7
Figure 3-B-2..8

Section C. Medical Examination Techniques and Lab Testing Standards

1. Scope..1
2. Speech Impediment..1
3. Head, Face, Neck, and Scalp (Item 17 of DD-2808)...1
4. Nose, Sinuses, Mouth, and Throat (Item 19, 20 of DD-2808)...........................2
5. Ears (General) and Drums (Item 21, 22 of DD-2808).......................................2
6. Eyes (General), Ophthalmoscopic, and Pupils (Item 23, 24, 25 of DD-2808)........3
7. Ocular Mobility (Item 26 of DD-2808)...5
8. Heart and Vascular System (Item 27 of DD-2808)...5
9. Lungs and Chest (Item 28 of DD-2808)..9
10. Anus and Rectum (Item 30 of DD-2808)..11
11. Abdomen and Viscera (Item 31 of DD-2808)...11
12. Genitourinary System (Item 32 of DD-2808)...11
13. Extremities (Item 33, 34, 35 of DD-2808)..12
14. Spine and Other Musculoskeletal (Item 36 of DD-2808)...............................14
15. Identifying Body Marks, Scars, and Tattoos (Item 37 of DD-2808)..............15
16. Neurologic (Item 39 of DD-2808)...16
17. Psychiatric (Item 40 of DD-2808)...17

18. Endocrine System.. 18
19. Dental (Item 43 of DD-2808).. 18
20. Laboratory Findings... 19
Figure 3-C-1..25
21. Height, Weight and Body Build... 26
22. Distant Visual Acuity and Other Eye Tests... 26
23. Audiometer.. 33
24. Psychological and Psychomotor.. 33
Figure 3-C-2..34
Figure 3-C-3..37
Figure 3-C-4..38

Section D. Medical Standards for Appointment, Enlistment and Induction in the Armed Forces

1. Scope...1
2. Medical Standards...1
3. Policy..2
4. Responsibilities of Commandant (CG-11)... 2
5. Height..3
6. Weight...3
7. Head..3
8. Eyes...3
9. Vision..7
10. Ears.. 8
11. Hearing...8
12. Nose, Sinuses, Mouth and Larynx... 9
13. Dental... 10
14. Neck..11
15. Lungs, Chest Wall, Pleura, and Mediastinum..................................... 11
16. Heart..13
17. Abdominal Organs and Gastrointestinal System................................. 16
18. Female Genitalia...19
19. Male Genitalia..20
20. Urinary System...21
21. Spine and Sacroiliac Joints...22
22. Upper Extremities..23
23. Lower Extremities..25
24. Miscellaneous Conditions of the Extremities......................................27
25. Vascular System...28
26. Skin and Cellular Tissues...29
27. Blood and Blood-Forming Tissues.. 31
28. Systemic..31
29. Endocrine and Metabolic..34
30. Neurologic..35
31. Learning, Psychiatric, and Behavioral...37
32. Tumors and Malignancies..40

33. Miscellaneous.. 40
    Figure 3-D-1 Evaluation for Risk OF Head Injury Sequelae............................ 42
    Figure 3-D-2 Classification and Comparative nomenclature of Cervical Smears......... 43

Section E. Physical Standards for Programs Leading to Commission

1. Appointment as Cadet, USCG Academy... 1
2. Commissioning of Cadets..2
3. Enrollment as an Officer Candidate..2
4. Commissioning of Officer Candidates...3
5. Coast Guard Direct Commission Program...4
6. Direct Commission in the CG Reserve..4
7. Direct Commission of Licensed Officers of U. S. Merchant Marine...................4
8. Appointment to Warrant Grade...4

Section F. Physical Standards Applicable to All Personnel (Regular and Reserve) For: Reenlistment; Enlistment of Prior Service USCG Personnel; Retention; Overseas Duty; and Sea Duty

1. General Instructions..1
2. Use of List of Disqualifying Conditions and Defects...................................1
3. Head and Neck..2
4. Esophagus, Nose, Pharynx, Larynx, and Trachea...................................... 2
5. Eyes.. 2
6. Ears and Hearing... 5
7. Lungs and Chest Wall...5
8. Heart and Vascular System...7
9. Abdomen and Gastrointestinal System..9
10. Endocrine and Metabolic Conditions (Diseases).......................................11
11. Genitourinary System.. 12
12. Extremities..14
13. Spine, Scapulae, Ribs, and Sacroiliac Joints.. 17
14. Skin and Cellular Tissues... 18
15. Neurological Disorders...19
16. Psychiatric Disorders. (See section 5-B concerning disposition).......................20
17. Dental...21
18. Blood and Blood-Forming Tissue Diseases..21
19. Systemic Diseases, General Defects, and Miscellaneous Conditions.................. 22
20. Tumors and Malignant Diseases... 23
21. Sexually Transmitted Disease... 23
22. Human Immunodeficiency Virus (HIV)... 23
23. Transplant recipient... 24

Section G. Physical Standards for Aviation

1. Classification of Aviation Personnel... 1
2. General Instructions for Aviation Examinations... 1

3. Restrictions Until Physically Qualified……………………………………………..4
4. Standards for Class 1……………………………………………………………....4
5. Candidates for Flight Training……………………………………………………..7
6. Requirements for Class 2 Aircrew………………………………………………..10
7. Requirements for Class 2 Medical Personnel……………………………………10
8. Requirements for Class 2 Technical Observers…………………………………11
9. Requirements for Class 2 Air Traffic Controllers……………………………….11
10. Requirements for Landing Signal Officer (LSO)………………………………...11
11. Refractive Surgery…………………………………………………………………12
12. Contact Lenses……………………………………………………………………13

Section H. Physical Examinations and Standards for Diving Duty

1. Examinations………………………………………………………………………..1
2. Standards……………………………………………………………………………2

Section A. Administrative Procedures

1. Applicability of Physical Standards..1
2. Prescribing of Physical Standard 1
3. Purpose of Physical Standards 1
4. Application of Physical Standards 1
5. Interpretation of Physical Standards 2
6. Definitions of Terms Used in this Chapter 2
7. Required Physical Examinations and Their Time Limitations 3
8. Waiver of Physical Standards 10
9. Substitution of Physical Examinations 12

This page intentionally left blank.

COMDTINST M6000.1E

CHAPTER THREE – PHYSICAL STANDARDS AND EXAMINATION

Section A. Administrative Procedures.

1. Applicability of Physical Standards.

    a. CG standards. The provisions of this chapter apply to all personnel of the CG and CG Reserve on active or inactive duty and to commissioned officers of the U.S. Public Health Service assigned to active duty with the CG.

    b. Armed Forces standards. Members of the other Armed Forces assigned to the CG for duty are governed by the applicable instructions of their parent Service for examination standards and for administrative purposes.

2. Prescribing of Physical Standards. Individuals to be enlisted, appointed, or commissioned in the CG or CG Reserve must conform to the physical standards prescribed by the Commandant. Separate standards are prescribed for various programs within the Service. All CG members are required to be medically ready for deployment. All Individual Medical Readiness (IMR) requirements, as delineated in the Coast Guard Periodic Health Assessment (PHA), COMTINST M6150.3, are required to be met by CG AD and SELRES members (to include Direct Commission Officers at point of accession). The CG clinic affiliated with the point of accession is responsible for inputting the IMR data into the applicable medical information system (MIS) database (i.e. Medical Readiness Reporting System (MRRS), etc.).

3. Purpose of Physical Standards. Physical standards are established for uniformity in procuring and retaining personnel who are physically fit and emotionally adaptable to military life. These standards are subject to change at the Commandant's direction when the needs of the CG dictate.

4. Application of Physical Standards.

    a. Conformance with Physical Standards Mandatory. To determine physical fitness, the applicant or member shall be physically examined and required to meet the physical standards prescribed in this chapter for the program or specialty and grade or rate involved. An examinee who does not meet the standards shall be disqualified.

    b. Evaluation of Physical Fitness. The applicant's total physical fitness shall be carefully considered in relation to the character of the duties to that the individual may be called upon to perform. Physical profiling is not a CG policy. Members shall be considered fit for unrestricted worldwide duty when declared physically qualified. The examiner must be aware of the different physical standards for various programs. Care shall be taken to ensure an examinee is not disqualified for minor deviations that are clearly of no future significance with regard to general health, ability to serve, or to cause premature retirement for physical disability. However, conditions that are likely to cause future disability or preclude completing a military career of at least twenty years, whether by natural progression or by recurrences, are also disqualifying. This policy shall be followed when an authentic history of such a condition is established, even though clinical signs may not be evident during the physical examination or periodic health assessment (PHA).

5. <u>Interpretation of Physical Standards</u>. Examiners are expected to use discretion in evaluating the degree of severity of any defect or disability. They are not authorized to disregard defects or disabilities that are disqualifying in accordance with the standards found in this Chapter.

6. <u>Definitions of Terms Used in this Chapter</u>.

   a. <u>Officers</u>. The term "officers" includes commissioned officers, warrant officers, and commissioned officers of the U.S. Public Health Service (USPHS).

   b. <u>Personnel</u>. The term "personnel" includes members of the CG and CG Reserve, and the USPHS on AD with the CG.

   c. <u>Medical and Dental Examiners</u>. Medical and dental examiners are medical and dental officers of the uniformed services, contract physicians and dentists, or civilian physicians or dentists who have been specifically authorized to provide professional services to the CG. Some USMTFs have qualified enlisted examiners who also conduct medical examinations and their findings require countersignature by a Medical Officer.

   d. <u>Flight Surgeons, Aviation Medical Officers and Aeromedical Physician Assistants</u>. Officers of a uniformed service who have been so designated because of special training.

   e. <u>Command/Unit</u>. For administrative action required on the Report of Medical Examination, DD-2808 the command/unit level is the unit performing personnel accounting services for the individual being physically examined.

   f. <u>Reviewing/Approving Authority</u>. Commander, Personnel Service Center (PSC-de) and HSWL SC are responsible for approval of physical examinations as outlined herein. Clinic Administrators may act as reviewing and/or approving authority for physical examinations performed in their AOR, including those performed by contract physicians and USMTF's as designated by HSWL SC, except for those that are aviation or dive related. Clinic Administrators may request physical examination review/approval authority for Clinic Supervisors assigned to their clinic from HSWL SC. Reviewing authority shall not be delegated below the HSC level. Upon approval or disapproval of the physical examination, an entry in the comments block of the Medical Readiness and Reporting System (MRRS) will be made stating where the physical was approved or disapproved and the reason for disapproval, if applicable. Clinic Administrators may review physical examinations performed by contract physicians and USMTFs within their AOR.

g. <u>Convening Authority</u>. Convening Authority is an individual authorized to convene a medical board as outlined in Physical Disability Evaluation System, COMDTINST M1850.2 (series).

h. <u>Time Limitation</u>. The time limitation is the period for which the physical examination remains valid to accomplish its required purpose. The time limitation period begins as of the day after the physical examination is conducted.

7. <u>Required Physical Examinations and Their Time Limitations</u>.

   a. <u>Enlistment</u>. A physical examination is required for original enlistment in the CG and the CG Reserve. This physical examination will usually be performed by Military Entrance Processing Stations (MEPS) and is valid for twenty-four months. Approved MEPS physicals do not require further review. Recommendations noted on separation physical examinations from other services must have been resolved with an indication that the individual meets the standards. A certified copy of that physical examination must be reviewed and endorsed by the reviewing authority CG Recruiting Command (CGRC). The reviewing authority must indicate that the applicant meets the physical standards for enlistment in the USCG.

   (1) Recruiters who believe that applicants have been erroneously physically disqualified by MEPS, may submit the Report of Medical Examination, DD-2808 and Report of Medical History, DD-2807-1 (original or clean copies) along with supporting medical documentation to Commander (CGRC) for review.

   (2) Waiver of physical standards for original enlistment may also be submitted as above, and in accordance with paragraph 3-A-8 of this Chapter.

   (3) Separation physical examinations from any Armed Service may be used for enlistment in the CG, provided the examination has been performed within the last twelve (12) months. The physical examination must be as complete as a MEPS exam, include an HIV antibody test date (within the last 24 months) and result, and a Type II dental examination. A Report of Medical History, DD-2807-1 must also be included with elaboration of positive medical history in the remarks section (item #25). Forward all documents for review to Commander (CGRC).

   (4) Prior Service enlisted aviation personnel must obtain an aviation physical examination from a currently qualified Uniformed Services Flight Surgeon or AMO within the previous 12 months. This physical examination will be submitted with the rate determination package to Commander (CGRC).

   (5) Occasionally, applicants for initial entry into the Coast Guard will need to be examined at CG MTFs. In these cases, the physical examination will be performed per section 3-C. The examining Medical Officer may defer item #46 of the Report of Medical Examination, DD-2808 to the Reviewing Authority. Otherwise, the physical standards for entry (sections 3-D, 3-E

and 3-G as appropriate) must be meticulously applied when completing this item. The completed Report of Medical Examination, DD-2808 and Report of Medical History, DD-2807-1 will be forwarded to the reviewing authority, Commander (CGRC).

b. Pre-Commissioning/Appointments. A physical examination is required within 12 months prior to original appointment as an officer in the CG or CG Reserve for personnel in the following categories:

(1) Appointments to Warrant Grade, except that physical examinations for members of the CG Ready Reserve must be within 24 months prior to the date of execution of the Acceptance and Oath of Office, CG-9556.

(2) Appointment of a Direct Commission Officer, prior to the date of execution of the Acceptance and Oath of office.

(3) Appointment of a Licensed Officer of the U. S. Merchant Marine as a commissioned officer (examination required within 6 months).

(4) Graduates of the CG Academy and Officer Candidates School, prior to the execution of the Acceptance and Oath of Office.

c. Separation from Active Duty.

(1) A complete physical examination is required within 12 months for retirement, involuntary separation, or release from any active duty (RELAD) of 30 days or longer into the Ready Reserves (selected drilling or IRR).

(2) Other members separating from the CG e.g., discharge or transfer to standby reserve (non-drilling) may request a medical and/or dental examination. The medical examination must include: notation of any current problems, a blood pressure measurement, and address items on the preventive medicine stamp. In addition to the above, the practitioner shall ascertain the health needs of the member and undertake measures deemed necessary to meet those needs. The dental examination, if requested, must at least be a Type III exam. These examinations may be annotated on a SF-600, and upon completion, do not require approval.

(3) For members enrolled in the Occupational Medical Surveillance and Evaluation Program (OMSEP), see Chapter 12 of this Manual for guidance.

(4) See Chapter 12 of the CG Personnel Manual, COMDTINST M1000.6 (series), for amplification on administrative discharge procedures.

d. Overseas Transfer, Sea Duty and Port Security Unit (PSU) Assignment, Modified Physical Screening.

COMDTINST M6000.1E

(1) To help identify and resolve health related issues prior to transfer a modified physical screening utilizing the Modified Screening For: Overseas Assignment and/or Sea Duty Health Screening, CG-6100 is required for all personnel if one of the following apply:

   (a) PCS transfer to vessel with a deployment schedule of 60 consecutive days or more (out of 365).

   (b) PCS transfer to an overseas assignment. (e.g., Alaska, Hawaii or Puerto Rico)

   (c) Transferring from one overseas assignment to another overseas assignment.

   (d) PSU personnel (Must be done annually).

(2) The Modified Screening For: Overseas Assignment and/or Sea Duty Health Screening, CG-6100 must be completed as follows: Section B must be completed and signed by the patient. Section C thru E must be completed and signed by either a civilian, DOD or CG medical or dental provider, or CG IDHS. Any responses of medical or dental significance requiring further clarification or evaluation need to be reviewed by either a civilian, DOD or CG medical or dental provider. Section F must be completed and signed by the cognizant clinic administrator for final approval or disapproval. The Modified Screening For: Overseas Assignment and/or Sea Duty Health Screening, CG-6100 must be placed in section 1 of the health record. The modified physical screening will include the following:

   (a) A health history completed by the evaluee. (The evaluee will certify by signature that all responses are true).

   (b) Documentation of the previous approved physical examination to include the status of recommendations and summary of significant health changes.

   (c) Review of the health record to ensure routine health maintenance items are up-to-date to include:

      1. Routine gynecologic examinations.

      2. Two pairs of glasses and gas mask inserts for PSU personnel if required to correct refractive error, DNA sampling, G-6-PD screening, immunizations, HIV testing and a Type 2 dental examination.

   (d) Review malaria chemoprophylaxis, TST and special health concern requirements. Contact the Center for Disease Control and Prevention (CDC) at http://www.cdc.gov or http://www.travel.state.gov for information. Questions regarding the appropriate preventive medical measures should be referred to Commandant (CG-1121).

    (e) If PCS transferring to a foreign country, HIV antibody test must have been conducted within the past 6 months with results noted prior to transfer.

    (f) If an evaluee is enrolled (or will be enrolled based on new assignment) in the Occupational Medical Surveillance and Evaluation Program (OMSEP), ensure appropriate periodic/basic examination is performed.

e. <u>Applicant</u>.

  (1) <u>Commissioning Programs</u>. A physical examination is required for applicants for entry into the CG as follows:

    (a) CG Academy: DODMERB physical examination within 24 months.

    (b) Officer Candidate School: MEPS physical within 24 months of entry date, except.

      1. CG personnel on active duty may obtain the physical examination at a USMTF within 24 months of entry date.

      2. Members of other Armed Services may submit a physical examination from a USMTF provided the examination has been performed within the past twelve (12) months and is as complete as a MEPS physical examination.

    (c) Direct commission: MEPS physical within 24 months of entry date or oath of office for Ready Reserve Direct Commission, except aviation programs, where examination by a Uniformed Service Flight Surgeon or AMO is required within 12 months of entry date.

    (d) Applicants for service academies, ROTC scholarship programs, and the Uniformed Services University School of Health Sciences (USUHS) are authorized to utilize MTFs for their initial physical examination and additional testing if necessary. (Office of Assistant Secretary of Defense Health Affairs, OASD (HA) policy memo 9900003/Physical Examinations for ROTC Applicants (notal)).

      1. Applicants for entry into these program and prospective flight personnel should be treated as mission related priorities with scheduling precedence associated with priority group 1.

      2. Scheduling of physical examinations, additional tests and evaluations are to be conducted in a timely manner.

(2) Aviation. An aviation physical examination is required for applicants for training in all categories of aviation specialties. This physical examination is valid for 24 months for Class II applicants and 12 months for pilot applicants.

(3) Diving. A dive applicant physical examination is required for all applicants for duty involving diving, and is valid for twelve months.

f. Pre-Training Screening Examinations. A screening examination is required within 1 week of reporting to the CG Academy, Officer Candidate School, Direct Commission Officer orientation, or the Recruit Training Center. This screening examination shall be sufficiently thorough to ensure that the person is free from communicable and infectious diseases, and is physically qualified. The results of this examination shall be recorded on a Chronological Record of Medical Care, SF-600 and filed in the health record.

g. Retired Members Recalled to Active Duty. A physical examination is required for retired personnel who are recalled to active duty. This physical examination is valid for 12 months. A physical examination performed for retirement may be used for recall providing the date of recall is within 6 months of the date of the physical examination.

h. Annual. An annual physical examination, consisting of the Report of Medical Examination, DD-2808, and Report of Medical History, DD-2807-1, and completion of the appropriate health risk assessment is required on all aviation personnel age 50 or older.

i. Biennial.

(1) Biennial physical examination is required every 2 years after initial designation, until age 48, for the following:

(a) All aviation personnel (including air traffic controllers) the initial physical examination (which will count as the PHA) will consist of the Report of Medical Examination, DD-2808 and Report of Medical History, DD-2807-1, and completion of the Navy Fleet and Marine Corps Health Risk Assessment (HRA). The subsequent annual aviation physical examination will be the PHA. These two exams will alternate every other year until age 50.

(b) All Landing Signal Officers (LSO).

(2) The biennial exam will be performed either within 2 months prior to the members birth month or during the members birth month. The period of validity of the biennial physical will be aligned with the last day of the service member's birth month. (Example: someone born on 3 October would have August, September, and October in which to accomplish his/her

physical. No matter when accomplished in that time frame, the period of validity of that exam is until 31 October two years later).

    (3) The requirement to perform a biennial exam will not be suspended in the event of training exercises or deployment. Aircrew with scheduled deployment during their 90 day window to accomplish their biennial exam may accomplish their biennial exam an additional 90 days prior and continue with the same valid end date. This may result in a member having a valid biennial for 30 months. Members unable to accomplish a biennial exam prior to being deployed will be granted an additional 60 days upon return in which to accomplish their physical.

    (4) Additionally, a comprehensive physical may be required during a post-mishap investigation, MEB, or as part of a work-up for a medical disqualification.

    (5) Personnel designated as aircrew are expected to maintain a biennial exam schedule regardless of current aviation duty status.

j. <u>Triennial</u>. A physical examination is required every three (3) years for all PHS officers detailed to the CG who are 50 years of age or older.

k. <u>Periodic Health Assessment (PHA)</u>. The PHA is a multi-component process that will ensure CG members are ready for deployment, ensure individual medical readiness (IMR) data is electronically recorded, and deliver evidence-based clinical preventive services. The PHA will address prevention of disease and injury by focusing on prevention strategies each member can incorporate into his/her lifestyle. As per Coast Guard Periodic Health Assessment (PHA), COMDTINST 6150.3 (series) the PHA has replaced the routine five year (quinquennial) physical examination. Every CG member will receive a PHA annually during the member's birth month period. For the purpose of this Instruction, a member's birth month period is defined as the actual month of birth and the preceding two (2) months. Specialty examinations (Department of Defense Medical Examination Review Board (DODMERB), Military Entrance Processing Station (MEPS), commissioning, appointment to Chief Warrant Officer (CWO), enlistment, retirement, confinement, release from AD (RELAD), aviation, landing signal officer (LSO), dive, and Medical Evaluation Board (MEB) will still be required.

l. <u>Quinquennial/Diving</u>. A physical examination is required every five (5) years for all personnel maintaining a current diving qualification (also note "Other" in item #15.c. of Report of Medical Examination, DD-2808) and for all PHS officers under age 50 detailed to the CG (per PHS policy).

m. <u>Occupational Medical Surveillance and Evaluation Program (OMSEP)</u>. Those individuals who are occupationally exposed to hazardous substances, physical energies, or employed in designated occupations must undergo physical examinations as required by Chapter 12 of this Manual.

n. Miscellaneous Physical Examinations.

   (1) Retention. This examination is done at the direction of the Commanding Officer when there is substantial doubt as to a member's physical or mental fitness for duty.

   (2) Pre-confinement Physical Screening. In general, personnel who are presented for this screening, who do not require acute medical treatment or hospitalization, are fit for confinement. Cases where a member requires more than routine follow-up medical care, or has certain psychiatric conditions, that may make them unfit for confinement, should be discussed with the chief Medical Officer (or his/her representative) at the confining facility. Personnel requiring detoxification for alcohol or drug dependency are not fit for confinement; however, members that have been detoxified or that may require rehabilitation alone are fit for confinement. This screening shall be recorded on a Chronological Record of Medical Care, SF-600 and together with a copy of the last complete and approved Report of Physical Examination Form, DD-2808 and Report of Medical History Form, DD-2807-1 shall be submitted to the Reviewing Authority.

   (3) Post Confinement Physical Examination. Ensure a separation physical examination has been completed prior to the member departing the confining facility. The separation physical shall meet the standards of section 3-F and must be approved by HSWL SC.

   (4) Reservists. A District Commander may require any reservist attached to a command within that area to undergo a complete physical examination if reasonable doubt exists as to the reservist's physical or mental fitness for duty.

   (5) Non-Fitness for Duty Determination Physical Examinations. The Senior Health Services Officer (SHSO) retains the authority and responsibility to determine capability and capacity to conduct non-fitness for duty physical examinations for all eligible beneficiaries.

   (6) Medical Evaluation Boards (MEB). Medical Evaluation Boards are convened to evaluate the present state of health and fitness for duty of any active duty/selected reserve member.

o. Annual Command Afloat Medical Screening. Officers and enlisted personnel scheduled to assume command afloat shall undergo a medical screening prior to assignment. The initial screening may be conducted by a Medical Officer where applicable, or an HS not in the prospective chain of command of the member being screened. Thereafter, all Commanding Officers and Officers-in-Charge of afloat units will have an annual command afloat medical screening. This screening will also be performed by a Medical Officer where available; otherwise, the screening may be performed by a Health Services Technician who IS NOT in the chain of command of the person being screened. The screening process will include a medical history completed by the member, a visual acuity check, blood pressure measurement, and a thorough review of interval history in the member's health record. Results are to be recorded on the Annual Command Afloat Medical Screening, CG-6000-2. The Annual Command Afloat Medical Screening, CG-6000-2 and a copy of the last PHA shall then be forwarded to the local approving authority or HSWL SC for review. HSWL SC will approve or disapprove the screening using section 3-F (retention standards) as the guiding directive. If a question arises as to the fitness of the individual, HSWL SC may request additional information from the examining unit. If HSWL SC is unable to render a decision as to the fitness for command, the entire command afloat screening package will be forwarded to Commandant (CG-112) for final action. The reviewed form shall be returned to the member's command for filing in the member's health record.

p. Dental Examinations. Annual Type II dental examinations are required for all active duty and SELRES members.

8. Waiver of Physical Standards.

a. Definition of Waiver. A waiver is an authorization to retain the member when an individual does not meet the physical standards prescribed for the purpose of the examination.

(1) Normally, a waiver will be granted when it is reasonably expected that the individual will remain fit for duty and the waiver is in the best interests of the CG. A service member will not be granted a waiver for a physical disability determined to be not fit for duty by a physical evaluation board approved by the Commandant. In these cases, the provisions for retention on active duty contained in the Physical Disability Evaluation System, COMDTINST M1850.2 (series) and the Personnel Manual, COMDTINST M1000.6 (series) apply.

(2) If a member is under consideration by the physical disability evaluation system, no medical waiver request shall be submitted for physical defects or conditions described in the medical board. All waiver requests received for conditions described in the medical board will be returned to the member's unit without action.

(3) A waiver of a physical standard is not required in a case where a Service Member's ability to perform on duty has been reviewed through the physical disability evaluation system and the approved finding of the Commandant is fit for duty.

b. Authority for Waivers. Commander PSC-epm (enlisted), PSC-opm (officers), and PSC-rpm (reserve) have the sole authority to grant waivers. The decision to authorize a waiver is based on many factors, including the recommendations of the Chief, Office of Health Services, Commandant (CG-112); the best interest of the Service; and the individual's training, experience, and duty performance. Waivers are not normally authorized but shall be reviewed by Commander (PSC) for the following:

(1) Original enlistment in the regular CG of personnel without prior military service.

(2) Appointment as a Cadet at the CG Academy.

(3) Training in any aviation or diving category specialty.

(4) A waiver can be terminated if there is appropriate medical justification.

c. <u>Types of Waivers</u>.

(1) <u>Temporary</u>. A temporary waiver may be authorized when a physical defect or condition is not stabilized and may either progressively increase or decrease in severity. These waivers are authorized for a specific period of time and require medical reevaluation prior to being extended.

(2) <u>Permanent</u>. A permanent waiver may be authorized when a defect or condition is not normally subject to change or progressive deterioration, and it has been clearly demonstrated that the condition does not impair the individual's ability to perform general duty, or the requirements of a particular specialty, grade, or rate.

d. <u>Procedures for Recommending Waivers</u>.

(1) <u>Medical Officer</u>. A Medical Officer who considers a defect disqualifying by the standards, but not a disability for the purpose for which the physical examination is required, shall:

(a) Enter a detailed description of the defect in Item 77 of the Report of Medical Examination, DD-2808.

(b) Indicate that either a temporary or permanent waiver is recommended.

(2) <u>Command/Unit Level</u>. When the command receives a Report of Medical Examination, DD-2808 indicating that an individual is not physically qualified, the command shall inform the individual that he/she is not physically qualified. The individual shall inform the command via letter of his/her intentions to pursue a waiver. The Medical Officer is required to give a recommendation on whether the waiver is appropriate and if the individual may perform his/her duties with this physical defect. This recommendation shall be completed on a Medical Record, SF-507. A cover letter stating the command's opinion as to the appropriateness of a waiver,

the individual's previous performance of duty, special skills, and any other pertinent information, shall accompany the Medical Officers report. The waiver request package shall be forwarded directly from the member's unit to Commander PSC-epm or opm, or Commandant (PSC-rpm) as appropriate.

   e. Command Action on Receipt of a Waiver Authorization. A command receiving authorization from the Commander PSC-epm/opm/rpm for the waiver of a physical standard shall carefully review the information provided to determine any duty limitation imposed and specific instructions for future medical evaluations. Unless otherwise indicated in the authorization, a waiver applies only to the specific category or purpose for which the physical examination is required. A copy of the waiver authorization shall be retained in both the service and health records for the period for which the waiver is authorized. Copies of future Report of Medical Examination, DD-2808 for the same purpose shall be endorsed to indicate a waiver is or was in effect.

9. Substitution of Physical Examinations.

   a. Rule for Substitution of Physical Examinations. In certain circumstances a physical examination performed for one purpose or category may be substituted to meet another requirement provided the following criteria are met:

      (1) The examinee was physically qualified for the purpose of the previous examination and all the required tests and recommendations have been completed.

      (2) The Report of Medical Examination, DD-2808 used for substitution bears an endorsement from the Reviewing Authority or Commandant (CG-112), as appropriate, indicating that the examinee was qualified for the purpose of the previous examination.

      (3) There has been no significant change in the examinee's medical status since the previous examination.

      (4) A review of the report of the previous examination indicates that the examinee meets the physical standards of the present requirement.

      (5) The date of the previous examination is within the validity period of the present requirement.

      (6) All additional tests and procedures to meet the requirements of the current physical examination have been completed.

   b. No substitutions are authorized for the following physical examinations:

      (1) Enlistment.

(2) Pre-training.

(3) Applicants for or designated personnel in special programs (aviation, diving, Academy).

(4) Command Afloat.

c. <u>Procedures for Reporting Substitution</u>. Substitutions of a physical examination shall be reported by submitting a copy of the Report of Medical Examination, DD-2808 and Report of Medical History, DD-2807-1 being used to meet the present requirements with the endorsement illustrated on the Modified Screening For: Overseas Assignment and/or Sea Duty Health Screening, CG-6100. Retain a copy of the substitution endorsement in the health record.

This page intentionally left blank

Section B. Report of Medical Examination Form, DD-2808 and Report of Medical History Form, DD-2807-1

1. Report of Medical Examination Form, DD-2808..1
2. Report of Medical History Form, DD-2807-1..1
3. Findings and Recommendations of Report of Medical Examination, DD-2808.....1
4. Correction of Defects Prior to Overseas Transfer or Sea Duty Deployment...........5
5. Objection to Assumption of Fitness for Duty at Separation....................................5
6. Separation Not Appropriate by Reason of Physical Disability...............................6
7. Procedures for Physical Defects Found Prior to Separation...................................6
    Figure 3-B-1...7
    Figure 3-B-2...8

This page intentionally left blank.

B. Report of Medical Examination, DD-2808 / Report of Medical History, DD-2807-1.

1. Report of Medical Examination, DD-2808.

   a. Report of Medical Examination, DD-2808. The Report of Medical Examination, DD-2808 is the proper form for reporting a complete physical examination. The Report of Medical Examination, DD-2808 can be obtained from the Commandant (CG-1121) Publications and Directives web site at http://www.uscg.mil/hq/cg1/cg112/pubs.asp or by http://www.dior.whs.mil/forms/DD2808.PDF directly from the DOD forms web site.

   b. Detailed instructions for the preparation and distribution of this form are contained in section 4-B of this Manual.

2. Report of Medical History, DD-2807-1.

   a. Report of Medical History, DD-2807-1. The Report of Medical History, DD-2807-1 is the proper form for reporting a member's medical history. The Report of Medical History, DD-2807-1 can be obtained from the Commandant (CG-1121) Publications and Directives web site at http://www.uscg.mil/hq/cg1/cg112/pubs.asp or by http://www.dior.whs.mil/forms/DD2807-1.PDF directly from the DOD forms web site.

   b. Detailed instructions. on the preparation and distribution of this form are contained in section 4-B of this Manual.

3. Findings and Recommendations of Report of Medical Examination, DD-2808.

   a. Action by the Medical Examiner.

      (1) Review of Findings and Evaluation of Defects. When the results of all tests have been received and evaluated, and all findings recorded, the examiner shall consult the appropriate standards of this chapter to determine if any of the defects noted are disqualifying for the purpose of the physical examination. When physical defects are found that are not listed in the standards as disqualifying, but that in the examiner's opinion would preclude the individual from performing military service or the duties of the program for which the physical examination was required, the examiner shall state that opinion on the report indicating reasons. If in the examiner's opinion, a defect listed as disqualifying is not disabling for military service, or a particular program, the examiner shall indicate the basis for this opinion and recommend a waiver in accordance with the provisions of Section A of this Chapter.

      (2) Remediable Defects. When the physical examination of active duty personnel indicates defects that are remediable or that may become potentially disabling unless a specific medical program is followed, the examiner shall clearly state any recommendations. If the examining facility has the capability of correcting the defect or providing extended outpatient follow-up or medical care, tentative arrangements for care

shall be scheduled, subject to the approval of the examinee's command. If the examining facility does not have the capabilities of providing the necessary care, tentative arrangements for admission or appointment at another facility shall be scheduled, again subject to the approval of the individual's command.

(3) Advising the Examinee. After completing the physical examination, the medical examiner will advise the examinee concerning the findings of the physical examination. At the same time, the examinee shall be informed that the examiner is not an approving authority for the purpose of the examination and that the findings must be approved by proper authorities.

(4) Disposition of Reports. The original Report of Medical Examination, DD-2808 and the original Report of Medical History, DD-2807-1, together with any reports of consultations or special testing reports not entered on the Report of Medical Examination, DD-2808 or Report of Medical History, DD-2807-1, shall be forwarded to the activity that referred the individual for the physical examination.

b. Review and Action on Reports of Physical Examination by Command.

(1) Command Responsibility.

(a) The command has a major responsibility in ensuring the proper performance of physical examinations on personnel assigned and that physical examinations are scheduled sufficiently far in advance to permit the review of the findings and correction of medical defects prior to the effective date of the action for which the examination is required. The command is also responsible to ensure that the individual complies with the examiner's recommendations and to initiate any administrative action required on a Report of Medical Examination.

(b) All Report of Medical Examination, DD-2808's shall be reviewed by Commanding Officers, or their designee, to determine that the prescribed forms were used and that all necessary entries were made.

(c) When the medical examiner recommends further tests or evaluation, or a program of medical treatment (such as hearing conservation, periodic blood pressure readings, etc.), the command will ensure that these tests or examinations are completed or that the individual is directed to and does comply with the recommended program. When a necessary test, evaluation, or program can be completed within a 60 day period, the unit may hold the Report of Medical Examination, DD-2808 to permit the forwarding of results. In all cases the command shall endorse the Report of Medical Examination, DD-2808 to indicate what action has been taken and forward the report to the reviewing authority if the 60 day period cannot be met or has elapsed.

    (d) Disposition of Reports.

        1. If a physical examination is accomplished for a purpose for which the command has administrative action, the original Report of Medical Examination, DD-2808 and Report of Medical History, DD-2807-1 and a return self-addressed envelope shall be forwarded to the reviewing authority. No action will be taken to accomplish the purpose for which the physical examination was taken until the endorsed original of the report is returned by the reviewing authority indicating the examinee meets the physical standards for the purpose of the examination.

        2. Approved MEPS physicals do not require further review. The original physical (Report of Medical Examination, DD-2808 and Report of Medical History, DD-2807-1) will be carried to the Training Center by the individual.

        3. If the physical examination is for a purpose requiring the consent or approval of either Commandant or HSWL SC, the procedures previously described for command review and action will be accomplished, except rather than forwarding the report of the examination directly to the reviewing authority, it will be included with other supporting documents (letters, recommendations, etc.) and forwarded through the chain of command.

        4. Units not using a CG health care facility shall send physical examinations to the appropriate CG clinic (as designated by HSWL SC or PSC (opm or epm) as appropriate.

c. Action by the Reviewing Authority.

    (1) The Commandant is the final reviewing authority for all physical examinations, except for applicants to the CG Academy.

    (2) Reviewing authorities are listed in Figure 3-B-2.

    (3) Flight physicals performed on aviators and aviation school students during training. Aviation physical exams that are reviewed and approved by the Navy Operational Medicine Institute (NOMI) or other armed services Flight Surgeons are considered valid. HSWL SC will not be the approving authority for these physicals. PSC will remain the waiver approval authority for these physicals, when a waiver is required prior to final approval. Upon completion of flight training and/or assignment to a CG unit, the approved physical will be considered valid until the last day of the member's next birth month.

The unit Flight Surgeon will clear the aviator for all flight related duties based on the approved flight physical.

(4) Commander, Personnel Service Center (PSC-cm) is the reviewing authority for aviator candidate, aircrew candidate, and diving candidate physical examinations. Commander, CGRC shall review disapproved MEPS physicals to ensure proper application of physical standards.

(5) The Department of Defense Medical Examination Review Board (DODMERB) is the reviewing authority for physical examinations performed on Academy applicants. MEPS is the reviewing authority for physical examinations performed in their facilities.

(6) Each Report of Medical Examination, DD-2808 shall be carefully reviewed to determine whether the findings reported indicate the examinee does or does not meet the appropriate physical standards. If further medical evaluation is required to determine that the examinee does meet the standards, or to resolve doubtful findings, the reviewing authority shall direct the Commanding Officer or recruiting station to obtain the evaluation and shall provide such assistance as may be required.

(7) The reviewing authority shall endorse the original of the Report of Medical Examination, DD-2808 indicating whether the examinee does or does not meet the physical standards required. This endorsement, if at all possible, should be placed in Item 44 of the Report of Medical Examination, DD-2808 (if there is no room, place endorsement in Item 73). See Figure 3-B-1 for an example of the endorsement. The date of the endorsement should be no more than 60 days from the start of the physical. If more than 60 days have elapsed, indicate why on the endorsement or disapprove the physical.

(8) The endorsed original of the physical examination shall be forwarded to the individual's unit for filing in the member's health record.

(9) Enter all approved physicals into the Medical Readiness Reporting System (MRRS). The date entered is the date the member received their physical (dated entered on the Report of Medical Examination, DD-2808). Do not enter an unapproved physical into MRRS.

d. <u>Disposition of Reports</u>.

(1) When the individual meets the appropriate physical standards, forward the physical examination as indicated in Figure 3-B-2.

(2) When the individual does not meet the appropriate physical standards and a waiver has been recommended, endorse the physical examination and forward it in accordance with section 3-A-8.

(3) When the individual is not physically qualified for the purpose of the examination and a waiver is not recommended, the reviewing authority will arrange for the examinee to be evaluated by a medical board and

provide administrative action as outlined in the Physical Disability Evaluation System, COMDTINST M1850.2 (series).

4. Correction of Defects Prior to Overseas Transfer or Sea Duty Deployment.

   a. Medical Defects. Before an individual departs for an overseas assignment for 60 consecutive days or greater , to permanent assignment aboard a Polar Icebreaker, or to a vessel deploying from its home port for 60 consecutive days or greater, all remediable medical defects, such as hernias, pilonidal cysts or sinuses requiring surgery, etc., must be corrected. Those defects that are not easily corrected will be referred to Commander PSC for consideration. These procedures also apply to personnel presently assigned to such vessels. In these cases all necessary corrective measures or waivers will be accomplished prior to the sailing date.

   b. Dental Defects. All essential dental treatment shall be completed prior to overseas transfer or sea duty deployment except those described in 4-C-3.c (3) (b). Essential dental treatment constitutes those procedures necessary to prevent disease and disabilities of the jaw, teeth, and related structures. This includes extractions, simple and compound restorations, and treatment for acute oral pathological conditions such as Vincent's stomatitis, acute gingivitis, and similar conditions that could endanger the health of the individual during a tour of duty. Missing teeth are to be replaced when occluding tooth surfaces are so depleted that the individual cannot properly masticate food. Elective dental procedures (those that may be deferred for up to twelve months without jeopardizing the patient's health, i.e., Class II patient need not be completed prior to overseas transfer providing both of the following conditions exist:

      (1) Completion of such elective procedures prior to transfer would delay the planned transfer.

      (2) Adequate Service dental facilities are available at the overseas base.

   c. Vision Defects. A refraction shall be performed on all personnel whose visual acuity is less than 20/20 in either eye (near or distant) or whose present eyewear prescription does not correct their vision to 20/20. All personnel requiring glasses for correction shall have a minimum of two pair prior to overseas transfer or sea duty deployment. All personnel requiring corrective lenses shall wear them for the performance of duty.

5. Objection to Assumption of Fitness for Duty at Separation.

   a. Member's responsibilities. Any member undergoing separation from the service that disagrees with the assumption of fitness for duty and claims to have a physical disability as defined in section 2-A-38 of the Physical Disability Evaluation System, COMDTINST M1850.2 (series), shall submit written objections within 10 days of signing the Chronological Record of Service, CG-4057 to Commander PSC. Such objections based solely on items of medical history or physical findings will be resolved at the local level. The member is responsible for submitting copies of the following information along with the written objections:

(1) Report of Medical Examination, DD-2808.

(2) Report of Medical History, DD-2807-1.

(3) Signed copy of the Chronological Record of Service, CG-4057.

(4) Appropriate consultations and reports.

(5) "Other pertinent documentation."

(6) The rebuttal is a member's responsibility and command endorsement is not required.

b. Rebuttal package. The package shall contain thorough documentation of the physical examination findings, particularly in those areas relating to the individual's objections. Consultations shall be obtained to thoroughly evaluate all problems or objections the examinee indicates. Consultations obtained at the examinee's own expense from a civilian source shall also be included with the report.

c. Commander (PSC) responsibility. Commander (PSC) will evaluate each case and based upon the information submitted take one of the following actions:

(1) Find separation appropriate, in which case the individual will be so notified and the normal separation process completed.

(2) Find separation inappropriate, in which case the entire record will be returned and appropriate action recommended.

(3) Request additional documentation before making a determination.

6. Separation Not Appropriate by Reason of Physical Disability. When a member has an impairment (in accordance with section 3-F of this Manual) an Initial Medical Board shall be convened only if the conditions listed in paragraph 2-C-2.(b), Physical Disability Evaluation System, COMDTINST M1850.2 (series), are also met. Otherwise the member is suitable for separation.

7. Procedures for Physical Defects Found Prior to Separation.

a. Policy. No person shall be separated from the Service with any disease in a communicable state until either rendered noninfectious, or until suitable provisions have been made for necessary treatment after separation.

b. Remediable Non-Disqualifying Defects. Remediable physical defects that would not normally prevent the individual from performing the duties of grade or rate shall be corrected only if there is reasonable assurance of complete recovery and sufficient time remaining prior to separation.

FIGURE 3-B-1   COMDTINST M6000.1E

DATE:_____ REVIEWERS UNIT _____

Does /does not meet the physical standards for (title or category or purpose of examination), as prescribed in (appropriate section of Medical Manual, COMDTINST M6000.1 (series)).

Disqualifying Defects:

Signature and Title of Reviewer

COMDTINST M6000.1E FIGURE 3-B-2

Physical Exam Purpose	Note:	Approving Authority	Reviewing Authority:
Aviator Candidate	(1,2)	PSC-opm	PSC-cm
Aircrew Candidate	(1,2)	PSC-epm	PSC-cm
Diving Candidate	(1,7)	NDSTC	HSWL SC
Physician Assistant Candidate	(1,5)	PSC-opm	PSC-cm
Flight Surgeon (FS)		PSC-PSD-med	PSC-PSD-med
FS Candidate	(1)(3)	PSC-PSD-med	PSC-PSD-med
Aviator	(1)	PSC-PSD-med	PSC-PSD-med
Aircrew	(1)	PSC-PSD-med	PSC-PSD-med
Diving	(1)(6)	Designated DMO	Designated DMO
Annual	(1)	HSWL SC or Clinic Administrator (CA)	HSWL SC or Clinic Administrator (CA)
LSO	(1)	HSWL SC or CA	HSWL SC or CA
Quinquennial	(1)	HSWL SC or CA	HSWL SC or CA
Overseas/Sea Duty	(1)	HSWL SC or CA	HSWL SC or CA
Retention	(1)	HSWL SC or CA	HSWL SC or CA
Retirement	(1,4)	HSWL SC or CA	HSWL SC or CA
Involuntary Separation	(1,4)	HSWL SC or CA	HSWL SC or CA
RELAD	(1,4)	HSWL SC or CA	HSWL SC or CA
Precom /Appts	(1)	HSWL SC or CA	HSWL SC or CA
Direct Commission	(1,5)	CGRC	CGRC
OCS	(1,5)	CGRC	CGRC
Enlistment	(2)	CGRC	CGRC

NOTES:

(1) The reviewing authority shall review, endorse and return the original to the member's unit for filing in the member's or applicant's health record.
(2) Forward the unendorsed physical to the appropriate office (as listed above) with the application/training request package. That office will forward the physical to CG PSC for review.
(3) Forward the original and one copy to Commandant (CG-1121) for review.
(4) Ensure that a completed Chronological Record of Care, CG-4057 accompanies the completed Report of Medical Examination, DD-2808 and Report of Medical History, DD-2807-1.
(5) Reviewing authority for current USCG or USCGR members only. For all others, Note (2) above applies. Forward a copy of the first/front page of the Report of Medical Examination, DD-2808 with endorsement to the appropriate office with the application package.

FIGURE 3-B-2 (cont.)   COMDTINST M6000.1E

(6) Diving Medical Officer (DMO) will be designated by Commandant (CG-1121). The currently designated DMO is listed on the Operational Medicine website.
(7) Diving candidate physicals shall be forwarded by HSWL SC to Coast Guard Liaison Office (CGLO) at COMMANDING OFFICER, NAVAL DIVING SALVAGE TRAINING CENTER, 350 CRAG RD, PANAMA CITY FL 32407-7016.

CGLO will notify member of status of physical exam. Physical exam will be retained at NDSTC until member commences training at which time the physical exam will be entered into the health record.

This page intentionally left blank.

COMDTINST M6000.1E

Section C. Medical Examination Techniques and Lab Testing Standards

1. Scope...1
2. Speech Impediment..1
3. Head, Face, Neck, and Scalp (Item 17 of DD-2808) 1
4. Nose, Sinuses, Mouth, and Throat (Item 19, 20 of DD-2808).....................................2
5. Ears (General) and Drums (Item 21, 22 of DD-2808) 2
6. Eyes (General), Ophthalmoscopic, and Pupils (Item 23, 24, 25 of DD-2808) 3
7. Ocular Mobility (Item 26 of DD-2808) 5
8. Heart and Vascular System (Item 27 of DD-2808) 5
9. Lungs and Chest (Item 28 of DD-2808) 9
10. Anus and Rectum (Item 30 of DD-2808) 11
11. Abdomen and Viscera (Item 31 of DD-2808) 11
12. Genitourinary System (Item 32 of DD-2808)..11
13. Extremities (Item 33, 34, 35 of DD-2808)...12
14. Spine and Other Musculoskeletal (Item 36 of DD-2808)..14
15. Identifying Body Marks, Scars, and Tattoos (Item 37 of DD-2808).........................15
16. Neurologic (Item 39 of DD-2808) 16
17. Psychiatric (Item 40 of DD-2808) 17
18. Endocrine System 18
19. Dental (Item 43 of DD-2808) 18
20. Laboratory Findings...19
Figure 3-C-1..25
21. Height, Weight and Body Build...26
22. Distant Visual Acuity and Other Eye Tests 26
23. Audiometer 33
24. Psychological and Psychomotor 33
Figure 3-C-2..34
Figure 3-C-3..37
Figure 3-C-4..38

This page intentionally left blank.

C. **Medical Examination Techniques and Lab Testing Standards.**

1. **Scope.** This section is a medical examination technique guide applicable for all physical examinations and periodic health assessments (PHA). Detailed instructions for the PHA are contained in the CG PHA, COMDTINST 6150.3.

2. **Speech Impediment.** Administer the "Reading Aloud Test" (RAT) as listed.

    a. **Procedure.** Have the examinee stand erect, face you across the room and read aloud, as if confronting a class of students.

    b. **Pauses.** If the individual pauses, even momentarily, on any phrase or word, immediately and sharply say, "What's that?", and require the examinee to start over again with the first sentence of the test.

    c. **Second trial.** The person who truly stammers usually will halt again at the same word phonetic combination often revealing serious stammering. Examinees who fail to read the test without stammering after three attempts will be disqualified.

    d. **Reading aloud test.** "You wished to know all about my grandfather. Well, he is nearly 93 years old; he dresses himself in an ancient black frock coat usually minus several buttons; yet he still thinks as swiftly as ever. A long, flowing beard clings to his chin, giving those who observe him a pronounced feeling of the utmost respect. When he speaks, his voice is just a bit cracked and quivers a trifle. Twice each day he plays skillfully and with zest upon our small organ. Except in the winter when the ooze or snow or ice is present, he slowly takes a short walk in the open air each day. We have often urged him to walk more and smoke less, but he always answers, 'Banana Oil.' Grandfather likes to be modern in his language."

3. **Head, Face, Neck, and Scalp (Item 17 of DD-2808).**

    a. **Head and Face.** Carefully inspect and palpate the head and face for evidence of injury, deformity, or tumor growth. Record all swollen glands, deformities, or imperfections noted. Inquire into the cause of all scars and deformities. If a defect is detected such as moderate or severe acne, cysts, or scarring, make a statement as to whether this defect will interfere with wearing military clothing and equipment.

    b. **Neck.** Carefully inspect and palpate for glandular enlargement, deformity, crepitus, limitations of motion, and asymmetry; palpate the parotid and submaxillary regions, the larynx for mobility and position, the thyroid for size and nodules, and the supraclavicular areas for fullness and masses. If enlarged lymph nodes are detected describe them in detail with a clinical opinion of their etiology.

    c. **Scalp.** Examine for deformities such as depressions and exostosis.

4. Nose, Sinuses, Mouth, and Throat (Item 19, 20 of DD-2808).

   a. Nasal or sinus complaints. If there are no nasal or sinus complaints, simple anterior rhinoscopy will suffice, provided that in this examination, the nasal mucous membrane, the septum, and the turbinates appear normal. If the examinee has complaints, a more detailed examination is required. Most commonly, these complaints are external nasal deformity, nasal obstruction, partial or complete on one or both sides; nasal discharge; postnasal discharge; sneezing; nasal bleeding; facial pain; and headaches.

   b. Abnormalities in the mucous membrane. Abnormalities in the mucous membrane in the region of the sinus ostia, the presence of pus in specific areas, and the cytologic study of the secretions may provide valuable information regarding the type and location of the sinus infection. Evaluate tenderness over the sinuses by transillumination or x-ray. Examination for sinus tenderness should include pressure applied over the anterior walls of the frontal sinuses and the floors of these cavities and also pressure over the cheeks. Determine if there is any tenderness to percussion beyond the boundaries (as determined by x-ray) of the frontal sinuses. Note any sensory changes in the distribution of the supra-orbital or infra-orbital nerves that may indicate the presence of neoplasm. Note any external swelling of the forehead, orbit, cheek, and alveolar ridge.

   c. Mouth and tongue. Many systemic diseases manifest themselves as lesions of the mouth and tongue; namely leukemia, syphilis, agranulocytosis, pemphigus, erythema multiform, and dermatitis medicamentosa. Note any abnormalities or lesions on lips or buccal mucous membrane, gums, tongue, palate, floor of mouth, and ostia of the salivary ducts. Note the condition of the teeth. Pay particular attention to any abnormal position, size, or the presence of tremors or paralysis of the tongue and the movement of the soft palate on phonation.

   d. Throat. Record any abnormal findings of the throat. If tonsils are enucleated, note possible presence and position of residual or recurrent lymphoid tissue and the degree of scarring. If tonsils are present, note size, presence of pus in crypts, and any associated cervical lymphadenopathy. Note presence of exudate, ulceration, or evidence of neoplasm on the posterior pharyngeal crypts. Describe any hypertrophied lymphoid tissue on the posterior pharyngeal wall or in the lateral angle of the pharynx and note if there is evidence of swelling that displaces the tonsils, indicating possible neoplasm or abscess. Perform direct or indirect laryngoscopy if the individual complains of hoarseness.

5. Ears (General) and Drums (Item 21, 22 of DD-2808). Inspect the auricle, the external canal, and the tympanic membrane using a speculum and good light. Abnormalities (congenital or acquired) in size, shape, or form of the auricles, canals, or tympanic membranes must be noted, evaluated, and recorded.

   a. Auricle. Note deformities, lacerations, ulcerations, and skin disease.

b. <u>External canal</u>. Note any abnormality of the size or shape of the canal and inspect the skin to detect evidence of disease. If there is material in the canal, note whether it is normal cerumen, foreign body, or exudate. Determine the source of any exudate in the canal. If this exudate has its origins in the middle ear, record whether it is serous, purulent, sanguinous, or mucoid; whether it is foul smelling; and, whether it is profuse or scanty.

c. <u>Tympanic membrane</u>. Remove all exudate and debris from the canal and tympanic membrane before examination. Unless the canal is of abnormal shape, visualize the entire tympanic membrane and note and record the following points.

  (1) List any abnormality of the landmarks indicating scarring, retraction, bulging, or inflammation.

  (2) Note whether the tympanum is air containing.

  (3) List any perforations, giving size and position, indicating whether they are marginal or central, which quadrant is involved, and whether it is the flaccid or the tense portion of the membrane that is included.

  (4) Attempt, if the tympanic membrane is perforated, to determine the state of the middle ear contents, particularly concerning hyperplastic tympanic mucosa, granulation tissue, cholesteatoma, and bone necrosis. Do the pathological changes indicate an acute or chronic process? This clinical objective examination should permit evaluating the infectious process in the middle ear and making a reasonably accurate statement regarding the chronicity of the infection; the extent and type of involvement of the mastoid; the prognosis regarding hearing; and, the type of treatment (medical or surgical) that is required.

  (5) Note, for all aviation and dive physical examinations, whether the examinee can properly auto insufflate tympanic membrane.

6. <u>Eyes (General), Ophthalmoscopic, and Pupils (Item 23, 24, 25 of DD-2808)</u>. External and ophthalmoscopic examinations of the eyes are required on all examinations. Contact lenses shall not be worn during any part of the eye examination, including visual acuity testing. It is essential that such lenses not be worn for 72 hours preceding examination. The strength of the contact that an examinee may possess shall not be accepted as the refraction nor will it be entered as such in Item 60, Report of Medical Examination Form DD-2808. The general examination shall include the following specific points and checks:

  a. <u>General</u>.

    (1) Bony abnormality or facial asymmetry.

    (2) Position of the eyes.

    (3) Exophthalmus.

(4) Manifest deviation of the visual axis.

(5) Epiphora or discharge.

(6) Position of puncta or discharge when pressure exerted over lacrimal sac.

b. Lids.

(1) Ptosis.

(2) Position of lashes, eversion or inversion.

(3) Inflammation of margins.

(4) Cysts or tumors.

c. Conjunctiva. Examine the palpebral and bulbar conjunctiva by:

(1) Eversion of upper lid.

(2) Depression and eversion of lower lid.

(3) Manually separating both lids.

d. Pupils.

(1) Size.

(2) Shape.

(3) Equality.

(4) Direct, consensual, and accommodative reactions.

e. Directly and obliquely examine.

(1) Cornea. For clarity, discrete opacities, superficial or deep scarring, pannus, vascularization, pterygium, and the integrity of the epithelium.

(2) Anterior Chamber. For depth, alteration of normal character of the aqueous humor, and retained foreign bodies.

(3) Iris. For abnormalities and pathologic changes.

(4) Crystalline Lens. For clouding or opacities.

f. Ophthalmoscopic.

(1) Media. Examine with a plano ophthalmoscopic lens at a distance of approximately 18 to 21 inches from the eye. Localize and describe any opacity appearing in the red reflex or direct examination or on eye movement.

(2) Fundus. Examine with the strongest plus or weakest minus lens necessary to bring optic nerve into sharp focus. Pay particular attention to the color, surface, and margin of the optic nerve, also record any abnormality of the pigmentation or vasculature of the retina.

(3) Macula. Examine for any change.

7. Ocular Motility (Item 26 of DD-2808).

   a. Ascertain the motility of the eyeballs by testing for binocular eye movement (ductions and versions) in the cardinal positions of gaze. If any abnormalities are suspected, verify with the cover/uncover test.

   b. Observe if the eyes move together and whether there is loss of motion in any direction (paralysis or paresis), or absence of muscle balance, whether latent (heterophoria) or manifest (strabismus / heterotropia). Have the examinee look at a test object and alternately cover and uncover one eye leaving the other uncovered and observe the movement, if any, in each eye. In heterotropia movement occurs only in the eye that is covered and uncovered; on being covered, it deviates and on being uncovered, it swings back into place to take up fixation with the other eye that has remained uncovered.

8. Heart and Vascular System (Item 27 of DD-2808).

   a. General. In direct light, have the examinee stand at ease, with arms relaxed and hanging by sides. Do not permit the examinee to move from side to side or twist to assist in the examination, as these maneuvers may distort landmarks: and increase muscular resistance of the chest wall. Examine the heart by the following methods: inspection, palpation, auscultation, and when considered necessary, by mensuration.

   b. Inspection. Begin from above and go downward, with special reference to the following:

      (1) Any malformation that might change the normal relations of the heart.

      (2) Pulsations in the suprasternal notch and in the second interspaces to the right and left of the sternum.

      (3) Character of the precordial impulse.

      (4) Epigastric pulsations.

   c. Palpation. First palpate to detect thrills over the carotids, thyroid glands, suprasternal notch, apex of the heart, and at the base. Use palms of hands in palpating and use light pressure, as hard pressure may obliterate a thrill. To locate the maximum cardiac impulse, have the examinee stoop and throw the shoulders slightly forward, thus bringing the heart into the closest possible relation with the chest wall. Palpate both radial arteries at the same time for equality in rate and volume. Run the finger along the artery to note any changes in its walls. Place the palm of one hand over the heart and fingers of the other over the radial artery to see if all ventricular contractions are transmitted. Palpate to determine the degree of tension or compression of the pulse. In an estimate of pulse rate, the excitement of undergoing a physical examination must be considered.

d. <u>Auscultation</u>. In auscultating the heart, bear in mind the four points where the normal heart sounds are heard with maximum intensity:

(1) Aortic area, second interspace to right of sternum. Here the second sound is distinct.

(2) Tricuspid area, junction of the fifth right rib with the sternum. Here the first sound is distinct.

(3) Pulmonic area, second interspace to left of sternum. Here the second sound is most distinct.

(4) Mitral area, fifth interspace to left of sternum. Here the first sound is most clearly heard.

e. <u>Blood Pressure</u>.

(1) Only the sitting blood pressure is required.

(2) Other positions required only if sitting blood pressure exceeds 139 mmHG systolic or 89 mmHG diastolic.

(3) Take the sitting blood pressure with the examinee comfortably relaxed in a sitting position with legs uncrossed and the arm placed on a rest at the horizontal level of the heart. The condition of the arteries, the tenseness of the pulse, and the degree of accentuation of the aortic second sound must be taken into consideration, as well as the relation between the systolic and diastolic pressure.

(4) Personnel recording blood pressure must be familiar with situations that result in spurious elevation. A Medical Officer shall repeat the determination in doubtful or abnormal cases and ensure that the proper recording technique was used.

(5) Artificially high blood pressure may be observed as follows.

(a) If the compressive cuff is too loosely applied.

(b) If the compressive cuff is too small for the arm size. Cuff width should be approximately one-half arm circumference. In a very large or very heavily muscled individual, this may require an "oversize" cuff.

(c) If the blood pressure is repetitively taken before complete cuff deflation occurs. Trapping of venous blood in the extremity results in a progressive increase in recorded blood pressure.

(6) At least five minutes of rest should precede the blood pressure recording. Due regard must be given to physiologic effects such as excitement, recent exercise, smoking or caffeine within the preceding thirty minutes, and illness.

(7) No examinee shall be rejected based on the results of a single recording. If 2 out of the 3 positions exceed 139 mmHG systolic or 89 mmHG diastolic, the disqualifying blood pressures will be rechecked for 3 consecutive days in the morning and afternoon of each day and averaged. The first determination shall be recorded in Item 58 and the repeat determinations in Item 73 of DD-2808. Patients being treated for HTN that have blood pressures less than 140 systolic and 90 diastolic do not require three-day blood pressure checks.

(8) While emphasizing that a diagnosis of elevated blood pressure not be prematurely made, it seems evident that a single "near normal" level does not negate the significance of many elevated recordings.

f. Blood Pressure Determination.

(1) Use procedures recommended by the American Heart Association.

(2) Take the systolic reading as either the palpatory or auscultatory reading depending on which is higher. In most normal subjects, the auscultatory reading is slightly higher.

(3) Record diastolic pressure as the level at which the cardiac tones disappear by auscultation. In a few normal subjects, particularly in thin individuals and usually because of excessive stethoscope pressure, cardiac tones may be heard to extremely low levels. In these instances, if the technique is correct and there is no underlying valvular defect, a diastolic reading will be taken at the change in tone.

(4) Note variations of blood pressures with the position change if there is a history of syncope or symptoms to suggest postural hypertension.

(5) Obtain blood pressure in the legs when simultaneous palpation of the pulses in upper and lower extremities reveals a discrepancy in pulse volume.

g. Pulse Rate.

(1) Determine the pulse rate immediately after the blood pressure. Only the sitting position is required.

(2) In the presence of a relevant history, arrhythmia, or a pulse of less than 50 or over 100, an electrocardiogram will be obtained.

h. Interpretation of Abnormal Signs and Symptoms. The excitement of the examination may produce violent and rapid heart action often associated with a transient systolic murmur. Such conditions may erroneously be attributed to the effects of exertion; they usually disappear promptly in the recumbent posture. Try to recognize the excitable individuals and take measures to eliminate psychic influences from the test.

i. Hypertrophy-Dilatation. An apex beat located at or beyond the left nipple line, or below the sixth rib, suggests an enlargement sufficient to disqualify for military service. Its cause, either valvular disease or hypertension in the majority of cases, should be sought. A horizontal position of the heart must be distinguished from left ventricular enlargement. EKG, ultrasound studies, fluoroscopy, and chest x-ray may be indicated for diagnosis.

j. Physiological Murmurs. Cardiac murmurs are the most certain physical signs by which valvular disease may be recognized and its location determined. The discovery of any murmur demands diligent search for other evidence of heart disease. Murmurs may occur, however, in the absence of valvular lesions or other cardiac disease. Such physiological murmurs are not causes for rejection.

   (1) Characteristics. The following characteristics of physiological murmurs will help differentiate them from organic murmurs:

   (a) They are always systolic in time.

   (b) They are usually heard over a small area, the most common place being over the pulmonic valve and mitral valve.

   (c) They change with position of the body, disappearing in certain positions. They are loudest usually in the recumbent position and are sometimes heard only in that position.

   (d) They are transient in character, frequently disappearing after exercise.

   (e) They are usually short, rarely occupying all of the systole, and are soft and of blowing quality.

   (f) There is no evidence of heart disease or cardiac enlargement.

   (2) Most Common Types. The most common types of physiological murmurs are:

   (a) Those heard over the second and third left interspaces during expiration, disappearing during forced inspiration. These are particularly common in individuals with flexible chests, who can produce extreme forced expiration. Under such circumstances, murmurs may be associated with a vibratory thrust.

   (b) Cardio-respiratory murmurs caused by movements of the heart against air in a part of the lung overlapping the heart. They usually vary in different phases of respiration and at times disappear completely when the breath is held.

   (c) Prolongations of the apical first sound that are often mistaken for murmurs.

(3) Diagnosis. An EKG, chest x-ray, and echocardiogram are usually indicated to firmly establish the true cause of a murmur and should be done if there is any question of abnormality.

k. Electrocardiograms. Use standard positions for precordial leads when completing electrocardiograms.

9. Lungs and Chest (Item 28 of DD-2808).

    a. History and x-ray studies. A thorough examination includes a complete history (DD-2807-1) careful physical examination, and necessary x-ray and laboratory studies. In screening examinations, the history and x-ray studies are the most immediately revealing examination techniques.

    b. Exam. Remember that several disqualifying diseases such as tuberculosis and sarcoidosis may not be detectable by physical examination and the absence of abnormal physical signs does not rule out disqualifying pulmonary disease. Such diseases, as well as others (neopasms and fungus infections), may be detected only by chest x-ray.

      (1) Conduct the physical examination in a thorough, systematic fashion. Take particular care to detect pectus abnormalities, kyphosis, scoliosis, wheezing, persistent rhonchi, basilar rales, digital clubbing, and cyanosis. Any of these findings require additional intensive inquiry into the patient's history if subtle functional abnormalities or mild asthma, bronchitis, or bronchiectasis are to be suspected and evaluated. The physical examination shall include the following:

         (a) Inspection. The examinee should be seated in a comfortable, relaxed position with the direct light falling upon the chest. Careful comparison of the findings elicited over symmetrical areas on the two sides of the chest gives the most accurate information regarding condition of the underlying structures. Observe for asymmetry of the thoracic cage, abnormal pulsation, atrophy of the shoulder girdle or pectoral muscles, limited or lagging expansion on forced inspiration. The large, rounded relatively immobile "barrel" chest suggests pulmonary emphysema.

         (b) Palpation.

            1. Observe for tumors of the breast or thoracic wall, enlarged cervical, supraclavicular, or axillary lymph nodes, suprasternal notch, and thrills associated with respiration or the cardiac cycle.

            2. A breast examination should also be performed based upon the Clinical Preventive Services guidance as contained in the Coast Guard Periodic Health Assessment, COMDTINST 6150.3.

Monthly self-examination is recommended for all adult female patients.

    (c) <u>Auscultation</u>. Instruct the examinee to breathe freely but deeply through the mouth. Listen to an entire respiratory cycle before moving the stethoscope bell to another area. Note wheezing, rales, or friction rubs. Compare the pitch and intensity of breath sounds heard over symmetrical areas of the two lungs. Instruct the examinee to exhale during this process. Note any rales, paying particular attention to moist rales that "break" with the cough or fine rales heard at the beginning of inspiration immediately after cough.

(2) Do not hesitate to expand the history if abnormalities are detected during examination or in repeating the examination if chest film abnormalities are detected.

c. <u>Asthma bronchiectasis, and tuberculosis</u>. There are three conditions that are most often inadequately evaluated and result in unnecessary and avoidable expense and time loss. These three are asthma (to include "asthmatic bronchitis"), bronchiectasis, and tuberculosis.

(1) <u>Asthma</u>. In evaluating asthma, a careful history is of prime importance since this condition is characteristically intermittent and may be absent at the time of examination. Careful attention to a history of episodic wheezing with or without accompanying respiratory infection is essential. Ask about the use of prescription or over-the-counter bronchodilators.

(2) <u>Bronchiectasis</u>. Individuals who report a history of frequent respiratory infections accompanied by purulent sputum or multiple episodes of pneumonia should be suspected of bronchiectasis. This diagnosis can be further supported by a finding of post-tussive rales at one or both bases posteriorly or by a finding of lacy densities at the lung base on the chest film. If bronchiectasis is considered on the basis of history, medical findings or chest film abnormalities, seek confirmatory opinion from the examinee's personal physician or refer the examinee to a pulmonologist for evaluation and recommendations.

(3) <u>Tuberculosis (TB)</u>.

    (a) Active TB is often asymptomatic and not accompanied by abnormal physical findings unless the disease is advanced. If only such manifestations as hemoptysis or draining sinuses are looked for, most cases of TB will be missed.

    (b) The QuantiFERON® - TB Gold test (QFT-G) or theTuberculin Skin Test (TST) can aid in diagnosing Mycobacterium tuberculosis infection, including latent tuberculosis infection (LTBI) and tuberculosis (TB) disease.

- (c) If positive, evaluate the chest film for any infiltrate, cavity, or nodular lesion involving the apical or posterior segments of an upper lobe or superior segment of a lower lobe. Many tuberculosis lesions may be partially hidden or obscured by the clavicles. When any suspicion of an apical abnormality exists, an apical lordotic view must be obtained for clarification.

- (d) It is neither practical nor possible, in most instances, to determine whether or not a TB lesion is inactive on the basis of a single radiologic examination. Therefore, refer any examinee suspected of TB to a pulmonologist or to an appropriate public health clinic for evaluation.

- (e) An initial TST is mandatory and shall be made a part of the physical examination for all personnel entering on active duty for a period of 30 days or more.

- (f) See www.cdc.gov/tb/ for additional information on Tuberculosis Management.

10. Anus and Rectum (Item 30 of DD-2808). All examinations shall include a visual inspection of the anus. Perform a digital rectal examination and test for fecal occult blood in accordance with the Clinical Preventive Service guidelines as contained in the CG Periodic Health Assessment, COMDTINST 6150.3. When anorectal disease is suspected a consultation with a gastroenterologist may be indicated.

11. Abdomen and Viscera (Item 31 of DD-2808).

    a. Examination. Examine the abdomen with the examinee supine, as well as standing to detect hernias.

    b. Methods. Use appropriate clinical laboratory, radiologic, and endoscopic examinations to confirm a diagnosis.

12. Genitourinary System (Item 32 of DD-2808).

    a. General. All physical examinations shall search for evidence of Sexually Transmitted Infections (STI) or malformation.

    b. Instructions for examination according to sex.

        (1) Females. The examination shall include:

            (a) Inspection of the external genitalia.

            (b) Either a vaginal or rectal bimanual palpation of the pelvic organs.

            (c) Papanicolaou (PAP) testing and visualization of the cervix and vaginal canal by speculum in accordance with 20.f. of this section.

(2) Males. The glans penis and corona will be exposed. The testes and scrotal contents will be palpated and the inguinal lymph nodes will be examined for abnormalities. Palpate the inguinal canals while having the patient perform a valsalva.

13. Extremities (Item 33, 34, 35 of DD-2808). Carefully examine the extremities for deformities, old fractures and dislocations, amputations, partially flexed or ankylosed joints, impaired functions of any degree, varicose veins, and edema. In general the examination shall include:

    a. Elbow. With the examinee holding the upper arms against the body with the forearms extended and fully supinated, observe for the presence of normal carrying angle. Have the examinee flex the elbows to a right angle and keeping the elbows against the body, note ability to fully supinate and pronate the forearms. Test medial and lateral stability by placing varus and valgus strain on the joint with the elbow extended. Test the power of the flexor, extensor, supinator, and pronator muscles by having the examinee contract these muscles against manual resistance. If indicated, x-rays should include antero-posterior and lateral views.

    b. Foot.

        (1) Examine the feet for conditions such as flatfoot, corns, ingrown nails, bunions, deformed or missing toes, hyperhidrosis, color changes, and clubfoot.

        (2) When any degree of flatfoot is found, test the strength of the feet by requiring the examinee to hop on the toes of each foot for a sufficient time and by requiring the examinee to alight on the toes after jumping up several times. To distinguish between disqualifying and nondisqualifying degrees of flatfoot, consider the extent, impairment of function, appearance in uniform, and presence or absence of symptoms. Remember, it is usually not the flatfoot condition itself that causes symptoms but an earlier state in which the arches are collapsing and the various structures are undergoing readjustment of their relationships. Report angles of excursion or limitation; comparative measurements; use of orthotics or other supports; and x-ray results if indicated.

    c. Hip.

        (1) With the examinee standing, observe the symmetry of the buttocks, the intergluteal clefts, and infragluteal fold. Palpate the iliac crest and greater trochanters for symmetry.

        (2) If abnormalities are suspected, have the examinee stand first on one foot and then the other, flexing the nonweight bearing hip and knee and observing for ability to balance as well as for instability of the joint, as indicated by dropping downward of the buttock and pelvis of the flexed (non-weight bearing) hip. A positive Trendelenburg sign necessitates x-ray evaluation.

(3) While supine have the examinee flex the hip, abduct and adduct the hip and rotate the leg inward. Observe for hesitancy in performing these motions, incomplete range of motion, or facial evidence of pain on motion. Test muscle strength in each position.

(4) With examinee prone, test for ability to extend each leg with knee extended and test for power in each hip in extension.

(5) If abnormalities are detected requiring x-rays, obtain an antero-posterior and a lateral view of each hip for comparison.

d. <u>Knee</u>.

(1) With trousers (skirt/dress), shoes, and socks removed, observe general muscular development of legs, particularly the thigh musculature.

(2) Have examinee squat, sitting on heels, and observe for hesitancy, weakness, and presence or absence of pain or crepitus.

(3) With examinee sitting, test for ability to fully extend the knee and test power in extension by applying pressure to the lower leg with knee extended. Compare equality of power in each leg. With knee flexed, test for hamstring power by attempting to pull leg into extension; compare equality of strength in each leg. Palpate entire knee for tenderness. With examinee still sitting on the table edge, sit and grasp the heel between the knees; then test for cruciate ligament stability by first pulling the tibia anteriorly on the femur and by then pushing the tibia posteriorly on the femur ("Drawer Sign").

(4) With the examinee supine, mark on each leg a distance of 1 inch above the patella and 6 inches above the patella, making sure this is done with muscles relaxed. Measure circumferences at these levels and note presence or absence of atrophy. Test the medial and lateral collateral ligaments by placing varus and valgus strain on the extended knee. Manipulate the knee through a complete range of flexion and extension, noting any difference between the sides and any abnormal restriction.

(5) If there is a history of knee injury assess muscular strength, ligamentous stability, and range of motion. Also look for evidence of inflammatory or degenerative processes.

(6) In the presence of any history of "locking," recurrent effusion, or instability, or when atrophy measured is more than 3/8 inch or when limitation of motion or ligamentous instability is detected, obtain x-rays including an antero-posterior, lateral, and intercondylar view.

(7) An orthopedic evaluation is required on all recruit physicals if there is evidence of any abnormality.

e. <u>Shoulder</u>.

   (1) With the examinee stripped to the waist, inspect both anteriorly and posteriorly for asymmetry, abnormal configuration, or muscle atrophy.

   (2) From the back, with the examinee standing, observe the scapulohumeral rhythm as the arms are elevated from the sides directly overhead, carrying the arms up laterally. Any arrhythmia may indicate shoulder joint abnormality and is cause for particularly careful examination. Palpate the shoulders for tenderness and test range of motion in flexion, extension, abduction, and rotation. Compare each shoulder in this respect.

   (3) Test muscle power of abductors, flexors, and extensors of the shoulder, as well as power in internal and external rotation. Have the examinee attempt to lift a heavy weight with arms at the side to establish integrity of the acromioclavicular joint.

f. <u>Wrist and Hand</u>.

   (1) Palpate the wrist for tenderness in the anatomical snuff box often present in undiscovered fractures of the carpal navicular. Observe and compare muscle strength and range of motion, flexion, extension, radial, and ulnar deviation.

   (2) Inspect the palms and extended fingers for excessive perspiration, abnormal color or appearance, and tremor, indicating possible underlying organic disease.

   (3) Have the examinee flex and extend the fingers making sure interphalangeal joints flex to allow the finger tips to touch the flexion creases of the palm.

   (4) With the hands pronated, observe the contour of the dorsum of the hands for atrophy of the soft tissues between the metacarpals seen in disease or malfunction of peripheral nerves.

   (5) With the fingers spread, test for strength, and interosseous muscle function by forcing the spread fingers against the resistance of the examinee.

   (6) If indicated, obtain antero-posterior and lateral x-rays of the wrist, as well as antero-posterior and oblique views of the hand.

14. <u>Spine and Other Musculoskeletal (Item 36 of DD-2808)</u>. Carefully examine for evidence of intervertebral disc syndrome, myositis, and traumatic lesions of the low back (lumbosacral and sacroiliac strains). If there is any indication of congenital deformity, arthritis, spondylolisthesis, or significant degree of curvature, obtain orthopedic consultation and x-rays.

   a. <u>Examination</u>. With the examinee stripped and standing, note the general configuration of the back, the symmetry of the shoulders, iliac crests and hips, and any abnormal curvature. Palpate the spinous processes and the erector spinae muscle masses for tenderness. Determine absence of pelvic tilt by palpating the iliac crests. Have examinee flex and extend spine and bend to each side, noting ease with which this is done and the presence or absence of pain on motion. Test rotary motion by gripping the pelvis on both sides and having the examinee twist to each side as far as possible.

    b. Reflexes. With the examinee sitting on the examining table, test patellar and ankle reflexes and fully extend the knee, note complaints of pain (this corresponds to a 90 degree straight leg raising test in supine position).

    c. Strength. With the examinee supine, test dorsiflexor muscle power of the foot and toes, with particular attention to power of the extensor hallucis longus. Weakness may indicate nerve root pressure on Sl. Flex hip fully on abdomen and knee flexed and determine presence or absence of pain on extremes of rotation of each hip with hip flexed to 90 degrees. Frequently, in lumbosacral sprains of chronic nature, pain is experienced on these motions. Place the heel on the knee of the opposite extremity and let the flexed knee fall toward the table. Pain or limitation indicates either hip joint and/or lumbosacral abnormality.

    d. Extension. While prone, have the examinee arch the back and test strength in extension by noting the degree to which this is possible.

    e. Abnormal findings. If pain is experienced on back motions in association with these maneuvers or if there is asymmetry or abnormal configuration, back x-rays, including pelvis, should be obtained. These should include antero-posterior, lateral, and oblique views.

15. Identifying Body Marks, Scars, and Tattoos (Item 37 of DD-2808).

    a. Examination. Carefully inspect the examinee's body, front and rear, on each side of the median line separately, commencing with the scalp and ending at the foot. Record under the "Notes" section on the face of the DD-2808 all body marks, tattoos, and scars useful for identification purposes. Also state if no marks or scars are found.

    b. Description of Body Marks, Scars, and Tattoos.

        (1) Indicate the size, location, and character of scars, moles, warts, birthmarks, etc.

        (2) When recording the location of a tattoo, include narrative description of the design. Tattoo transcriptions of words or initials shall be recorded in capital letters. Describe the size of a tattoo regarding its general dimensions only. A statement relative to color or pigment is not required.

        (3) Note amputations and losses of parts of fingers and toes showing the particular digit injured and the extent or level of absence.

c. <u>Abbreviations for Body Marks, Scars, and Tattoos</u>.

   (1) The following are authorized abbreviations for the descriptions or conditions indicated:

Amp.- amputation	m. - mole	w. -wart
f. -flat	p. -pitted	VSULA-
fl. -fleshy	r. -raised	vaccination scar
s. -scar smooth	l. -linear	upper left arm
v. -vaccination	o. -operative	h. -hairy

   (2) Combinations of the above abbreviations are permissible: p.s. 1/2d. - pitted scar 1/2 inch diameter, f.p.s. 1x1/2 - flat pitted scar 1 inch long and 1/2 inch wide, r.h.m. 1/4d. - raised hairy mole 1/4 inch diameter.

   (3) Do not use abbreviations when describing tattoos since they are likely to be mistaken as signifying tattooed letters.

16. <u>Neurologic (Item 39 of DD-2808)</u>. Conduct a careful neurological examination being attentive to the following:

   a. <u>Gait</u>. The individual shall: walk a straight line at a brisk pace with eyes open, stop, and turn around. Look for spastic, ataxic, incoordination, or limping gait, absence of normal associated movements, deviation to one side or the other, the presence of abnormal involuntary movement, undue difference in performance with the eyes open and closed.

      (1) Stand erect, feet together, arms extended in front. Look for unsteadiness and swaying, deviation of one or both of the arms from the assumed position, tremors, or other involuntary movements.

      (2) Touch the nose with the right and then the left index finger, with the eyes closed. Look for muscle atrophy or pseudohypertrophy, muscular weakness, limitation of joint movement, and spine stiffness.

   b. <u>Pupils</u>. Look for irregularity, inequality, diminished or absent contraction to light or lack of accommodation.

   c. <u>Deep Sense (Romberg)</u>. Negative, slightly positive, or pronouncedly positive.

   d. <u>Deep Reflexes: Patellar, Biceps, etc</u>. Record as absent (o), diminished (-), normal (+), hyperactive (++), and exaggerated (+++).

   e. <u>Sensory Disturbances</u>. Examine sensation by lightly pricking each side of the forehead, bridge of the nose, chin, across the volar surface of each wrist, and dorsum of each foot. Look for inequality of sensation right and left. If these sensations are abnormal, vibration sense should be tested at ankles and wrists with a tuning fork. With eyes closed, the examinee shall move each heel down the other leg from knee to ankle. Test sense of movement of great toes and thumb. Look for diminution or loss of vibration and plantar reflexes. When indicated, perform appropriate laboratory tests and x-ray examinations.

- f. <u>Motor Disturbances</u>. Evidence of muscle weakness, paresis, or any other abnormality.

- g. <u>Muscular Development</u>. Evidence of atrophy, compensatory hypertrophies, or any other abnormality.

- h. <u>Tremors</u>. State whether fine or coarse, intentional or resting, and name parts affected.

- i. <u>Tics</u>. Specify parts affected. State whether they are permanent or due to fatigue or nervous tension.

- j. <u>Cranial Nerves.</u> Examine carefully for evidence of impaired function or paresis. Remember that some of the cranial nerves are subject to frequent involvement in a number of important diseases, such as syphilis, meningitis, encephalitis lethargica, and injuries to the cranium.

- k. <u>Psychomotor Tension</u>. Test the ability to relax voluntarily by having the examinee rest the forearm upon your palm then test the forearm tendon reflexes with a percussion hammer.

- l. <u>Peripheral Circulation</u>. Examine for flushing, mottling, and cyanosis of face, trunk, and extremities. Question as to the presence of localized sweating (armpits and palms) and cold extremities. Carefully study any abnormalities disclosed on the neurological examination and express an opinion as to their cause and significance and whether they are sufficient cause for rejection.

17. <u>Psychiatric (Item 40 of DD-2808)</u>.

    a. <u>Personality Evaluation</u>. In order to evaluate the adequacy of the examinee's personality for adjustment to the conditions of military service:

    (1) Estimate the examinee's capacity coupled with real respect for personality and due consideration for feelings.

    (2) Conduct the examination in private to encourage open and honest answers.

    (3) Attempt to discover any difficulties that the examinee may have had with interpersonal relationships at work or during leisure activities.

    b. <u>Diagnosis of Psychiatric Disorders</u>. The diagnosis of most psychiatric disorders depends upon an adequate longitudinal history, supplemented by information obtained from other sources, such as family, physicians, schools, churches, hospitals, social service or welfare agencies, and courts.

c. Telltale Signs of Psychiatric Disorders. Be watchful for any of the following: inability to understand and execute commands promptly and adequately, lack of normal response, abnormal laughter, instability, seclusiveness, depression, shyness, suspicion, over boisterousness, timidity, personal uncleanliness, stupidity, dullness, resentfulness to discipline, a history of enuresis persisting into late childhood or adolescence, significant nail biting, sleeplessness or night terrors, lack of initiative and ambition, sleep walking, suicidal tendencies, whether bona fide or feigned. Abnormal autonomic nervous system responses (giddiness, fainting, blushing, excessive sweating, shivering or goose flesh, excessive pallor, or cyanosis of the extremities) are also occasionally significant. Note also the lack of responses as might reasonably be expected under the circumstances.

d. Procedures for Psychiatric Examination.

(1) Mental and personality difficulties are most clearly revealed when the examinee feels relatively at ease. The most successful approach is one of straightforward professional inquiry, coupled with real respect for the individual's feelings and necessary privacy. Matters of diagnostic significance are often concealed when the examinee feels the examination is being conducted in an impersonal manner or without due concern for privacy.

(2) Pay close attention to the content and implication of everything said and to any other clues, in a "matter-of-fact manner". Follow-up whatever is not self evident or commonplace.

e. Aviation only: Although this phase of the examination is routinely performed only on candidates for flight training, it may be made part of any aviation physical examination. The objective is to determine the examinee's basic stability, motivation, and capacity to react favorably to the special stresses encountered in flying. Report any significant personality change in an experienced aviator. Following the completion of the general examination:

(1) Study carefully the examinee's family history.

(2) Determine the family's attitude towards flying and the examinee's reaction to the stresses of life in general and emotional response and control.

18. Endocrine System. Evaluate endocrine abnormalities during the general clinical examination. Palpate the thyroid for abnormality and observe the individual for signs of hyperthyroidism or hypothyroidism. Observe general habitus for evidence of endocrine dysfunction.

19. Dental (Item 43 of DD-2808).

a. Who May Conduct Dental Examinations.

(1) For Academy, OCS, and direct commission applicants: a Uniformed Services Dental Officer.

(2) For all aviation, diving, and overseas/sea duty physical examinations: a Uniformed Services Dental Officer or a contract dentist.

(3) For all others: a Uniformed Services dental officer, a contract dentist, or a medical examiner if a dentist is unavailable.

b. Procedures for Conducting Dental Examinations.

(1) Applicants for Original Entry. Whenever practical, applicants for original entry into the Service shall be given a Type II dental examination. Otherwise, the Dental Officer shall determine the type of examination that is appropriate for each examinee.

(2) Active Duty Personnel. Members on active duty, who are assigned to locations where CG, USMTF, or civilian contract dental clinics are available, shall be required to have an annual Type II dental examination.

(3) Reserve Personnel.

(a) Type II dental examination is required annually for all SELRES.

1. Members who are unable to be screened by a CG or DOD Dental Clinic or who do not participate in the TRICARE Dental Plan or have private dental insurance may use a civilian dentist provided they follow HSWL SC direction.

2. HSWL SC is authorized to provide payment of SELRES dental exams obtained from civilian sources. Payment for dental cleaning and follow-up care is not authorized.

3. The results from dental exams provided by DOD or civilian dentists shall be submitted on an Active Duty Reserve Forces Dental Examination, DD Form 2813.

c. Dental Restorations and Prostheses. The minimum number of serviceable teeth prescribed for entry in various programs of the Service is predicated on having retentive units available to provide for the reception of fixed bridges or partial dentures that may be necessary for satisfactory masticatory or phonetic function. Prostheses already present should be well-designed, functional, and in good condition.

20. Laboratory Findings.

a. Required Tests. Personnel undergoing physical examinations are required to have the following tests performed, except where obtaining them is not possible or expeditious, or incurring charges for them is not authorized. In such cases, these tests shall be obtained at the first duty station where facilities are available. All Labs must be performed within 180 days of the physical exam or they will be considered out of date. The normal values listed below are for guidance. Abnormal laboratory values alone are not disqualifying; however, the causative underlying condition may be. Minimal deviations may not require further evaluation and this should be noted as NCD (not considered disqualifying) in item 74 by the examiner. Normal variants should be noted as such.

b. <u>Hematology/Serology</u>.

(1) <u>Hematology</u>. Perform a hemoglobin (HGB) or hematocrit (HCT) on all examinees. Perform other hematological studies only as indicated.

(a) Hemoglobin - Males 13-18 gm/100ml Females 11.7-16 gm/100ml.

(b) Hematocrit - Males 40-54%, Females 35-47%.

If any of these parameters are abnormal, an RBC and indices shall be done. Normal indices are:

RBC-Males	4.3 to 6.2 million
Females	3.8 to 5.4 million
MCV-	82-92 cubic microns
MCH-	27-32 picograms
MCHC -	30-36%

(2) <u>Serological Test for Syphilis (RPR/STS)</u>.

(a) Required for all aviation physicals and diving candidate physicals.

(b) Unless there is a documented history of adequately treated syphilis, all examinees testing positive shall have repeat testing three or more days later. Ensure that at the time of obtaining serum the examinee neither has, nor is convalescing from, any acute infectious disease or recent fever. If available at no charge, the facilities of local or state health departments may be used for performing serological tests. Examinees with a history of treated syphilis should have declining or low titer positive reaction.

(c) If the second test is positive then obtain an FTA/ABS. If the FTA/ABS is positive, further evaluation may be required to determine the appropriate therapy.

(d) Several conditions that are known to give false RPR/STS are infectious mononucleosis, malaria, yaws, pinta, chicken pox, infectious hepatitis, immunization, and atypical pneumonia. The cause of a false positive serological test for syphilis should be explored since many diseases giving a false positive are also disqualifying.

(e) New diagnosis of syphilis requires disease reporting per local governmental requirements and IAW Chapter 7-B-3 of this Manual.

(f) Diagnosis of syphilis requires testing for other sexually transmitted infections (gonorrhea, chlamydia, HIV and Hepatitis B).

(3) <u>Sickle Cell Preparation Test</u>. Applicants for aviation and diving training shall be tested for sickling phenomenon, if not previously tested. Evaluate positive sickledex results by a quantitative hemoglobin electrophoresis. Greater than 40 percent Hbs is disqualifying for aviation and diving. Once the test has been completed, the results will be filed in the health record and recorded on the Problem Summary List. This is a one time test that never needs to be repeated and the results shall be filed in the health record.

(4) <u>Lipid Testing</u>.

   (a) Lipid screening should be performed based upon the Clinical Preventive Services guidelines as contained in CG Periodic Health Assessment, COMDTINST 6150.3.

(5) <u>HIV Antibody</u>.

   (a) All HIV testing should be performed in accordance with the Coast Guard Human Immunodeficiency Virus (HIV) Program, COMDTINST 6230.9.

(6) <u>Tuberculosis (TB) Surveillance/Screening</u>. CG members are required to have a baseline Tuberculin skin test (TST) or Quantiferon Gold Test (QFT) per the Centers for Disease Control and Prevention (CDC) guidance. No group of CG personnel is at high risk for TB. Individuals whose duties include alien migrant interdiction, marine safety operations, and health care personnel are not at increased risk unless they work in facilities that regularly care for persons with active TB disease. Therefore, periodic screening for TB is not warranted. Members whose last recorded TST reaction was reactive shall be screened during the PHA for indicators of active disease. This involves reviewing the HR and asking the member about the following: persistent and/or productive cough (especially coughing up blood), chest pain, fever, chill, night sweats, appetite loss, and unintended weight loss. Routine evaluation of old TST reactors by chest radiograph is not authorized nor warranted. A Medical Officer may order a TST and/or chest radiograph on a patient with clinical signs/symptoms of active TB or an individual TST on a patient with risk factors listed below:

(a) Close contacts of persons known or suspected to have active TB (sharing the same household or other enclosed environments).

(b) Foreign-born persons from areas where TB is common (Asia, Africa, Latin America, Eastern Europe, Russia).

http://www.cdc.gov/tb/education/Mantoux/guide.htm.

c. Chest X-ray (Item 52 of DD-2808).

   (1) Will be accomplished as part of the physical examinations for application for aviation or diving programs. Chest X-rays previously performed within eighteen (18) months of application, with normal results, are acceptable if there is no change in clinical presentation.

   (2) Will not be performed for routine screening purposes without a prior clinical evaluation and a specific medical indication. The Senior Medical Executive may authorize an exception to this policy when there are obvious medical benefits to be gained by routine screening x-ray examination (e.g., Asbestos Medical Surveillance Program). Such exceptions should be authorized only after careful consideration of the diagnostic yield and radiation risk of the x-ray study, as well as other significant or relevant costs or social factors. X-ray examinations will not be ordered solely for medical-legal reasons.

d. Electrocardiogram (Item 52 of DD-2808).

   (1) Electrocardiograms (ECG) shall be accomplished routinely on the following individuals:

      (a) Those in whom medical history or clinical findings are suggestive of cardiac abnormalities.

      (b) Examinees with a sitting pulse rate of less than 50 or more than 100.

      (c) Applicants for aviation and diving training.

      (d) All designated aviation personnel every four (4) years until age 40, then biennially. For designated aviation personnel on physical examinations where no EKG is required, place the date and results of the last EKG in block #52 (Other) of Report of Medical Examination, DD-2808.

   (2) All student and designated aviation personnel shall have an ECG on file in their health record.

   (3) All tracings will be compared to the baseline reading in the health record, if one is present. If significant changes are present, obtain a cardiac consultation. A report of the consult shall be submitted for

review along with the DD-2808. It is imperative then that proper techniques for recording the ECG be followed.

(a) The routine ECG will consist of 12 leads, namely standard leads 1, 2, 3, AVR, AVL, AVF, and the standard precordial leads V1 through V6.

(b) Take care to properly place the precordial electrodes. It is important that the electrodes across the left precordium are not carried along the curve of the rib but are maintained in a straight line. Be particular in placing the first precordial lead so as to avoid beginning placement in the third interspace rather than the fourth. Do not smear electrode paste from one precordial position to another. Include a standardization mark on each recording.

e. Urinalysis. A urinalysis is required on all physical examinations. The urine shall be tested for specific gravity, glucose, protein, blood, leukocyte esterase, and nitrite by an appropriate dipstick method. A microscopic examination is required only if any of these dipstick tests is abnormal.

(1) Specific Gravity. Normal values are 1.005-1.035. Specific gravity varies with fluid intake, time of day, climate, and medication. As a rule, elevation of the specific gravity reflects only the state of hydration, while a low specific gravity may reflect kidney disease. In evaluating abnormalities, a repeat is generally sufficient, provided the factors above are considered and explained to the individual. Where possible, the repeat should be a first morning specimen which is usually the most concentrated.

(2) Glucose. Any positive test is abnormal. A false positive for glucose may occur in individuals who take Vitamin C or drink large quantities of fruit juice. As soon as practical after discovery of the glycosuria, obtain a fasting blood glucose. If glycosuria persists or if the fasting blood glucose exceeds 125 mg/100 ml, evaluate the individual for diabetes.

(3) Protein. A trace positive protein is often associated with a highly concentrated (specific gravity 1.024 or greater) early morning specimen and is considered normal and need not be repeated. A one plus or greater protein, or a trace positive in the presence of a dilute urine, should be evaluated by a 24-hour specimen (normal range 10-200 mg protein/24 hours).

(4) Microscopic.

(a) Normal: 0-5 WBC

  0-5 RBC (clean catch specimen)

  Occasional epithelial cells (more may be normal

in an otherwise normal urinalysis)

No casts occasional bacteria

    (b) Pyuria usually indicates an infection or improper collection techniques. Appropriate follow-up is required, including a repeat after the infection has cleared.

    (c) Hematuria may normally occur following heavy exercise or local trauma and as a false positive in menstruating females. It always requires evaluation with the minimum being a repeat showing no hematuria.

    (d) Casts, heavy bacteria, other organisms, and abnormal cells require further evaluation.

f. PAP Test (Item 52 a. of DD-2808).

  (1) A PAP test is required at the following times on female members:

    (a) On the pre-training physical examination at time of initial entry into the CG.

    (b) In accordance with the Clinical Preventive Services guidelines as contained in CG Periodic Health Assessment, COMDTINST 6150.3.

  (2) PAP tests and pelvic examinations (by civilian or military practitioners) that have been performed within one year of periodic examinations are acceptable. In any case, results of the pelvic examination and PAP test will be recorded in Item 52 a. The practitioner is responsible for communicating the result of the PAP smear (either positive or negative) to the patient.

  (3) To reduce false-negative smears, endocervical sampling shall be done using a cytobrush, provided no contraindication is present (as in pregnancy or cervical stenosis). Laboratories to which smears are sent for interpretation must, as a matter of routine, indicate on their reports whether endocervical sampling was adequate. Where endocervical cell sampling is reported as inadequate, the smear shall be repeated.

g. Pulmonary Function Test (PFT). Perform a PFT on all applicable Occupational Medical Surveillance and Evaluation Program (OMSEP) examinations and when clinically indicated.

  (1) Screening spirometry should not be performed if the subject falls into one of the following catagories:

    (a) Is acutely ill from any cause.

(b) Has smoked or used an aerosolized bronchodilator within the past hour.

(c) Has eaten a heavy meal within the previous two hours.

(d) Has experienced an upper or lower respiratory tract infection during the past three weeks.

(e) Administer the PFT by following the manufacturers' instructions.

FIGURE 3-C-1

	SPIROMETRIC GUIDELINES	
	OBSTRUCTIVE DISEASE FEV-1/FVC	RESTRICTIVE DISEASE FCV% FCV PREDICTED
NORMAL	> 0.69	> .80
MILD TO MODERATE	0.45 -0.69	0.51-0.80
SEVERE	< 0.45	<0.51

h. Special Tests. In some cases, information available should be supplemented by additional tests or diagnostic procedures (eye refractions, x-rays, repeated blood pressure readings, etc.), in order to resolve doubts as to whether the examinee is or is not physically qualified. If facilities are available to perform such tests at no cost, they should be obtained as indicated in individual cases. Otherwise, applicants for original entry in the Service will be required to obtain such tests at their own expense, if they desire further consideration.

i. Laboratory Values (OMSEP). All laboratory values not previously discussed but that accompany a physical examination (e.g., chemistry profiles, etc.,) must have accompanying normals for the laboratory that performed the tests.

j. Mammography. Breast cancer screening via mammography should be performed in accordance with the Clinical Preventive Services guidelines as continue in CG Periodic Health Assessment, COMDTINST 6150.3. Results should be documented on the routine physical exams. Mammograms done between the required screening ages can be used to satisfy the periodic requirement. This judgment is left to the practitioner. If mammography is not done at the required ages, the reason must be supplied in item 73 of the Report of Medical Examination, DD-2808 and should include date and result of the last mammogram. Practitioners are responsible for communicating mammography results (either positive or negative) to the patient.

   k. <u>Glucose-6-Phosphate Dehydrogenase (G-6-PD)</u>. Qualitative testing (present or not) for G-6-PD deficiency is required for all AD and SELRES members. The results of testing shall be annotated on the Adult Preventive and Chronic Care Flowsheet, DD-2766 as well as in MRRS. Once testing is accomplished, it need never be repeated.

21. <u>Height, Weight, and Body Build</u>.

    a. <u>Height</u>. Measure the examinee's height in both meters and to the nearest inch, without shoes.

    b. <u>Weight</u>.

        (1) Weights are with underwear/undergarments only.

        (2) Weigh the examinee on a standard set of scales calibrated and accurate. Record the weight both kilograms and pounds. Do not record fractions of pounds, such as ounces.

    c. <u>Frame Size</u>. Using a cloth tape, measure the wrist of the dominant hand, measure all the way around from lateral to medial styloid process. Measure in centimeters and inches including fraction of inches.

    d. <u>Body Fat Percentage</u>. Determined by MEPS.

22. <u>Distant Visual Acuity and Other Eye Tests</u>.

    a. <u>Distant Visual Acuity, General</u>. Visual defects are one of the major causes for physical disqualification from the armed services. Methods of testing vision have varied greatly among the armed services and from place to place in each Service. Consequently, visual test results are not always comparable. An examinee presenting for examination at one place might be qualified for visual acuity, while at another place, disqualified. Although this is an undesirable situation, no practical solution, such as prescribing standards for equipment and conditions (room size, ventilation, paint colors, room illumination, etc.), is available to the CG as the examinations are obtained from various sources over which the CG has no control. It is therefore imperative that examiners be especially painstaking to obtain the most accurate results possible.

    b. <u>Examination Precautions</u>.

        (1) Make every effort to conduct the examination when the examinee is in normal physical condition. Follow the examination routine in the order prescribed in the following instructions. Record the vision for each eye when determined so that errors and omissions will be avoided.

(2) It may be extremely difficult to obtain an accurate measure of visual acuity. Bear in mind those individuals who are anxious to pass visual acuity tests may resort to deception. Similarly, other individuals may attempt to fail a visual acuity test to avoid undesirable duties. Hence, be prepared to cope with either possibility in order to uncover and recognize visual defects without the cooperation of the person being tested.

(3) Refer uncooperative examinees to a Medical Officer.

c. Examination Procedures.

(1) In order to obtain a more valid evaluation, inform examinees that contact lenses will not be worn during the evaluation and for 72 hours before. Orthokeratotic lenses shall be removed for 14 days or until vision has stabilized for 3 successive examinations.

(2) If the examinee wears glasses, they must be removed before entering the exam room. Test each examinee without unnecessary delay after entering the examining room. In order to prevent personnel from memorizing the charts, permit only one examinee to view the test charts at a time. Ensure other examinees cannot hear the examination.

(3) Follow manufactures instructions on how to conduct a visual acuity test for the piece of equipment you are using. Visual acuity may also be determined with the Armed Forces Vision Tester (AFVT). Follow manufactures instruction on how to administer this test.

d. Score recording. Record vision test scores as a fraction in that the upper number is the distance in feet from the chart and the lower number is the value of the smallest test chart line read correctly. Thus, a person reading at a distance of 20 feet, the 30 foot test chart line is given a score of 20/30. 20/20 indicates that a person reads at a distance of 20 feet the test chart line marked 20. Similarly, 20/200 means a person can read at a distance of 20 feet only the test chart line marked 200.

e. Refraction.

(1) Eye refractions are required:

(a) When applying for flight training (SNA) (This must include cycloplegic.).

(b) When visual acuity falls below 20/20 in either eye (near or distant).

(2) Subsequent refractions are required only if the visual acuity deteriorates further.

(3) If a cycloplegic is used during the course of refraction, then the examinee must wear dark glasses until the effects disappear. The

installation of 1 drop into each eye of 1% solution of pilocarpine hydrochloride in distilled water after completing the examination will constrict the pupil and thus relieve the photophobia.

f. Near Vision. Test near vision on all examinees and record results in Item 61 of DD-2808 using Snellen notations. The examinee should be positioned so that the light source is behind him/her and the near vision test card is well illuminated. See manufacturer's instructions on how to administer the test. Record near vision both with and without corrective lenses if glasses are worn or required. Record corrections worn in Item 73. See the chart below for conversion from the various near point letter nomenclatures to Snellen notations.

CONVERSION TABLE FOR VARIOUS NEAR POINT LETTER NOMENCLATURE

Standard Test Chart	Snellen English Linear	Snellen Metric	Jaegar
14/14	20/20	0.50	J-1
14/17.5	20/25	.62	J-2
14/21	20/30	.75	J-4
14/28	20/40	1.00	J-6
14/35	20/50	1.25	J-8
14/49	20/70	1.75	J-12
14/70	20/100	2.25	J-14
14/140	20/200		

g. Heterophoria.

(1) Except for aviation personnel, special tests for heterophoria are not required unless medically indicated.

(2) Heterophoria is a condition of imperfect muscle balance in which the eyes have a constant tendency to deviate and latent deviation is overcome by muscular effort (fusion to maintain binocular single vision). Fusion is responsible for the two eyes working together in harmony and when anything prevents this, fusion is disrupted and one eye deviates. Since heterophoria is only a tendency of the eyes to deviate, no actual deviation is apparent when the eyes are being used

together under ordinary conditions. The deviation becomes visible only when fusion control is weakened or abolished. When deviation occurs, its exact amount can be estimated with some accuracy by neutralizing the deviation with prisms of varying strength. If the eye deviates toward its fellow, the deviation is known as esophoria; if it deviates away from its fellow, the deviation is known as exophoria; if it deviates up or down, the deviation is known as hyperphoria. The condition of perfect muscle balance (no deviation) is orthophoria.

    (3) The vertical and horizontal phorias may be tested with the Phoropter or AFVT.

h. Accommodation. There is no requirement to test accommodation unless medically indicated.

i. Color Perception Tests. Examinees are qualified if they pass either the Pseudoisochromatic Plates (PIP) or the Farnsworth Lantern (FALANT) test. The testing for color vision must be unaided or with standard corrective lenses only. Use of any lenses (such as Chromagen) or other device to compensate for defective color vision is prohibited. Examinees may be found qualified, "on record", if a previous certified physical examination has a passing PIP or FALANT score available for review. Exception: At the time of accession medical screening (e.g. CG Academy (including cadets and OCS candidates), Cape May recruits) the PIP color vision test will be repeated and normal color vision confirmed under controlled conditions as described below. Examinees failing the PIP will be administered the FALANT test. Examinees who fail the PIP are qualified if they pass the FALANT.

    (1) Farnsworth Lantern Test (FALANT).

        (a) Administration and Scoring.

            1 Instruct the examinee: "The lights you will see in this lantern are either, red, green, or white. They look like signal lights at a distance. Two lights are presented at a time--in any combination. Call out the colors as soon as you see them, naming first the color at the top and then the color at the bottom. Remember, only three colors--red, green, and white-- and top first".

            2 Turn the knob at the top of the lantern to change the lights; depress the button in the center of the knob to expose the lights. Maintain regular timing of about two seconds per exposure.

COMDTINST M6000.1E

        3   Expose the lights in random order, starting with RG or GR combinations (Nos. 1 or 5), continuing until each of the 9 combinations have been exposed.

        4   If no errors are made on the first run of nine pairs of lights, the examinee passes.

        5   If any errors are made on the first run, give two more complete exams with one done in the opposite direction (to prevent memorization). Passing score is at least 16 out of 18 correct for the two runs.

        6   An error is considered the miscalling of one or both of a pair of lights; if an examinee changes responses before the next light is presented, record the second response only.

        7   If an examinee uses glasses for distance, they shall be worn.

        8   If an examinee says "yellow," "pink," etc., state, "There are only 3 colors--red, green, and white".

        9   If an examinee takes a long time to respond, state, "As soon as you see the lights call them".

    (b) Operation of Lantern.

        1   Give the test in a normally lighted room, screen from glare, exclude sunlight. The examinee should face the source of room illumination.

        2   Test only one examinee at a time (do not allow others to watch).

        3   Station the examinee 8 feet from the lantern.

        4   The examinee may stand or sit, tilt the lantern so that the aperture in the face of the lantern is directed at examinee's head.

(2) <u>Pseudoisochromatic Plates (PIP)</u>. When Pseudoisochromatic Plates are used to determine color perception, a color vision test lamp with a daylight filter or a fluorescent light with a daylight tube shall be used for illumination. Do not allow the examinee to trace the patterns or otherwise touch test plates. Show the plates at a distance of 30 inches and allow 2 seconds to identify each plate. If the examinee hesitates, state "read the numbers." If the examinee fails to respond, turn to the next plate without comment. Qualification is ascertained as follows:

Chapter 3. C. Page 30

(a) 20 plate test set. Examinee must correctly read at least 17, excluding demonstration plates.

(b) 18 plate test set. Examinee must correctly read at least 14 excluding demonstration plates.

(c) 15 plate test set (one demo). Examinee must correctly read 10 plates.

j. <u>Depth Perception</u>. Depth perception may be determined by the Armed Forces Vision Tester (AFVT) or OPTEC 2300, the Random Dot Circles Test (RANDOT), or the Titmus Graded Circles Stereo Acuity Test (TITMUS). When doing a physical on the DD-2808, if you do not use the AFVT, line through the pre-printed entry and record the test used with the proper score. If you use the AFVT and then also use another depth perception test, record the AFVT in block 67 and then record the additional depth perception test findings in block 60 (other vision test) or block 73 (notes). Required for all aviation personnel and when medically indicated.

(1) If the AFVT or OPTEC 2300 is used, have the patient seated comfortably. If the patient wears a habitual spectacle prescription they may be tested without the prescription, but if they fail, retest with the prescription. Test emulates distance test (optical infinity). Refer to manual for correct settings for model being used. The following guidelines must be adhered to when testing:

(a) Group A is for demonstration purposes only and should not be used as part of the actual test (see manual).

(b) Group B is at the level of the new overall standard of 40 seconds of arc, there are three presentations of five circles each within group b. The patient identifies the circle within each presentation that appears "closest".

(c) Patient must correctly identify all presentations within group b to pass.

(d) You may test beyond group b if desired but it is not necessary. Record as "AFVT group b - pass".

(e) If patient fails any in the group, retest using RANDOT and/or Titmus below.

(2) RANDOT. If the patient wears habitual spectacle prescription they may test without the prescription, but if the patient fails, retest with the prescription. Polaroid spectacles may also be worn (over habitual prescription if requested). Test distance is 40 cm (16 inches). Provide adequate light but avoid reflections from the tests surface. Hold test upright to maintain the proper axis of polarization. Do not permit the patients head to tilt during testing. The following guidelines must be adhered to when testing:

(a) There are ten presentations of three circles each in the RANDOT, you must test all ten presentations, do not stop after number seven.

(b) You must test all presentation in order, do not jump around since each level is progressively more difficult.

(c) Patient identifies the circle that appears "closest".

(d) Test until the patient misses two levels in a row.

(e) Record the last level passed successfully.

(f) For RANDOT, a minimum passing score is correctly identifying presentations 1 through 7 which equal 40 seconds of arc.

(g) Record as the number missed over the number possible. For example, "RANDOT 3/10 pass" or "RANDOT 4/10 fail".

(h) If the patient fails the RANDOT, the patient may be retested using AFVT / OPTEC 2300 or TITMUS.

(3) TITMUS. If the patient wears habitual spectacle prescription they may test without the prescription, but if they fail, retest with the prescription. Polaroid spectacles may also be worn (over habitual prescription if requested). Test distance is 40 cm (16 inches). Provide adequate light but avoid reflections from the tests surface. Hold test upright to maintain the proper axis of polarization. Do not permit the patients head to tilt during testing. The following guidelines must be adhered to when testing:

(a) There are nine presentations of four circles each in the Titmus.

(b) You must test all nine presentations.

(c) You must test all presentations in order. Do not jump around since each level is progressively more difficult.

(d) Patient identifies the circle that appears "closest".

(e) Test until the patient misses two levels in a row (or the last presentation).

(f) Record the last level passed successfully.

(g) For Titmus, a minimum passing score is correctly identifying all of the presentation 1 through 9 which equals 40 seconds of arc.

(h) Record the number missed over the number possible. For example "Titmus 0/9 PASS" or "1/9 FAIL"

k. <u>Field of Vision</u>. Except for aviation personnel, special tests for field of vision are not required unless medically indicated. Exact procedures on how to perform this test can be obtained from the HS required references.

l. Night Vision. A test for night vision (dark adaptation) is not required unless indicated for medical or special reasons.

m. Red Lens Test. The red lens test is required on DODMERB examinations and when medically indicated. See manufactures instruction on how to perform this test.

n. Intraocular Tension.

  (1) General. Determine intraocular tension each time an eye refraction is performed, during all annual physical examinations, all aviation physicals, and when medically indicated. Above normal tension is a sign of glaucoma; below normal tension of ten exists in degenerated eyeballs or as a normal finding; alterations in tension are sometimes found in cyclitis. Questionable findings on palpation and ophthalmoscopic examination shall be further evaluated.

  (2) Testing Intraocular Tension.

    (a) General. Routine tonometry shall be performed by a Medical Officer, optometrist, or a technician who has received instruction in properly performing and interpreting this test.

    (b) Instrument. The tonometer estimates the intraocular pressure (IOP) or tension within the eyeball.

    (c) Precaution. Determine intraocular tension after all other eye examinations have been completed. Because of corneal denuding by tonometric measurement, a refraction (cycloplegic or manifest) shall not be performed for at least 24 hours following this procedure.

    (d) Readings. Intraocular pressure consistently above 21mm Hg in either eye or a difference of 4 or more between the two eyes, shall be referred for ophthalmologic evaluation.

23. Audiometer.

  a. An audiometric examination is required on all physical examinations using frequencies 500, 1000, 2000, 3000, 4000, and 6000 hertz.

  b. Obtain reference audiograms on all personnel upon initial entry into the CG at recruit training and all officer accession points (Academy, OCS, Direct Commission, etc.,), and at first duty station for all others.

24. Psychological and Psychomotor. Psychological and psychomotor testing is not required unless medically indicated.

FIGURE 3-C-2

The following chart enumerates certain conditions, defects, and items of personal history that require thorough evaluation and sets forth the special test, examination, or report desired in each instance.

ITEM:	EXAMINATION AND INFORMATION DESIRED:
ALBUMINURIA, findings of	Repeat test on a second specimen. If still positive do a quantitative 24 hr urine protein.
ASTHMA history of,	Detailed report of asthma and other allergic conditions and a statement from cognizant physician on (1) number and approximate dates of attacks of asthmatic bronchitis or other allergic manifestations; (2) signs, symptoms, and duration of each attack; (3) type and amount of bronchodilating drugs used, and history of any attacks requiring hospitalization.
BACKACHE, back injury	Current orthopedic consultation and report on or wearing of back strength, stability, mobility, and functional brace, history of capacity of back. Report of appropriate x-rays. Transcript of any treatment from cognizant physician.
BLOOD PRESSURE, elevated	Repeat blood pressure (all positions) a.m. and p.m. for 3 consecutive days. Prolonged bed rest shall not precede blood pressure determinations.
CONCUSSIONS	See Head Injury
CONVULSIONS OR SEIZURE	Neurological consultation and electroencephalogram. Transcript of any treatment from cognizant physician.
DIABETES, family history of parent, sibling, or more than one grandparent	Fasting glucose (normal diet with 10-12 but less than 16 hours fast). If elevated, repeat and include 2 hr post prandial.
DIZZINESS or FAINTING SPELLS, history of	Neurological consultation
ENURESIS or history of into late childhood or adolescence (age 12)	Comment on applicant's affirmative reply to question "bed wetting" to include number of past incidents and age at last episode.
FLATFOOT, symptomatic	Current orthopedic consultation with history. Detailed report on strength, stability, mobility, and functional capacity of foot. Report of appropriate x-rays.
GLYCOSURIA, finding or History	See Diabetes.

FIGURE 3-C-2 (cont.)

HAY FEVER, history of	Detailed report of hay fever and other allergic conditions and a statement from personal physician on (1) number, severity, and duration of attacks of hay fever or any other allergic manifestations, and (2) type and amount of drugs used in treatment thereof.
HEADACHES, frequent or severe, history of	Neurological consultation.
HEAD INJURY with loss of consciousness in past 5 years, history of	Neurological consultation; clinical abstract of treatment from physician.
HEMATURIA, history of or finding of	Medical consultation with evaluation report, including appropriate laboratory studies and/or complete urological evaluation if indicated.
HEPATITIS, history of	Serum Bilirubin, SGOT, SGPT, SGT, Anti-HCV, and HB_SAg.
JAUNDICE, history of in past 5 years	Serum Bilirubin, SGOT, SGPT, and SGT.
JOINT, KNEE, internal derangement, history of	Current orthopedic consultation and report of strength, stability, mobility, and functional capacity of knee. Report of appropriate x-rays together with comparative measurement of the thighs, knees, and legs.
JOINT, SHOULDER, dislocation, history of	Current orthopedic consultation and report on strength, stability, mobility, and functional capacity of shoulder. Report of appropriate x-rays.
MALOCCLUSION, TEETH, history of	Report of examination by a dentist with comment as to whether incisal and masticatory function is sufficient for satisfactory ingestion of the ordinary diet, statement as to presence and degree of facial deformity with jaw in natural position and clarity of speech.
MASTOIDECTOMY, bilateral, history of	Current ENT consultation to include audiogram.
MOTION SICKNESS, history of	Detailed report of all occurrences of motion sickness (such as air, train, sea, swing, carnival-ride), and the age at the time of the last occurrence.
NASAL POLYPS, history of	ENT consultation, with comment as to date polyps removed if no longer present. Detailed report by physician on allergic history and manifestation to include required medication.
SKULL FRACTURE, in past 5 years, history of	See Head Injury.
SLEEPWALKING, beyond childhood, history of (age 12)	Detailed comment by physician. Comment on applicant's affirmative reply to question "been a sleepwalker" to include number of incidents and age at last episode.

FIGURE 3-C-2 (cont.)

SQUINT (cross eyed)	Examination for degree of strabismus and presence of complete and continuous 3rd degree binocular fusion. Request completion of DD-2808 Items 62 and 65 and notation of degree of strabismus.
STUTTERING or, STAMMERING	Report of Reading Aloud Test in Section 3-C-2.
VERTEBRA, fracture or dislocation, history of	Current orthopedic consultation and report on strength, stability, mobility, and functional capacity of spine. Report of appropriate x-rays.

Figure 3-C-3

HEIGHT STANDARDS

Category	Minimum (cm/inches)	Maximum (cm/inches)
AVIATION PERSONNEL:		
Candidate for Flight Training	157.4/62	198/78
Class 1 Pilot	157.4/62	198/78
Aircrew Candidate	152.5/60	198/78
Designated Aircrew	152.5/60	198/78
ENLISTED PERSONNEL:		
Enlistment in USCG	152.5/60	198/78*
Enlistment in USCG Reserve	152.5/60	198/78*
CANDIDATES FOR:		
USCG Academy	152.5/60	198/78*
Officer Candidate School	152.5/60	198/78*
Appointment of Licensed Officers of U.S. Merchant Marines in the USCG	152.5/60	198/78*
Direct Commission in USCG	152.5/60	198/78*

- MAXIUM HEIGHTS WAIVERABLE TO 203 CM/ 80 INCHES BY COMMANDER PERSONNEL SERVICE CENTER (PSC-adm-1)

NOTES:

1. Heights are without shoes.
2. Metric conversion: 1 inch = 2.54 cm

Figure 3-C-4

MINIMUM DISTANT VISUAL ACUITY REQUIREMENTS

CATEGORY		VISION
A. Aviation Personnel:	Uncorrected	Corrected
1. Candidates for Flight Training	20/50	20/20
2. Pilot, Class	20/200	20/20
3. Pilot, Class 1R	(as waivered)	20/20
4. Flight Surgeon, Aviation Medical Examiner or Aviation Mission Specialist	20/400	20/20
5. Candidate for Aircrew	20/100	20/20
6. Designated Aircrew	20/200	20/20
7. Landing Signal Officer (LSO)	20/200	20/20
8. Air Traffic Controller Candidate	20/100	20/20
9. Designated Air Traffic Controller	20/200	20/20
B. Officers (Note 1):		
1. Commissioned or Warrant in the USCG or USCGR	20/400	20/20
2. Appt in the USCG of Licensed Officers of the Merchant Marine	20/400	20/20
3. Direct Commission in the USCGR	20/400	20/20
4. Appointment as Cadet	20/400	20/20
5. Precommissioning of Cadets	20/400	20/20
6. OCS Candidates	20/400	20/20
7. Precommissioning of Officer Candidates	20/400	20/20
8. Diving Candidates	20/100	20/20
9. Designated Diver	20/200	20/20
C. Enlisted Personnel:		
1. Enlistment in the USCG or USCGR	See 3.D.9	(Note 2)
2. Diving Candidates	(Note 3)	20/20
3. Designated Diver	(Note 3)	20/20

Notes:

1. Refractive error does not exceed plus or minus 8.0 diopters spherical equivalent (sphere + 1/2 cylinder) and that astigmatism does not exceed 3.00 diopters and anisometropia does not exceed 3.50 diopters.

2. Corrected vision shall be 20/40 in the better eye and 20/70 in the other or 20/30 in the better eye and 20/100 in the other, or 20/20 in the better and 20/400 in the other. (Note that near visual acuity must correct to at least 20/40 in the better eye.) Refractive error does not exceed plus or minus 8.00 diopters spherical equivalent (sphere + 1/2 cylinder) and ordinary spectacles do not cause discomfort by reason of ghost images, prismatic displacement, etc.; error must not have been corrected by orthokeratology or keratorefractive surgery.

3. 20/100 in the better eye and 20/200 in the worse eye.

COMDTINST M6000.1E

Section D. Medical Standards for Appointment, Enlistment and Induction in the Armed Forces

1. Scope...1
2. Medical Standards...1
3. Policy..2
4. Responsibilities of Commandant (CG-11)..2
5. Height..3
6. Weight...3
7. Head...3
8. Eyes..3
9. Vision...7
10. Ears..8
11. Hearing..8
12. Nose, Sinuses, Mouth and Larynx...9
13. Dental...10
14. Neck...11
15. Lungs, Chest Wall, Pleura, and Mediastinum..11
16. Heart...13
17. Abdominal Organs and Gastrointestinal System.......................................16
18. Female Genitalia..19
19. Male Genitalia...20
20. Urinary System..21
21. Spine and Sacroiliac Joints..22
22. Upper Extremities..23
23. Lower Extremities...25
24. Miscellaneous Conditions of the Extremities..27
25. Vascular System..28
26. Skin and Cellular Tissues..29
27. Blood and Blood-Forming Tissues..31
28. Systemic..31
29. Endocrine and Metabolic..34
30. Neurologic...35
31. Learning, Psychiatric, and Behavioral..37
32. Tumors and Malignancies...40
33. Miscellaneous..40
Figure 3-D-1 Evaluation for Risk of Head Injury Sequelae..............................42
Figure 3-D-2 Classification & Comparative Nomenclature of Cervical Smears...........43

This page intentionally left blank.

COMDTINST M6000.1E

D. **Medical Standards for Appointment, Enlistment and Induction in the Armed Forces.**

1. **Scope.** This section applies to the Office of the Secretary of Defense, the Military Departments (including the CG at all times, including when it is a service in the Department of Homeland Security by agreement with that Department), the United States Merchant Marine Academy by agreement with the Secretary of Commerce, the Office of the Chairman of the Joint Chiefs of Staff and the Joint Staff, the Combatant Commands, the Office of the Inspector General of the Department of Defense, the Defense Agencies, the DoD Field Activities, and all other organizational entities in the DoD (hereinafter referred to collectively as the "DOD Components"). The term "Armed Forces," as used herein, refers to the Army, Navy, Air Force, Marine Corps, and the CG.

2. **Medical Standards.** This section establishes medical standards, which if not met, are grounds for rejection for military service. Other standards may be prescribed for a mobilization for a national emergency. The medical standards in this section apply to the following personnel:

    a. **Applicants for appointment as commissioned or warrant officers in the active and reserve components.**

    b. **Applicants for enlistment in the Armed Forces.** For medical conditions or defects predating original enlistment, these standards apply to enlistees' first six (6) months of active duty.

    c. **During training.** Applicants for enlistment in the Reserve and federally recognized units or organizations of the National Guard. For medical conditions or defects predating original enlistment, these standards apply during the enlistees' initial period of active duty for training until their return to Reserve or National Guard units.

    d. **After 12 months.** Applicants for reenlistment in Regular and Reserve components and in federally recognized units or organizations of the National Guard when after a period of more than twelve (12) months have elapsed since discharge.

    e. **Schools.** Applicants for the Scholarship or Advanced Course Reserve Officers Training Corps (ROTC), and all other Armed Forces' special officer personnel procurement programs.

    f. **Retention of cadets and midshipmen at the U.S. Service Academies and students enrolled in ROTC scholarship programs.**

    g. **Individuals on the Temporary Disability Retired List (TDRL).** Individuals on the TDRL who have been found fit on reevaluation and wish to return to active duty. The prior disabling condition(s) and any other medical conditions identified before placement on the TDRL, that shall not have prevented reenlistment, are exempt from this Instruction.

  h. All individuals being inducted into the Armed Forces.

3. Policy.

   a. International Classification of Disease (ICD) codes. It is CG policy, by agreement with DoD Directive 6130 (series) Physical Standard for Appointment, to utilize the ICD codes in this Section, in all records pertaining to a medical condition that results in a personnel action, such as separation or medical waiver. In addition, when a medical condition standard is waived or results in a separation, written clarification of the personnel action should be provided using standard medical terminology.

   b. Standards. The standards in this section shall be for the acquisition of personnel in the programs in 3.D.2 of this Manual.

   c. Disqualifying standards. Unless otherwise stipulated, the conditions listed in this section are those that would be disqualifying by virtue of current diagnosis, or for which the candidate has a verified past medical history. The medical standards for appointment, enlistment or induction into the Armed Forces are classified by the following general systems.

4. Responsibilities of Commandant (CG-11).

   a. Review CG policies. Review CG policies to conform with the standards contained in DoD Directive 6130 (series) Physical Standard for appointment.

   b. Recommend changes. Recommend to the Office of the Assistant Secretary of Defense (Health Affairs) [OASD (HA)] suggested changes in the standards after service coordination has been accomplished.

   c. Review all the standards on a quinquennial basis. Review all the standards on a quinquennial basis and recommend changes to the OASD (HA). This review will be initiated and coordinated by the DoD Medical Examination Review Board.

   d. Implement standards. Ensure that implementation of the standards in this section are accomplished throughout the U.S. Military Entrance Processing Command.

   e. Direct clinics. Under the provisions of DoD Directive 6130 (series), Medical Standards for Appointment, Enlisted or Induction, direct the clinics to apply and uniformly implement the standards contained in this section.

   f. Authorize waivers. Commandant (CG-11) delegates to CG PSC and the CG Recruiting Command the authority to implement waiver procedures that ensures the uniform application of appointment, enlistment, induction and retention standards.

  g. <u>Authorize changes in visual standards</u>. Authorize the changes in Service-specific visual standards (particularly for officer accession programs) and establish other standards for special programs. Notification of any proposed changes in standards shall be provided to the ASD (HA) at least 60 days before implementation.

  h. <u>Ensure that accurate ICD codes are assigned</u>. Ensure that accurate ICD codes are assigned to all medical conditions resulting in a personnel action, such as separation, waiver, or assignment limitation, and that such codes are included in all records of such actions.

  i. <u>Eliminate inconsistencies and inequities based on race, sex, or examination location in the application of these standards by the Armed Forces</u>.

5. <u>Height</u>. The causes for rejection for appointment, enlistment, and induction in relation to height standards are established by each of the military services. Height standards for the CG are:

  a. <u>Men</u>: Height below 152.5 cm (60 inches) or over 198 cm (78 inches).

  b. <u>Women</u>: Height below 152.5 cm (60 inches) or over 198 cm (78 inches).

6. <u>Weight</u>. The causes for rejection for appointment, enlistment, and induction in relation to weight standards are contained in Weight /Physical Fitness Standards for CG Military Personnel, COMDTINST M1020.8 (series).

7. <u>Head</u>.

  a. <u>Deformities</u>. Deformities of the skull, face, or mandible (754.0) of a degree that shall prevent the individual from the proper wearing of a protective mask or military headgear are disqualifying.

  b. <u>Bone loss</u>. Loss, or absence of the bony substance of the skull (756.0 or 738.1) not successfully corrected by reconstructive materials, or leaving residual defect in excess of one (1) square inch (6.45cm2), or the size of a 25-cent piece is disqualifying.

8. <u>Eyes</u>.

  a. <u>Lids</u>.

   (1) Current Blepharitis (373.0), chronic or acute, until cured (373.00) is disqualifying.

   (2) Current Blepharospasm (333.81) is disqualifying.

(3) Current Dacryocystitis, acute (375.32), chronic (375.42), or unspecified (375.30) is disqualifying.

(4) Deformity of the lids or other disorders affecting eyelid function (374.4), complete or extensive lid deformity, or significant ptosis, sufficient to interfere with vision or impair protection of the eye from exposure is disqualifying.

(5) Current growths or tumors of the eyelid, other than small, non-progressive, asymptomatic, benign lesions, are disqualifying.

b. Conjunctiva.

(1) Current chronic conjunctivitis (372.1), including but not limited to trachoma (076) and chronic allergic conjunctivitis (372.14), is disqualifying.

(2) Current or recurrent Pterygium (372.4) if condition encroaches on the cornea in excess of three (3) millimeters, interferes with vision, is a progressive peripheral Pterygium (372.42), or is a recurring Pterygium after two (2) operative procedures (372.45) is disqualifying.

(3) Current Xerophthalmia (372.53) or other manifestations of Vitamin A deficiency xerophthalmia (264.7) is disqualifying.

c. Cornea.

(1) Current or history of corneal dystrophy or degeneration of any type (371.5), including but not limited to keratoconus (371.6) of any degree, is disqualifying.

(2) History of refractive surgery, including but not limited to: Lamellar (P11.7) and/or penetrating keratoplasty (P11.6), Radial Keratotomy, and Astigmatic Keratotomy is disqualifying. Refractive surgery performed with an Excimer Laser, including but not limited to, Photorefractive Keratectomy (commonly known as PRK), Laser Epithelial Keratomileusis (commonly known as LASEK), and laser-assisted in situ Keratomileusis (commonly known as LASIK) (ICD-9 code for each is P11.7) is disqualifying if any of the following conditions are met:

(a) Pre-surgical refractive error in either eye exceeded a spherical equivalent of +8.00 to -8.00 diopters.

(b) For initial LASIK, at least 90 days recovery period has not occurred between last refractive surgery or augmenting procedure and accession medical examination. For all other laser refractive corneal surgery, at least 180 days recovery period has not occurred between last refractive or augmenting procedure and accession medical examination.

(c) There have been complications and/or medications or ophthalmic solutions, or any other therapeutic interventions such as sunglasses, are required.

(d) Post-surgical refraction in each eye is not stable as demonstrated by at least two (2) separate refractions at least one (1) month apart, with one refraction at least 90 days post-procedure, and the most recent of which demonstrates more than +/- 0.50 diopters difference for spherical vision and/or more than +/- 0.50 diopters for cylinder vision.

(3) Current keratitis (370), acute or chronic, including but not limited to recurrent corneal ulcers (370.0), erosions (abrasions), or herpetic ulcers (054.42) is disqualifying.

(4) Current corneal neovascularization, unspecified (370.60), or corneal opacification (371) from any cause that is progressive or reduces vision below the prescribed visual acuity standards is disqualifying.

(5) Current or history of Uveitis or Iridocyclitis (364.3) is disqualifying.

(6) Implantable Contact Lenses (ICL) may be considered for an accession waiver into the CG as long as the following conditions are met: (This does not apply to aviation personnel)

(a) Accession vision standards are met.

(b) Six (6) months has elapsed since the procedure was performed.

d. Retina.

(1) Current or history of retinal conditions that impair visual function or are progressive, including retinal defects and dystrophies, Angiomatoses (759.6), retinoschisis and retinal cysts (361.1), phakomas (362.89), and other congenito-retinal hereditary conditions (362.7).

(2) Current or history of any chorioretinal or retinal inflammatory conditions, including but not limited to conditions leading to neovascularization, chorioretinitis, histoplasmosis, toxoplasmosis, or vascular conditions of the eye, to include Coat's Disease or Eales Disease.

(3) Current or history of degenerative changes of any part of the retina (362.60) is disqualifying.

(4) Current or history of detachment of the retina (361), history of surgery for same, or peripheral retinal injury, defect (361.3), or degeneration that may cause retinal detachment is disqualifying.

e. Optic Nerve.

(1) Current or history of optic neuritis (377.3), including but not limited to Neuroretinitis, secondary optic atrophy, or documented history of retrobulbar neuritis is disqualifying.

(2) Current or history of optic atrophy (377.1) or cortical blindness (377.75) is disqualifying.

(3) Current or history of Papilledema (377.0) is disqualifying.

f. <u>Lens</u>.

(1) Current Aphakia (379.31), history of lens implant, or current or history of dislocation of a lens is disqualifying.

(2) Current or history of opacities of the lens (366), including cataract (366.9), are disqualifying.

g. <u>Ocular Mobility and Motility</u>.

(1) Current or recurrent Diplopia (368.2) is disqualifying.

(2) Current nystagmus (379.50) other than physiologic "end-point nystagmus" is disqualifying.

(3) Esotropia (378.0), exotropia (378.10), and hypertropia (378.31): For entrance into Service academies and officer programs, the individual Military Services may set additional requirements. The Military Services shall determine special administrative criteria for assignment to certain specialties.

h. <u>Miscellaneous Defects and Diseases</u>.

(1) Current or history of abnormal visual fields due to diseases of the eye or central nervous system (368.4), or trauma (368.9) is disqualifying.

(2) Absence of an eye, clinical anophthalmos, unspecified congenital (743.00) or acquired, current, or history of other disorders of globe (360.8) is disqualifying.

(3) Current asthenopia (368.13) is disqualifying.

(4) Current unilateral or bilateral non-familial exophthalmoses (376) are disqualifying.

(5) Current or history of glaucoma (365), including but not limited to pre-glaucoma (365.0 -365.04) as evidenced by

intraocular pressure above 21 millimeters of mercury (mmHg) on two (2) or more determinations using applanation tonometry, or changes in the optic disc, or visual field loss associated with glaucoma is disqualifying.

    (6) Current loss of normal pupillary reflex, reactions to accommodation (367.5) or light (379.4), including Adie's Syndrome is disqualifying.

    (7) Current night blindness (368.60) is disqualifying.

    (8) Current or history of intraocular foreign body (360) is disqualifying.

    (9) Current or history of ocular tumors (190) is disqualifying.

    (10) Current or history of any organic disease of the eye (360) or adnexa (376, 379.9), not specified in paragraph E1.2.1. through subparagraph E1.2.9.8. above, which threatens vision or visual function is disqualifying.

9. <u>Vision</u>. The Secretaries of the Military Departments shall, under the provisions of DoD Directive 6130 (series), Medical Standards for Appointment, Enlistment, or Induction in the Armed Forces have authority to change Service-specific vision standards and establish other standards for special programs.

    a. <u>Distant visual acuity</u>. Current distant visual acuity of any degree that does not correct to at least one of the following (367) is disqualifying.

        (1) 20/40 in one eye and 20/70 in the other eye.

        (2) 20/30 in one eye and 20/100 in the other eye.

        (3) 20/20 in one eye and 20/400 in the other eye.

    b. <u>Near visual acuity</u>. Current near visual acuity of any degree that does not correct to 20/40 in the better eye (367) is disqualifying.

    c. <u>Refractive error</u>. Current refractive error [hyperopia (367.0), myopia (367.1), astigmatism (367.2)] or history of refractive error prior to any refractive surgery manifest by any refractive error in spherical equivalent of worse than -8.00 or +8.00 diopters is disqualifying. Waivers may be considered on a case by case basis for non-aviation new accessions who have up to -10.00 diopters of myopia if the following conditions are met: a) the potential accession has had a retinal evaluation performed by an ophthalmologist in the twelve months prior to requesting the waiver; b) the retinal evaluation yields normal results and there is no evidence of ocular pathology including but not limited to retinal detachments, retinal tears or lattice degeneration and; c) there is no history of prior ocular pathology or retinal surgery. This waiver consideration should also be applied to potential accessions who otherwise meet accession post-refractive surgery criteria as outlined in chapter 3-D.8.c(2) of ref (a).

    d. <u>Cases requiring contact lenses</u>. Current complicated cases requiring contact lenses for adequate correction of vision, such as corneal scars and opacities (370.00) and irregular astigmatism (367.22) are disqualifying.

    e. <u>Color vision (368.5)</u>. Failure to pass a color vision test is not an automatic disqualification. For entrance into U.S. Service Academies, ROTC, and special programs, color vision requirements may be set by the individual Services.

10. <u>Ears</u>.

    a. <u>External ear</u>. Current atresia of the external ear (744.02) or severe microtia (744.23), congenital or acquired stenosis (380.5), chronic otitis externa (380.2), or severe external ear deformity (744.3) that prevents or interferes with the proper wearing of hearing protection is disqualifying.

    b. <u>Mastoiditis</u>. Current or history of mastoiditis (383.9), residual with fistula (383.81), chronic drainage or conditions requiring frequent cleaning of the mastoid bone is disqualifying.

    c. <u>Ménière's Syndrome</u>. Current or history of Ménière's Syndrome or other chronic diseases of the vestibular system (386) are disqualifying.

    d. <u>Inner ear</u>. Current or history of chronic otitis media (382) beyond the thirteenth (13th) birthday, cholesteatoma (385.3), or history of any inner (P20) or middle (P 19) ear surgery (including cochlear implantation) is disqualifying. Myringotomy or successful tympanoplasty is NOT disqualifying.

    e. <u>Perforation of the tympanic membrane</u>. Current perforation of the tympanic membrane (384.2) or history of surgery to correct perforation during the preceding 120 days (P 19) is disqualifying.

11. <u>Hearing</u>. All hearing defects are coded with ICD-9 code 389.

    a. <u>Audiometric Hearing Levels</u>.

        (1) Audiometric hearing levels are measured by audiometers calibrated to the standards in American National Standards Institute (ANSI S3.6-2004) and shall be used to test the hearing of all applicants.

        (2) Current hearing threshold level in either ear greater than that described below is disqualifying:

            (a) Pure tone at 500, 1000, and 2000 cycles per second for each ear of not more than 30 decibels (dB) on the average with no individual level greater than 35 dB at those frequencies.

(b) Pure tone level not more than 45 dB at 3000 cycles per second or 55 dB at 4000 cycles per second for each ear.

(c) There is no standard for 6000 cycles per second.

b. Current or history of hearing aid use (V53.2) is disqualifying.

12. <u>Nose, Sinuses, Mouth and Larynx</u>.

   a. <u>Rhinitis</u>.

   (1) Current allergic rhinitis due to pollen (477.0), other allergen (477.8), or cause unspecified (477.9), if not controlled by oral medication or topical corticosteroid medication is disqualifying. History of allergic rhinitis immunotherapy within the previous year is disqualifying.

   (2) Current chronic non-allergic rhinitis (472.0) if not controlled by oral medication or topical corticosteroid medication is disqualifying.

   b. <u>Cleft lip or palate</u>. Current cleft lip or palate defects (749) not satisfactorily repaired by surgery **or** that interferes with the use of wear of military equipment, or that prevents drinking from a straw is disqualifying.

   c. <u>Leukoplakia</u>. Current leukoplakia of oral mucosa, including tongue (528.6) is disqualifying.

   d. <u>Chronic conditions of larynx</u>. Current chronic conditions of larynx including vocal cord paralysis (478.3), chronic hoarseness (784.49), chronic laryngitis (476.0), larynx ulceration (478.79), polyps (478.4), granulation tissue (478.5), or other symptomatic disease of larynx or vocal cord dysfunction not elsewhere classified (478.7) are disqualifying.

   e. <u>Anosmia or parosmia</u>. Current anosmia or parosmia (781.1) is disqualifying.

   f. <u>Epistaxis</u>. History of recurrent epistaxis with more than one episode per week of bright red blood from the nose occurring over a three (3) month period (784.7) is disqualifying.

   g. <u>Nasal polyp or history of nasal polyps</u>. Current nasal polyp or history of nasal polyps (471), unless more than twelve (12) months have elapsed since nasal polypectomy and asymptomatic is disqualifying.

h. Perforation of nasal septum. Current perforation of nasal septum (478.1) is disqualifying.

i. Chronic sinusitis. Current chronic sinusitis (473) or current acute sinusitis (461.9) is disqualifying. Such conditions exist when evidenced by chronic purulent discharge, hyperplastic changes of nasal tissue, symptoms requiring frequent medical attention, or X-ray findings.

j. Trachea. Current or history of tracheostomy (V44.0) or tracheal fistula (530.84) is disqualifying.

k. Anomalies of upper alimentary tract. Current or history of deformities, or conditions or anomalies of upper alimentary tract (750.9), of the mouth, tongue, palate, throat, pharynx, larynx, and nose that interfere with chewing, swallowing, speech, or breathing is disqualifying.

l. Pharyngitis. Current chronic pharyngitis (472.1) and chronic nasopharyngitis (472.2) are disqualifying.

13. Dental.

a. Diseases of the jaw. Current diseases or pathology of the jaws or associated tissues that prevent normal functioning are disqualifying. Those diseases or conditions include but are not limited to temporomandibular disorders (524.6) and/or myofascial pain. A minimum of six (6) months healing time must elapse for any individual completing surgical treatment of any maxillofacial pathology lesions.

b. Severe malocclusion. Current severe malocclusion (524), which interferes with normal mastication or requires early and protracted treatment, or a relationship between the mandible and maxilla that prevents satisfactory future prosthodontic replacement is disqualifying.

c. Insufficient natural healthy teeth. Current insufficient natural healthy teeth, six (6) or more grossly (visually) cavitated and/or carious teeth (521.0) is disqualifying. Lack of a serviceable prosthesis that prevents adequate incision and mastication of a normal diet is disqualifying. Applicants with multiple complex dental fixtures and/or implant plant systems with associated complications are disqualifying. Individuals undergoing endodontic care are acceptable for entry in the Delayed Entry Program (DEP) only if a civilian or military dentist or endodontist provides documentation that active endodontic treatment shall be completed prior to being sworn into active duty.

d. Current orthodontic appliances. Current orthodontic appliances for continued treatment (V53.4) are disqualifying. Permanent or removable retainer appliances are permissible, provided all active orthodontic treatment has been satisfactorily completed. Individuals undergoing active orthodontic care are acceptable for accession (including DEP) only if a civilian or military orthodontist provides documentation that active orthodontic treatment shall be completed prior to being sworn into active duty. Entrance into active duty will not occur until all orthodontic treatment is documented to be completed.

14. Neck.

    a. Current symptomatic cervical ribs (756.2) are disqualifying.

    b. History of congenital cyst(s). Current or history of congenital cyst(s) (744.4) of branchial cleft origin or those developing from the remnants of the thyroglossal duct, with or without fistulous tracts, is disqualifying.

    c. Contraction of the neck muscles. Current contraction (723) of the muscles of the neck, spastic or non-spastic, or cicatricial contracture of the neck to the extent it interferes with the proper wearing of a uniform or military equipment, or is so disfiguring as to interfere with or prevent satisfactory performance of military duty is disqualifying.

15. Lungs, Chest Wall, Pleura, and Mediastinum.

    a. Elevation of the diaphragm. Current abnormal elevation of the diaphragm (either side) is disqualifying. Any nonspecific abnormal findings on radiological and other examination of body structure, such as lung field (793.1) or other thoracic or abdominal organ (793.2) is disqualifying.

    b. Current abscess of the lung or mediastinum (513) are disqualifying.

    c. Acute infection of the lungs. Current or history of recurrent acute infectious processes of the lung, including but not limited to viral pneumonia (480), pneumococcal pneumonia (481), bacterial pneumonia (482), pneumonia due to other specified organism (483), pneumonia infectious disease classified elsewhere (484), bronchopneumonia (organism unspecified) (485), pneumonia (organism unspecified) (486), are disqualifying.

    d. Asthma. Airway hyper responsiveness including asthma (493), reactive airway disease, exercise-induced bronchospasm or asthmatic bronchitis, reliably diagnosed and symptomatic after the 13th birthday is disqualifying.

        (1) Reliable diagnostic criteria may include any of the following elements: Substantiated history of cough, wheeze, chest tightness and/or dyspnea

which persists or recurs over a prolonged period of time, generally more than twelve (12) months.

> (2) Individuals meet the standard if within the past three (3) years there is or are:
>
> (a) No use of controller or rescue medications, including but not limited to inhaled corticosteroids, leukotriene receptor antagonists, or short-acting beta agonists.
>
> (b) No exacerbations requiring acute medical treatment.
>
> (c) No use of oral steroids, and a current normal spirometry (within the past ninety (90) days) performed in accordance with American Thoracic Society (ATS) guidelines and as defined by current National Heart, Lung, and Blood Institute (NHLBI) standards.

e. Current bronchitis (490), acute or chronic symptoms over three (3) months occurring at least twice a year (491) is disqualifying.

f. Current or history of bronchiectasis (494) is disqualifying. Bronchiectasis during the first year of life is not disqualifying if there are no residual or sequelae.

g. Current or history of bronchopleural fistula (510), unless resolved with no sequelae is disqualifying.

h. Current or history of Chronic Obstructive Pulmonary Disease (491), or bullous or generalized pulmonary emphysema (492) is disqualifying.

i. Current chest wall malformation (754.89), including but not limited to pectus excavatum (754.81) or pectus carinatum (754.82), if these conditions interfere with vigorous physical exertion is disqualifying.

j. History of emphysema (510.9) is disqualifying.

k. Pulmonary fibrosis (515) is disqualifying.

l. Current foreign body in lung (934.8, 934.9), trachea (934.0), or bronchus (934.1) is disqualifying.

m. History of thoracic surgery (P 32-33), including open and endoscopic procedures is disqualifying.

n. Current or history of pleurisy with effusion (511.9) within the previous two (2) years is disqualifying.

o. Current or history of pneumothorax (512) occurring during the year preceding examination if due to trauma (860) or surgery, or occurring during the two (2) years preceding examination from spontaneous (512.8) origin is disqualifying.

p. Recurrent spontaneous pneumothorax (512.8) is disqualifying.

q. History of chest wall surgery (34-34.9), including breast (85-85.9), during the preceding six (6) months, or with persistent functional limitations is disqualifying.

16. <u>Heart</u>.

    a. <u>Valvular heart diseases</u>. History of valvular repair or replacement is disqualifying.

    (1) Current or history of the following valvular conditions as defined by the current American College of Cardiology and American Heart Association guidelines does not meet the standard:

    (a) Severe pulmonic regurgitation.

    (b) Severe tricuspid regurgitation.

    (c) Moderate pulmonic regurgitation unless documented mean pulmonary artery pressure <25mm Hg.

    (d) Moderate tricuspid regurgitation unless documented mean pulmonary artery pressure <25mm Hg.

    (e) Moderate or severe mitral regurgitation.

    (f) Mild, moderate or severe aortic regurgitation.

    (2) The following are considered normal variants that meet the standards:

    (a) Trace or mild pulmonic regurgitation.

    (b) Trace or mild tricuspid regurgitation.

    (c) Trace or mild mitral regurgitation in the absence of mitral valve prolapse.

    (d) Trace Aortic insufficiency.

    b. Mitral valve prolapse with normal exercise tolerance not requiring medical therapy meets the standard.

c. Bicuspid aortic valve (746.4), in the absence of stenosis or regurgitation as in 16.a.(1) above, meets the standard.

d. All valvular stenosis.

e. Current or history of atherosclerotic coronary heart disease (410).

f. Current history of pacemaker or defibrillator implantation.

g. History of supraventricular tachycardia.

(1) Supraventricular tachycardia (427.0) associated with an identifiable reversible cause and no recurrence during the preceding two (2) years while off all medications meets the standard.

(2) Those with identified atrioventricular nodal reentrant tachycardia (AVNRT) or atrioventricular reentrant tachycardia (AVRT) Wolff-Parkinson-White syndrome (WPW) who have undergone successful ablative therapy with no recurrence of symptoms after three (3) months and with documentation of normal electrocardiograph (ECG) meet the standard.

(3) History of recurrent atrial fibrillation or flutter.

h. Premature atrial or ventricular contractions sufficiently symptomatic to require treatment, or result in physical or physiological impairment.

i. Abnormal ECG patterns:

(1) Long QT.

(2) Brugada pattern.

(3) WPW pattern does not meet the standard unless associated with low risk accessory pathway by appropriate diagnostic testing.

j. Current or history of ventricular arrhythmias (427.1) including ventricular fibrillation, tachycardia, or multifocal premature ventricular contractions. Occasional asymptomatic unifocal premature ventricular contractions meet the standard.

k. Current or history of conduction disorders, including but not limited to disorders of sinus arrest, asystole, Mobitz type II second-degree atrioventricular (AV) block (426.12), and third-degree AV block (426.0).

l. In the absence of cardiovascular symptoms the following meet the standard:

   (1) Sinus arrhythmia.

   (2) First degree AV block.

   (3) Left axis deviation of < -45 degrees.

   (4) Early repolarization.

   (5) Incomplete right bundle branch block.

   (6) Wandering atrial pacemaker or ectopic atrial rhythm.

   (7) Sinus bradycardia.

   (8) Mobitz type I second-degree AV block (426.13)

m. Current or history of conduction disturbances such as left anterior hemiblock (426.2), right or left bundle branch block (426.4) do not meet the standard unless asymptomatic with a normal echocardiogram.

n. Current or history of cardiomyopathy (425), cardiomegaly, hypertrophy (defined as septal wall thickness of 15mm or greater), dilation (429.3) or congestive heart failure (428).

o. History of myocarditis (422) or pericarditis (420) does not meet the standard unless the individual is free of all cardiac symptoms, does not require medical therapy, and has normal echocardiography for at least one year.

p. Current persistent tachycardia (785.0) (as evidenced by average heart rate of 100 beats per minute or greater over a 24 hour period of continuous monitoring).

q. Current or history of congenital anomalies of heart and great vessels (746). The following conditions meet the standard with an otherwise normal current (within 6 months) echocardiogram.

   (1) Dextrocardia with Situs inversus without any other anomalies.

   (2) Ligated or occluded patent ductus arteriosus.

   (3) Corrected atrial septal defect/patent foramen ovale without residual.

(4) Corrected ventricular septal defect without residual.

r. History of recurrent syncope and/or presyncope (780.2), to include black out, fainting, loss of alteration of level of consciousness (excludes vasovagal reactions with identified trigger such as venipuncture) does not meet standard unless there has been no recurrence during the preceding two (2) years while off all medications.

17. Abdominal Organs and Gastrointestinal System.

    a. Esophageal Disease.
        (1) Current or history of esophageal disease (530.0-530.9), including but not limited to ulceration, varices, fistula, achalasia is disqualifying.
        (2) Gastro-Esophageal Reflux Disease (GERD) (530.81), with complications including stricture, or maintenance on acid suppression medication, other dysmotility disorders; or chronic or recurrent esophagitis (530.1), is disqualifying.
        (3) Current or history of reactive airway disease associated with GERD (530.81) is disqualifying.
        (4) History of surgical correction for GERD within six (6) months (P42 esophageal correction, P43 stomach correction, and P45 intestinal correction.) is disqualifying.
        (5) Current or history of dysmotility disorders and chronic or recurrent esophagitis (530) is disqualifying.

(Waivers will not be granted for surgeries performed to control weight including all forms of bariatric surgery)

    b. Stomach and Duodenum.

        (1) Current gastritis, chronic or severe (535), or non-ulcerative dyspepsia that requires maintenance medication is disqualifying.

        (2) Current or history of ulcer of stomach or duodenum confirmed by X-ray or endoscopy (533) is disqualifying.

        (3) History of surgery for peptic ulceration or perforation (533.0-599.9) is disqualifying.

c. Small and Large Intestine.

   (1) Current or history of inflammatory bowel disease, including but not limited to unspecified (558.9), regional enteritis or Crohn's disease (555), ulcerative colitis (556), or ulcerative proctitis (556.2), is disqualifying.

   (2) Current or history of intestinal malabsorption syndromes, including but not limited to post-surgical and idiopathic (579), is disqualifying. Lactase deficiency is disqualifying only if of sufficient severity to require frequent intervention, or to interfere with normal function.

   (3) Current or history of gastrointestinal functional and motility disorders within the past two (2) years, including but not limited to pseudo-obstruction, megacolon, history of volvulus, or chronic constipation and/or diarrhea (787.91), regardless of cause, persisting or symptomatic in the past two (2) years, is disqualifying.

   (4) History of gastrointestinal bleeding (578), including positive occult blood (792.1), if the cause has not been corrected is disqualifying. Meckel's diverticulum (751.0), if surgically corrected greater than six (6) months prior is not disqualifying.

   (5) Current or history of irritable bowel syndrome (564.1) of sufficient severity to require frequent intervention or to interfere with normal function is disqualifying.

   (6) History of bowel resection is disqualifying.

   (7) Current or history of symptomatic diverticular disease of the intestine (562) is disqualifying.

d. Hepatic-Biliary Tract.

   (1) Current acute or chronic hepatitis, hepatitis carrier state (070), hepatitis in the preceding six (6) months or persistence of symptoms after six (6) months, or objective evidence of impairment of liver function is disqualifying.

   (2) Current or history of cirrhosis (571), hepatic cysts (573.8), abscess (572.0), or sequelae of chronic liver disease (571.3) is disqualifying.

   (3) Current or history of symptomatic cholecystitis, unless successfully surgically corrected, acute or chronic, with or without cholelithiasis (574); postcholecystectomy syndrome; or other disorders of the gallbladder and biliary system (576) is disqualifying. Cholecystectomy is not disqualifying if performed greater than six (6) months prior to examination and patient remains asymptomatic. Fiberoptic procedure to correct sphincter dysfunction or cholelithiasis, if performed greater than six (6)

months prior to examination and patient remains asymptomatic may not be disqualifying.

(4) Current or history of pancreatitis, acute (577.0) or chronic (577.1) is disqualifying.

(5) Current or history of metabolic liver disease, including but not limited to hemochromatosis (275.0), Wilson's disease (275.1), or alpha-1 anti-trypsin deficiency (273.4) is disqualifying.

(6) Current enlargement of the liver from any cause (789.1) is disqualifying.

e. <u>Anorectal</u>.

(1) Current anal fissure or anal fistula (565) is disqualifying.

(2) Current or history of anal or rectal polyp (569.0), prolapse (569.1), stricture (569.2), or fecal incontinence (787.6) within the last two (2) years is disqualifying.

(3) Current hemorrhoid (internal or external), when large, symptomatic, or with a history of bleeding (455) within the last sixty (60) days, is disqualifying.

f. <u>Spleen</u>.

(1) Current splenomegaly (789.2) is disqualifying.

(2) History of splenectomy (P41.5) is disqualifying, except when resulting from trauma.

g. <u>Abdominal Wall</u>.

(1) Current hernia (except for small or asymptomatic umbilical hernias), including but not limited to uncorrected inguinal (550) and other abdominal wall hernias (553) are disqualifying.

(2) History of open or laparoscopic abdominal surgery (P54) during the preceding six (6) months is disqualifying.

h. <u>Obesity</u>.

(1) History of any gastrointestinal procedure for the control of obesity is disqualifying. Artificial openings, including but not limited to ostomy (V44) are disqualifying.

18. Female Genitalia.

    a. Uterine bleeding. Current or history of abnormal uterine bleeding (626.2), including but not limited to menorrhagia, metrorrhagia, or polymenorrhea is disqualifying.

    b. Amenorrhea. Current unexplained amenorrhea (626.0) is disqualifying.

    c. Dysmenorrhea. Current or history of dysmenorrhea (625.3) that is incapacitating to a degree recurrently necessitating absences of more than a few hours from routine activities is disqualifying.

    d. Endometriosis. Current or history of endometriosis (617) is disqualifying.

    e. Major abnormalities or defects of the genitalia. History of major abnormalities or defects of the genitalia such as change of sex (P64.5), hermaphroditism, pseudohermaphroditism, or pure gonadal dysgenesis (752.7) is disqualifying.

    f. Ovarian cyst(s). Current or history of ovarian cyst(s) (620.2) when persistent or symptomatic is disqualifying.

    g. Pelvic inflammatory disease. Current pelvic inflammatory disease (614) or history of recurrent pelvic inflammatory disease is disqualifying. Current or history of chronic pelvic pain or unspecified symptoms associated with female genital organs (625.9) is disqualifying.

    h. Pregnancy. Current pregnancy (V22) is disqualifying until six (6) months after the end of the pregnancy.

    i. Uterine absence/enlargement. History of congenital uterine absence (752.3) is disqualifying. Current uterine enlargement due to any cause (621.2) is disqualifying.

    j. Genital infection or ulceration. Current or history of genital infection or ulceration, including but not limited to herpes genitalis (054.11) or condyloma acuminatum (078.11), if of sufficient severity requiring frequent intervention or to interfere with normal function is disqualifying.

    k. Abnormal gynecologic cytology. Current or history of abnormal gynecologic cytology, including but not limited to unspecified abnormalities of the Papanicolaou smear of the cervix (795.0), excluding Atypical Squamous Cells of Undetermined Significance without Human Papilloma Virus (HPV) (079.4) and confirmed Low-Grade Squamous Intraepithelial Lesion (LGSIL) (622.9) is disqualifying. For the purposes of this Instruction, confirmation is by colposcopy or repeat cytology.

(1) A temporary waiver for one (1) year may be considered for cervical intraepithelial neoplasia (CIN)-2/3 if the following conditions are met:

   (a) It is the first occurrence of CIN-2/3;

   (b) The woman has an excisional or ablative procedure for CIN-2/3;

   (c) There is no evidence of invasive/micro-invasion and no involvement of endocervical glandular components;

(2) A permanent waiver may be considered after one (1) year if the member meets the accession standards in ref (a) at each of the quarterly follow-up examinations during the temporary waiver period.

19. Male Genitalia.

   a. Testicles absent. Absence of one or both testicles, congenital (752.89) or undescended (752.51) is disqualifying. Unilateral loss of testis, unrelated to cancer is not disqualifying.

   b. Epispadias or hypospadias. Current epispadias (752.62) or hypospadias (752.61), when accompanied by evidence of urinary tract infection, urethral stricture, or voiding dysfunction, is disqualifying.

   c. Testicle enlargement or epididymis. Current enlargement or mass of testicle or epididymis (608.9) is disqualifying.

   d. Orchitis or epididymitis. Current orchitis or epididymitis (604.90) is disqualifying.

   e. Penis amputation. History of penis amputation (878.0) is disqualifying.

   f. Genital infection or ulceration. Current or history of genital infection or ulceration, including but not limited to herpes genitalis (054.13) or condyloma acuminatum (078.11), if of sufficient severity to require frequent intervention or to interfere with normal function is disqualifying.

   g. Prostatitis. Current acute prostatitis (601.0) or chronic prostatitis (601.1) is disqualifying.

   h. Hydrocele. Current hydrocele (603) with greatest dimension of four (4) centimeters or greater or symptomatic, is disqualifying.

   (1) Left varicocele (456.4), if symptomatic, or associated with testicular atrophy, or varicocele larger than the testis, is disqualifying.

   (2) Any right varicocele is disqualifying.

i. Scrotal pain. Current or history of chronic scrotal pain or unspecified symptoms associated with male genital organs (608.9) is disqualifying.

j. Genitalia abnormalities or defects. History of major abnormalities or defects of the genitalia such as change of sex (P64.5), hermaphroditism, pseudohermaphroditism, or pure gonadal dysgenesis (752.7) is disqualifying.

20. Urinary System.

    a. Cystitis. Current cystitis, or history of chronic or recurrent cystitis (595) is disqualifying.

    b. Urethritis. Current urethritis, or history of chronic or recurrent urethritis (597.80) is disqualifying.

    c. Enuresis. History of enuresis (788.30) or incontinence of urine (788.30), or the control of it with medication or other treatment past the fifteenth (15th) birthday is disqualifying.

    d. Urinary tract disease. Current hematuria (599.7), pyuria, or other findings indicative of urinary tract disease (599) is disqualifying.

    e. Urethral stricture or fistula. Current urethral stricture (598) or fistula (599.1) is disqualifying.

    f. Kidney.

        (1) Current absence of one kidney, congenital (753.0) or acquired (V45.73), is disqualifying.

        (2) Current pyelonephritis (590.0) (chronic or recurrent), or any other unspecified infections of the kidney (590.9) is disqualifying.

        (3) Current or history of polycystic kidney (753.1) is disqualifying.

        (4) Current or history of horseshoe kidney (753.3) is disqualifying.

        (5) Current or history of hydronephrosis (591) is disqualifying.

        (6) Current or history of acute (580) or chronic (582) nephritis of any type is disqualifying.

        (7) Current or history of proteinuria (791.0) greater than 200 milligrams in 24 hours; or a protein-to-creatinine ratio greater than 0.2 in a random urine sample, if greater than 48 hours after strenuous activity is disqualifying, unless consultation determines the condition to be benign orthostatic proteinuria.

(8) Current of history of urolithiasis (592) within the preceding twelve (12) months is disqualifying. Recurrent calculus, nephrocalcinosis, or bilateral renal calculi at any time is disqualifying.

21. Spine and Sacroiliac Joints.

    a. Ankylosing spondylitis. Ankylosing spondylitis or other inflammatory spondylopathies (720) is disqualifying.

    b. Sacroiliac joints. Current or history of any condition, including but not limited to the spine or sacroiliac joints, with or without objective signs, are disqualifying if:

        (1) It prevents the individual from successfully following a physically active vocation in civilian life (724), or is associated with local or referred pain to the extremities, muscular spasms, postural deformities, or limitation in motion.

        (2) Requires external support.

        (3) Requires limitation of physical activity or frequent treatment.

    c. Spine deviation or curvature. Current deviation or curvature of spine (737) from normal alignment, structure, or function is disqualifying if:

        (1) It prevents the individual from following a physically active vocation in civilian life.

        (2) It interferes with the proper wearing of a uniform or military equipment.

        (3) It is symptomatic.

        (4) There is lumbar or thoracic scoliosis greater than 30 degrees, or kyphosis and lordosis greater than 50 degrees when measured by the Cobb Method.

    d. Fusion vertebral bodies. History of congenital fusion (756.15) involving more than two vertebral bodies or any surgical fusion of spinal vertebrae (P81.0) is disqualifying.

    e. Vertebra fracture or dislocation. Current or history of fracture or dislocation of the vertebra (805) is disqualifying. A compression fracture involving less than 25 percent of a single vertebra is not disqualifying if the injury occurred more than one (1) year before examination and the applicant is asymptomatic. A history of fractures of the transverse or spinous processes is not disqualifying if the applicant is asymptomatic.

        (1) Vertebral fractures that do not meet the standards:

(a) Compression fractures involving more than or equal to 25 percent of a single vertebra,

(b) Compression fractures involving less than 25 percent of a single vertebra occurring within the past twelve (12) months or it is symptomatic,

(c) Any compression fracture that is symptomatic.

(2) Vertebral fractures that meet the standard:

(a) Compression fractures involving less than 25 percent of a single vertebra if it occurred more than twelve (12) months before the accession exam and the applicant is asymptomatic,

(b) Fractures of the transverse or spinous process that are not symptomatic.

f. Epiphysitis. History of juvenile epiphysitis (732.6) with any degree of residual change indicated by X-ray or kyphosis is disqualifying.

g. Herniated nucleus pulposus. Current herniated nucleus pulposus (722) or history of surgery to correct is disqualifying. A surgically corrected asymptomatic single level lumbar or thoracic diskectomy with full resumption of unrestricted activity meets the standard.

h. Spina bifida. Current or history of spina bifida (741) when symptomatic, when there is more than one vertebral level involved or with dimpling of the overlying skin is disqualifying. History of surgical repair of spina bifida is disqualifying.

i. Spondylolysis. Current or history of spondylolysis congenital (756.10-756.12), or acquired (738.4) and spondylolisthesis congenital (756.12) or acquired (738.4) are disqualifying.

22. Upper Extremities.

a. Limitation of motion. Current active joint ranges of motion less than the measurements listed in paragraphs below are disqualifying.

(1) Shoulder (726.1)

(a) Forward elevation to 90 degrees.

(b) Abduction to 90 degrees.

(2) Elbow (726.3)

(a) Flexion to 130 degrees.

(b) Extension to 15 degrees.

(3) <u>Wrist</u> (726.4). A total range of 60 degrees (extension plus flexion), or radial and ulnar deviation combined arc 30 degrees.

(4) <u>Hand</u> (726.4)

(a) Pronation to 45 degrees.

(b) Supination to 45 degrees.

(5) <u>Fingers and Thumb</u> (726.4). Inability to clench fist, pick up a pin, grasp an object, or touch tips of at least three fingers with thumb.

b. <u>Hand and Finger</u>.

(1) Absence of the distal phalanx of either thumb (885) is disqualifying.

(2) Absence of any portion of the index finger is disqualifying.

(3) Absence of distal and middle phalanx of the middle, or ring finger of either hand irrespective of the absence of little finger (886) is disqualifying.

(4) Absence of more than the distal phalanx of any two of the following: index, middle, or ring finger of either hand (886) is disqualifying.

(5) Absence of hand or any portion thereof (887) is disqualifying, except for specific absence of fingers as noted above.

(6) Current polydactyly (755.0) is disqualifying.

(7) Intrinsic paralysis or weakness of upper limbs, including but not limited to nerve paralysis, carpal tunnel and cubital syndromes, lesion of ulnar, median, or radial nerve (354) sufficient to produce physical findings in the hand such as muscle atrophy and weakness is disqualifying.

c. <u>Residual Weakness and Pain</u>. Current disease, injury, or congenital condition with residual weakness or symptoms that prevents satisfactory performance of duty, including but not limited to chronic joint pain associated with the shoulder (719.41), the upper arm (719.42), the forearm (719.43), and the hand (719.44); or chronic joint pain as a late effect of fracture of the upper extremities (905.2), as a late effect of sprains without mention of injury (905.7), and as late effects of tendon injury (905.8) are disqualifying.

23. Lower Extremities.

   a. Limitation of Motion. Current active joint ranges of motion less than the measurements listed in the subparagraphs below are disqualifying:

   (1) Hip (due to disease (726.5) or injury (905.2)).

      (a) Flexion to 90 degrees.

      (b) No demonstrable flexion contracture.

      (c) Extension to 10 degrees (beyond 0 degrees).

      (d) Abduction to 45 degrees.

      (e) Rotation of 60 degrees (internal and external combined).

   (2) Knee (due to disease (726.6) or injury (905.4)).

      (a) Full extension to 0 degrees.

      (b) Flexion to 110 degrees.

   (3) Ankle (due to disease (726.7) or injury (905.4) or congenital).

      (a) Dorsiflexion to 10 degrees.

      (b) Planter flexion to 30 degrees.

      (c) Subtalar eversion and inversion totaling 5 degrees.

   b. Foot and Ankle.

   (1) Current absence of a foot or any portion thereof (896) is disqualifying.

   (2) Absence of a single lesser toe or any portion thereof that is symptomatic and does not impair function meets the standard.

   (3) Deformity of the toes that prevents the proper wearing of military footwear or impairs walking, marching, running, maintaining balance or jumping is disqualifying.

   (4) Symptomatic deformity of the toes (acquired (735) or congenital (755.66)), including but not limited to conditions such as hallux valgus (735.0), hallux varus (735.1), hallux rigidicus (735.2), hammer toe(s) (735.4), claw toe(s) (735.5), or overriding toe(s) (735.8) are disqualifying.

(5) Clubfoot (754.70) or pes cavus (754.71) that prevents the proper wearing of military footwear or causes symptoms when walking, marching, running, or jumping is disqualifying.

(6) Rigid or symptomatic pes planus (acquired (734), congenital (754.61)).

(7) Current ingrown toenails (703.0), if infected or symptomatic are disqualifying.

(8) Current or history of plantar fasciitis (728.71) is disqualifying.

(9) Symptomatic neuroma (355.6) is disqualifying.

c. <u>Leg, Knee, Thigh, and Hip</u>.

(1) Current loose or foreign body in the knee joint (717.6) is disqualifying.

(2) History of uncorrected anterior (717.83) or posterior (717.84) cruciate ligament injury is disqualifying.

(3) History of surgical reconstruction of knee ligaments (P81.4) meets the standard if twelve (12) months has elapsed since reconstruction, and the knee is asymptomatic and stable.

(4) Recurrent ACL reconstruction is disqualifying.

(5) Symptomatic medial (717.82) or lateral (717.42) meniscal injury is disqualifying. The following meets the standard if asymptomatic and released to full and unrestricted activity:

(a) Meniscal repair, at greater than six (6) months after surgery.

(b) Partial meniscectomy at greater than three (3) months after surgery.

(6) Meniscal transplant is disqualifying.

(7) Symptomatic medial and lateral collateral ligament instability is disqualifying.

(8) Current or history of congenital dislocation of the hip (754.3), osteochondritis of the hip (Legg-Perthes Disease) (732.1), or slipped capital femoral epiphysis of the hip (732.2) is disqualifying.

(9) Hip dislocation (835) within two (2) years preceding examination is disqualifying. Hip dislocation after two (2) years meets the standard if asymptomatic and released to full unrestricted activity.

(10) Symptomatic osteochondritis of the tibial tuberosity (Osgood-Schlatter Disease) (732.4) within the past twelve (12) months is disqualifying.

(11) Stress fractures, recurrent or single episode during the past twelve (12) months are disqualifying.

d. General.

(1) Current deformities, disease, or chronic joint pain of pelvic region, thigh (719.45), lower leg (719.46), knee (717.9), ankle and/or foot (719.47) that have interfered with function to such a degree as to prevent the individual from following a physically active vocation in civilian life, or that would interfere with walking, running, weight bearing, or the satisfactory completion of training or military duty are disqualifying.

(2) Current leg-length discrepancy resulting in a limp (736.81) is disqualifying.

24. Miscellaneous Conditions of the Extremities.

a. Chondromalacia. Current or history of chondromalacia (717.7), including but not limited to chronic patello-femoral pain syndrome and retro-patellar pain syndrome, osteoarthritis (715.3), or traumatic arthritis (716.1) is disqualifying.

b. Dislocations of any major joints. Current joint dislocation if unreduced, or history of recurrent dislocations/subluxations or instability of the hip (835), elbow (832), ankle (837), or foot is disqualifying.

c. History of any dislocation/subluxations or instability of the knee (718.86) or shoulder (831).

d. Osteoarthritis. Current or history of chronic osteoarthritis (715.3) or traumatic arthritis (716.1) of isolated joints that has interfered with a physically active lifestyle, or that prevents the satisfactory performance of military duty is disqualifying.

e. Fractures.

(1) Current malunion or non-union of any fracture (733.8) (except asymptomatic ulnar styloid process fracture) is disqualifying.

(2) Current retained hardware (including plates, pins, rods, wires, or screws) used for fixation that is symptomatic or interferes with proper wearing of protective equipment or military uniform. Retained hardware is not disqualifying if fractures are healed, ligaments are stable, and there is no pain.

f. Orthopedic implants. Current orthopedic implants or devices to correct congenital or post-traumatic orthopedic abnormalities (V43) are disqualifying.

g. Bone or joint contusion. Current or history of contusion of bone or joint; an injury of more than a minor nature which shall interfere or prevent performance of military duty, or shall require frequent or prolonged treatment, without fracture, nerve injury, open wound, crush or dislocation, which occurred in the preceding six (6) months and recovery has not been sufficiently completed or rehabilitation resolved are disqualifying.

h. Joint replacement. History of joint replacement of any site (V43.6) is disqualifying.

i. Muscular paralysis, contracture, or atrophy. Current or history of neuromuscular paralysis, weakness, contracture, or atrophy (728), of sufficient degree to interfere with or prevent satisfactory performance of military duty, or requires frequent or prolonged treatment, is disqualifying.

j. Osteochondroma or osteocartilaginous exostoses. Current symptomatic osteochondroma or history of multiple osteocartilaginous exostoses (727.82) are disqualifying.

k. Osteoporosis. Current osteoporosis (733.0) as demonstrated by a reliable test such as a DEXA scan is disqualifying.

l. Osteopenia. Current osteopenia (733.9) until resolved is disqualifying.

m. Osteomyelitis. Current osteomyelitis (730.0) or history of recurrent osteomyelitis is disqualifying.

n. Osteochondritis desiccans. Current or history of osteochondritis desiccans (732.7) is disqualifying.

o. History of cartilage surgery to include but not limited to cartilage debridement, chondroplasty, microfracture, or cartilage transplant procedure are disqualifying.

p. Compartment Syndrome. Current or history of any post-traumatic (958.9) or exercise induced (729.7-79) compartment syndrome is disqualifying.

q. Avascular Necrosis. Current or history of avascular necrosis of any bone is disqualifying.

r. Tendon Disorders. Current or history of recurrent tendon disorder including but not limited to tendonitis, tendonopathy, or tenosynovitis are disqualifying.

25. Vascular System.

a. Arteries and blood vessels. Current or history of abnormalities of the arteries (447), including but not limited to aneurysms (442), arteriovenous malformations, atherosclerosis (440), or arteritis (such as Kawasaki's disease) (446), are disqualifying.

b. Vascular disease. Current or medically managed hypertension (401) is disqualifying. Hypertension is defined as systolic pressure greater than 140 mmHg and/or diastolic pressure greater than 90 mmHg confirmed by manual blood pressure (BP) cuff averaged over two or more properly measured, seated, blood pressure readings on each of two or more consecutive days (isolated, single day BP elevation is not disqualifying unless confirmed on two or more consecutive days).

c. Peripheral vascular disease. Current or history of peripheral vascular disease (443.9), including but not limited to diseases such as Raynaud's Disease (443.0), and vasculidities are disqualifying.

d. Venous diseases. Current or history of venous diseases, including but not limited to recurrent thrombophlebitis (451), thrombophlebitis during the preceding year, or evidence of venous incompetence, such as large or symptomatic varicose veins, edema, or skin ulceration (454) are disqualifying.

26. Skin and Cellular Tissues.

    a. Sebaceous glands. Current diseases of sebaceous glands including severe and/or cystic acne (706), or hidradenitis, suppurativa (705), scalp perifollicular (704) if extensive involvement of the neck, scalp, axilla, groin, shoulders, chest, or back is present or shall be aggravated by or interfere with the proper wearing of military equipment are disqualifying. Applicants under treatment with systemic retinoids, including but not limited to isotretinoin (Accutane ®), are disqualified until eight (8) weeks after completion of therapy.

    b. Current or history of atopic dermatitis (691) or eczema (692.9) after the twelfth (12th) birthday.

        (1) Atopic Dermatitis. Active or history of residual or recurrent lesions in characteristic areas (face, neck, antecubital and/or popliteal fossae, occasionally wrists and hands) are disqualifying.

        (2) Non-Specific Dermatitis. Current or history of recurrent or chronic non-specific dermatitis to include contact dermatitis (692) (irritant/allergic), or dyshydrotic dermatitis (705.81) requiring more treatment than with over the counter medications is disqualifying.

    d. Cysts.

(1) Current cyst (706.2) (other than pilonidal cyst) is of such a size or location as to interfere with the proper wearing of military equipment is disqualifying.

(2) Current pilonidal cyst (685) is evidenced by the presence of a tumor mass or a discharging sinus, or is a surgically resected pilonidal cyst that is symptomatic, unhealed, or less than six (6) months post-operative is disqualifying.

e. Bullous dermatoses. Current or history of bullous dermatoses (694), including but not limited to dermatitis herpetiformis, pemphigus, and epidermolysis bullosa (757.39), is disqualifying. Resolved bullous impetigo meets the standards.

f. Lymphedema. Current or chronic lymphedema (457.1) is disqualifying.

g. Furunculosis or carbuncle. Current or history of furunculosis or carbuncle (680) if extensive, recurrent, or chronic is disqualifying.

h. Hyperhidrosis of hands or feet. Current or history of severe hyperhidrosis of hands or feet (705.2, 780.8), unless controlled by topical medications is disqualifying.

i. Skin anomalies congenital or acquired. Current or history of congenital (757) or acquired (216) anomalies of the skin, such as nevi or vascular tumors that interfere with function, or are exposed to constant irritation are disqualifying. History of Dysplastic Nevus Syndrome is disqualifying (232).

j. Keloid formation. Current or history of keloid formation (701.4), including pseudofolliculitis and keloidalis nuchae (706.1), if that tendency is marked or interferes with the proper wearing of military equipment is disqualifying.

k. Lichen planus. Current lichen planus (cutaneous and/or oral) (697.0) is disqualifying.

l. Neurofibromatosis. Current or history of neurofibromatosis (Von Recklinghausen's Disease) (237.7) is disqualifying.

m. Photosensitivity. History of photosensitivity (692.72), including but not limited to any primary sun-sensitive condition, such as polymorphous light eruption or solar urticaria, or any dermatosis aggravated by sunlight, such as lupus erythematosus is disqualifying.

n. Psoriasis, Radiodermatitis, scleroderma. Current or history of psoriasis (696.1) is disqualifying. Current or history of radiodermatitis (692.82) is disqualifying. Current or history of scleroderma (710.1) is disqualifying.

o. Urticaria. Current or history of chronic urticaria lasting longer than six (6) weeks or recurrent episodes of urticaria (708.8) within the past two (2) years not associated with angioedema, hereditary angioedema (277.6) or maintenance therapy for chronic urticaria, even if not symptomatic is disqualifying.

p. Plantar wart(s). Current symptomatic plantar wart(s) (078.19) is disqualifying.

q. Scars or any other chronic skin disorder. Current scars (709.2), or any other chronic skin disorder of a degree or nature that requires frequent outpatient treatment or hospitalization, which in the opinion of the certifying authority shall interfere with proper wearing of military clothing or equipment, or which exhibits a tendency to ulcerate or interferes with the satisfactory performance of duty is disqualifying.

r. Prior burn (949) injury involving 18 percent or more of the body surface area (including graft sites), or resulting in functional impairment to such a degree, due to scarring, as to interfere with the satisfactory performance of military duty to decreased range of motion, strength, or agility.

s. Fungus infections. Current localized types of fungus infections (117), interfering with the proper wearing of military equipment or the performance of military duties are disqualifying. For systemic fungal infections, refer to paragraph 28.v.

27. Blood and Blood-Forming Tissues.

    a. Anemia. Current hereditary or acquired anemia, which has not been corrected with therapy before appointment or induction is disqualifying. For the purposes of this Instruction, anemia is defined as a hemoglobin of less than 13.5 for males and less than 12 for females. Use the following ICD-9 codes for diagnosed anemia: hereditary hemolytic anemia (282), sickle cell disease (282.6), acquired hemolytic anemia (283), aplastic anemia (284), or unspecified anemias (285).

    b. Coagulation defects. Current or history of coagulation defects (286) including but not limited to von Willebrand's Disease (286.4), idiopathic thrombocytopenia (287), Henoch-Schönlein Purpura (287.0) are disqualifying.

    c. Agranulocytosis and/or leukopenia. Current or history of diagnosis of any form of chronic or recurrent agranulocytosis and/or leukopenia (288.0) is disqualifying.

28. Systemic.

    a. Immunodeficiencies. Current or history of disorders involving the immune mechanism, including immunodeficiencies (279) is disqualifying. Presence of

Human Immunodeficiency Virus or serologic evidence of infection (042) is disqualifying. False positive screening test(s) with ambiguous results on confirmatory immunologic testing is disqualifying.

b. <u>Lupus</u>. Current or history of lupus erythematosus (710.0) or mixed connective tissue disease variant (710.9) is disqualifying.

c. <u>Sclerosis</u>. Current or history of progressive systemic sclerosis (710.1), including CRST Variant is disqualifying. A single plaque of localized Scleroderma (morphea) that has been stable for at least two (2) years is not disqualifying.

d. <u>Reiter's disease</u>. Current or history of Reiter's disease (099.3) is disqualifying.

e. <u>Rheumatoid arthritis</u>. Current or history of rheumatoid arthritis (714.0) is disqualifying.

f. <u>Sjögren's syndrome</u>. Current or history of Sjögren's syndrome (710.2) is disqualifying.

g. <u>Vasculitis</u>. Current or history of vasculitis, including but not limited to polyarteritis nodosa and allied conditions (446.0), arteritis (447.6), Behçet's (136.1), and Wegner's granulomatosis (446.4) is disqualifying.

h. <u>Tuberculosis (010)</u>.

   (1) Current active tuberculosis or substantiated history of active tuberculosis in any form or location, regardless of past treatment, in the previous two (2) years is disqualifying.

   (2) Current residual physical or mental defects from past tuberculosis that shall prevent the satisfactory performance of duty are disqualifying.

   (3) Individuals with a past history of active tuberculosis greater than two (2) years before appointment, enlistment, or induction are qualified if they have received a complete course of standard chemotherapy for tuberculosis.

   (4) Current or history of untreated latent tuberculosis (positive Purified Protein Derivative with negative chest x-ray) (795.5) is disqualifying. Individuals with a tuberculin reaction in accordance with American Thoracic Society (ATS) and U.S. Public Health Service (USPHS) guidelines are eligible for enlistment, induction, and appointment, provided they have received chemoprophylaxis in accordance with ATS and USPHS guidelines. A negative QuantiFERON®-TB Gold (QFT®-G) with a positive tuberculin skin test meets the standard.

i. <u>Syphilis</u>. Current untreated syphilis is disqualifying (097).

j. <u>Anaphylaxis</u>. History of anaphylaxis (995.0) is disqualifying.

(1) History of anaphylaxis to stinging insects (989.5) is disqualifying. A cutaneous only reaction to a stinging insect under the age of sixteen (16) meets the standard. Applicants who have been treated for 3-5 years with maintenance venom immunotherapy meet the standard.

(2) History of systemic allergic reaction to food or food additives (995.60-995.69) are disqualifying. Systemic allergic reaction may be defined as a temporally related, systemic, often multi-system, reaction to a specific food. The presence of a food-specific immunoglobulin E antibody without a correlated clinical history meets the standard.

(3) Oral allergy syndrome is disqualifying.

(4) Hypersensitivity to latex is disqualifying.

(5) Exercise induced anaphylaxis (with or without food) is disqualifying.

(6) Idiopathic anaphylaxis is disqualifying.

(7) Acute, early, or immediate anaphylactic onset is disqualifying.

(8) History of angioedema or urticaria is disqualifying.

k. <u>Tropical fevers</u>. Current residual of tropical fevers, including but not limited to fevers, such as malaria (084) and various parasitic or protozoan infestations that prevent the satisfactory performance of military duty is disqualifying.

l. <u>Sleep disturbances</u>. Current sleep disturbances (780.5), including but not limited to sleep apneas or narcolepsy or history of narcolepsy is disqualifying.

m. <u>Malignant hyperthermia</u>. History of malignant hyperthermia (995.86) is disqualifying.

n. <u>Industrial solvent or other chemical intoxication</u>. History of industrial solvent or other chemical intoxication (982) with sequelae is disqualifying.

o. <u>Motion sickness</u>. History of motion sickness (994.6) resulting in recurrent incapacitating symptoms or of such a severity to require pre-medication in the previous three (3) years is disqualifying.

p. <u>Rheumatic fever</u>. History of rheumatic fever (390) is disqualifying.

q. <u>Muscular dystrophies</u>. Current or history of muscular dystrophies (359) or myopathies is disqualifying.

r. <u>Amyloidosis</u>. Current or history of amyloidosis (277.3) is disqualifying.

s. Granuloma. Current or history of eosinophilic granuloma (277.8) is disqualifying. Healed eosinophilic granuloma, when occurring as a single localized bony lesion and not associated with soft tissue or other involvement meets the standard. All other forms of the Histiocytosis (202.3) are disqualifying.

t. Polymyositis /dermatomyositis. Current or history of polymyositis (710.4) /dermatomyositis complex (710.3) with skin involvement is disqualifying.

u. Rhabdomyolysis / Sarcoidosis. History of rhabdomyolysis (728.88) is disqualifying. Current or history of sarcoidosis (135) is disqualifying.

v. Fungus infections. Current systemic fungus infections (117) are disqualifying. For localized fungal infections, refer to paragraph 26.s.

29. Endocrine and Metabolic.

   a. Adrenal dysfunction. Current or history of adrenal dysfunction (255) is disqualifying.

   b. Diabetes mellitus. Current or history of diabetes mellitus (250) is disqualifying.

   c. Pituitary dysfunction. Current or history of pituitary dysfunction (253) is disqualifying.

   d. Gout. Current or history of gout (274) is disqualifying.

   e. Hyperparathyroidism or hypoparathyroidism. Current or history of hyperparathyroidism (252.0) or hypoparathyroidism (252.1) is disqualifying.

   f. Thyroid Disorders.

      (1) Current goiter (240) is disqualifying.

      (2) Current hypothyroidism (244) uncontrolled by medication is disqualifying.

      (3) Current or history of hyperthyroidism (242.9) is disqualifying.

      (4) Current thyroiditis (245) is disqualifying.

   g. Nutritional deficiency diseases. Current nutritional deficiency diseases, including but not limited to beriberi (265), pellagra (265.2), and scurvy (267) are disqualifying.

h. Glycosuria. Current persistent Glycosuria, when associated with impaired glucose tolerance (250) or renal tubular defects (271.4) is disqualifying.

i. Acromegaly. Current or history of Acromegaly, including but not limited to gigantism (253.0), or other disorders of pituitary function (253) is disqualifying.

30. Neurologic.

    a. Cerebrovascular conditions. Current or history of cerebrovascular conditions, including but not limited to subarachnoid (430) or intracerebral (431) hemorrhage, vascular insufficiency, aneurysm or arteriovenous malformation (437) are disqualifying.

    b. Central nervous system anomalies. History of congenital or acquired anomalies of the central nervous system (742) or meningocele (741.9) is disqualifying.

    c. Meninges disorders. Current or history of disorders of meninges, including but not limited to cysts (349.2) is disqualifying.

    d. Hereditodegenerative disorders. Current or history of degenerative and hereditodegenerative disorders, including but not limited to those disorders affecting the cerebrum (330), basal ganglia (333), cerebellum (334), spinal cord (335), or peripheral nerves (337) are disqualifying.

    e. Headaches. History of recurrent headaches (784.0), including but not limited to migraines (346) and tension headaches (307.81) that interfere with normal function in the past three (3) years, or of such severity to require prescription medications are disqualifying.

    f. Head Injury. (854.0)

        (1) History of severe head injury shall be disqualifying if associated with any of the following:

            (a) Post-traumatic seizure(s) occurring more than 30 minutes after injury.

            (b) Persistent motor or sensory deficits.

            (c) Impairment of intellectual function.

            (d) Alteration of personality.

            (e) Unconsciousness, amnesia, or disorientation of person, place, or time of 24-hours duration or longer post-injury.

(f) Multiple fractures involving skull or face (804).

(g) Cerebral laceration or contusion (851).

(h) History of epidural, subdural, subarachnoid, or intracerebral hematoma (852).

(i) Associated abscess (326) or meningitis (958.8).

(j) Cerebrospinal fluid rhinorrhea (349.81) or otorrhea (388.61) persisting more than seven (7) days.

(k) Focal neurologic signs.

(l) Radiographic evidence of retained foreign body or bony fragments secondary to the trauma and/or operative procedure in the brain.

(m) Leptomeningeal cysts or Arteriovenous Fistula (447.0).

(2) History of moderate head injury (854.03) is disqualifying. After two (2) years post-injury, applicants may be qualified if neurological consultation shows no residual dysfunction or complications. Moderate head injuries are defined as unconsciousness, amnesia, or disorientation of person, place, or time alone or in combination, of more than 1 and less than 24-hours duration post-injury, or linear skull fracture.

(3) History of mild head injury (854.02) is disqualifying. After 1 month post-injury, applicants may be qualified if neurological evaluation shows no residual dysfunction or complications. Mild head injuries are defined as a period of unconsciousness, amnesia, or disorientation of person, place, or time, alone or in combination of 1 hour or less post-injury.

(4) History of persistent post-traumatic symptoms (310.2) that interfere with normal activities or have duration of greater than 1 month is disqualifying. Such symptoms include, but are not limited to headache, vomiting, disorientation, spatial disequilibrium, impaired memory, poor mental concentration, shortened attention span, dizziness, or altered sleep patterns.

g. Infectious Diseases of the Central Nervous System.

(1) Current or history of acute infectious processes of the central nervous system, including but not limited to meningitis (322), encephalitis (323), or brain abscess (324), are disqualifying if occurring within one (1) year before examination, or if there are residual neurological defects.

(2) History of neurosyphilis (094) of any form, including but not limited to general paresis, tabes dorsalis, or meningovascular syphilis, is disqualifying.

h. Paralysis, weakness, lack of coordination, chronic pain, or sensory disturbance. Current or history of paralysis, weakness, lack of coordination, chronic pain, or sensory disturbance or other specified paralytic syndromes (344) is disqualifying.

i. Epilepsy. Any seizure occurring beyond the 6th birthday, unless the applicant has been free of seizures for a period of 5 years while taking no medication for seizure control, and has a normal electroencephalogram (EEG) is disqualifying. All such applicants shall have a current neurology consultation with current EEG results (345).

j. Nervous system disorders. Chronic nervous system disorders, including but not limited to myasthenia gravis (358.0), multiple sclerosis (340), and tic disorders (307.20) (e.g., Tourette's (307.23)) are disqualifying.

k. Central nervous system shunts. Current or history of retained central nervous system shunts of all kinds (V45.2) are disqualifying.

l. Narcolepsy or cataplexy. Current or history of narcolepsy or cataplexy (347) is disqualifying.

31. Learning Psychiatric and Behavioral.

    a. Attention Deficit Hyperactivity Disorder. Attention Deficit Hyperactivity Disorder (ADHD) (314) does not meet the standard unless the following criteria are met:

    (1) The applicant has not required an Individualized Education Program or work accommodations since the age of 14.

    (2) There is no history of comorbid mental disorders.

    (3) The applicant has never taken more than a single daily dosage of medication or has not been prescribed medication for this condition for more than 24 cumulative months after the age of 14.

    (4) During periods off of medication after the age of 14, the applicant has been able to maintain at least a 2.0 grade point average without accommodations.

    (5) Documentation from the applicant's prescribing provider that continued medication is not required for acceptable occupational or work performance.

    (6) Applicant is required to enter Service and pass Service specific training periods with no prescribed medication for ADHD.

b. Learning Disorders. History of learning disorders (315), including but not limited to dyslexia (315.02), do not meet the standard unless the applicants demonstrated passing academic and employment performance without utilization or recommendation of academic and/or work accommodations at any time since age 14.

c. Pervasive Developmental Disorders. Pervasive Developmental Disorders (299 series) including Asperger Syndrome, Autistic Spectrum Disorders, and Pervasive Developmental Disorder-Not Otherwise Specified (299.9) is disqualifying.

d. Psychotic features. Current or history of disorders with psychotic features such as schizophrenic disorders (295), delusional disorders (297), or other and unspecified psychoses (298) is disqualifying.

e. Bipolar Disorders/Psychoses. History of bipolar disorders (296.4-7) and affective psychoses (296.8) are disqualifying.

f. Depressive disorders. History of depressive disorders (296), Dysthymic (300.4), Cyclothymic (301.11) requiring outpatient care for longer than twelve (12) months by a physician or other mental health professional (to include V65.40), or any inpatient treatment in a hospital or residential facility is disqualifying.

g. Depressive disorders not otherwise specified (311), or unspecified mood disorder (296.90), does not meet the standards unless:

(1) Outpatient care was not required for longer than twenty-four (24) months (cumulative) by a physician or other mental health professional (V65.40).

(2) Has been stable without treatment for the past thirty-six (36) continuous months.

(3) Did not require any inpatient treatment in a hospital or residential facility.

h. Adjustment disorders. History of a single adjustment disorder (309) within the previous three (3) months, or recurrent episodes of adjustment disorders are disqualifying.

i. Conduct or behavior disorders. Current or history of disturbance of conduct (312), impulse control (312.3), oppositional defiant (313.81), other behavior disorders (313), or personality disorder (301) are disqualifying.

(1) History (demonstrated by repeated inability to maintain reasonable adjustment in school, with employers or fellow workers, or social groups), interview, psychological testing revealing that the degree of immaturity, instability, of personality inadequacy, impulsiveness, or dependency shall interfere with adjustment in the Armed Forces.

(2) Recurrent encounters with law enforcement agencies (excluding minor traffic violations) or antisocial behaviors are tangible evidence of impaired capacity to adapt to military service.

j. Other behavior disorders. Current or history of other behavior disorders is disqualifying, including but not limited to conditions such as the following:

(1) Enuresis (307.6) as defined in current edition of Diagnostic and Statistical Manual of Mental Disorders, after 15th birthday.

(2) Encopresis (307.7) after 13th birthday.

(3) Somnambulism (sleepwalking) (307.4) or a single episode of sleepwalking after 15th birthday.

k. Eating Disorders. History of anorexia nervosa (307.1) or bulimia (307.51) are disqualifying. Other eating disorders (307.50; 52-54) including unspecified disorders of eating (307.59) occurring after the 13th birthday are disqualifying.

l. Receptive or expressive language disorder. Any current receptive or expressive language disorder, including but not limited to any speech impediment, stammering and stuttering (307.0) of such a degree as to significantly interfere with production of speech or to repeat commands is disqualifying.

m. Suicidal behavior. History of suicidal behavior, including gesture(s) or attempt(s) (300.9), or history of self-mutilation or injury used as a way of dealing with life and emotions is disqualifying.

n. Obsessive-compulsive/Posttraumatic Stress Disorder. History of obsessive-compulsive disorder (300.3), or posttraumatic stress disorder (309.81) are disqualifying.

o. Anxiety disorders. History of anxiety disorders (300.01), anxiety order not otherwise specified (300.00), panic disorder (300.2), agoraphobia (300.21, 300.22), social phobia (300.23), simple phobias (300.29), other acute reactions to stress (308) are disqualifying unless:

(1) The applicant did not require any treatment in an inpatient or residential facility.

(2) Outpatient care was not required for longer than twelve (12) months (cumulative) by a physician or other mental health professional (to include V65.40).

(3) The applicant has not required treatment (including medication) for the past 24 continuous months.

Chapter 3. D. Page 39

(4) The applicant has been stable without loss of time from normal pursuits for repeated periods even if of brief duration; and without symptoms or behavior of a repeated nature which impaired social, school, or work efficiency for the past 24 continuous months.

p. <u>Dissociative disorders</u>. Current or history of dissociative disorders, conversion, or factitious disorders (300.1), or depersonalization (300.6) are disqualifying.

q. <u>Somatoform disorders</u>. Current or history of somatoform disorders (300.8), hypochondriasis (300.7), or pain disorder related to psychological factors (307.80 and .89) are disqualifying.

r. <u>Psychosexual conditions</u>. Current or history of psychosexual conditions (302), including but not limited to transsexualism, exhibitionism, transvestism, voyeurism, and other paraphilias are disqualifying.

s. <u>Alcohol dependence, abuse</u>. Current or history of alcohol dependence (303), drug dependence (304), alcohol abuse (305), or other drug abuse (305.2 thru 305.9) is disqualifying.

t. <u>Mental disorders</u>. Current or history of other mental disorders (all 290-319 not listed above) that, in the opinion of the civilian or military provider, shall interfere with or prevent satisfactory performance of military duty are disqualifying.

u. <u>Prior psychiatric hospitalization for any cause</u>.

32. <u>Tumors and Malignancies</u>.

    a. <u>Tumors</u>. Current benign tumors (M8000) or conditions that interfere with function, prevent the proper wearing of the uniform or protective equipment, shall require frequent specialized attention, or have a high malignant potential, such as Dysplastic Nevus Syndrome are disqualifying.

    b. <u>Malignant tumors</u>. Current or history of malignant tumors (V10) is disqualifying. Skin cancer (other than malignant melanoma) removed with no residual is not disqualifying.

33. <u>Miscellaneous</u>.

    a. <u>Parasitic diseases</u>. Current or history of parasitic diseases, if symptomatic or carrier state, including but not limited to filariasis (125), trypanosomiasis (086), schistosomiasis (120), hookworm (uncinariasis) (126.9), unspecified infectious and parasitic disease (136.9) are disqualifying.

b. <u>Frequent or prolonged treatment</u>. Current or history of other disorders, including but not limited to cystic fibrosis (277.0), or porphyria (277.1), that prevent satisfactory performance of duty or require frequent or prolonged treatment are disqualifying.

c. <u>Cold-related disorders</u>. Current or history of cold-related disorders, including but not limited to frostbite, chilblain, immersion foot (991), or cold urticaria (708.2), are disqualifying. Current residual effects of cold-related disorders, including but not limited to paresthesias, easily traumatized skin, cyanotic amputation of any digit, ankylosis, trench foot, or deep-seated ache are disqualifying.

d. <u>Angioedema</u>. History of angioedema, including hereditary angioedema (277.6) is disqualifying.

e. <u>Organ or tissue transplantation</u>. History of receiving organ or tissue transplantation (V42) is disqualifying.

f. <u>Pulmonary or systemic embolization</u>. History of pulmonary (415) or systemic embolization (444) is disqualifying.

g. <u>Metallic poisoning</u>. History of untreated acute or chronic metallic poisoning, including but not limited to lead, arsenic, silver (985), beryllium, or manganese (985) is disqualifying. Current complications or residual symptoms of such poisoning are disqualifying.

h. <u>Heat pyrexia heatstroke or sunstroke</u>. History of heat pyrexia (992.0), heatstroke (992.0), or sunstroke (992.0) is disqualifying. History of three or more episodes of heat exhaustion (992.3) is disqualifying. Current or history of a predisposition to heat injuries, including disorders of sweat mechanism, combined with a previous serious episode is disqualifying. Current or history of any unresolved sequelae of heat injury, including but not limited to nervous, cardiac, hepatic or renal systems is disqualifying.

i. <u>Interference of performance of duty</u>. Current or history of any condition that in the opinion of the Medical Officer shall significantly interfere with the successful performance of military duty or training is disqualifying (should use specific ICD code whenever possible, or 796.9).

j. <u>Pathological conditions</u>. Any current acute pathological condition, including but not limited to acute communicable diseases, until recovery has occurred without sequelae is disqualifying.

Evaluation for Risk of Head Injury Sequelae

DEGREE OF HEAD INJURY	MINIMUM REQUIRED WAITING PERIOD	EVALUATION REQUIREMENTS
MILD	ONE MONTH	COMPLETE NEUROLOGICAL EXAMINATION BY A PHYSICIAN
MODERATE	TWO YEARS	COMPLETE NEUROLOGICAL EVALUATION BY A NEUROLOGIST OR INTERNIST CT SCAN
SEVERE	PERMANENT DISQUALIFICATION	COMPLETE NEUROLOGICAL EVALUATION BY NEUROLOGIST OR NEUROSURGEON CT SCAN NEUROPSYCHOLOGICAL EVALUATION

Classification and Comparative Nomenclature of Cervical Smears

Original Classification	CIN System	Bethesda System
Class I: No abnormal cells	Normal smear;	
Class II: Atypical cells present below the level of cervical neoplasia		Atypical squamous cells of undetermined significance
Class III: Smear contains abnormal cells consistent with dysplasia	Mild dysplasia = CIN1 Moderate dysplasia = CIN2	Low-grade SIL (Changes associated with HPV & CIN1)
Class IV Smear contains abnormal cells consistent with carcinoma-in-situ	Severe dysplasia and carcinoma-in-situ = CIN3	High-grade SIL (CIN2, CIN3, and carcinoma-in-situ)
Class V: Smear contains abnormal 1. cells consistent with carcinoma 2. squamous cell carcinoma		Squamous cell carcinoma

Abbreviations: CIN = cervical intraepithelial neoplasia
SIL = squamous intraepithelial lesion

This page intentionally left blank

Section E. Physical Standards for Programs Leading to Commission

1. Appointment as Cadet, United States CG Academy 1
2. Commissioning of Cadets 2
3. Enrollment as an Officer Candidate 2
4. Commissioning of Officer Candidates 3
5. CG Direct Commission Program 4
6. Direct Commission in the CG Reserve 4
7. Direct Commission of Licensed Officers of U. S. Merchant Marine 4
8. Appointment to Warrant Grade 4

This page intentionally left blank.

E. Physical Standards for Programs Leading to Commission.

1. Appointment as Cadet, USCG Academy.

   a. Physical Examinations.
      (1) Applicants are encouraged to review the physical standards as published in the Academy Bulletin with their private physician prior to submitting their application for cadet candidate. This review serves to rule out, at this stage of the potential cadet's processing, applicants who obviously will not meet the required physical standards for appointment. In some cases, the physician may recommend a complete physical examination. Inaccuracy in ascertaining defects and determining the candidate's physical status at the time of this review results in unnecessary work for the CG and disappointment to the candidate when defects are subsequently found during the formal physical examination.

      (2) Candidates and their parents and sponsors are urged to refrain from requesting waivers for medical defects. The CG bases its decision to disqualify an individual on medical facts revealed in a thorough physical examination. Candidates unable to satisfy the minimum requirements are not suited for commission in the Regular CG, and consequently are not eligible for training at the Academy. A request for waiver for a medical defect invariably results in disappointment to all concerned.

      (3) Two physical examinations are required:

          (a) Formal physical examination before appointment is tendered.

          (b) Pre-training examination at the time of reporting to the Academy.

      (4) Formal physical examinations prior to accepting of candidates must be performed by a U. S. Public Health Service, Navy, Army, Air Force, or Veteran's Administration Medical Officer authorized to perform each exam by Department of Defense Medical Examination Review Board (DODMERB). All candidates are instructed where to report for such examinations.

   b. Physical Standards. All candidates for the CG Academy must meet the physical standards for enrollment as an officer candidate. DODMERB is reviewing authority.

   c. Retention. The standards for retention of a cadet at the Academy are the same as those for enrollment as an officer candidate, except that the Superintendent of the Academy is authorized to establish physical fitness and weight control programs designed to have cadets maintain weight closer to the ideal than the standards stipulated elsewhere for Service personnel. These stricter goals during cadet years are intended to take advantage of the Academy's unique environment of rigorous physical activity combined with opportunities for diet control and weight monitoring. These programs will instill lifelong behavior patterns to support the Service weight control standards.

2. <u>Commissioning of Cadets</u>. The pre-appointment physical examination of cadets in the graduating class should be held at least 6 months prior to acceptance of the commission. This physical examination should be conducted to determine physical fitness for commission in the Regular Service (section 3-D and 3-E) with recommendations made accordingly. Cadets should not be summarily disqualified for commissioning merely because they do not meet the standards for appointment as cadets provided that they may reasonably be expected to be physically capable of completing a full and effective CG career. In general, relatively minor defects that would be disqualifying for original commission direct from civilian life are not disqualifying for commission of a cadet in whom the Government has a considerable investment.

3. <u>Enrollment as an Officer Candidate</u>.

   a. <u>Physical Examination</u>. The physical examination for an officer candidate must be conducted by a Medical Officer and a Dentist. Particular care must be exercised during the examination in order that candidates may not be rejected later as a result of reexamination at Officer Candidate School. A complete physical examination is given officer candidates upon arrival at OCS to determine medical fitness and freedom from disease. Physician Assistant Officer Candidates will only receive an initial OCS candidate physical.

   b. <u>Physical Standards for Enrollment</u>. The standards contained in section 3-D (section 3-F for enlisted OCS candidates), as modified below, are applicable for enrollment as an officer candidate. Conditions not enumerated, that in the medical examiner's opinion will not permit a full productive career, shall be recorded in detail with appropriate recommendations.

      (1) Distant Visual Acuity. Uncorrected visual acuity shall be not worse than 20/400 in either eye provided that vision is correctable to 20/20 and that refractive error does not exceed plus or minus 8.0 diopters spherical equivalent (sphere + 1/2 cylinder), astigmatism does not exceed 3.00 diopters, and anisometropia does not exceed 3.50 diopters. Eyes must be free from any disfiguring or incapacitating abnormality and from acute or chronic disease. All personnel requiring corrective lenses shall wear them for the performance of duty.

      (2) Near visual acuity of any degree that does not correct to 20/40 in the better eye.

      (3) Normal color perception.

      (4) Teeth.

(a) All candidates shall be given a Type II dental examination by a dental officer, as part of the pre-training physical examination.

(b) Caries. No more than four teeth may exhibit multi-surface caries.

(c) Endodontics. The need for endodontic intervention on seven or more canals is disqualifying.

(d) Maxillary and Mandibular Bones. Malunited fractures of maxillary or mandibular bones and deformities of maxillary or mandibular bones interfering with mastication or speech are disqualifying. The presences of extensive necrosis or osseous lesions requiring surgical intervention are also disqualifying.

(e) Oral Tissues. Extensive loss of oral tissues that would prevent the replacement of missing teeth with a satisfactory prosthetic appliance is disqualifying. Unresolved oral inflammatory diseases are disqualifying. Hypertrophic, hyperplastic, or leukoplakic conditions of the soft tissue of the oral cavity may be disqualifying and will be considered on a case-by-case basis.

(f) Periodontal Disease. The presence of advanced periodontal disease is disqualifying.

(g) Serviceable Teeth. A sufficient number of teeth, natural or artificial, in functional occlusion to assure satisfactory incision, mastication, and phonation are required. The minimum requirement is edentulous upper and lower jaws corrected by full dentures. A requirement for placement of a prosthesis to meet the above requirements is disqualifying.

(h) Temporomandibular Joint. Current symptoms and/or history of chronic temporomandibular joint dysfunction is disqualifying (see also section 3-D-16.b).

(i) Orthodontics. Candidates with active appliances will need to submit a waiver request for continuing active orthodontic treatment as described in Chapter 2 Section A. 3. e. of this Manual.

4. Commissioning of Officer Candidates.

   a. The physical examination given upon arrival at OCS precludes the need for a commissioning physical examination providing there has been no intervening change in physical status and a visual acuity and color perception examination are given prior to actual commissioning.

b. The physical standards for commissioning are the same as for enrollment as an officer candidate. Final determination as to physical fitness for commissioning is made by the Commandant.

5. CG Direct Commission Program. Physical standards for CG active duty members (CWO's, Enlisted) that apply for the Direct Commission program are the same as for retention of officers in the regular CG. Refer to Section F of this Manual for the standards. Physical standards for all other applicants are the same as for enrollment of officer candidates.

6. Direct Commission in the CG Reserve.

   a. Non-aviator. The physical examination and standards for direct commission in the Reserve are the same for enrollment of officer candidates, except that Ready Reserve Direct Commission (RRDC) examinations must be within 24 months prior to the date of execution of the Acceptance and Oath of Office (CG-9556).

   b. Aviator. Candidates for direct commission in the Reserve as aviators must obtain an aviation physical examination from a currently qualified uniformed services Flight Surgeon or AMO within the last 12 months. The candidate must meet the standards for Class I, contained in section 3-G.

7. Direct Commission of Licensed Officers of U. S. Merchant Marine.

   a. Physical Examination. Two physical examinations are required: a preliminary physical at the time of the written examination; and a pre-appointment physical examination taken by successful candidates within six months of actual commission. The physical examination must be conducted by a Medical Officer of the uniformed services on active duty. Final determination of physical fitness will be made by the Commandant.

   b. Physical Standards. The physical standards for direct commission of Licensed Officers of the U. S. Merchant Marine are the same as for enrollment of officer candidates. All these standards must be met without waiver.

8. Appointment to Warrant Grade.

   a. Physical Examination. A complete physical examination is required within 12 months prior to appointment to Warrant Officer, except that physical examinations for members of the CG Ready Reserve must be within 24 months prior to the date of execution of the Acceptance and Oath of Office (CG-9556).

b. <u>Physical Requirements</u>. The physical standards for appointment of CG members to Warrant Officer are the same as for retention of officers in the regular CG. Refer to Section 3-F of this Manual for the standards. Physical standards for all other applicants are the same as for enrollment of officer candidates.

This page intentionally left blank.

Section F. Physical Standards Applicable to All Personnel (Regular and Reserve) For: Reenlistment; Enlistment of Prior Service USCG Personnel; Retention; Overseas Duty; and Sea Duty

1. General Instructions 1
2. Use of List of Disqualifying Conditions and Defects 1
3. Head and Neck 2
4. Esophagus, Nose, Pharynx, Larynx, and Trachea 2
5. Eyes 2
6. Ears and Hearing 5
7. Lungs and Chest Wall 5
8. Heart and Vascular System 7
9. Abdomen and Gastrointestinal System 9
10. Endocrine and Metabolic Conditions (Diseases) 11
11. Genitourinary System 12
12. Extremities 14
13. Spine, Scapulae, Ribs, and Sacroiliac Joints 17
14. Skin and Cellular Tissues 18
15. Neurological Disorders 19
16. Psychiatric Disorders. (see section 5-B concerning disposition) 20
17. Dental 21
18. Blood and Blood-Forming Tissue Diseases 21
19. Systemic Diseases, General Defects, and Miscellaneous Conditions 22
20. Tumors and Malignant Diseases 23
21. Sexually Transmitted Infection 23
22. Human Immunodeficiency Virus (HIV) 23
23. Transplant recipient 24

This page intentionally left blank.

F. Physical Standards Applicable to All Personnel (Regular and Reserve) For: Reenlistment; Enlistment of Prior Service USCG Personnel; Retention; Overseas Duty; and Sea Duty.

1. General Instructions.

    a. Scope. This section establishes specific physical standards applicable to all personnel (regular and reserve) for:

    (1) Enlistment/reenlistment of prior service USCG personnel within 6 months of discharge from active duty in the regular CG.

    (2) Retention.

    (3) Overseas duty.

    (4) Sea duty.

    b. Physical Examinations. Physical examinations should be conducted by at least one Medical and one Dental Officer of the uniformed services or by contract physician/dentist.

    c. Fitness for Duty. Members are ordinarily considered fit for duty unless they have a physical impairment (or impairments) that interferes with the performance of the duties of their grade or rating. A determination of fitness or unfitness depends upon the individual's ability to reasonably perform those duties. Active duty or reserves on extended active duty considered permanently unfit for duty shall be referred to a Medical Evaluation Board (MEB) for appropriate disposition. Reservists in any status not found 'fit for duty' six months after incurring/aggravating an injury or illness, or reservists who are unlikely to be found 'fit for duty' within six months after incurring/aggravating an injury or illness shall be referred to a Medical Evaluation Board. See Reserve Policy Manual, COMDTINST M1001.28 (series), Chapter 6, "Reserve Incapacitation System".

2. Use of List of Disqualifying Conditions and Defects. This section lists certain medical conditions and defects that are normally disqualifying. However, it is not an all-inclusive list. Its major objective is to achieve uniform disposition of cases arising under the law, but it is not a mandate that possession of one or more of the listed conditions or physical defects (and any other not listed) means automatic retirement or separation. If the member's condition is disqualifying but he/she can perform his/her duty, a waiver request could be submitted in lieu of immediate referral to a Medical Evaluation Board. If the request is denied, then a Medical Evaluation Board is required. The only exception is HIV infection, which may not require waiver or referral to MEB if the member continues to fully perform duties. (see Chapter 3- F-22 of this Manual).

3. Head and Neck.

   a. Loss of substance of the skull. With or without prosthetic replacement when accompanied by moderate residual signs and symptoms.

   b. Torticollis (wry neck). Severe fixed deformity with cervical scoliosis, flattening of the head and face, and loss of cervical mobility.

4. Esophagus, Nose, Pharynx, Larynx, and Trachea.

   a. Esophagus.

      (1) Achalasia. Manifested by dysphagia (not controlled by dilation), frequent discomfort, inability to maintain normal vigor and nutrition, or requiring frequent treatment.

      (2) Esophagitis. Persistent and severe.

      (3) Diverticulum of the esophagus. Of such a degree as to cause frequent regurgitation, obstruction and weight loss, that does not respond to treatment.

      (4) Stricture of the esophagus. Of such a degree as to almost restrict diet to liquids, require frequent dilation and hospitalization, and cause difficulty in maintaining weight and nutrition.

   b. Larynx.

      (1) Paralysis of the larynx. Characterized by bilateral vocal cord paralysis seriously interfering with speech or adequate airway.

      (2) Stenosis of the larynx. Causing respiratory embarrassment upon more than minimal exertion.

      (3) Obstruction edema of glottis. If chronic, not amenable to treatment and requiring tracheotomy.

   c. Nose, Pharynx, Trachea.

      (1) Rhinitis. Atrophic rhinitis characterized by bilateral atrophy of nasal mucous membrane with severe crusting and concomitant severe headaches.

      (2) Sinusitis. Severe and chronic that is suppurative, complicated by polyps, and does not respond to treatment.

      (3) Trachea. Stenosis of trachea that compromises airflow to more than a mild degree.

5. Eyes.

   a. Diseases and Conditions.

      (1) Active eye disease or any progressive organic disease regardless of the stage of activity, that is resistant to treatment and affects the distant visual acuity or visual field so that the member fits into one of the following:

(a) Distant visual acuity does not meet the standards.

(b) The diameter of the field of vision in the better eye is less than 20°.

(2) Aphakia, bilateral. Regardless of lens implant(s).

(3) Atrophy of optic nerve.

(4) Glaucoma. If resistant to treatment, or affecting visual fields, or if side effects of required medications are functionally incapacitating.

(5) Diseases and infections of the eye. When chronic, more than mildly symptomatic, progressive and resistant to treatment after a reasonable period.

(6) Ocular manifestations of endocrine or metabolic disorders. Not disqualifying, per se; however, residuals or complications, or the underlying disease may be disqualifying.

(7) Residuals or complications of injury. When progressive or when reduced visual acuity or fields do not meet the standards.

(8) Retina, detachment of.

(a) Unilateral.

1. When visual acuity does not meet the standards.

2. When the visual field in the better eye is constricted to less than 20°.

3. When uncorrectable diplopia exists.

4. When detachment results from organic progressive disease or new growth, regardless of the condition of the better eye.

(b) Bilateral. Regardless of etiology or results of corrective surgery.

b. <u>Vision</u>.

(1) Aniseikonia. Subjective eye discomfort, neurologic symptoms, sensations of motion sickness and other gastrointestinal disturbances, functional disturbances and difficulties in form sense, and not corrected by iseikonic lenses.

(2) Binocular diplopia. Which is severe, constant, and in zone less than 20° from the primary position.

(3) Hemianopsia. Of any type, if bilateral, permanent, and based on an organic defect. Those due to a functional neurosis and those due to transitory conditions, such as periodic migraine, are not normally disqualifying.

(4) Night blindness. Of such a degree that the individual requires assistance in any travel at night.

(5) Visual Acuity.

(a) Visual acuity that cannot be corrected to at least 20/50 in the better eye.

(b) Complete blindness or enucleation of an eye.

(c) When vision is correctable only by the use of contact lenses or other corrective device (telescope lenses, etc.).

(6) Visual Fields. When the visual field in the better eye is constricted to less than 20°.

(7) Color Perception. Normal color perception is required for retention of commissioned officers (certain warrant officer specialties do not require normal color perception) and selected ratings [See the Personnel Manual, COMDTINST M1000.6(series) Chapter 5-B]. The testing for color vision must be unaided or with standard corrective lenses only. Use of any lenses (such as Chromagen) or other device to compensate for defective color vision is prohibited. Retesting for color perception is normally not required if results of previous tests are documented in the health record, and there has been no history of a change in color vision. Exception: At the time of accession medical screening (e.g. CG Academy (including cadets and OCS candidates), Cape May recruits) the PIP color vision test will be repeated and normal color vision confirmed under controlled conditions as described in Chapter 3 Section C 22.i of this manual. Examinees are qualified if they pass either the Pseudoisochromatic Plates (PIP) or the Farnsworth Lantern (FALANT) test. Examinees who fail the PIP are qualified if they pass the FALANT.

c. Corneal Refractive Surgery.

(1) The refractive surgery procedures radial keratotomy (RK), and intracorneal rings (ICR) are disqualifying.

(2) Corneal Refractive Surgery for aviation personnel and candidates is discussed in Chapter 3. Section G.13 of this Manual.

(3) Photorefractive keratectomy (PRK) or Laser Assisted in situ Keratomileusis (LASIK) is not disqualifying for non-aviation members, including diving personnel, and does not require a waiver if the following conditions are met:

(a) Must follow guidelines for elective health care contained in 2.A.6. Note: Personnel having any type of corneal refractive surgery shall not perform duties requiring stable eyesight (e.g. deck watch, boat crew, etc.) until medically cleared.

(b) There must be post surgical refractive stability defined as less than 0.50 diopter changes over two separate exams at least three months apart.

(c) Must meet all vision standards in 3-F.5.b (divers must meet vision standards in 3-H.2.h). If the member is unable to meet these standards they will be considered for separation as outlined in the Physical Disability Evaluation System, COMDTINST M1850.2 (series).

(4) Implantable Contact Lenses (ICL) are not disqualifying and do not need a waiver if the following conditions are met: (Does not apply to aviation personnel)

    (a) Must follow guidelines for elective health care contained in 2.A.6

    (b) Must meet retention vision standards by three months post operatively.

6. Ears and Hearing.

   a. Ears.

      (1) Infections of the external auditory canal. Chronic and severe, resulting in thickening and excoriation of the canal, or chronic secondary infection requiring frequent and prolonged medical treatment and hospitalization

      (2) Malfunction of the acoustic nerve. Evaluate hearing impairment.

      (3) Mastoiditis, chronic. Constant drainage from the mastoid cavity, requiring frequent and prolonged medical care.

      (4) Mastoidectomy. Followed by chronic infection with constant or recurrent drainage requiring frequent or prolonged medical care.

      (5) Meniere's syndrome. Recurring attacks of sufficient frequency and severity as to interfere with satisfactory performance of military duty, or require frequent or prolonged medical care.

      (6) Otitis Media. Moderate, chronic, suppurative, resistant to treatment, and necessitating frequent or prolonged medical care.

   b. Hearing. Retention will be determined on the basis of ability to perform duties of grade or rating.

7. Lungs and Chest Wall.

   a. Tuberculous (TB) Lesions. See www.cdc.gov/tb/.

      (1) Pulmonary tuberculosis.

         (a) When an active duty member's disease is found to be not incident to military service, or when treatment and return to useful duty will probably require more than 15 months, including an appropriate period of convalescence, or if expiration of service will occur before completion of period of hospitalization. (Career members who express a desire to reenlist after treatment may extend their enlistment to cover period of hospitalization.)

         (b) When a Reservist not on active duty has TB that will probably require treatment for more that 12 to 15 months including an appropriate period of convalescence before being able to perform full-time military duty. Individuals who are retained in the Reserve while undergoing treatment may not be called or ordered to active duty (including mobilization), active duty for training, or inactive duty training during the period of treatment and convalescence.

b. <u>Non-tuberculous Conditions</u>. Pulmonary diseases, other than acute infections, must be evaluated in terms of respiratory function, manifested clinically by measurements that must be interpreted as exertional or altitudinal tolerance. Symptoms of cough, pain, and recurrent infections may limit a member's activity. Many of the conditions listed below may coexist and in combination may produce unfitness.

(1) Atelectasis, or massive collapse of the lung. Moderately symptomatic with paroxysmal cough at frequent intervals throughout the day, or with moderate emphysema, or with residuals or complications that require repeated hospitalization.

(2) Bronchial Asthma. Associated with emphysema of sufficient severity to interfere with the satisfactory performance of duty, or with frequent attacks not controlled by inhaled or oral medications, or requiring oral corticosteroids more than twice a year.

(3) Bronchiectasis or bronchiolectasis. Cylindrical or saccular type that is moderately symptomatic, with productive cough at frequent intervals throughout the day, or with moderate other associated lung disease to include recurrent pneumonia, or with residuals or complications that require repeated hospitalization.

(4) Bronchitis. Chronic, severe persistent cough, with considerable expectoration, or with moderate emphysema, or with dyspnea at rest or on slight exertion, or with residuals or complications that require repeated hospitalization.

(5) Cystic disease of the lung, congenital. Involving more than one lobe of a lung.

(6) Diaphragm, congenital defect. Symptomatic.

(7) Hemopneumothorax, hemothorax, or pyopneumothorax. More than moderate pleuritic residuals with persistent underweight, or marked restriction of respiratory excursion and chest deformity, or marked weakness and fatigability on slight exertion.

(8) Histoplasmosis. Chronic and not responding to treatment.

(9) Pleurisy, chronic or pleural adhesions. Severe dyspnea or pain on mild exertion associated with definite evidence of pleural adhesions and demonstrable moderate reduction of pulmonary function.

(10) Pneumothorax, spontaneous. Repeated episodes of pneumothorax not correctable by surgery.

(11) Pneumoconiosis. Severe with dyspnea on mild exertion.

(12) Pulmonary calcification. Multiple calcifications associated with significant respiratory embarrassment or active disease not responsive to treatment.

(13) Pulmonary emphysema. Marked emphysema with dyspnea on mild exertion and demonstrable moderate reduction in pulmonary function.

(14) Pulmonary fibrosis. Linear fibrosis or fibrocalcific residuals that cause dyspnea on mild exertion and demonstrable moderate reduction in pulmonary function.

(15) Pulmonary sarcoidosis. If not responding to therapy and complicated by demonstrable moderate reduction in pulmonary function.

(16) Stenosis, bronchus. Severe stenosis associated with repeated attacks of bronchopulmonary infections requiring frequent hospitalization.

c. Surgery of the Lungs and Chest. Lobectomy. If pulmonary function (ventilatory tests) is impaired to a moderate degree or more.

8. Heart and Vascular System.

   a. Heart.

      (1) Arrhythmias. Associated with organic heart disease, or if not adequately controlled by medication or if they interfere with satisfactory performance of duty.

      (2) Arteriosclerotic disease. Associated with congestive heart failure, repeated anginal attacks, or objective evidence of myocardial infarction.

      (3) Endocarditis. Bacterial endocarditis resulting in myocardial insufficiency or associated with valvular heart disease.

      (4) Heart block. Associated with other symptoms of organic heart disease or syncope (Stokes-Adams Syndrome).

      (5) Myocarditis and degeneration of the myocardium. Myocardial insufficiency resulting in slight limitation of physical activity.

      (6) Pericarditis.

         (a) Chronic constrictive pericarditis unless successful remedial surgery has been performed.

         (b) Chronic serous pericarditis.

      (7) Rheumatic valvulitis and valvular heart disease. Cardiac insufficiency at functional capacity and therapeutic level of class IIC or worse, American Heart Association. A diagnosis made during the initial period of service or enlistment that is determined to be a residual of a condition that existed prior to entry in the service is disqualifying regardless of severity.

   b. Vascular System.

      (1) Arteriosclerosis obliterans. When any of the following pertain:

(a) Intermittent claudication of sufficient severity to produce pain and inability to complete a walk of 200 yards or less on level ground at 112 steps per minute without a rest.

(b) Objective evidence of arterial disease with symptoms of claudication, ischemic chest pain at rest, or with gangrenous or permanent ulcerative skin changes in the distal extremity.

(c) Involvement of more than one organ system or anatomic region (the lower extremities comprise one region for this purpose) with symptoms of arterial insufficiency.

(2) Congenital anomalies. Coarctation of aorta and other congenital anomalies of the cardiovascular system unless satisfactorily treated by surgical correction.

(3) Aneurysms. Aneurysm of any vessel not correctable by surgery and producing limiting symptomatic conditions precluding satisfactory performance of duty. Aneurysm corrected by surgery but with residual limiting symptomatic conditions that preclude satisfactory performance of duty.

(a) Satisfactory performance of duty is precluded because of underlying recurring or progressive disease producing pain, dyspnea, or similar symptomatic limiting conditions.

1. Reconstructive surgery including grafts, when prosthetic devices are attached to or implanted in the heart.

2. Unproven procedures have been accomplished and the patient is unable to satisfactorily perform duty or cannot be returned to duty under circumstances permitting close medical supervision.

(4) Periarteritis nodosa. With definite evidence of functional impairment.

(5) Chronic venous insufficiency (postphlebitic syndrome). When more than mild and symptomatic despite elastic support.

(6) Raynaud's phenomenon. Manifested by trophic changes of the involved part characterized by scarring of the skin or ulceration.

(7) Thrombophlebitis. When repeated attacks require such frequent treatment as to interfere with satisfactory performance of duty.

(8) Varicose veins. Severe and symptomatic despite therapy.

(9) Any condition requiring anti-thrombotic medication other than aspirin.

c. Miscellaneous.

(1) Erythromelalgia. Persistent burning pain in the soles or palms not relieved by treatment.

(2) Hypertensive cardiovascular disease and hypertensive vascular disease.

(a) Diastolic pressure consistently more than 90 mm Hg following an adequate period of therapy on an ambulatory status; or

(b) Any documented history of hypertension regardless of the pressure values if associated with one or more of the following:

1. Cerebrovascular symptoms.

2. Arteriosclerotic heart disease if symptomatic and requiring treatment.

3. Kidney involvement, manifested by unequivocal impairment of renal function.

4. Grade III (Keith-Wagener-Barker) changes in the fundi.

(3) Rheumatic fever, active, with or without heart damage. Recurrent attacks.

(4) Residual of surgery of the heart, pericardium, or vascular system under one or more of the following circumstances:

(a) When surgery of the heart, pericardium, or vascular system results in inability of the individual to perform duties without discomfort or dyspnea.

(b) When the surgery involves insertion of a pacemaker, reconstructive vascular surgery employing exogenous grafting material.

(c) Similar newly developed techniques or prostheses, the individual is unfit.

9. <u>Abdomen and Gastrointestinal System</u>.

   a. <u>Defects and Diseases</u>.

   (1) Achalasia. Manifested by dysphagia not controlled by dilation with frequent discomfort, or inability to maintain normal vigor and nutrition.

   (2) Amebic abscess residuals. Persistent abnormal liver function tests and failure to maintain weight and normal vigor after appropriate treatment.

   (3) Biliary dyskinesia. Frequent abdominal pain not relieved by simple medication, or with periodic jaundice.

   (4) Cirrhosis of the liver. Recurrent jaundice or ascites; or demonstrable esophageal varices or history of bleeding there from.

   (5) Gastritis. Severe, chronic gastritis with repeated symptomatology and hospitalization and confirmed by gastroscopic examination.

   (6) Hepatitis, chronic. When, after a reasonable time (1 to 2 years) following the acute stage, symptoms persist, and there is objective evidence of impaired liver function.

(7) Hernia.

   (a) Hiatus hernia. Severe symptoms not relieved by dietary or medical therapy, or recurrent bleeding in spite of prescribed treatment.

   (b) Other. If operative repair is contraindicated for medical reasons or when not amenable to surgical repair.

(8) Ileitis, regional (Crohn's disease). Except when responding well to ordinary treatment other than oral corticosteroids or immune-suppressant medications.

(9) Pancreatitis, chronic. Frequent severe abdominal pain; or steatorrhea or disturbance of glucose metabolism requiring hypoglycemic agents.

(10) Peritoneal adhesions. Recurring episodes of intestinal obstruction characterized by abdominal colicky pain, vomiting, and intractable constipation requiring frequent hospital admissions.

(11) Proctitis, chronic. Moderate to severe symptoms of bleeding, or painful defecation, tenesmus, and diarrhea, with repeated hospital admissions.

(12) Ulcer, peptic, duodenal, or gastric. Repeated incapacitation or absences from duty because of recurrence of symptoms (pain, vomiting, or bleeding) in spite of good medical management, and supported by laboratory, x-ray, and endoscopic evidence of activity.

(13) Ulcerative colitis. Except when responding well to ordinary treatment.

(14) Rectum, stricture of. Severe symptoms of obstruction characterized by intractable constipation, pain on defecation, difficult bowel movements requiring the regular use of laxatives or enemas, or requiring repeated hospitalization.

b. <u>Surgery</u>.

   (1) Colectomy, partial. When more than mild symptoms of diarrhea remain or if complicated by colostomy.

   (2) Colostomy. When permanent.

   (3) Enterostomy. When permanent.

   (4) Gastrectomy.

      (a) Total.

      (b) Subtotal, with or without vagotomy, or gastrojejunostomy, when, in spite of good medical management, the individual develops one of the following:

         1. "Dumping syndrome" that persists for 6 months postoperatively.

         2. Frequent episodes of epigastric distress with characteristic circulatory symptoms or diarrhea persisting 6 months postoperatively.

3. Continues to demonstrate significant weight loss 6 months postoperatively. Preoperative weight representative of obesity should not be taken as a reference point in making this assessment.

4. Not to be confused with "dumping syndrome," and not ordinarily considered as representative of unfitness are: postoperative symptoms such as moderate feeling of fullness after eating; the need to avoid or restrict ingestion of high carbohydrate foods; the need for daily schedule of a number of small meals with or without additional "snacks."

(5) Gastrostomy. When permanent.

(6) Ileostomy. When permanent.

(7) Pancreatectomy.

(8) Pancreaticoduodenostomy, pancreaticogastrostomy, pancreaticojejunostomy. Followed by more than mild symptoms of digestive disturbance, or requiring insulin.

(9) Proctectomy.

(10) Proctopexy, proctoplasty, proctorrhaphy, or proctotomy. If fecal incontinence remains after appropriate treatment.

(11) Bariatric Surgery and all other forms of weight loss surgery are not authorized. A waiver may be granted for individuals who have had surgery prior to July 01, 2007 and remain world wide deployable. Any complications arising from this surgery that would compromise fitness for duty or world wide deployment may result in separation as a result of PDES action or administrative separation regardless of previously granted waivers

10. Endocrine and Metabolic Conditions (Diseases).

   a. Acromegaly. With function impairment.

   b. Adrenal hyperfunction. That does not respond to therapy satisfactorily or where replacement therapy presents serious problems in management.

   c. Adrenal hypofunction. Requiring medication for control.

   d. Diabetes Insipidus. Unless mild, with good response to treatment.

   e. Diabetes Mellitus. When requiring insulin or not well controlled by oral medications. Diabetes is considered well controlled when the glycohemoglobin is within the normal range. Waivers will be considered on a case-by-case basis for the use of non-insulin injectable medications e.g. Exenatide.

   f. Goiter. With symptoms of breathing obstruction with increased activity, unless correctable.

   g. Gout. With frequent acute exacerbations in spite of therapy, or with severe bone, joint, or kidney damage.

h. Hyperinsulinism. When caused by a malignant tumor, or when the condition is not readily controlled.

i. Hyperparathyroidism. When residuals or complications of surgical correction such as renal disease or bony deformities preclude the reasonable performance of military duty.

j. Hyperthyroidism. Severe symptoms, with or without evidence of goiter, that do not respond to treatment.

k. Hypoparathyroidism. With objective evidence and severe symptoms not controlled by maintenance therapy.

l. Hypothyroidism. With objective evidence and severe symptoms not controlled by medication.

m. Osteomalacia. When residuals after therapy preclude satisfactory performance of duty.

11. Genitourinary System.

   a. Genitourinary conditions.

      (1) Cystitis. When complications or residuals of treatment themselves preclude satisfactory performance of duty.

      (2) Dysmenorrhea. Symptomatic, irregular cycle, not amenable to treatment, and of such severity as to necessitate recurrent absences of more than 1 day/month.

      (3) Endometriosis. Symptomatic and incapacitating to degree that necessitates recurrent absences of more than 1 day/month.

      (4) Hypospadias. Accompanied by chronic infection of the genitourinary tract or instances where the urine is voided in such a manner as to soil clothes or surroundings, and the condition is not amenable to treatment.

      (5) Incontinence of urine. Due to disease or defect not amenable to treatment and so severe as to necessitate recurrent absences from duty.

      (6) Menopausal syndrome, physiologic or artificial. With more than mild mental and constitutional symptoms.

      (7) Strictures of the urethra or ureter. Severe and not amenable to treatment.

      (8) Urethritis, chronic. Not responsive to treatment and necessitating frequent absences from duty.

   b. Kidney.

      (1) Calculus in kidney. Bilateral, recurrent, or symptomatic and not responsive to treatment.

      (2) Congenital abnormality. Bilateral, resulting in frequent or recurring infections, or when there is evidence of obstructive uropathy not responding to medical or surgical treatment.

(3) Cystic kidney (polycystic kidney). When symptomatic and renal function is impaired, or if the focus of frequent infection.

(4) Glomerulonephritis, chronic.

(5) Hydronephrosis. More than mild, or bilateral, or causing continuous or frequent symptoms.

(6) Hypoplasia of the kidney. Associated with elevated blood pressure or frequent infections and not controlled by surgery.

(7) Nephritis, chronic.

(8) Nephrosis.

(9) Perirenal abscess. With residuals that preclude satisfactory performance of duty.

(10) Pyelonephritis or pyelitis. Chronic, that has not responded to medical or surgical treatment, with evidence of persistent hypertension, eyeground changes, or cardiac abnormalities.

(11) Pyonephrosis. Not responding to treatment.

c. <u>Genitourinary and Gynecological Surgery</u>.

(1) Cystectomy.

(2) Cystoplasty. If reconstruction is unsatisfactory or if residual urine persists in excess of 50 cc or if refractory symptomatic infection persists.

(3) Nephrectomy. When, after treatment, there is infection or pathology in the remaining kidney.

(4) Nephrostomy. If drainage persists.

(5) Oophorectomy. When, following treatment and convalescent period, there remain incapacitating mental or constitutional symptoms.

(6) Penis, amputation of.

(7) Pyelostomy. If drainage persists.

(8) Ureterocolostomy.

(9) Ureterocystostomy. When both ureters are markedly dilated with irreversible changes.

(10) Ureterocystostomy, cutaneous.

(11) Ureteroplasty.

(a) When unilateral procedure is unsuccessful and nephrectomy is necessary, consider on the basis of the standard for a nephrectomy.

(b) When bilateral, evaluate residual obstruction or hydronephrosis and consider unfitness on the basis of the residuals involved.

(12) Ureterosigmoidostomy.

(13) Ureterostomy. External or cutaneous.

(14) Urethrostomy. When a satisfactory urethra cannot be restored.

12. <u>Extremities</u>.

   a. <u>Upper</u>.

      (1) Amputations. Amputation of part or parts of an upper extremity equal to or greater than any of the following:

         (a) A thumb proximal to the interphalangeal joints.

         (b) Two fingers of one hand.

         (c) One finger, other than the little finger, at the metacarpophalangeal joint and the thumb of the same hand at the interphalangeal joint.

      (2) Joint ranges of motion. Motion that does not equal or exceed the measurements listed below. Measurements must be made with a goniometer and conform to the methods illustrated in 3-F-EXHIBIT 1.

         (a) Shoulder.

            1. Forward elevation to 90°.

            2. Abduction to 90°.

         (b) Elbow.

            1. Flexion to 100°.

            2. Extension to 60°.

         (c) Wrist. A total range, extension plus flexion, of 15°

         (d) Hand. For this purpose, combined joint motion is the arithmetic sum of the motion at each of the three finger joints.

            1. An active flexor value of combined joint motions of 135° in each of two or more fingers of the same hand.

            2. An active extensor value of combined joint motions of 75° in each of the same two or more fingers.

            3. Limitation of motion of the thumb that precludes apposition to at least two finger tips.

      (3) Recurrent dislocations of the shoulder. When not repairable or surgery is contraindicated.

b. <u>Lower</u>.

   (1) Amputations.

      (a) Loss of a toe or toes that precludes the ability to run, or walk without a perceptible limp, or to engage in fairly strenuous jobs.

      (b) Any loss greater than that specified above to include foot, leg, or thigh.

   (2) Feet.

      (a) Hallux valgus. When moderately severe, with exostosis or rigidity and pronounced symptoms; or severe with arthritic changes.

      (b) Pes Planus. Symptomatic more than moderate, with pronation on weight bearing that prevents wearing military shoes, or when associated with vascular changes.

      (c) Talipes cavus. When moderately severe, with moderate discomfort on prolonged standing and walking, metatarsalgia, or that prevents wearing a military shoe.

   (3) Internal derangement of the knee. Residual instability following remedial measures, if more than moderate; or with recurring episodes of effusion or locking, resulting in frequent incapacitation.

   (4) Joint ranges of motion. Motion that does not equal or exceed the measurements listed below. Measurements must be made with a goniometer and conform to the methods illustrated in 3-F-EXHIBIT 2.

      (a) Hip.

         1. Flexion to 90°.

         2. Extension to 0.

      (b) Knee.

         1. Flexion to 90°.

         2. Extension to 15°.

      (c) Ankle.

         1. Dorsiflexion to 10°.

         2. Plantar Flexion to 10°.

   (5) Shortening of an extremity, which exceeds two inches.

c. Miscellaneous.

   (1) Arthritis.

      (a) Due to infection. Associated with persistent pain and marked loss of function with x-ray evidence and documented history of recurring incapacity for prolonged periods.

      (b) Due to trauma. When surgical treatment fails or is contraindicated and there is functional impairment of the involved joint that precludes satisfactory performance of duty.

      (c) Osteoarthritis. Severe symptoms associated with impaired function, supported by x-ray evidence and documented history of recurrent incapacity for prolonged periods.

      (d) Rheumatoid arthritis or rheumatoid myositis. Substantiated history of frequent incapacitating and prolonged periods supported by objective and subjective findings.

      (e) Seronegative Spondylarthropaties. Severe symptoms associated with impaired function, supported by X-ray evidence and documented history of recurrent incapacity for prolonged periods.

   (2) Chondromalacia or Osteochondritis Dessicans. Severe, manifested by frequent joint effusion, more than moderate interference with function or with severe residuals from surgery.

   (3) Fractures.

      (a) Malunion. When, after appropriate treatment, there is more than moderate malunion with marked deformity or more than moderate loss of function.

      (b) Nonunion. When, after an appropriate healing period, the nonunion precludes satisfactory performance of military duty.

      (c) Bone fusion defect. When manifested by more than moderate pain or loss of function.

      (d) Callus, excessive, following fracture. When functional impairment precludes satisfactory performance of duty and the callus does not respond to adequate treatment.

   (4) Joints.

      (a) Arthroplasty. With severe pain, limitation of motion and function.

      (b) Bony or fibrous ankylosis. Severe pain involving major joints or spinal segments in an unfavorable position, or with marked loss of function.

(c) Contracture of joint. Marked loss of function and the condition is not remediable by surgery.

(d) Loose bodies within a joint. Marked functional impairment complicated by arthritis that precludes favorable treatment or not remediable by surgery.

(5) Muscles.

(a) Flaccid paralysis of one or more muscles, producing loss of function that precludes satisfactory performance of duty following surgical correction or if not remediable by surgery.

(b) Spastic paralysis of one or more muscles producing loss of function that precludes satisfactory performance of duty.

(6) Myotonia congenita.

(7) Osteitis deformans. Involvement of single or multiple bones with resultant deformities, or symptoms severely interfering with function.

(8) Osteoarthropathy, hypertrophic, secondary. Moderately severe to severe pain present with joint effusion occurring intermittently in one or multiple joints and with at least moderate loss of function.

(9) Osteomyelitis, chronic. Recurrent episodes not responsive to treatment, and involving the bone to a degree that interferes with stability and function.

(10) Tendon transplant. Fair or poor restoration of function with weakness that seriously interferes with the function of the affected part.

13. <u>Spine, Scapulae, Ribs, and Sacroiliac Joints</u>.

   a. <u>Congenital anomalies</u>.

   (1) Spina bifida. Demonstrable signs and moderate symptoms of root or cord involvement.

   (2) Spondylolysis or spondylolisthesis. With more than mild symptoms resulting in repeated hospitalization or significant assignment limitation.

   b. <u>Coxa vara</u>. More than moderate with pain, deformity, and arthritic changes.

   c. <u>Herniation of nucleus pulposus</u>. More than mild symptoms following appropriate treatment or remediable measures, with sufficient objective findings to demonstrate interference with the satisfactory performance of duty.

   d. <u>Kyphosis</u>. More than moderate, or interfering with function, or causing unmilitary appearance.

   e. <u>Scoliosis</u>. Severe deformity with over two inches of deviation of tips of spinous processes from the midline.

14. Skin and Cellular Tissues.

    a. Acne. Severe, unresponsive to treatment, and interfering with the satisfactory performance of duty or wearing of the uniform or other military equipment.

    b. Atopic dermatitis. More than moderate or requiring periodic hospitalization.

    c. Amyloidosis. Generalized.

    d. Cysts and tumors. See section 3-F-20.

    e. Dermatitis herpetiformis. If fails to respond to therapy.

    f. Dermatomyositis.

    g. Dermographism. Interfering with satisfactory performance of duty.

    h. Eczema, chronic. Regardless of type, when there is more than minimal involvement and the condition is unresponsive to treatment and interferes with the satisfactory performance of duty.

    i. Elephantiasis or chronic lymphedema. Not responsive to treatment.

    j. Epidermolysis bullosa.

    k. Erythema multiforme. More than moderate and chronic or recurrent.

    l. Exfoliative dermatitis. Chronic.

    m. Fungus infections, superficial or systemic. If not responsive to therapy and interfering with the satisfactory performance of duty.

    n. Hidradenitis suppurative and folliculitis decalvans.

    o. Hyperhydrosis. Of the hands or feet, when severe or complicated by a dermatitis or infection, either fungal or bacterial, and not amenable to treatment.

    p. Leukemia cutis and mycosis fungoides.

    q. Lichen planus. Generalized and not responsive to treatment.

    r. Lupus erythematous. Chronic with extensive involvement of the skin and mucous membranes and when the condition does not respond to treatment.

    s. Neurofibromatosis. If repulsive in appearance or when interfering with satisfactory performance of duty.

    t. Panniculitis. Relapsing febrile, nodular.

u. Parapsoriasis. Extensive and not controlled by treatment.

v. Pemphigus. Not responsive to treatment, and with moderate constitutional or systemic symptoms, or interfering with satisfactory performance of duty.

w. Psoriasis. Extensive and not controllable by treatment.

x. Radiodermatitis. If resulting in malignant degeneration at a site not amenable to treatment.

y. Scars and keloids. So extensive or adherent that they seriously interfere with the function of an extremity.

z. Scleroderma. Generalized, or of the linear type that seriously interferes with the function of an extremity or organ.

aa. Ulcers of the skin. Not responsive to treatment after an appropriate period of time or if interfering with satisfactory performance of duty.

bb. Urticaria. Chronic, severe, and not amenable to treatment.

cc. Xanthoma. Regardless of type, but only when interfering with the satisfactory performance of duty.

dd. Other skin disorders. If chronic, or of a nature that requires frequent medical care or interferes with satisfactory performance of military duty.

15. Neurological Disorders.

    a. Amyotrophic sclerosis, lateral.

    b. Atrophy, muscular, myelopathic. Includes severe residuals of poliomyelitis.

    c. Atrophy, muscular. Progressive muscular atrophy.

    d. Chorea. Chronic and progressive.

    e. Convulsive disorders. (This does not include convulsive disorders caused by, and exclusively incident to the use of, alcohol.) Following a seizure, the member is NFFD, and will remain unfit until he/she is controlled with medications with no seizures for twelve months. A medical board is not required if the convulsive disorder is well controlled.

    f. Friedreich's ataxia.

    g. Hepatolenticular degeneration.

    h. Migraine. Manifested by frequent incapacitating attacks or attacks that last for several consecutive days and unrelieved by treatment.

i. <u>Multiple sclerosis</u>.

j. <u>Myelopathy transverse</u>.

k. <u>Narcolepsy, cataplexy, and hypersomnolence</u>.

l. <u>Obstructive Sleep Apnea</u>. When not correctable by use of CPAP or surgical means.

m. <u>Paralysis, agitans</u>.

n. <u>Peripheral nerve conditions</u>.

   (1) Neuralgia. When symptoms are severe, persistent, and not responsive to treatment.

   (2) Neuritis. When manifested by more than moderate, permanent functional impairment.

o. <u>Syringomyelia</u>.

p. <u>General</u>. Any other neurological condition, regardless of etiology, when after adequate treatment, there remain residuals, such as persistent severe headaches, convulsions not controlled by medications, weakness or paralysis of important muscle groups, deformity, incoordination, pain or sensory disturbance, disturbance loss of consciousness, speech or mental defects, or personality changes of such a degree as to definitely interfere with the performance of duty.

16. <u>Psychiatric Disorders</u>. (See Chapter 5 Section B of this manual concerning disposition.)

    a. <u>Disorders with Psychotic Features</u>. Recurrent psychotic episodes, existing symptoms or residuals thereof, or recent history of psychotic reaction sufficient to interfere with performance of duty or with social adjustment.

    b. <u>Affective disorders; anxiety, post-traumatic stress disorder or somatoform disorders</u>. Persistence or recurrence of symptoms sufficient to require treatment (medication, counseling, psychological or psychiatric therapy) for greater than twelve (12) months. Prophylactic treatment associated with significant medication side effects such as sedation, dizziness, or cognitive changes or requiring frequent follow-up that limit duty options is disqualifying. Prophylactic treatment with medication may continue indefinitely as long as the member remains asymptomatic following initial therapy. Any member requiring medication for any of the above disorders must be removed from aviation duty. (Incapacity of motivation or underlying personality traits or disorders will be processed administratively. See Personnel Manual, COMDTINST M1000.6 (series) for further guidance.)

    c. <u>Mood disorders</u>. Bipolar disorders or recurrent major depression do not require the six (6) month evaluation period prior to initiating a medical board. All other mood disorders associated with suicide attempt, untreated substance abuse, requiring hospitalization, or requiring treatment (including medication, counseling, psychological or psychiatric therapy) for more than twelve (12) months.

Prophylactic treatment associated with significant side effects such as sedation, dizziness, or cognitive changes, or frequent follow-up that limit duty options is disqualifying. Prophylactic treatment with medication(s) may continue indefinitely as long as the member remains asymptomatic following initial therapy. Any member requiring medication for any of the above disorders must be removed from aviation duty. (Incapacity of motivation or underlying personality traits or disorders will be processed administratively. See Personnel Manual, COMDTINST M1000.6 (series) for further guidance.)

 d. <u>Personality; sexual; factitious; psychoactive substance use disorders; personality trait(s); disorders of impulse control not elsewhere classified</u>. These conditions may render an individual administratively unfit rather than unfit because of a physical impairment. Interference with performance of effective duty will be dealt with through appropriate administrative channels (see Chapter 5 Section B).

 e. <u>Adjustment Disorders</u>. Transient, situational maladjustment due to acute or special stress does not render an individual unfit because of physical impairment. However, if these conditions are recurrent and interfere with military duty, are not amenable to treatment, or require prolonged treatment, administrative separation should be recommended (see Chapter 5 Section B).

 f. <u>Disorders usually evident in infancy, childhood, or adolescence, disorders of intelligence</u>. These disorders, to include developmental disorders, may render an individual administratively unfit rather than unfit because of a physical impairment. Anorexia Nervosa and Bulimia are processed through PDES, while the remaining are handled administratively, if the condition significantly impacts, or has the potential to significantly impact performance of duties (health, mission, and/or safety). Use of non-controlled medications such as Atomoxetine or Buproprion to treat, control, or improve performance for individuals diagnosed with Attention Deficit Disorder (either ADD or ADHD) may be allowed in individuals when a good prognosis is present. Individuals with Attention Deficit Disorder that significantly impacts performance despite treatment, or if treatment is refused or due to non-compliance, have a disqualifying condition and are processed administratively as per Chapter 12 of the CG Personnel Manual, COMDTINST M1000.6 (series).

17. <u>Dental</u>. Diseases and abnormalities of the jaws or associated tissues when, following restorative surgery, there remain residual conditions that are incapacitating or interfere with the individual's satisfactory performance of military duty, or deformities that are disfiguring. Personnel must be in a Class 1 or Class 2 (see 4.C.3.c.(3)) dental status to execute sea duty or overseas duty orders. Prior service personnel must meet the enlistment dental standards contained in section 3-D.

18. <u>Blood and Blood-Forming Tissue Diseases</u>. When response to therapy is unsatisfactory, or when therapy requires prolonged, intensive medical supervision.

 a. <u>Anemia</u>.

 b. <u>Hemolytic disease, chronic and symptomatic</u>.

c. <u>Leukemia, chronic</u>.

d. <u>Polycythemia</u>.

e. <u>Purpura and other bleeding diseases</u>. Any condition requiring long-term coumadin.

f. <u>Thromboembolic disease</u>.

g. <u>Splenomegaly, chronic</u>.

19. <u>Systemic Diseases, General Defects, and Miscellaneous Conditions</u>.

   a. <u>Systemic Diseases</u>.

      (1) Blastomycosis.

      (2) Brucellosis. Chronic with substantiated recurring febrile episodes, severe fatigability, lassitude, depression, or general malaise.

      (3) Leprosy. Any type.

      (4) Myasthenia gravis.

      (5) Porphyria Cutanea Tarda.

      (6) Sarcoidosis. Progressive, with severe or multiple organ involvement and not responsive to therapy.

      (7) Tuberculosis (TB).

         (a) Meningitis, tuberculosis.

         (b) Pulmonary TB, tuberculous empyema, and tuberculous pleurisy.

         (c) TB of the male genitalia. Involvement of the prostate or seminal vesicles and other instances not corrected by surgical excision, or when residuals are more than minimal, or are symptomatic.

         (d) TB of the female genitalia.

         (e) TB of the kidney.

         (f) TB of the larynx.

         (g) TB of the lymph nodes, skin, bone, joints, eyes, intestines, and peritoneum or mesentery will be evaluated on an individual basis considering the associated involvement, residuals, and complications.

      (8) Symptomatic neurosyphilis. In any form.

   b. <u>General Defects</u>.

      (1) Visceral, abdominal, or cerebral allergy. Severe or not responsive to therapy.

(2) Cold injury. Evaluate on severity and extent of residuals, or loss of parts as outlined in section 3-F-12.

c. Miscellaneous Conditions or circumstances.

(1) Chronic Fatigue Syndrome, Fibromyalgia, and Myofascial Syndrome when not controlled by medication or with reliably diagnosed depression.

(2) The individual is precluded from a reasonable fulfillment of the purpose of employment in the military service.

(3) The individual's health or well-being would be compromised if allowed to remain in the military service.

(4) The individual's retention in the military service would prejudice the best interests of the Government.

(5) Required chronic and continuous DEA controlled (Class I-V) medications, such as Ritalin, Amphetamine, Cylert, Modafanil.

(6) Required chronic anti-coagulant, other than aspirin, such as Coumadin.

(7) Chronic (greater than 30 days per year) use of immunosuppressive medications including steroids.

20. Tumors and Malignant Diseases.

a. Malignant Neoplasms. If they are unresponsive to therapy or when the residuals of treatment are in themselves disqualifying under other provisions of this section or in individuals on active duty when they preclude satisfactory performance of duty.

b. Neoplastic Conditions of Lymphoid and Blood Forming Tissues. Render an individual unfit for further military service.

c. Benign Neoplasms. Except as noted below, benign neoplasms are not generally a cause of unfitness because they are usually remediable. Individuals who refuse treatment are unfit only if their condition precludes satisfactory performance of military duty. However, the following normally render the individual unfit for further military service:

(1) Ganglioneuroma.

(2) Meningeal fibroblastoma. When the brain is involved.

21. Sexually Transmitted Infection. Complications or residuals of such chronicity or degree of severity that the individual is incapable of performing useful duty.

22. Human Immunodeficiency Virus (HIV). CG personnel who demonstrate no evidence of unfitting conditions of immunologic deficiency, neurologic deficiency, and progressive clinical or laboratory abnormalities associated with HIV or AIDS-defining condition shall be retained in the service unless some other reason for separation exists. Military personnel who are HIV antibody positive and retained shall not be assigned to

deployable billets (e.g. cutters, Patrol Force South West Asia, Deployable Operations Group units), or small boat stations or outside the continental United States. COMDTINST M6230.9, Coast Guard Human Immunodeficiency Virus (HIV) Program provides detailed guidance on identification, surveillance and administration of CG personnel infected with HIV.

23. <u>Transplant recipient</u>. Any organ or tissue except hair or skin.

3-F – EXHIBIT 1
MEASUREMENT OF ANKYLOSIS AND JOINT MOTION
UPPER EXTREMITIES

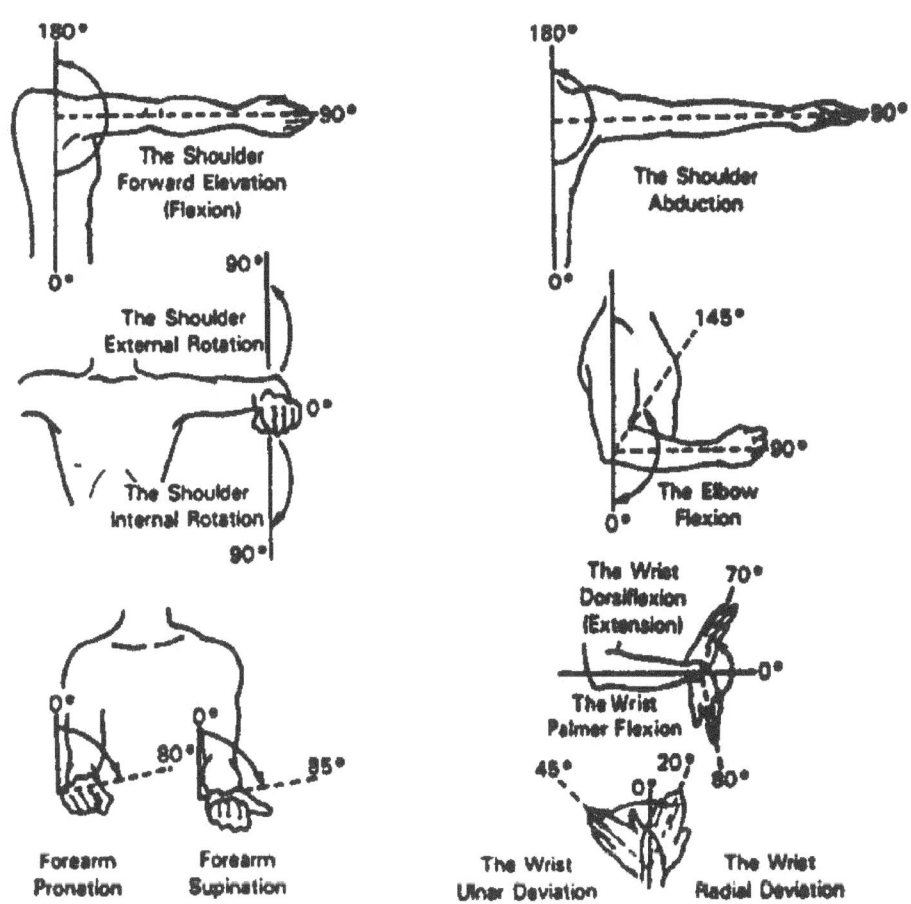

This Exhibit provides a standardized description of ankylosis and joint motion measurement of the upper extremities. The anatomical position is considered as 0° with two major exceptions: (1) in measuring shoulder rotation, the arm is abducted to 90° and the elbow is flexed to 90° so that the forearm reflects the midpoint (0°) between internal and external rotation of the shoulder; and (2) in measuring pronation and supination, with the arm next to the body and the elbow flexed to 90°, the forearm is in mid position (0°) between pronation and supination when the thumb is uppermost.

3-F — EXHIBIT 2
MEASUREMENT OF ANKYLOSIS AND JOINT MOTION
LOWER EXTREMITIES

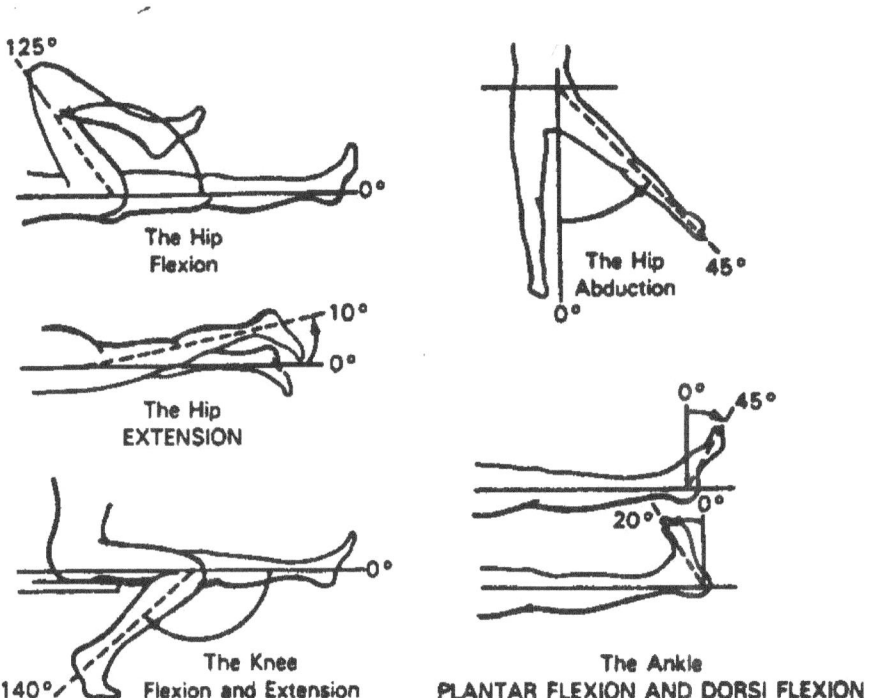

This Exhibit provides a standardized description of ankylosis and joint motion measurement of the lower extremities. The anatomical position is considered as 0°.

Section G. Physical Standards for Aviation

1. Classification of Aviation Personnel. 1
2. General Instructions for Aviation Examinations. 1
3. Restrictions Until Physically Qualified. 4
4. Standards for Class 1. 4
5. Candidates for Flight Training...7
6. Requirements for Class 2 Aircrew...10
7. Requirements for Class 2 Medical Personnel. 10
8. Requirements for Class 2 Technical Observers...11
9. Requirements for Class 2 Air Traffic Controllers...11
10. Requirements for Landing Signal Officer (LSO). 11
11. Refractive Surgery. 12
12. Contact Lenses...13

This page intentionally left blank.

G. Physical Standards for Aviation.

1. Classification of Aviation Personnel.

   a. Aviation Personnel in General. Classification of CG aviation personnel is similar to that prescribed for Navy aviation personnel. The term "aviation personnel" includes all individuals who, in the performance of their duty, are required to make frequent aerial flights. Aviation personnel are divided into two classes: Class 1 and Class 2.

   b. Class 1. Class 1 consists of aviation personnel engaged in actual control of aircraft, which includes aviators, student aviators, and student Flight Surgeons that are chosen to perform solo flights.

   c. Changing Classes. Except for changes in class due solely to age, individuals requiring a change in their classification for more than two months must submit the following to Commander PSC:

      (1) Medical Record, SF-507 completed by a Flight Surgeon/Aviation Medical Officer stating the need for the class change and whether a permanent or temporary change is requested; and

      (2) Command endorsement.

   d. Class 2. Class 2 consists of aviation personnel not engaged in actual control of aircraft. This includes aviation observers, technical observers, Flight Surgeons, Aviation Medical Officers, Aviation Mission Specialists, aircrew members, Air Traffic Controllers, and other persons ordered to duty involving flying.

2. General Instructions for Aviation Examinations.

   a. Object of Aviation Physical Examinations.

      (1) The examination for flying shall be limited to members of the aeronautical organization and authorized candidates. The object of an aviation physical examination is to ensure individuals involved in aviation are physically and mentally qualified for such duty, and to remove from aviation those who are temporarily or permanently unfit because of physical or mental defect.

      (2) The main objective in examining candidates for flight training is selecting individuals who can fly safely and continue to do so for at least 20 years.

      (3) For designated aviators, the objective is to determine if the individual can fly safely during the next 24 months.

b. <u>Performance of Aviation Physical Examinations</u>. To promote safety and to provide uniformity and completeness, an aviation physical examination must be performed by a currently qualified Flight Surgeon (FS), Flight Surgeon Trainee (FST), Aviation Medical Officer (AMO), or Aeromedical Physician Assistant (APA) authorized by the Commandant or currently serving in the DOD. Only physicians or physician assistants who have successfully passed a course at a school of aviation medicine of the U. S. Armed Forces leading to the designation of "Flight Surgeon", "Aviation Medical Officer" or "Aeromedical Physician Assistant" are so authorized. Civilian physicians who were military Flight Surgeons and who are currently certified by the Federal Aviation Administration as aviation medical examiners may also be authorized. Flight physicals performed by a DOD Flight Surgeon and approved through Army or Navy channels will be accepted as an approved flight physical.

c. <u>Scope of Aviation Physical Examination</u>. In addition to the general service requirements specified in section 3-D, certain special requirements must be met by the various categories of individuals concerned with aviation. The extent of the examination and the physical standards vary for the several categories of aviation personnel. The term "flight or aviation physical examination" is therefore incomplete unless the character of the duty that the examinee is to perform is specified--this incomplete term shall not be used in item #16 of Report of Medical Examination, DD-2808 as the purpose of the examination. Examiners shall conduct aviation physical examinations in accordance with the general procedures specified in this section and in section 3-C.

d. <u>Required Aviation Physical Examinations</u>. Each individual in the Service who is assigned to duty requiring performance of frequent aerial flights, regardless of classification, must have passed an aviation physical within the preceding 24 months. In some cases, more frequent examinations are required. Aviation physical examinations are required as indicated in this section. They may also be ordered whenever needed to determine an individual's physical fitness for the type aviation duty to which assigned.

   (1) <u>Entry on Active Duty</u>. Reserve aviation personnel who perform frequent aerial flights must have passed an aviation physical examination, commensurate with the type of duty to be performed, within the 24 months preceding active duty or active duty for training. Aviators who are not members of aviation reserve units must have satisfactorily passed an aviation physical examination within six months immediately preceding the actual control of aircraft.

   (2) <u>Biennial</u>. All aviation personnel, including Reservists on inactive duty for training, who will actually control aircraft or perform frequent aerial flights must obtain a biennial aviation physical examination commensurate with the type of duty to be performed. The examination

is required every two (2) years after initial designation. Upon reaching age 50, the examinations become annual.

(3) <u>Direct Commission</u>. An aviation physical examination is required prior to direct commissioning of aviators in the Reserve. The aviator is required to meet Class I standards.

(4) <u>Candidates for Designation as Class 1</u>. All candidates for flight training, whether or not they are already in the Service, must pass a physical examination for flight training duty. The examination date must not precede the application date by more than 12 months.

(5) <u>Candidates for Designation as Class 2</u>. An approved aviation physical examination less than 24 months old is required both when applying for a Class 2 aviation training program and prior to a Class 2 designation.

(6) <u>FAA Airmen Medical Certificate</u>. After receiving Federal Aviation Administration (FAA) Aviation Medical Examiner (AME) training, CG Flight Surgeons/AMOs may request authorization from Commandant (CG-1121) to perform Second and Third Class physical examinations and issue FAA Medical Certificates to all military personnel on active duty including active duty for training. The FAA Administrator furnishes AME's with the necessary instructions, guides, and forms required for this purpose. Except in those instances where there is a military requirement for FAA certification, examination and issuance of medical certificates shall not interfere with the Flight Surgeon's primary duties. Whenever possible, certificates should be obtained in conjunction with a required aviation physical examination.

(7) <u>Aircraft Accidents</u>. Any CG member involved in a Class A or B aircraft mishap in which damage to the aircraft or injury to any crewmember occurs shall undergo a complete aviation physical examination as part of the mishap investigation. Examinations after other mishaps are left to the discretion of the Flight Surgeon/AMO.

(8) <u>Quinquennial</u>. The quinquennial examination of a Reserve aviation special duty officer must be an aviation physical examination.

(9) <u>Separation</u>. An aviation physical examination is not required of aviation personnel being separated from active duty. The requirements for examination are the same as those for the separation from active duty of non-aviation personnel.

e. <u>Boards</u>. Assignment to and continuation of duty involving flying is an administrative process. Except for enlisted personnel in aviation ratings, fitness to perform aviation duties is a determination independent of the determination of fitness for continued service. The process regarding physical disqualifications and waivers for aviation personnel is outlined in the Coast Guard Aviation Medicine Manual, COMDTINST 6410.3 (series).

    f. Reporting Fitness for Flying Duties. The process for reporting fitness for duty for aviation personnel is outlined in the Coast Guard Aviation Medicine Manual, COMDTINST 6410.3.

    g. Reporting Aviation Physical Examinations. The process for reporting aviation physical examinations for aviation personnel is outlined in the CG Aviation Medicine Manual, COMDTINST 6410.3.

3. Restrictions Until Physically Qualified. The process regarding restrictions until physically qualified for aviation personnel is outlined in the CG Aviation Medicine Manual, COMDTINST 6410.3 (series).

4. Standards for Class 1.

    a. General. The physical examination and physical standards for Class 1 are the same as those prescribed in sections 3-C and 3-D of this Manual, as modified by the following subparagraphs.

    b. History.

        (1) History of any of the following is disqualifying: seizures, isolated or repetitive (grand mal, petit mal, psychomotor, or Jacksonian); head injury complicated by unconsciousness in excess of 12 hours or post traumatic amnesia or impaired judgment exceeding 48 hours; malaria, until adequate therapy has been completed and there are no symptoms while off all medication for 3 months.

        (2) For persons already in the CG a complete review of their health record is most important. Flight Surgeons are authorized to postpone the examination of persons who fail to present their health record at the time of examination. In exercising this prerogative, due consideration must be made in cases where access to the individual's health record is administratively impracticable.

    c. Therapeutics and General Fitness. Note on the Report of Medical Examination, DD-2808 if the individual received medication or other therapeutic procedures within 24 hours of the examination. In general, individuals requiring therapeutics or who have observed lowering of general fitness (dietary, rest, emotional, etc.,) which might affect their flying proficiency shall not be found qualified for duty involving flying.

    d. Each aviation physical will have a Valsalva, and AA (Aeronautical Adaptability) performed and noted.

    e. Height. Minimum 157.4 cm (62 inches). Maximum 198 cm (78 inches).

f. <u>Chest</u>. Any condition that serves to impair respiratory function may be cause for rejection. Pulmonary function tests are recommended to evaluate individuals with a history of significant respiratory system problems.

g. <u>Skin</u>. Psoriasis unless mild by degree, not involving nail-pitting and not interfering with the wearing of military equipment or clothing.

h. <u>Cardiovascular System</u>.

   (1) Cardiac arrhythmia, heart murmur, or other evidence of cardiovascular abnormalities shall be carefully studied. Evidence of organic heart disease, rhythm disturbances or vascular diseases, if considered to impair the performance of flying duties, is cause for rejection.

   (2) Sinus Bradycardia. Extreme sinus bradycardia may be a reflection of an underlying conduction system abnormality. There may be an inability to increase the heart rate in response to increased demand.

   (a) <u>Waiver: If the heart rate increases with exercise, the bradycardia is NCD, and no waiver is required.</u>

   1. If the resting HR is less than 50, supply a current EKG demonstrating a sinus rhythm without evidence of prolonged QT, pre-excitation (ie WPW etc) cardiac hypertrophy, heart block, or ischemic changes. Any such changes require further work up.

   2. Provide a rhythm strip demonstrating a rise of at least 10 bpm from baseline with exercise in less than 2 minutes.

   (b) <u>Treatment: No treatment is indicated if the rate increases with exercise; the condition is NCD.</u>

   (c) <u>Discussion: A resting HR<50 bpm in our population is almost usually caused by excellent physical conditioning.</u>

i. <u>Teeth</u>. The following are disqualifying:

   (1) Any carious teeth that would react adversely to sudden changes in barometric pressure or produce indistinct speech by direct voice or radio transmission.

   (2) Any dental defect that would react adversely to sudden changes in barometric pressure or produce indistinct speech by direct voice or radio transmission.

   (3) Fixed active orthodontic appliances require a waiver from PSC (opm or epm). Fixed retainers are exempts.

(4) Routine crown and temporary dental work is not disqualifying for aviation missions. Recommend that temporary crowns be cemented with permanent cement like polycarboxylate or zinc oxyphosphate cement until the permanent crown is delivered. Recommend temporary grounding of 6-12 hours after procedures. Such work may be disqualifying for deployment.

j. Distant Visual Acuity. Distant visual acuity shall be not less than 20/200 in either eye and if less than 20/20 must be correctable to 20/20 with standard lenses. When the visual acuity of either eye is less than 20/20 correction shall be worn at all times while flying.

k. Oculomotor Balance. The following are disqualifying:

(1) Esophoria greater than 10 prism diopters.

(2) Exophoria greater than 10 prism diopters.

(3) Hyperphoria greater than 1.5 prism diopters.

(4) Prism divergence at 20 feet and 13 inches is optional. These tests shall be accomplished only on designated aviators who have sustained significant head injury, central nervous system disease, or who have demonstrated a change in their phorias.

l. Eyes. Any pathologic condition that may become worse or interfere with proper eye function under the environmental and operational conditions of flying disqualifies. History of radial keratotomy is disqualifying. Intraocular pressures shall be tested and reported with each periodic exam.

m. Near Visual Acuity. Uncorrected near vision (both eyes) shall be not less than 20/200 correctable to 20/20, with correction worn in multivision lenses while flying if uncorrected near vision is less than 20/40 in either eye.

n. Color Vision. Normal color perception is required. The testing for color vision must be unaided or with standard corrective lenses only. Use of any lenses (such as Chromagen) or other device to compensate for defective color vision is prohibited. See Chapter 3 Section C. 22. i. for details on how to perform the test.

o. Depth Perception. Normal depth perception is required. When any correction is required for normal depth perception it must be worn at all times. See Chapter 3 Section C. 22. j. for details on how to perform the test.

p. Field of Vision. The field of vision for each eye shall be normal as determined by the finger fixation test. When there is evidence of abnormal contraction of the field of vision in either eye, the examinee shall be subjected to perimetric study for form. Any contraction of the form field of 15 degrees or more in any meridian is disqualifying.

q. Refraction. There are no refractive limits.

r. Ophthalmoscopic Examination. Any abnormality disclosed on ophthalmoscopic examination that materially interferes with normal ocular function is disqualifying. Other abnormal disclosures indicative of disease, other than those directly affecting the eyes, shall be considered with regard to the importance of those conditions.

s. Ear. The examination shall relate primarily to equilibrium and the patency of eustachian tubes. A perforation or evidence of present inflammation is disqualifying. The presence of a small scar with no hearing deficiency and no evidence of inflammation does not disqualify. Perforation, or marked retraction of a drum membrane associated with chronic ear disease, is disqualifying.

t. Sickle Cell Preparation Test. Quantitative hemoglobin electrophoreses greater than 40% Hemoglobin-s is disqualifying because of the risk of hypoxia induced red blood cell deformation in the aviation environment.

5. Candidates for Flight Training.

    a. Standards. Candidates for flight training shall meet all the requirements of Class 1, with the following additions or limitations:

        (1) Cardiovascular.

            (a) Candidates with accessory conduction pathways (Wolff-Parkinson-White (WPW), other ventricular pre-excitation patterns) are CD. No waiver is recommended for candidates with this condition.

            (b) Candidates with WPW Syndrome who have had definitive treatment via Radio Frequency (RF) ablation with demonstrable non-conduction on follow-up Electrophysiologic Studies (EPS) are considered for waiver on a case-by-case basis.

            (c) Asymptomatic candidates: When incidentally noted accessory bypass tracts, proven incapable of sustained rapid conduction as demonstrated by EPS, is discovered in a candidate, the candidate (if asymptomatic), will be considered qualified. In general, EPS is not recommended in asymptomatic individuals.

        (2) Height. Candidates for Class I training must also satisfy the following anthropometric requirements: Refer to figure 3-G-1 through figure 3-G-4 for guidelines on measurements.

            (a) Sitting height: 33 inches to 40.9 inches. Record in parentheses in Item 73, Report of Medical Examination, DD-2808 (SH_____), see figure 3-G-1 for proper measurements.

(b) <u>Sitting eye height</u>: 28.5 inches or greater. Record in parentheses in Item 73, Report of Medical Examination, DD-2808 (SEH_____), see figure 3-G-2 for proper measurements.

(c) <u>Thumb tip reach</u>: 28.5 inches or greater. Record in parentheses in Item 73, Report of Medical Examination, DD-2808 (TTR_____), see figure 3-G-3 for proper measurements.

(d) <u>Buttock-knee length</u>: 21 inches to 27.9 inches. Record in parentheses in Item 73, Report of Medical Examination, DD-2808 (BKL_____), see figure 3-G-3 for proper measurements.

(e) <u>Add</u>: sitting eye height (SEH) and thumb tip reach (TTR), 57 inches or greater. Record in parentheses in Item 73, Report of Medical Examination, DD-2808 (SEH + TTR = _____).

(3) <u>Vision</u>.

(a) Uncorrected distant visual acuity must be not less than 20/50 each eye and correctable 20/20 each eye. Uncorrected near visual acuity must be not less than 20/20 each eye (may be waiverable).

(b) While under the effects of a cycloplegic, the candidate must read 20/20 each eye. The following are disqualifying:

1. Total myopia greater than (minus) -2.00 diopters in any meridian.

2. Total hyperopia greater than (plus) +3.00 diopters in any meridian.

3. Astigmatism greater than (minus) -0.75 diopters. (Report the astigmatic correction in terms of the negative cylinder required.)

4. The purpose of this cycloplegic examination is to detect large latent refractive errors that could result in a change of classes during an aviation career. Therefore, the maximum correction tolerated at an acuity of 20/20 shall be reported. Cycloplegics reported as any other acuity, e.g., 20/15 will be returned.

(c) Refractive Surgery: The CG will consider sending candidates to Navy Flight School who have had photorefractive keratectomy, (anterior corneal stromal surface laser ablation), and meet all of the enrollment criteria. Refractive surgery may be done by a DOD or a civilian provider. (This is an elective procedure. Guidelines for elective procedures are outlined in Chapter 2 Section A 6. of this manual.) Candidates must have demonstrated refractive stability as confirmed by clinical records. Neither the spherical or cylindrical portion of the refraction may have changed more than 0.50 diopters during the two most recent postoperative manifest refractions separated by at least one month. The final manifest shall be performed no sooner than the end of the minimum waiting period (3 or 6 months depending on the degree of preoperative refractive error). The member must have postoperative uncorrected visual acuity of at least 20/50 correctable with spectacles to at least 20/20 for near and distance vision. Detailed enrollment criteria may be obtained by contacting PSC-opm-2.

(4) Hearing. Audiometric loss in excess of the limits set forth in the following table is disqualifying:

FREQUENCY	500	1000	2000	3000	4000
EITHER EAR	30	25	25	45	55

(5) Personality. Must demonstrate, in an interview with the Flight Surgeon, a personality make-up of such traits and reaction that will indicate that the candidate will successfully survive the rigors of the flight training program and give satisfactory performance under the stress of flying.

(6) Chest x-ray. Aviation trainees must have had a chest x-ray within the past three years.

(7) Report of Medical History, DD-2807-1. In addition to the normal completion of the Report of Medical History, DD-2807-1, the following statement shall be typed in block 29 and signed by the applicant: "I certify that I do not now use, nor have I ever used, contact lens for any purpose, and that I am not aware that my uncorrected vision has ever been less than 20/50." If the applicant cannot sign this statement, include a full explanation by the examining Flight Surgeon, and an ophthalmology consultation.

b. Reporting.

(1) The importance of the physical examination of a candidate should be recognized not only by the examining Flight Surgeon but also by health services personnel assisting in the procedure and preparing the report. Candidates often come from a great distance or from isolated ships. If the examination cannot be completed in one working day, seek the Commanding Officer's help in making it possible for the candidate to remain available for a second working day. Careful planning should keep such cases to a minimum. If a report, upon reaching Commandant (CG-112), is found to be incomplete and must be returned, the candidate will suffer undue delay in receiving orders and in some cases

will be completely lost to the CG as a candidate. The preparation of the Report of Medical Examination, DD-2808 in the case of a candidate requires extreme care by all concerned.

(2) In a report of the examination of a candidate, rigid adherence to set standards is expected. The examining officers are encouraged to use freely that portion of the report that provides for "remarks" or "notes." Comments made under "remarks" are the examiner's opinion. Information from any source may be molded into an expression of professional opinion. A final recommendation of the examiner must be made. When such recommendation is not consistent with standards set by Commandant (CG-11) the examiner shall note that fact on the form under "remarks" or "notes" and a reasonable explanation made. When space on a Report of Medical Examination, DD-2808 is inadequate, use a Medical Record, SF-507.

6. Requirements for Class 2 Aircrew.

   a. Aircrew Candidates. Unless otherwise directed by Commander PSC (epm), personnel will not be permitted to undergo training leading to the designation of aircrewmen unless a Flight Surgeon/aviation Medical Officer has found them physically qualified for such training. Should it be desirable, for exceptional reasons, to place in training a candidate who does not meet the prescribed physical standards, the Commanding Officer may submit a request for a waiver, with the Report of Medical Examination, DD-2808 and Report of Medial History, DD-2807-1, to Commander PSC, justifying the request. Aircrew candidates shall meet the standards for Class 1, except that minimum height is 152.5 cm/60 inches and uncorrected distant visual acuity must be not less than 20/100 each eye, correctable to 20/20 each eye. Cycloplegic refraction and anthropometric measurements are not indicated. A chest x-ray is required within the previous 3 years.

   b. Designated Aircrew. Aircrew shall meet the standards for Class 1, except the minimum height is 152.5 cm/60 inches.

7. Requirements for Class 2 Medical Personnel.

   a. Flight Surgeon (FS)/Aviation Medical Officer (AMO)/Aeromedical Physician Assistants (APA), FS Candidates. While assigned to a Duty Involving Flight Operations billet, FS/AMOs/APAs shall meet the standards for Class II Aircrew, except that minimum height is 152.5 cm (60 inches).

   b. Aviation Mission Specialists (AMS)/AMS Candidates. Aviation Mission Specialists (Health Services Technicians (HS) who are assigned to flight orders), shall meet the standards for Class II Aircrew, except that minimum height is 152.5 cm (60 inches).

8. Requirements for Class 2 Technical Observers. The term "technical observer" is applied to personnel who do not possess an aviation designation but who are detailed to duty involving flying. The examination shall relate primarily to equilibrium and the patency of eustachian tubes. They shall meet the standards prescribed for general duty. These personnel are not required to undergo a physical examination for flying provided a complete physical examination, for any purpose, has been passed within the preceding 60 months and intervening medical history is not significant. The physical examination need not be conducted by an FS/AMO. Technical observers who are required to undergo egress training must have a current (general purpose) physical examination and a status profile chit indicating "OK DIF/Dunker/Chamber."

9. Requirements for Class 2 Air Traffic Controllers. Air traffic controllers, tower controllers, and ground control approach operators shall meet the general physical standards for Class 1, except:

   a. Articulation. Must speak clearly and distinctly without accent or impediment of speech that would interfere with radio communication. Voice must be well modulated and pitched in medium range. Stammering, poor diction, or other evidence of speech impediments that become manifest or aggravated under excitement are disqualifying.

   b. Height. Same as general service.

   c. Visual Acuity.

      (1) Candidate's visual acuity shall be no worse than 20/100 for each eye correctable to 20/20 each eye and the correction shall be worn while on duty.

      (2) Personnel already designated shall have distant visual acuity no worse than 20/200 each eye correctable to 20/20 each eye and the correction shall be worn while on duty.

      (3) Air Traffic Controllers whose vision becomes worse than 20/200 either eye may not engage in the control of air traffic in a control tower but may be otherwise employed in the duties of their rating.

   d. Depth Perception. Normal depth perception is required.

   e. Heterophoria. The following are disqualifying:

      (1) esophoria or exophoria greater than 6 prism diopters; and

      (2) hyperphoria greater than 1 prism diopter.

10. Requirements for Landing Signal Officer (LSO).

    a. Physical Examinations for Landing Signal Officer (LSO).

       (1) Candidates. Officer and enlisted candidates for training as LSO's shall have a physical examination prior to the training leading to

qualification. LSO duties for flight deck require stricter visual acuity standards than those for general duty in the CG. Examination by a FS/AMO is not required.

   (2) Reexamination. Biennial reexamination is required of all currently qualified LSO's.

  b. Physical Standards for LSO's. In addition to the physical standards required for officer and enlisted personnel, the following standards apply:

   (1) Distant Visual Acuity. The uncorrected distant visual acuity shall be no worse than 20/200 in each eye and must be correctable to 20/20 in each eye. If the uncorrected distant visual acuity is less than 20/20 in either eye, corrective lenses must be worn while performing LSO duties.

   (2) Depth Perception. Normal depth perception is required.

   (3) Color Vision. Normal color perception is required.

11. Refractive Surgery. All Classes: Certain Corneal refractive surgery can be waived for all classes. NOTE: Class 1 can only undergo refractive surgery while serving in a non-flying status. Only PRK and variants of custom wave form, LASEK and epi-LASIK are approved. Procedures with a corneal stromal flap will be considered for aviation personnel on a case by case basis. Other corneal refractive surgery, rings or implants are disqualifying and will not be considered. The PRK procedure, which is approved, must be performed at a MTF for all aviation classes. (Exception: see Chap 3.Section G. 5. a(3)(c) for SNA candidate requirements)

  a. All pre-operative, operative and post operative medical records must be submitted for review by the waiver authority.

  b. Preoperative refractive limits: Sphere: -8.00 to +6.00 diopters. Cylinder: -3.00 to +3.00 diopters. Anisometropia: 3.5 diopters.

  c. Post-operative refractive stability. Demonstration of post-operative refractive stability shall be demonstrated by 2 consecutive manifest refractions, obtained at least 30 days apart. For those with a pre-operative refraction of plano to -5.50 diopters of sphere the initial post operative refraction should be no sooner than 30 days after the surgery. A follow up refraction shall be done no sooner than 30 days after the initial post refraction. For those with a pre-operative refraction of -5.75 to -8.00 diopters of sphere or +0.25 to +6.00 diopters of sphere, the earliest manifest refraction is at 6 months post-op.

  d. Refractive stability. If refractive stability is demonstrated as evidenced by less than a 0.50 diopters change over two separate exams at least four weeks apart, then the member can apply to PSC for a waiver 3 months after surgery. The post-operative manifest refractions can vary by no more than 0.50 diopters. Waiver consideration will not be made until this is achieved.

e. <u>Quality of vision questionnaire</u>. The member must not have any visual complaints post operatively per the quality of vision questionnaire which is to be included in the waiver package. This form can be found on the following Commandant (CG-112) Web Site: http://www.uscg.mil/hq/cg1/cg11/.

f. <u>Post operative standards</u>. Post operatively the member must meet all aviation visual standards in this section. (Member must have 20/20 vision or vision correctable to 20/20 in both eyes)

g. Submission of a waiver request and follow up will be IAW applicable message or COMDTINST. All required follow up exams will be accomplished on time and be within guidelines or conditions of the waiver will be deemed not met and the member will be grounded and required to re-submit the waiver request.

h. A quality of vision questionnaire and visual acuity check is to be done every three months for one year after the surgery. This information is to be noted in the member's medical record and reviewed by the Flight Surgeon.

12. <u>Contact Lenses</u>.

   a. Class 1 personnel may be authorized by their local Flight Surgeon to wear contact lenses while flying, provided the following conditions are met:

   (1) Only gas permeable disposable soft lenses may be used.

   (2) The lenses are to be removed during the hours of sleep.

   (3) The lenses are disposed of after 2 weeks of use.

   (4) All prescribed optometry follow-up visits are adhered to. After routine safe use has been established and documented by the prescribing optometric authority, an annual optometric recheck is the minimum required. A copy of the record of any visit to an eye care professional will be furnished by the member to the local Flight Surgeon for review and placement in the member's health record.

   (5) Following any change in the refractive power of the contact lens, the member must be checked on the AFVT to ensure that CG Class I standards for acuity and depth perception are met. In addition, the Flight Surgeon shall document that there is no lens displacement, when user moves his/her eyes through all 8 extreme ranges of gaze.

(6) Contact lens case, saline for eye use, and an appropriate pair of eyeglasses are readily accessible (within reach) to the lens wearer while in-flight.

(7) Contact lens candidate submits request to the command agreeing to abide the above conditions.

(8) The Flight Surgeon authorizes use of contact lenses after ensuring that such use is safe and the user fully understands the conditions of use. This authorization expires after one year. Initial and any annual re-authorizations shall be documented by an entry in the health record.

(9) Contact lens use is not a requirement for aviation operations. The decision to apply for authorization is an individual option. Accordingly, lens procurement and routine optometric care related to contact lens use at government expense are not authorized.

b. The optional wearing of contact lenses by Class 2 personnel performing duty involving flying and by air control personnel in the actual performance of their duties is authorized under the following circumstances:

(1) Individuals are fully acclimated to wearing contact lenses and visual acuity is fully corrected by such lenses;

(2) Individuals wearing contact lenses while performing flight or air control duties have on their person, at all times, an appropriate pair of spectacles;

(3) A Flight Surgeon has specifically authorized the wearing of contact lenses while performing flight or air control duties (An entry shall be made on a Chronological Record of Care, SF-600 in the individual's health record authorizing wearing of contact lenses.); and

(4) Wearing contact lenses while performing aviation duties is an individual option. Accordingly, procuring contact lenses at government expense is not authorized.

COMDTINST M6000.1E

Sitting Height

Purpose

This measurement is important in the design and layout of work stations occupied by Navy personnel. Controls must be placed in numerous locations, and the minimum acceptable space between the helmet and the canopy of cockpits must be considered.

Equipment Required

Anthropometer

Measurement Procedure

1. The subject sits erect facing forward with the head level (see illustration below), the shoulders and upper arms relaxed, and the forearms and hands extended forward horizontally with the palms facing each other. The thighs are parallel, and the knees are flexed 90° with the feet in line with the thighs.

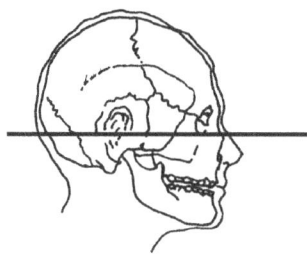

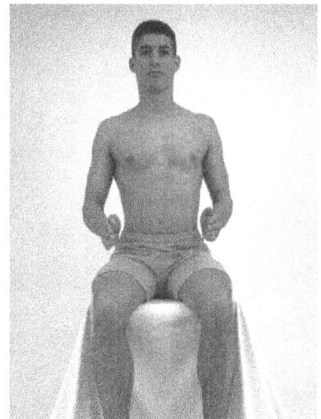

2. Measure the vertical distance between the sitting surface and the top of the head with an anthropometer. The shoulders and upper extremities should be relaxed. Measure at the maximum point of quiet respiration.

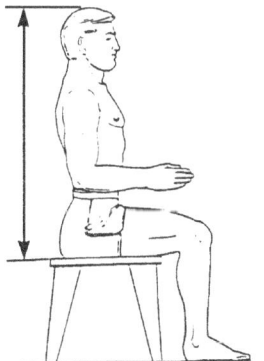

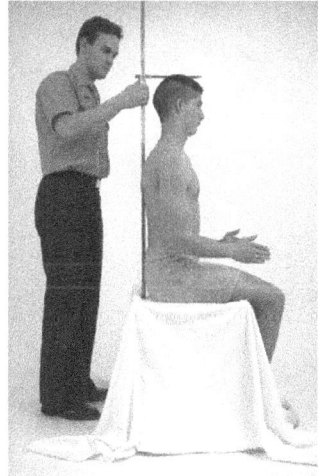

NOTE: *Measurements are to be taken to the nearest eighth of an inch. The measurement should be taken at least twice. If there is a large variation between the two measurements, recheck the body position and repeat measurements.*

COMDTINST M6000.1E

Eye Height, Sitting

Purpose

Sitting Eye Height plays a decisive role in instrument panel layout, viewing angles, and seat adjustment, since the pilot must have optimum vision both inside and outside of the cockpit.

Equipment Required

Anthropometer

Measurement Procedure

1. The subject sits erect facing forward with the head level (see illustration below), the shoulders and upper arms relaxed, and the forearms and hands extended forward horizontally with the palms facing each other. The thighs are parallel and the knees are flexed 90° with the feet in line with the thighs.

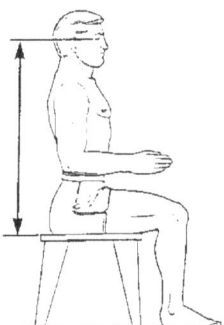

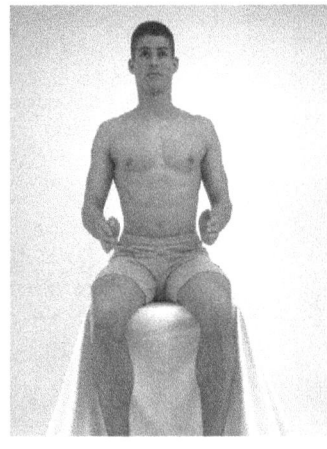

2. Measure the vertical distance between the sitting surface and the corner or angle formed by the meeting of the eyelids on the outer corner of the right eye with an anthropometer.

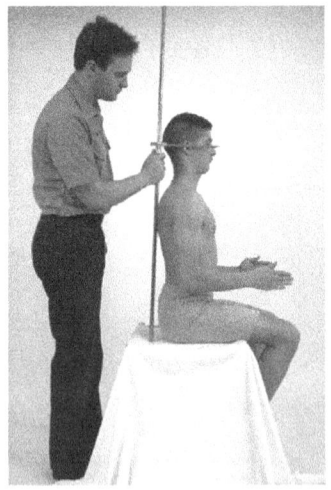

NOTE: Measurements are to be taken to the nearest eighth of an inch. Measurements should be taken at least twice. If there is a large variation between the two measurements, recheck body position and repeat measurements.

COMDTINST M6000.1E

Thumbtip Reach

Purpose

This measurement is important in the design and layout of work stations occupied or used by Navy personnel. Thumbtip reach is particularly useful for the placement of controls in various locations within cockpits.

Equipment Required

Wall--mounted linear scale.

Measurement Procedure

1. The subject stands erect in a corner looking straight ahead with the feet together and heels 7.87 inhes (20 cm) from the back wall.
2. With the buttocks and shoulder placed against the wall, the right arm and hand (palm down) are stretched horizontally along the scale while the thumb continues along the horizontal line of the arm with the index finger curving around to touch the pad at end of the thumb.

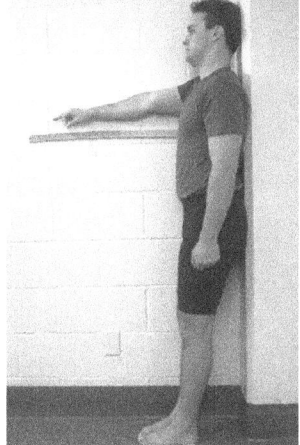

3. The subject's right shoulder is held against the rear wall. The horizontal distance from the back wall to the tip of the right thumb is measured.

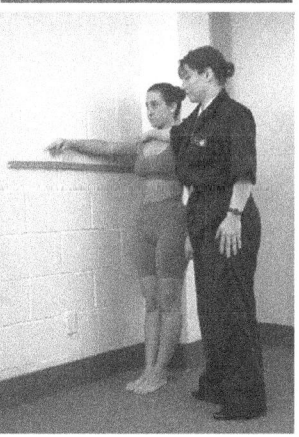

NOTE 1: *Measurements are to be taken to the nearest eighth of an inch. Measurements should be taken at least twice. If there is a large variation between the two measurements, recheck body position and repeat measurements.*

Chapter 3. G. Page 17

Buttock-Knee Length

Purpose

This measurement is usually associated with ejection seat clearance and threshold values between the knee and the glare shield (or canopy bow).

Equipment Required

Anthropometer

Measurement Procedure

1. While the subject sits erect, draw a landmark on the bottom tip of the right knee cap. The subject's thighs should be parallel, with the knees flexed at 90°. The feet should be in line with the thighs, and lying flat on the surface of a footrest or the floor.

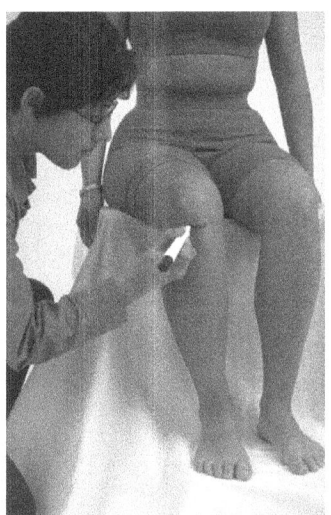

2. The anthropometer is placed flush against the buttock plate at the most posterior point on either buttock, and the anterior point to the right knee is measured with an anthropometer.

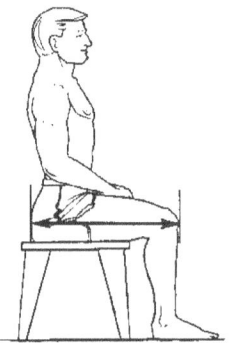

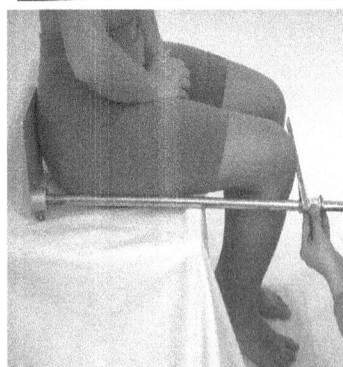

Section H. Physical Examinations and Standards for Diving Duty

1. Examinations..1
2. Standards...2

This page intentionally left blank.

H. Physical Examinations and Standards for Diving Duty. To promote safety and to provide uniformity and completeness, a diving physical examination must be performed by a currently qualified Dive Medical Officer (DMO). Any health care provider can recommend to the command a limited duty status based upon medical illness or injury. An ill or injured diver may only be returned to diving duties by a qualified DMO.

1. Examinations.

    a. Candidates. Personnel whose duty exposes them to a hyperbaric environment must conform to the physical standards for diving duty. The Physical standards for diving duty are a combination of standards contained in section 3-D and the additional standards listed in this section. It is therefore critical that the HCP evaluating divers and candidates for diver training be familiar with these physical standards.

    b. Dive Physical Examinations. Dive physical examinations should be performed by a Medical Officer who has successfully completed the diving Medical Officer (DMO) course at the Naval Diving Salvage training Center (NDSTC). However, any credentialed CG HCP may perform a Dive Physical but final approval can only be made by review and countersignature of a qualified Dive Medical Officer (DMO).

    c. Frequency of examination. The diving physical is performed on candidates when applying for initial dive training. Subsequent examinations are performed on designated divers on birth date at ages 20, 25, 30, 35, 40, 45, 50, and annually thereafter, and in support of waiver requests when a diver's physical condition requires a determination of fitness for diving duty. All members on diving duty will have an annual periodic health assessment (PHA) to maintain diving duty qualification. This will include recommended preventive health examinations. For divers the annual PHA will include documentation of skin cancer screening. Additionally, all designated divers require an audiogram every 5 years. If at anytime a significant threshold shift is documented, follow up per OMSEP requirements outlined in Chapter 12, section 7, of this manual will be completed. When a members hearing falls outside the diving duty standards, a waiver is required.

    d. Documentation. A dive physical will consist of a completed Report of Medical History, DD-2807-1 and Report of Medical Examination, DD-2808. All applicants for initial and follow-on dive training must have a valid Diver/Buds/s Medical Screening Questionnaire, CG-6000-3 (formally known as Exhibit 8), completed and signed no later than 30 days prior to commencing training. This form serves as an interval medical history from the time the original dive physical was performed up to the member's training date as well as a medical screening for any missed or new condition that may be considered disqualifying. Any condition found to be disqualifying needs to be addressed prior to the member's transfer to dive training. The U.S. Military Diving Medical Screening Questionnaire should be added to the member's medical record.

e. Waivers. Waivers for initial application or continuance of duty may be requested if a disqualifying condition exists. The request is routed from the examining HCP to HSWL SC then on to a DMO. Initial applicant waivers must also be approved by NDSTC prior to the member commencing training. Appropriate documentation for the waiver request includes:

   (1) A Chronological Record of Care, SF-600 prepared by the examining HCP requesting the waiver referencing the specific standard for which the member is not physically qualified, a clinical synopsis including history, focused examination, clinical course, appropriate ancillary studies, and appropriate specialty consultation, followed by a recommendation of "waiver recommended" or "waiver not recommended" with supporting rationale.

   (2) Endorsement by the member's CO.

   (3) Enclosure documentation of pertinent studies supporting the waiver or recommending disqualification.

   (4) Specialty consult supporting the waiver or recommending disqualification.

f. Fitness for diving duty. Any credentialed CG health care provider can recommend to the command a limited duty status based upon medical illness or injury. An ill or injured diver may only be returned to diving duty by a qualified DMO.

2. Standards.

   a. Age Requirements. Candidates beyond the age of 35 shall not be considered for initial training in diving.

   b. Ear, Nose and Throat. Chronic Eustachian tube dysfunction or inability to equalize middle ear pressure is disqualifying. Any persistent vertigo, dysequilibrium, or imbalance with inner ear origin is disqualifying. Maxillofacial or crainiofacial abnormalities precluding the comfortable use of diving headgear, mouthpiece, or regulator is disqualifying. Hearing must meet standards for initial acceptance for active duty. Hearing standards are:

      (1) 1000Hz -30dB, 2000Hz-35dB, 3000Hz- 45dB, 4000Hz-55dB

      (2) Results greater than the above listed dB require a waiver. Designated divers with full recovery from either tympanic membrane perforation or acute sinusitis may be returned to diving duties after evaluation by a DMO.

   c. Eyes and Vision. All divers must have corrected visual acuity not worse than 20/25 in one eye. For Second Class Divers (DV2) assigned to diving duty and Diving Medical Technicians (DMT): 20/20 in each eye. History of refractive corneal surgery is not considered disqualifying. However, candidates must wait 3 months following their most recent surgery (PRK or LASIK), have satisfactory improvement in visual acuity, and be fully recovered from any surgical procedure. A designated diver must wait 1 month post-LASIK/PRK and be fully recovered from any surgical procedure with satisfactory improvement in their visual acuity prior to resumption of diving. Corneal complications lasting 6 months or longer after cessation of hard contact lens wear is disqualifying. Lack of adequate color vision is disqualifying. Waivers will be considered on a case-by-case basis.

d. Pulmonary. History of spontaneous pneumothorax is disqualifying. Traumatic Pneumothorax (other than caused by a diving-related pulmonary barotrauma) is disqualifying. A waiver request will be considered for a candidate or designated diver after a period of at least 6 months and must include: a normal pulmonary function test, standard, non-contrast chest CT, favorable recommendation from a pulmonologist, and final evaluation and approval by a DMO. Chronic obstructive or restrictive pulmonary disease is disqualifying. Candidates and designated divers undergoing drug therapy for a positive Tuberculin Skin Test (TST) must complete a full course of chemoprophylaxis prior to the start of diver training or reinstatement to diving duty. Designated divers who experience mediastinal or subcutaneous emphysema resulting from a dive are restricted from diving duty for 1 month. They may be returned to diving duty following completion of the waiver process if the diver is asymptomatic and is determined to have a normal, standard, non-contrast chest CT. A history of pulmonary barotrauma in a diver candidate is disqualifying. Designated divers who experience a second pulmonary barotrauma are considered permanently disqualified for diving duty.

e. Skin and Lymphatics. Skin cancer or severe chronic or recurrent skin conditions exacerbated by sun exposure, diving, the hyperbaric environment or the wearing of occlusive attire (e.g., a wetsuit) are disqualifying.

f. Gastrointestinal. Gastroesophageal reflux disease that interferes with or is aggravated by diving duty is considered disqualifying. Designated divers with full recovery from acute infections of abdominal organs may be returned to diving duties at the discretion of a DMO. Designated divers with a history of symptomatic or bleeding hemorrhoids may be returned to diving duties at the discretion of a DMO. Designated divers with a full recovery from abdominal surgery (including hernia repair) may apply for a waiver after 3 months of post-operative recovery.

g. Genitourinary. Invasive cancer is disqualifying. Designated divers with a full recovery from acute infections of genitourinary organs may be returned to diving duties at the discretion of a DMO. Pregnancy is disqualifying. Post-partum members are eligible for diving duties 6 months after delivery. Return to earlier duty requires a waiver.

h. Dental. All divers must be dental class 1 or 2. Fixed active orthodontic appliances require a waiver from PSC-opm or epm (fixed retainers are exempt).

i. Musculoskeletal. Any musculoskeletal condition that is chronic or recurrent which predisposes to diving injury, limits performance of diving duties, or may confuse the diagnosis of a diving injury is disqualifying. Any fracture (including stress fractures) is disqualifying if it is less than 3 months post injury, and if there are any residual symptoms. Designated divers with full recovery from uncomplicated fractures with no residual pain may be reinstated at the discretion of a DMO. Bone or joint surgery is disqualifying if it is within 6 months and there is any significant or functional residual symptoms. Retained hardware is not disqualifying unless it results in limited range of motion.

j. Psychiatric. The special nature of diving duties requires a careful appraisal of the candidate's emotional, temperamental, and intellectual fitness. Past or recurrent symptoms of neuropsychiatric disorder or organic disease of the nervous system are disqualifying. No individual with a history of personality disorder shall be accepted. Neurotic trends, emotional immaturity or instability and antisocial traits, if of sufficient degree to militate against satisfactory adjustment are disqualifying. Stammering or other speech impediment that might become manifest under excitement is disqualifying. Treatment of any emotional, psychological, behavioral, or mental dysfunction should be completed and the diver asymptomatic before return to duty is supportable by a waiver. No time limit is required post treatment but the recommendation of the attending mental health professional of fitness for full duty and concurrent assessment of fitness for duty by a DMO is sufficient to begin the waiver process. Use of psychotropic medication for any purpose including those that are not psychiatric such as smoking, migraine headaches, pain syndromes, is not prohibited with diving duty but must be approved by a DMO. Diagnosis of alcohol dependence will result in disqualification until successful completion of a treatment program and a 1-year aftercare program. A diagnosis of alcohol abuse or alcohol incident will result in disqualification from diving duty until all recommended treatment courses or course mandated by the members CO have been completed.

k. Neurological. Idiopathic seizures are disqualifying except for febrile convulsions before age 5. Two years of non-treated seizure-free time is necessary before a waiver will be considered. Seizures with known cause may be returned earlier to duty by waiver. Syncope, if recurrent, unexplained, or not responding to treatment is disqualifying. All dive physicals require documentation of a full neurologic examination and tympanic membrane mobility in blocks 44 and 72b respectively on the Report of Medical Examination, DD 2808.

l. Decompression Sickness / Arterial Gas Embolism. In a diving duty candidate, any prior history of decompression sickness or arterial gas embolism is disqualifying and requires a waiver. Designated divers diagnosed with any decompression sickness (including symptoms of joint pain or skin changes) shall: have an entry made in their medical record describing the events and treatment of the injury, signed by the attending DMO and be evaluated by a cardiologist for presence of a patent foramen ovale (PFO) with results documented in health record. Designated divers diagnosed with AGE or DCS type II presenting with neurological, pulmonary, or shock symptoms will be disqualified for diving duty pending work-up and evaluation by a DMO and waiver approval.

m. Required Labs and Special Studies. For candidates applying for initial dive duty and for designated diver physical examinations the following labs and special studies are required in support of Report of Medical Examination, DD-2808: Serology, CBC with Diff, Lipid panel, Fasting blood glucose, HIV, Urinalysis, Hepatitis C screening, G6PD, Sickle Cell, Blood type, Chest x-ray (PA and lateral), Audiogram, EKG, and PPD. In addition to the Immunization and Chemoprophylaxis (Joint Publication), COMDTINST M6230.4 (series) requirements, all diver candidates and designated divers must be immunized against both Hepatitis A and B. Diver candidates must have two doses of Hepatitis A immunization and at least the first two of three doses of Hepatitis B immunization prior to the start of diver training.

n. Miscellaneous. The use of Bupropion for tobacco cessation is not disqualifying for diving duty, but requires approval by a DMO. Qualified divers or dive candidates are not fit for diving duty when they are taking INH for positive TST testing. Waiver must be obtained to return to diving duty.

This page intentionally left blank

COMDTINST M6000.1E

CHAPTER 4

HEALTH RECORDS AND FORMS

Section A. Health Records.

1. Purpose and Background 1
2. Contents of the Health Record 1
3. Custody of Health Records 4
4. Opening Health Records 6
5. Checking out the Health Record 7
6. Terminating Health Records 10
7. Creating an Additional Volume 13
8. Lost, Damaged, or Destroyed Health Records 13
9. Accuracy and Completeness Check 14

Section B. Health Record Forms.

FORM	TITLE	
1. CG-3443	Health Record Cover	1
2. CG-5266	Drug Sensitivity Sticker	2
3. DD-2766	Adult Preventive and Chronic Care Flowsheet Form	2
4. SF-513	Consultation Sheet	3
5. SF-507	Medical Record	4
6. DD-2795	Pre-Deployment Health Assessment	4
7. DD-2796	Post-Deployment Health Assessment	4
8. DD-2900	Post-Deployment Health Re-Assessment	4
9. CG-6020	Medical Recommendation for Flying	5
10. DD-2808	Report of Medical Examination	5
11. DD-2807-1	Report of Medical History	11
12. CG-5447	History and Report of OMSEP Examination	15
13. CG-5447A	Periodic History and Report of OMSEP Examination	18
14. CG-5684	Medical Board Report Cover Sheet	19
15. SF-600	Chronological Record of Medical Care	19
16. SF-558	Emergency Care and Treatment	22
17. CG-5214	Emergency Medical Treatment Report	23
18. SF-519	Radiographic Reports	25
19. Laboratory Reports		26
20. DD-771	Eyewear Prescription	26
21. SF-602	Syphilis Record	28
22. OF-522	Authorization for Anesthesia, Operations, etc.	28
23. DD-1141	Record of Occupational Exposure to Ionizing Radiation	28
24. Audiogram Results		30
25. DD-2215	Reference Audiogram	30

26. DD-2216   Hearing Conservation Data 30
27. CG-4057   Chronological Record of Service 30
28. DD-2870   Authorization for Disclosure of Medical or Dental Information 31
29. DD-2871   Request to Restrict Medical or Dental Information 31
30. PHS-731   International Certificate of Vaccination 31
31. SF-515   Tissue Examination 32
32. DD-877   Request for Medical/Dental Records or Information 32
33. CG-6100   Modified Screening For: Overseas Assignment and/or Sea Duty Health Screening 33
34. CG-6201   Bloodborne Pathogens Exposure Guidelines 33
35. CG-6202   Examination Protocol for Exposure to: CHROMIUM COMPOUNDS 33
36. CG-6203   Examination Protocol for Exposure to: ASBESTOS 33
37. CG-6204   Examination Protocol for Exposure to: BENZENE 33
38. CG-6205   Examination Protocol for Exposure to: NOISE 33
39. CG-6206   Examination Protocol for Exposure to: HAZARDOUS WASTE 33
40. CG-6207   Examination Protocol for Exposure to: LEAD 33
41. CG-6208   Examination Protocol for Exposure to: RESPIRATOR WEAR 33
42. CG-6209   Examination Protocol for Exposure to: PESTICIDES 34
43. CG-6210   Examination Protocol for Exposure to: RESPIRATORY SENSITIZERS 34
44. CG-6211   Examination Protocol for Exposure to: BLOODBORNE PATHOGENS 34
45. CG-6212   Examination Protocol for Exposure to: TUBERCULOSIS 34
46. CG-6213   Examination Protocol for Exposure to: SOLVENTS 34
47. CG-6214   Examination Protocol for Exposure to: RADIATION 34
48. CG-6215   How to Calculate a Significant Threshold Shift 34

Section C. Dental Records Forms

FORM   TITLE

1. CG-3443-2 Dental Record Cover 1
2. NAVMED 6600/3 Dental Health Questionnaire 2
3. SF-603   Dental Record 2
4. SF-603-A   Dental Continuation 14
5. SF-513   Consultation Sheet 14
6. Lost Dental Records 14
7. Special Dental Records Entries 14
8. Dental Examination Requirements 14
9. Recording of Dental Treatments on Chronological Record of Care, SF-600 15

Section D. Dental Records Forms.

1. Purpose and Background 1
2. Contents of Clinical Records 2
3. Extraneous Attachments 3
4. Opening Clinical Records 3
5. Terminating Clinical Records 4
6. Custody of Clinical Records 4
7. Safekeeping of Clinical Records 4
8. Transfer of Clinical Records 4
9. Lost Damaged or Destroyed Clinical Records...5

Section E. Employee Medical Folders.

1. Purpose and Background 1
2. Custody of Employee Medical Folders (EMF's) 1
3. Contents of the Employee Medical Folders..2
4. Accountability of Disclosures 3
5. Opening Employee Medical Folder 3
6. Terminating Employee Medical Folders 3
7. Transferring to Other Government Agencies 4
8. Lost, Damaged, or Destroyed Employee Medical Folders 4
9. Employee Medical Folder, SF-66 D 4

Section F. Inpatient Medical Records.

1. Purpose and Background 1
2. Maintenance and Storage..2
3. Disposition of IMRs..3
4. Inpatient Medical Record Forms and Required Entries...4

Section G. Mental Health Records.

1. Active duty..1
2. Non-active duty 1
3. Psychiatric Evaluation Format..1
4. Custody of Mental Health Records...1

COMDTINST M6000.1E

This page intentionally left blank

Chapter 4 Contents

COMDTINST M6000.1E

Section A. Health Records.

1. Purpose and Background 1
2. Contents of the Health Record 1
3. Custody of Health Records 4
4. Opening Health Records 6
5. Checking Out the Health Record 7
6. Terminating Health Records 10
7. Creating an Additional Volume 13
8. Lost, Damaged, or Destroyed Health Records 13
9. Accuracy and Completeness Check 14

This page intentionally left blank.

CHAPTER FOUR – HEALTH RECORDS AND FORMS

Section A. Health Records.

1. Purpose and Background.

    a. Introduction. The health record is the chronological medical and dental record of an individual while a member of the CG or the CG Reserve. The primary reasons for compiling a health record are listed below.

        (1) To develop an accurate clinical history that will help in future diagnosis and treatment.

        (2) To protect the Government, the individual concerned, and the individual's dependents. It may be used in adjudicating veterans claims by making permanently available in a single record all entries relative to physical examinations, medical and dental history, preliminary to entry and throughout the individual's entire CG career. This is accomplished by opening or maintaining medical and dental records:

            (a) Upon entry into the Service.

            (b) As required to maintain concise, yet complete, records during period of service.

            (c) At time of separation.

        (3) To facilitate appraisal of the physical fitness or eligibility for benefits by making selected, necessary information contained in the health record available to CG selection boards, disability evaluation system, Board of Correction of Military Records, for income tax purposes, and for claims to the Department of Veterans Affairs.

        (4) To furnish a basis for collecting statistical information.

        (5) To identify deceased persons through dental records when other means are inadequate.

        (6) To facilitate communication among health care providers, utilization managers, quality assurance and medical records personnel.

    b. Value of accuracy. As an individual's service career progresses, the health record increases in value to the Government, the individual, and the individual's family and dependents. Accuracy, therefore, is of the utmost importance in making entries, including entries regarding minor ailments or injuries which appear trivial at the time, but which must be recorded to protect the Government and the individual.

2. Contents of the Health Record. Each member's health record shall consist of a Health Record Cover, CG-3443 with medical records and dental records arranged as follows:

a. SECTION I - HISTORY OF CARE. All forms in this Section shall be arranged in the following order, (1) being the top and (9) being the bottom. Additionally, the forms should be grouped by date with the most recent on top. Do not separate corresponding Report of Medical Examination, DD-2808 forms and Report of Medical History, DD-2807-1.

   (1) Adult Preventive and Chronic Care Flowsheet DD-2766.

   (2) Consultation Sheet, SF-513.

   (3) Medical Record, SF-507.*

   (4) Pre-Deployment Health Assessment, DD-2795.*

   (5) Post-Deployment Health Assessment, DD-2796.*

   Post-Deployment Health Assessment, DD-2900.*
   (DD-2900 on top of the DD-2796 which is on top of the DD-2795, most recent on top, see Chapter 6 of this Manual for details on when to fill out these forms).

   (6) Medical Recommendation for Flying, CG-6020 (aviation personnel only)*. A copy of every CG-6020 completed for a member should be filed in the record with the most recent just below the DD-2766.

   (7) Report of Medical Examination, DD-2808, and Report of Medical History DD-2807-1.

   (8) History and Report of Occupational Medical Surveillance and Evaluation Program (OMSEP) Examination, CG-5447, and Periodic History and Report of OMSEP Examination, CG-5447A.

   (9) Medical Record, SF-507*. Attached to and filed after the form they continue.

   (10) Medical Board Report Cover Sheet, CG-5684*.

   * Annotates when required

b. SECTION II - RECORDS OF CARE. All forms in this Section (and their civilian equivalents) shall be arranged in the following order, (1) being the top and (3) being the bottom. Additionally, the forms should be grouped by date with the most recent on top.

   (1) Chronological Record of Care, SF-600. Command Medical Referral Form for weight evaluation shall be placed in chronological order with the SF 600's. See Coast Guard Weight and Body Fat Standards Program Manual, COMDTINST M1020.8 (series)

   (2) Emergency Care and Treatment, SF-558.

   (3) Emergency Medical Treatment Report, CG-5214.

c. SECTION III - RADIOLOGICAL REPORTS. All forms in this Section (and their civilian equivalents) shall be arranged in the following order, (1) being the top (2) being the bottom. Additionally, the forms should be grouped by date with the most recent on top.

   (1) Radiographic Consultation Request/Report, SF-519A.

   (2) Medical Record - Radiographic Reports, SF-519.

d. SECTION IV - LABORATORY REPORTS AND ECG REPORTS. All forms in this Section (and their civilian equivalents) should be grouped by date with the most recent on top.

e. SECTION V - MISCELLANEOUS. All forms in this Section shall be arranged in the following (1) being on top (11) being on the bottom. Additionally, the forms should be grouped by date with the most recent on top.

   (1) Request for Restriction of Information, DD-2871.

   (2) Authorization for Disclosure, DD-2870.

   (3) Eyewear Prescription, DD-771.

   (4) Hearing Conservation Program microprocessor test result strips. Reference Audiogram, DD- 2215 and Hearing Conservation Data Sheet, DD-2216 will also be place in section V in sequential order.

   (5) Request for Administration of Anesthesia and for Performance of Operations and other Procedures, OF-522.*

   (6) Syphilis Record, SF-602.*

   (7) Occupational Health Surveillance Questionnaire, CG-5197.*

   (8) Record of Occupational Exposure to Ionizing Radiation, DD-1141.*

   (9) Special Duty Medical Abstract, NAVMED 6150/2.*

   (10) Chronological Record of Service, CG-4057.*

   * Annotates when required

f. SECTION VI - DENTAL RECORD AND INTERNATIONAL VACCINATION RECORD. All forms in this Section shall be arranged in the following (1) being the top and (2) being the bottom.

   (1) U.S. Coast Guard Dental Record, CG-3443-2. If needed a Sensitivity Sticker, CG-5266 shall be placed on outside of Dental Record. All forms in the Dental Record shall be arranged in the following order (a) being the top and (d) being the bottom. Additionally, the forms should be grouped by date with the most recent on top.

      (a) Dental Health Questionnaire, CG-5605.

COMDTINST M6000.1E

- (b) Health Record - Dental (Continuation), SF-603A.*
- (c) Health Record – Dental, SF-603.
- (d) Request for Anesthesia, OF-522.

(2) International Certificate of Vaccination, PHS-731 *(This form is optional and only required when needed).

* Annotates when required

g. <u>Filing forms</u>. File forms of the same number in their assigned sequence, with the most recent on top of each previous form, e.g., Chronological Record of Care, SF-600 dated 94/02/15 is filed on top of SF-600 dated 94/02/14.

h. <u>Recording dates</u>. Record all dates on the Health Record Cover, CG-3443 in the following sequence (all numerals): year/month/day (e.g., 51/02/07).

i. <u>Review reports before filing</u>. Reports, including laboratory, X-ray, and consultations, shall be reviewed and initialed by the responsible MO, DO, PA, or NP before they are filed in the health record. IDHS's are authorized and required to sign negative HIV results (electronically or pen and ink) before hard copies are placed in the Health Record.

j. <u>The health record is a legal document</u>. As such, legibility of all information is essential. Patient ID information shall be typed, printed, or stamped. All entries shall be neat and legible. All signatures shall be accompanied by the stamped or typed name and rank of the practitioner.

3. <u>Custody of Health Records</u>. The following are the general responsibilities for keeping health records.

a. <u>Security</u>. Health records are the property of the Federal government and must be handled in accordance with the provisions of the HIPAA Regulations, the Privacy Act of 1974 and the Freedom of Information Act. Guidance in this area is contained in The Coast Guard Freedom of Information (FOIA) and Privacy Acts Manual, COMDTINST M5260.3 (series). Health record custody, privacy, confidentiality and security requirements are applicable to all documents and electronic files that contain protected health information, whether or not filed in the health record, such as Inpatient Medical Records and mental health treatment records. Disposal of all health record documents shall be in accordance with Information and Life Cycle Management Manual, COMDTINST M5212.12 (series).

(1) Since health records contain personal information of an extremely critical or sensitive nature, they are considered For Official Use Only requiring maximum security (high security locked cabinets or areas). All clinic personnel and all individuals who are designated as health record custodians are to ensure the protection of patients' SSN at all

times. Health records that are not filed while the patient is awaiting care shall be protected, ensuring the SSN is not visible. When a patient signs out their health record, records shall be placed in a large envelope, sealed, and shall not be opened until given to the appropriate clinic personnel or health record custodian.

(2) Except as contained in HIPAA and The Coast Guard Freedom of Information (FOIA) and Privacy Acts Manual, COMDTINST M5260.3 (series) the information contained in health records shall not be disclosed by any means of communication to any person, or to any agency unless requested in writing by or with the prior written authorization of the individual to whom the record pertains. It is the requestor's responsibility to obtain the written authorization.

b. Custody. Health records shall be retained in the custody of the Senior Health Services Officer of the unit to which the individual is attached. At units where there is no Medical Officer attached, the health record will become the responsibility of the Executive Officer in accordance with United States Coast Guard Regulations 1992, COMDTINST M5000.3 (series), who may delegate custody to the senior health services department representative. At units without a Health Services Technician the custody of the health record is the responsibility of the unit's Executive Officer. Maintenance of these health records may be delegated to health services personnel of another unit (e.g., Sectors). At no time shall individual members keep or maintain their own health record. If there is a need to check out a health record for an appointment at another health care facility, the health record custodian shall have the member complete and sign the Health Record Receipt Form, NAVMED 6150/7. The health record custodian shall place the record in an envelope, hand it to the member, and tell the member to return the record as soon as possible following the appointment. The envelope used for record transportation shall bear a printed request reminding outside providers to treat the contents as confidential and requesting providers to include copies of their consultations or case notes for placement in the health record. The responsibilities contained herein are also applicable to Reserve components.

c. Patient's right to examine record. Individuals may examine their own health record in the presence of a health services department representative, providing.

(1) Such examination does not interrupt the unit's scheduled mission.

(2) There is no information contained therein that would be detrimental to the individual's mental well-being, as determined by the member's attending physician.

d. Disclosure of information. The protected health information necessary for fitness-for-duty determinations, status for deployment and special operational duty, separations from duty, convalescent leave recommendations, inpatient admission and casualty notifications, and other routine disclosures for the military mission, is subject to inspection by the Commanding Officer, their delegate designated in writing, duly appointed counsel in the case of formal hearings, or duly appointed CG officials who are conducting authorized investigations. Such inspections will be conducted in the presence of a health services department representative to aid in the interpretation of health information.

    e. Signatures and stamps. Health services personnel making entries in health records shall ensure all entries, including signatures, are neat and legible. Signature information shall include the stamped or printed name and grade or rate of the signer.

    f. Erroneous entry. If an erroneous entry is made in a health record, the author of the entry shall draw a diagonal line through the complete entry, make an additional entry showing wherein and to what extent the original entry is in error, and initial clearly next to the correction.

    g. Responsibility of record. Health services personnel are responsible for the completeness of the entries made on any medical or dental form while the health record is in their custody. No sheet shall be removed from the health record except under conditions specified in this Manual.

    h. Member's authorization. Members are not authorized to write in, alter, remove documents from, or otherwise change their health record or its contents. Request for changes to health record contents shall be made in writing in accordance with procedures contained in the HIPAA Privacy Regulation and in Chapter 16 of the Coast Guard Freedom of Information and Privacy Acts Manual, COMDTINST M5260.3.

4. Opening Health Records.

    a. General.

        (1) A health record will be opened at the recruiting office for each individual upon entering the CG.

        (2) A new health record will be opened upon reenlistment of personnel with prior CG service when such enlistment is not effected the day following discharge. In all cases, request the individual's health record covering prior military service from the Department of Veteran Affairs (VA), Records Management Center, St. Louis, MO.

(3) Other specific occasions for opening a Health Record.

OCCASION	OPENED BY
Officer appointed from civilian status	First duty station
Reserve Officer	Unit where procured
Cadet	Academy
Retired Personnel recalled to Active Duty	First duty station
Original Record Lost or Destroyed	Responsible Custodian

5. <u>Checking out the Health Record</u>. Whenever a Health Record is checked out the Health Record Receipt Form, NAVMED 6150/7 shall be used as a permanent record of receipt and disposition of health records which are maintained at CG health care treatment facilities. For each health record maintained at CG facilities, complete the first four lines of a Health Record Receipt form and place into the health record folder. Whenever the health record is temporarily removed from the files, complete the charge-out information required on the bottom half of the Health Record Receipt, and retain in the health record file where that record is normally kept. Return the Health Record Receipt to the record when it is returned to the file. General Instructions for checking out the Health Record for appointments, Temporary Assigned Duty (TAD) and Permanent Change of Station (PCS) are as follows:

   a. <u>Medical Appointments</u>. When the member is permitted to hand carry their health record, the health record custodian shall:

      (1) Explain to the member their responsibility in the care of the Health Record as outlined in Chapter 4 Section A of this Manual. Make sure the member knows to return the record as soon as possible after the appointment.

      (2) Fill out the Health Record Receipt Form, NAVMED 6150\7.

      (3) Place the record in a sealed envelope.

(4) Attach the following information to the outside of the envelope:

> **For Official Use Only**
> **Information Enclosed**
>
> In accordance with public law and the U.S. Coast Guard Medical Manual COMDTINST M6000.1 (series) the contents of medical records are considered For Official Use Only.
>
> **Health Care Professional**
>
> Please enclose copies of consultations, procedures, or case notes of care rendered to the patient.
>
> **Patient**
>
> The enclosed records remain the property of the United States Government. You must return the Health Record as soon as possible to your command's Health Record Custodian. If you wish to review the enclosed information you may do so only in the presence of a health department representative.

b. <u>TAD</u>. When a member departs for a TAD assignment they will normally not carry any form of Health Record. If the member's TAD is such that they may require routine medical assistance (sickcall) the medical representative shall complete an Adult Preventive & Chronic Care Flowsheet, DD-2766, and the member will take a copy of this. Types of assignments which may require this type of "Health Record" is a TAD assignment aboard a cutter. The exception to this is when a member is going TAD to a facility that can provide additional medical support (example flight physicals) or is in receipt of orders to "A" school, the Chiefs Academy or Officer Candidate School. When a member departs to any of these assignments listed above, the member shall either hand carry their health record as per 5.a. above or their record shall be mailed, along with a DD-877 to the servicing clinic via traceable means (e.g. DHS authorized Commercial Carriers FedEx or UPS); US Postal Service (USPS): 1) Express Mail or 2) Proof of Delivery using Extra Services which are either Certified, Delivery Confirmation, or Signature Confirmation.

c. <u>PCS</u>.

(1) Upon notification that an individual will be transferred, an Accuracy and Completeness Check will be performed and all identified deficiencies corrected. All required entries shall be made in MRRS. Both the detaching unit and the receiving unit shall inspect the health record for Accuracy and Completeness Check as per Chapter 4 Section A. 9 of this Manual.

COMDTINST M6000.1E

(2) When a member is due to transfer, the Servicing Personnel Office (SPO) shall notify the medical custodian where to send the medical records as per Military Personnel Data Records (PDR) System, COMDTINST M1080.10 (series). (TO ENSURE THAT HEALTH RECORDS GET TO THE RIGHT LOCATION IN A TIMELY MANNER IT IS IMPERATIVE THAT THE SPO AND MEDICAL WORK TOGETHER). At the discretion of the health record custodian the health record of the member may be transferred in two ways. The departing member may be permitted to hand carry their medical record to their new unit or the record can be mailed.

   (a) When the member is permitted to hand carry their health record, the health record custodian shall:

       1. Fill out a Health Record Receipt Form (NAVMED 6150/7) with the date and where the members will be taking their record. Have the member sign the Health Record Receipt Form, NAVMED 6150/7. Cut the form at the double lines above the "INSTRUCTIONS" section and maintain the top section on file for two years.

       2. Place the record in a sealed envelope and instruct the member to give his health record to the health record custodian when they get to their new unit. Attach the same information to the outside of the envelope as you would in 5.a. (4) of this section.

       3. Inform the receiving unit via a Request for Medical/Dental Records or Information, DD-877 (this form can be e-mailed) that the member has departed with their health record and their estimated time of arrival. The new unit should inform the old unit that the record has been received via the DD-877 and perform an Accuracy and Completeness Check.

   (b) The records may also be mailed. The health record custodian will:

       1. In accordance with Military Personnel Data Records (PDR) System, COMDTINST M1080.10 (series), the health record custodian will receive the Medical/Dental Disposition Instructions from the SPO. The health record custodian will follow the disposition instruction and mail the health record by traceable means (e.g. DHS authorized Commercial Carriers FedEx or UPS); US Postal Service (USPS): 1) Express Mail or 2) Proof of Delivery using Extra Services which are either Certified, Delivery Confirmation, or Signature Confirmation. For the purpose of this manual, the term "traceable means" is defined as the use of services provided by either USPS or DHS authorized Commercial Carriers (FedEx or UPS) that can be tracked through the providers' web based shipping/tracking system. (Note: Be advised that USPS First Class mail less than 1 inch in thickness, destined for government agencies, with a

Chapter 4. A. Page 9

beginning ZIP Code range between 202XX-205XX is irradiated, which can destroy many important documents. Shipments sent via FedEx or UPS are not irradiated. Contact the receiving unit to determine the best way to send a record).

2. Inform the receiving unit via a Request for Medical/Dental Records or Information, DD-877 (this form can be e-mailed) that the member has departed with their health record and their estimated time of arrival. The new unit should inform the old unit that the record has been received via the DD-877 and perform an Accuracy and Completeness Check.

3. Fill out a Health Record Receipt Form, NAVMED 6150/7 with the date and where the member's record will be mailed. Have the member sign the Health Record Receipt Form, NAVMED 6150/7. Cut the form at the double lines above the "INSTRUCTIONS" section and maintain the top section on file for two years.

6. <u>Terminating Health Records</u>.

   a. <u>Discharge/Release from Active Duty (RELAD)</u>. Upon discharge, RELAD, the unit terminating the health record will inspect the health record, correct all errors, fill in omissions, and make sure the patient identification information is completed on all forms. The health record custodian (in accordance with Military Personnel Data Records (PDR) System, COMDTINST M1080.10 (series)) will receive the Medical/Dental Disposition Instructions from the SPO. The health record custodian will follow the disposition instruction and mail the health record by traceable means to the appropriate office. Via traceable means (e.g. DHS authorized Commercial Carriers FedEx or UPS); US Postal Service (USPS): 1) Express Mail or 2) Proof of Delivery using Extra Services which are either Certified, Delivery Confirmation, or Signature Confirmation. <u>DO NOT GIVE THE ORIGINAL HEALTH RECORD TO THE MEMBER UPON FINAL SEPARATION</u>. The member is entitled to a copy of the original health record. Cite the reason for separation on the reverse side of Chronological Record of Service, CG-4057 before mailing.

   b. <u>Disappearance, other than desertion</u>. Whenever an individual disappears and the facts regarding such disappearance are insufficient to justify a conclusion of death, enter a complete account of the circumstances on an SF-600 in the health record. Do not terminate the health record until final disposition.

   c. <u>Desertion</u>. When an individual is officially declared a deserter, enter an explanatory note on a Chronological Record of Care, SF-600. As per Military Personnel Data Records (PDR) System, COMDTINST M1080.10 (series) the SPO will instruct the health record custodian where to mail the health record. Once notified the health record custodian should mail the health record, via traceable means (e.g. DHS authorized Commercial

Carriers FedEx or UPS); US Postal Service (USPS): 1) Express Mail or 2) Proof of Delivery using Extra Services which are either Certified, Delivery Confirmation, or Signature Confirmation, within 2 working days.

d. Return of a deserter. Upon return of a deserter to his/her own command, a physical examination shall be performed and recorded on the Report Of Medical Examination, DD-2808. Retain the original for incorporation into the health record, and forward a copy to Commander (PSC) or Commander (PSC-rpm) for Reservists with a request for the deserter's health record.

e. Discharge of personnel convicted by civilian authorities. When the Commandant directs the discharge of personnel convicted by civilian authorities, the CO will make arrangements for their physical examination, to be recorded on a Report of Medical Examination, DD-2808. In the event no Medical Officer is available, obtain a statement signed by the warden of the penitentiary or reformatory that the person to be discharged from the CG is physically and mentally qualified for discharge and is not in need of hospitalization. The unit will take the warden's statement, accompanied by the health record, and follow the disposition instruction and mail the health record to the appropriate office via traceable means (e.g. DHS authorized Commercial Carriers FedEx or UPS); US Postal Service (USPS): 1) Express Mail or 2) Proof of Delivery using Extra Services which are either Certified, Delivery Confirmation, or Signature Confirmation.

f. Discharge of Courts-Martial Prisoners Confined in Federal Penitentiaries, Reformatories, and the Naval Disciplinary Command. When the Commandant directs the discharge of a courts-martial prisoner confined in a Federal penitentiary, reformatory, or the Naval Disciplinary Command, the command to which the prisoner has been administratively assigned shall arrange with the warden for physical examination of the prisoner. Results of this physical examination will be entered on the Report of Medical Examination, DD-2808 and signed by the Medical Officer of the designated penal institution. The command to which the prisoner has been administratively assigned will terminate the health record, using the information furnished on the Report of Medical Examination, DD-2808 and the account of medical, dental, and first aid treatments supplied by the penal institution. The unit will terminate health record, include the Report of Medical Examination, DD-2808, follow the disposition instruction from the SPO and mail the health record to the appropriate site via traceable means (e.g. DHS authorized Commercial Carriers FedEx or UPS); US Postal Service (USPS): 1) Express Mail or 2) Proof of Delivery using Extra Services which are either Certified, Delivery Confirmation, or Signature Confirmation.

g. Retired Personnel (Includes Temporary Retirement). Upon notification of retirement, make an entry on the Chronological Record of Service, CG-4057 under "Remarks" indicating place, date, and category under which retired. The command having custody of the health record will sign the CG-4057. The health record custodian will follow the instructions of the

SPO and mail the record to the appropriate office via traceable means (e.g. DHS authorized Commercial Carriers FedEx or UPS); US Postal Service (USPS): 1) Express Mail or 2) Proof of Delivery using Extra Services which are either Certified, Delivery Confirmation, or Signature Confirmation.

h. <u>Cadets</u>. When a cadet's service is terminated, the health record will be terminated and forwarded to the Cadet Record Office, for processing. Following this procedure, the record will be forwarded to the Registrar's Office and held until the departing cadet's class graduates. When this occurs, the record will be forwarded to the Federal Personnel Records Center, St. Louis, MO. This includes cadets who graduate from the Academy but do not accept or are not tendered a commission.

i. <u>Officers (Reserve) to Inactive Duty and Officers (Regular) who Resign to Accept a Reserve Commission</u>. In the case of reserve officers being released to inactive duty the health record will be terminated. The health record custodian will follow the instructions of the SPO and mail the record to the appropriate office via traceable means (e.g. DHS authorized Commercial Carriers FedEx or UPS); US Postal Service (USPS): 1) Express Mail or 2) Proof of Delivery using Extra Services which are either Certified, Delivery Confirmation, or Signature Confirmation.

j. <u>Death</u>. Upon notification of death, make an entry on a Chronological Record of Service, CG-4057 under "Remarks" indicating place, time, date, and a short explanation of the circumstances surrounding death. Verbal briefs are provided to those on a need to know basis (i.e. Commandant (CG-112), HSWL, etc.). CG Investigative Service (CGIS) may also inquire and request to review the health record. The health record shall be forwarded to the HSWL SC for a Quality Improvement (QI) review upon conclusion of local review(s). Findings of the review are forwarded to Commandant (CG-11) via Commandant (CG-112) to determine if additional investigation, process improvement, or adverse privileging action is warranted. The HSWL SC shall forward the original health record to Commander PSC (adm-3).

k. <u>Transfer to Federal Penitentiaries, Reformatories, or the Naval Disciplinary Command</u>. A letter of transmittal and a copy of the health record shall accompany a member who is being transferred under sentence of a courts-martial (who has not been or will not be discharged immediately) to a penal institution for execution of the unexpired sentence. The original health record, with a letter of transmittal stating the name of the penal institution to which the prisoner is being transferred and the length of the sentence, shall be forwarded to the command to which the member has been administratively assigned which shall maintain the health record until the prisoner has been discharged from the Service. A copy of the letter of transmittal shall also be forwarded to Commander (PSC).

l. Separation from service. Upon separation of the individual from the Service, the unit terminating the health record will inspect the health record, correct all errors, fill in omissions, and make sure the patient identification information is completed on all forms. The health record custodian will follow the instructions of the Servicing Personnel Office and mail the record by traceable means to the appropriate office.

7. Creating an Additional Volume. Due to chronic medical conditions, long narrative summaries, medical boards, etc., the record may fill to capacity which may cause the loss or damage to new records. Procedures for creating a second volume are as follows:

   a. Obtain a new Health Record, CG-3443 and transcribe the information from the original jacket.

   b. Write "VOLUME II" in bold print in the lower left corner of the new jacket cover. Insert forms required by this chapter.

   c. Write "VOLUME I" in bold print in the lower left corner of the original jacket cover.

   d. Transfer all documents pertaining to current or chronic illness to the new record.

   e. Remove the most recent Chronological Record of Care, SF-600 from VOLUME I and place it in VOLUME II. Insert a blank SF-600 on top of the remaining forms in VOLUME I and draw a diagonal line across the page. Enter the following on this line: CLOSED NO FURTHER ENTRIES IN THIS RECORD. REFER TO VOLUME II.

   f. Insert the most recent Report of Medical Examination, DD-2808 and the Report of Medical History, DD-2807-1 into VOLUME II.

   g. Problem summary list. Place the original Problem Summary List, NAVMED 6150/20 into VOLUME II and a copy of this form in VOLUME I with the annotation, "CLOSED. NO FURTHER ENTRIES.", below the last entry.

   h. Place the original Chronological Record of Service, CG-4057 in VOLUME II and a copy in VOLUME I.

8. Lost, Damaged, or Destroyed Health Records.

   a. Lost or destroyed. If a health record is lost or destroyed, a complete new health record shall be opened by the unit health record custodian. The designation "REPLACEMENT" shall be stamped or marked on the cover. If the missing health record should be recovered, any additional information or entries in the replacement record shall be inserted in the old record.

   b. Illegible. Health records which become illegible, thus destroying their value as permanent records, shall be restored and duplicated. The duplicate shall, as nearly as possible, be an exact copy of the original record before such record becomes illegible. Take particular care in transcribing the date onto the Report of Medical Examination, DD-2808 into the new record as such information may be required by the Department of Veterans Affairs to determine the individual's right to pension or other Federal benefits. Stamp or mark "DUPLICATE" on the cover of the new record. Explain the circumstances necessitating the duplication on a Chronological Record of Care, SF-600. Forward health records replaced by duplicate records to PSC-adm-3.

9. <u>Accuracy and Completeness Check</u>. Upon notification that an individual will be transferred, the detaching unit shall conduct an Accuracy and Completeness Check and all identified deficiencies corrected prior to transfer. The receiving unit shall inspect the health record for accuracy and completeness within 30 days of receiving the health record, in accordance with the following guidelines:

   a. <u>Immunizations</u>. That all immunizations are up-to-date (See Immunizations and Chemoprophylaxis, COMDTINST 6230.4 (series)).

   b. <u>Tuberculin Skin Test (TST)</u>. That TST screening is current in accordance with Chapter 7 Section D of this Manual.

   c. <u>HIV</u>. That HIV screening is current (every 2 years) in accordance with Chapter 3 Section C 20.b.(7) of this Manual.

   d. <u>Audiograms</u>. That all required audiograms are completed, especially on personnel involved in the hearing conservation program.

   e. <u>Forms completed and in the right order</u>. That required forms have been properly completed and are in the correct order.

   f. <u>Deficiencies corrected</u>. That all deficiencies in physical requirements shall be scheduled for correction, all missing forms shall be replaced, and all other clerical or administrative errors corrected.

   g. That all OMSEP requirements are met.

   h. That everything is properly recorded in the MRRS.

COMDTINST M6000.1E

Section B. Health Record Forms.

FORM	TITLE	
1. CG-3443	Health Record Cover	1
2. CG-5266	Drug Sensitivity Sticker	2
3. DD-2766	Adult Preventive and Chronic Care Flowsheet Form	2
4. SF-513	Consultation Sheet	3
5. SF-507	Medical Record	4
6. DD-2795	Pre-Deployment Health Assessment	4
7. DD-2796	Post-Deployment Health Assessment	4
8. DD-2900	Post-Deployment Health Re-Assessment	4
9. CG-6020	Medical Recommendation for Flying	5
10. DD-2808	Report of Medical Examination	5
11. DD-2807-1	Report of Medical History	11
12. CG-5447	History and Report of OMSEP Examination	15
13. CG-5447A	Periodic History and Report of OMSEP Examination	18
14. CG-5684	Medical Board Report Cover Sheet	19
15. SF-600	Chronological Record of Medical Care	19
16. SF-558	Emergency Care and Treatment	22
17. CG-5214	Emergency Medical Treatment Report	23
18. SF-519	Radiographic Reports	25
19. Laboratory Reports		26
20. DD-771	Eyewear Prescription	26
21. SF-602	Syphilis Record	28
22. OF-522	Authorization for Anesthesia, Operations, etc.	28
23. DD-1141	Record of Occupational Exposure to Ionizing Radiation	28
24. Audiogram Results		30
25. DD-2215	Reference Audiogram	30
26. DD-2216	Hearing Conservation Data	30
27. CG-4057	Chronological Record of Service	30
28. DD-2870	Authorization for Disclosure of Medical or Dental Information	31
29. DD-2871	Request to Restrict Medical or Dental Information	31
30. PHS-731	International Certificate of Vaccination	31
31. SF-515	Tissue Examination	32
32. DD-877	Request for Medical/Dental Records or Information	32
33. CG-6100	Modified Screening For: Overseas Assignment and/or Sea Duty Health Screening	33
34. CG-6201	Bloodborne Pathogens Exposure Guidelines	33
35. CG-6202	Examination Protocol for Exposure to: CHROMIUM COMPOUNDS	33
36. CG-6203	Examination Protocol for Exposure to: ASBESTOS	33
37. CG-6204	Examination Protocol for Exposure to: BENZENE	33
38. CG-6205	Examination Protocol for Exposure to: NOISE	33
39. CG-6206	Examination Protocol for Exposure to: HAZARDOUS WASTE	33
40. CG-6207	Examination Protocol for Exposure to: LEAD	33
41. CG-6208	Examination Protocol for Exposure to: RESPIRATOR WEAR	33

42. CG-6209   Examination Protocol for Exposure to: PESTICIDES 34
43. CG-6210   Examination Protocol for Exposure to: RESPIRATORY
                SENSITIZERS..34
44. CG-6211   Examination Protocol for Exposure to: BLOODBORNE
                PATHOGENS...34
45. CG-6212   Examination Protocol for Exposure to: TUBERCULOSIS........................34
46. CG-6213   Examination Protocol for Exposure to: SOLVENTS. 34
47. CG-6214   Examination Protocol for Exposure to: RADIATION. 34
48. CG-6215   How to Calculate a Significant Threshold Shift 34

COMDTINST M6000.1E

B. Health Record Forms.

1. Health Record Cover, CG-3443. Each patient's health record shall be maintained in a Health Record Cover, CG-3443. The CG-3443 shall be completed according to the following instructions:

   a. Last Name. Record in all capital letters.

   b. Given Name(s). Record given name(s) in full without abbreviations. If the individual has no middle name or initial then use the lower case letter "n" in parentheses (n). If the individual has only a middle initial(s) record each initial in quotation marks. When "Jr." or "II" or other similar designations are used they shall appear after the middle name or initial.

   DOE   John   Buck   Jr.
   Surname   First Name   Middle Name

   c. Beneficiary. Enter the appropriate beneficiary code to describe the patient (enter "20" for active duty members).

      (1) 01 to 19 - Dependent children in order of birth
      (2) 20 - Sponsor
      (3) 30 - Spouse
      (4) 31-39 - Unremarried former spouse
      (5) 40 - Dependent mother (active duty)
      (6) 45 - Dependent father (active duty)
      (7) 50 - Dependent mother-in-law (active duty)
      (8) 55 - Dependent father-in-law (active duty)
      (9) 60 - Other dependents
      (10) 80 - Humanitarian (non-eligible)
      (11) 90 - Civilian employee
      (12) 99 - Other eligible

   d. Sponsor's Social Security Number. Enter.

   e. Blood Type and Rh Factor. Enter the blood-type and Rh factor in the appropriate boxes. Use utmost caution when recording this information. If not known, complete a blood-type and Rh factor test as required.

   f. Special Status. Check the appropriate block to indicate whether the individual is in aviation or diving status, has a waiver, requires occupational monitoring, or has an allergy.

g. Date of Birth. Enter year, month and day (e.g., 51/02/07).

h. Local Use. Use the spaces provided below the sensitivity sticker location for local use information such as rank, unit, etc. as needed, and/or for the HIPAA Notice of Privacy Practices Acknowledgement sticker.

2. Drug Sensitivity Sticker, CG-5266.

    a. General. The Drug Sensitivity Sticker, CG-5266 should be initiated for anyone having documented history of sensitivity or hypersensitivity to specific drugs, serums, or vaccines, including PPD converters. Other non-drug allergies should be indicated on this form only if they will affect potential therapy (e.g., egg yolks). Every effort shall be made to verify the reported sensitivity and to confirm that it is allergic in nature.

    b. Detailed Instructions.

        (1) Prepare two originals. (One each for the health and dental records).

        (2) List the name of each drug, serum, vaccine, or anesthetic indicated on the Adult Preventive and Chronic Care Flowsheet, DD-2766.

        (3) Affix the Drug Sensitivity Sticker, CG-5266 vertically to the indicated location on the Health Record Cover, CG-3443 and vertically to the lower left corner on the front of the Dental Record Cover, CG-3443-2.

3. Adult Preventive and Chronic Care Flowsheet, DD-2766.

    a. General. The Adult Preventive and Chronic Care Flowsheet, DD-2766 shall be used as a temporary Health Record during TAD Deployments. It documents significant/chronic health problems, allergies, chronic medications, hospitalizations/surgeries, health counseling, immunizations, Purified Protein Derivative (PPD), DNA & HIV testing, (immunizations can be printed from Composite Health Care System (CHCS) data base and stapled in the form) placed in the screening (preventive medicine) exams, other medical readiness items (such as blood type, G6PD, sickle cell, glasses, dental exam, etc), and chart audits. It is advised that a copy of the completed DD-2766 remain in the record when the member goes TAD. In-house training sessions should be conducted prior to the implementation of this form.

    b. Detailed Instructions. The DD-2766 should be inserted as the first page of the medical record and all sections completed by the health care provider with the following guidelines exceptions:

        (1) Information from previous Problem Summary Lists should be copied and updated onto the DD-2766 as it is placed in the health record.

COMDTINST M6000.1E

(2) If the patient is not allergic to any drugs, indicate NKDA (no known drug allergies), in block 1.a.

(3) Sections 8.a., 10.e. and 10.i. are not required to be completed.

(4) Use a pencil to darken the circles on Section 7, Screening Exam.

(5) The Medical Officer should enter the date and location of every deployment the member participates in Section11, Pre/Post Deployment History. Pre and post deployment questionnaires are documented in Section 11 for participants in DOD deployment.

4. Consultation Sheet, SF-513.

   a. Purpose. A Consultation Sheet, SF-513 is used whenever a patient is referred to another facility for evaluation.

   b. Detailed Instructions. Complete the form as follows:

      (1) To. Facility or department to which the patient is being referred.

      (2) From. Unit referring the patient.

      (3) Date of Request. Self-explanatory.

      (4) Reason for Request. Specify the reason for referring the patient, i.e., chest pains, infected sebaceous cyst, etc.

      (5) Provisional Diagnosis. Self-explanatory.

      (6) Doctor's Signature. Must be signed by a Medical Officer, dental officer, or health services department representative. Accompanying this signature should be the qualifying degree of the individual requesting the consult.

      (7) Approved. Leave Blank.

      (8) Place of Consultation. Check the appropriate block.

      (9) Emergency/Routine. Check the appropriate block.

      (10) Identification No. Enter the patient's SSN.

      (11) Organization. Enter patient's branch of service.

      (12) Register No. If inpatient, enter the appropriate register number. If outpatient, leave d blank.

      (13) Ward No. If outpatient enter "OP." If inpatient, enter appropriate ward number.

      (14) Patient's Identification. Enter the appropriate patient identification information.

      (15) The remainder of the form is completed by the consultant.

COMDTINST M6000.1E

    c. <u>Completed Consultation Sheet, SF-513</u>. When the Consultation Sheet, SF-513 is completed and returned by the consultant the following actions are required:

        (1) Originator shall review and sign the SF-513.

        (2) The SF-513 shall then be filed in the appropriate dental or medical section of the health record.

5. <u>Medical Record, SF-507</u>. If received subsequent to the individual's discharge from the hospital, it shall be inserted in the health record immediately upon receipt. SF-507's are used for a variety of purposes, such as:

    a. <u>Patient's hospitalization</u>. To summarize the important facts about a patient's hospitalization.

    b. <u>Medical board</u>. To summarize the findings of a medical board.

    c. <u>Board of Flight Surgeons</u>. To report the results of a Board of Flight Surgeons.

6. <u>Pre-Deployment Health Assessment, DD-2795</u>. This form should be completed electronically using the Electronic Health Deployment Assessment (EDHA). The completed form should be printed out and placed in the health record. This form is used to assess the patient's health before possible deployment outside of the United States in support of military operations (and certain specified domestic deployments) and to assist military healthcare providers in identifying and providing present and future medical care. Directions for filling out this form can be found in Chapter 6. For questions concerning this form contact Operational Medicine at Commandant (CG-1121) http://www.uscg.mil/hq/cg1/cg11/.

7. <u>Post-Deployment Health Assessment, DD-2796</u>. This form should be completed electronically using the EDHA. The completed form should be printed out and placed in the health record. This form is used to assess the patient's health after deployment outside of the United States in support of military operations (and certain specified domestic deployments) and to assist military healthcare providers in identifying and providing present and future medical care. Direction for filling out this form can be found in Chapter 6 of this manual. For questions concerning this form contact Operational Medicine at Commandant (CG-1121) http://www.uscg.mil/hq/cg1/cg11/.

8. <u>Post-Deployment Health Re-Assessment, DD-2900</u>. This form should be completed electronically using the EDHA. The completed form should be printed out and placed in the health record. This form is designed to identify and address health concerns, with specific emphasis on mental health, that have emerged over time since deployment. Directions for filling out this form can be found in Chapter 6 of this Manual. For questions concerning this form contact

Operational Medicine at Commandant (CG-1121)
http://www.uscg.mil/hq/cg1/cg11/.

9. <u>Medical Recommendation for Flying, CG-6020</u>. Refer to the Aviation Medical Manual for instructions.

10. <u>Report of Medical Examination, DD-2808</u>.

   a. <u>Purpose</u>. The Report of Medical Examination, DD-2808 is used to record physical examination results to determine whether an examinee does, or does not, meet the standards established for the type of physical examination administered (e.g., initial enlistment, officer programs, retention, release from active duty, diving, aviation, retirement, etc.). The Report of Medical Examination, SF-88 is no longer applicable.

   b. <u>Preparation</u>.

      (1) When Prepared. A Report of Medical Examination, DD-2808 shall be prepared and submitted to the reviewing authority whenever a complete physical examination is required.

      (2) Required Entries. Certain groups of personnel are required to meet physical standards somewhat different from other groups. Accordingly, the use of all the spaces or use of the same spaces on the DD-2808 is not necessarily required for reporting the results of the various categories of physical examinations. If a certain item of the medical examination is required and facilities for accomplishing it are not available, an entry "NFA" (No Facilities Available) shall be made in the appropriate space. An entry "NE" (Not Evaluated) shall be made in the appropriate space for any item of the clinical evaluation (Items 17-42) which was not evaluated. For other items listed on the DD-2808 which were not required for a particular category of physical examination, an entry "NI" (Not Indicated) or "NA" (Not Applicable), shall be made in the appropriate space. Reference should be made to other provisions of Chapter 3, which prescribe the nature and scope of each physical examination and indicate the applicability of items of the DD-2808 to the particular program. Unless otherwise indicated by such provisions, the minimum requirements for completing the DD-2808 are:

         (a) All Examinations. Items 1-44, 45-63, 66, and 71a, shall be completed for all physical examinations, if facilities are available. Item 41 shall be completed for all female personnel.

         (b) Aviation Personnel. Additionally, Items 64, 65, and 66-70 and 72b shall be completed for physical examinations of aviation personnel.

COMDTINST M6000.1E

    (3) A physical examination must be thorough, recorded accurately, and contain sufficient information to substantiate the final recommendation. Before signing and forwarding, the examiner shall review the completed DD-2808 for completeness and accuracy. Failure to do so reflects significantly on the examiner's clinical and/or administrative attention to detail. Remember that the reviewing authority does not have the advantage of a direct examination and must rely on the examiner's written record and appropriate additional information in arriving at a decision.

  c. <u>Details for Entries on the Report of Medical Examination, DD-2808</u>.

    (1) Item 1: Date of Examination. Enter date in format - 02Aug15.

    (2) Item 2: Social Security Number. Enter the nine digits of their SSN.

    (3) Item 3: Last Name. Last Name - First Name - Middle Name. Record the surname in all capital letters. Record the given name(s) in full without abbreviation. If the individual's first or middle name consists only of an initial, enclose each initial in quotation marks (e.g., BAUR, Cheryl "W"). If the individual has no middle name, enter the letter "(n)" in parenthesis [e.g.., COFIELD, Bernie (n)]. Designations, such as, "Jr." or "II" shall appear after the middle name or initial. In the absence of a middle name or initial, these designations shall appear after the "(n)."

    (4) Item 4: Home Address. Enter the evaluee's present residence and not the home of record.

    (5) Item 5: Home Telephone Number. NA.

    (6) Item 6: Grade. Use official abbreviation of the current grade or rate. Example: HSCS; LTJG. If not a service member, enter "civilian."

    (7) Item 7: Date of Birth. (e.g. 57Sep04).

    (8) Item 8: Age. Enter age.

    (9) Item 9: Sex. Mark one or the other of the boxes.

    (10) Item 10: Race. Mark the box next to the racial or ethnic group of which member belongs.

    (11) Item 11: Total Years of Government Service. Enter years and months (e.g., 06 yrs 04 mo's).

    (12) Item 12: Agency. Enter the OPFAC number of the unit to which the examinee is attached.

    (13) Item 13: Organization and UIC/Code. List name of ship or station to which the examinee is assigned. Initial entry into Service; enter recruiting office concerned.

    (14) Item 14a: Rating or Specialty. NA

(15) Item 14b: Total Flying Time. Aviators only or NA.

(16) Item 14c: Last six months. Aviators only or NA.

(17) Item 15a: Service. Mark a box next to appropriate service.

(18) Item 15b: Component. Mark a box next to appropriate component.

(19) Item 15c: Purpose of Examination. Mark the box and corresponds to the appropriate purpose(s) of the examination. If not listed, mark "Other," and explain above the box such as: Diving Applicant; Biennial Aircrew; Medical Evaluation Board etc. Do not use the incomplete terms "flight physical," "diving physical," or "aviation physical." Rather, use specific terms such as "Class I Aviation,"

"Candidate for Flight Training," "Class II Aircrew," "Dive Candidate," "Quinquennial Diving," etc. Avoid nonstandard abbreviations. Differentiate between an applicant for a special program and a biennial physical for the same program. When necessary, continue under Item 73, Notes.

(20) Item 16: Examining Facility or Examiner. For civilian or contract physician, enter the full name and address. For USMTF, enter only the facility name, city and state in which located.

(21) Item 17-42: Clinical Evaluation. Check each item in appropriate column.

   (a) Item 35: Is continued on lower right side (Feet), circle appropriate category.

(22) Item 43: Dental Defects and Disease. For an oral examination as part of an accession physical, record whether or not the applicant is 'Acceptable' or 'Not Acceptable'. Refer to the standards described in Chapter 3 Section D-5 Physical standards for enlistment, appointment, and induction. Enter disqualifying defects in detail in Item 73. Record the Dental Classification. Refer to Chapter 4 Section C-3-c for definitions of dental classes. For routine physical examinations, record only the Dental Classification. When oral disease or dental defects are discovered on examination of active duty member personnel, suitable recommendations will be made for instituting corrective measures. A copy of the Dental Record, SF-603 does not need to be attached to the Report of Medical Examination, DD-2808.

(23) Item 44: Notes.

   (a) Approving official will endorse (stamp is authorized) in this box (if no room is available place in item 73 or add a separate endorsement) with the following information:

1. Date. This is the date that the member received their physical. For approved physicals this is also the date from which you will start counting to the next PE and the date of MRRS entry. (An unapproved physical shall not be entered into MRRS).

2. Does / Does Not meet physical standards.

3. What the physical was for.

4. Signature of approving authority and date. The signature is not necessary if the same person has signed in item 84. The date of the Approving authority should be no more than 60 days from the start of the physical, without written explanation for the delay.

Example: Date _____ Does / Does Not meet the physical standards for _____
as prescribed in Chapter 3.C of COMDT INST M6000.1 (series)
Signed _____ Date:_____
The disqualifying defects are:

(b) Describe every abnormality from Items 17-43 in detail. Enter pertinent item number before each comment. Continue in Item 73 and use a Continuation Sheet, SF-507 if necessary.

(24) Item 45: Laboratory Findings. Enter all laboratory results in quantitative values.

(a) Urinalysis. Enter specific gravity and results of albumin, sugar and if required, microscopic tests in the indicated spaces.

(b) Item 46: Urine HCG. If applicable.

(c) Item 47; H/H Enter either the hematocrit or the hemoglobin results.

(d) Item 48: Blood Type. If applicable.

(e) Item 49: HIV. Enter date drawn only in the results section.

(f) Item 50: Drugs Test Specimen ID Label. NA.

(g) Item 51: Alcohol. NA.

(h) Item 52: Other. Enter all other tests performed and their results which are not indicated on the form and which were performed in connection with the physical examination (e.g., sickle cell test, Papanicolaou (PAP) test, Tuberculin Skin Test (TST), Electrocardiogram (EKG), Chest X-ray results, etc.). The results will be continued in Item 73 or on a Medical Record, SF 507 if necessary. If provided on the lab report, include "normal" range values for all tests performed by a civilian or military lab. Use quantitative values and avoid vague terms such as "WNL" or other such qualitative forms.

(25) Item 53: Height. Measure without shoes and record to the nearest one-half centimeter (one-half inch).

(26) Item 54: Weight. Measure with the evaluee in under garments and record results to the nearest kilogram (pound).

(27) Item 55: Min Weight-Max weight, Max BF%. NA.

(28) Item 56: Temperature.

(29) Item 57: Pulse. Record the actual pulse rate.

(30) Item 58: Blood Pressure. Record the actual value in numerals for both systolic and diastolic.

(31) Item 59: Red/Green. NA

(32) Item 60: Other Vision Test. If applicable.

(33) Item 61: Distant Vision. Test and record using the Snellen scale. Record vision in the form of a fraction and in round numbers, such as 20/20, 20/40, not 20/20-2 or 20/40-3.

(34) Item 62: Refraction. Enter the lens prescription when the evaluee wears (or requires) lenses for correction of visual acuity. Do not enter the term "lenses".

(35) Item 63: Near Vision. Test and record using the Snellen scale. (See item 61).

(36) Item 64: Heterophoria. Enter when indicated.

(37) Item 65: Accommodation. Enter when indicated.

(38) Item 66: Color Vision. Color Vision. Enter the test used and the results.

  (a) Farnsworth Lantern (FALANT). Record the results as "Passed FALANT" or "Failed FALANT" followed by the fraction of correct over total (i.e., 9/9 or 17/18).

  (b) Pseudoisochromatic Plates (PIP). Record results as "Passed PIP" or "Failed PIP" followed by the fraction of correct over total (i.e., 12/14 or 14/14).

  (c) Enter "Passed on record" or "failed on record" if the results of a previous PIP or FALANT examination are available on record for review.

(39) Item 67: Depth Perception. When indicated, enter test used in left portion of Item 67.

COMDTINST M6000.1E

- (a) Armed Forces Vision Tester (AFVT). In the appropriate space in the right-hand portion of Item 65, record the letter designation of the highest group passed (i.e., Passed F).

- (b) Verhoeff. In the appropriate space in right-hand portion of Item 34, record perfect score as 16/16.

(40) Item 68: Field of Vision. Enter when indicated.

(41) Item 69: Night Vision. Enter when indicated.

(42) Item 70: Intraocular Tension. When indicated, enter the results in millimeters of mercury.

(43) Item 71: Audiometer. Required on ALL physical examinations. Use ANSI 1969 standards; do not use ISO or ASA standards.

- (a) Item 71a: Current.

- (b) Item 71b: If applicable.

(44) Item 72a: Reading Aloud Test. If applicable.

(45) Item 72b: Valsalva. When indicated mark either satisfactory (SAT) or unsatisfactory (UNSAT).

(46) Item 73: Notes and Significant or Interval History. Use this space for recording items such as:

- (a) Any pertinent medical history.

- (b) Summary of any condition which is likely to recur or cause more than minimal loss of duty time.

- (c) Wrist measurements.

- (d) Most recent HIV antibody test date (see Chapter 3-C-20.b.(5) of this Manual).

- (e) Date of TST and results.

(47) Item 74a: Examinee's Qualification. State whether or not the examinee is qualified for the purpose of the examination. If the purpose for the examination is an MEB, state whether or not the examinee is qualified or not qualified for retention and to perform the duties of his/her rank/rate at sea and foreign shores.

(48) Item 74b: Physical profile. Leave blank.

(49) Item 75: I have been advised of my disqualifying condition. If indicated, have evaluee sign and date.

(50) Item 76: Significant or Disqualifying Defects. Leave Blank

(51) Item 77: Summary of Defects and Diagnoses. List ALL defects in order to protect both the Government, and evaluee, in the event of future disability compensation claims. All defects listed which are not

COMDTINST M6000.1E

considered disqualifying shall be so indicated by the abbreviation NCD (Not Considered Disqualifying). When an individual has a disease or other physical condition that, although not disqualifying, requires medical or dental treatment clearly state the nature of the condition and the need for treatment. If a medical or dental condition is disqualifying, and treatment is scheduled to be completed prior to transfer to overseas or sea duty, indicate the date the member is expected to be fully qualified, e.g., "Dental appointment(s) scheduled, patient will be class I (dentally qualified) by (date)". Leave Profile Serial, RBJ, Qualified, and Waiver blocks blank.

(52) Item 78: Recommendations. Indicate any medical or dental recommendations. Specify the particular type of further medical or dental specialist examination indicated (use a Continuation Sheet, SF-507 if necessary).

(53) Item 79: Military Entrance Processing Station (MEPS) Workload. Leave Blank.

(54) Item 80: Medical Inspection Date. Leave Blank.

(55) Item 81-84: Names and Signature of Examiners. The name, grade, branch of Service, and status of each medical and dental examiner shall be typewritten, printed, or stamped in the left section. Each examiner shall sign using ballpoint pen or ink pen (black or blue-black ink only) in the appropriate section. Do not use facsimile signature stamps. When attachment sheets are used as a supplement or continuation to the report, they shall be serially number (both sides); however, indicate only the actual number of attached sheets in the bottom right block 87 on DD-2808.

(56) Item 85: Administrative Review. The person who reviews the PE for accuracy, prior to submitting for approval shall sign and date.

(57) Item 86: Waiver Granted. Leave Blank.

(58) Item 87: Number of attached Sheets. Fill in with appropriate number of forms attached.

11. Report of Medical History, DD-2807-1.

   a. Purpose. Report of Medical History, DD-2807-1 provides a standardized report of the examinee's medical history to help the examiner evaluate the individual's total physical condition, and to establish the presence of potentially disabling conditions which are not immediately apparent upon physical examination. In preparing the form, encourage the examinee to enter all medical problems or conditions experienced, no matter how minor they may be. The examiner must investigate and evaluate all positive medical history indicated on the form.

COMDTINST M6000.1E

b. <u>Preparation and Submission of Report of Medical History, DD-2807-1</u>. Prepare and submit DD-2807-1 with all physical examinations except: Periodic OMSEP and Substitution/Overseas/Sea Duty Modified Physical Examination.

c. <u>Preparation Procedures</u>. Report of Medical History, DD-2807-1 shall be prepared by the examinee and the examining Medical Officer.

   (1) The examinee shall furnish a true account of all injuries, illnesses, operations, and treatments since birth. False statements or willful omissions in completing the Report of Medical History, DD-2807-1 may result in separation from the Service upon arrival at the Academy, Recruit Training Center, Officer Candidate School, or later in the individual's career.

   (2) A copy of the Report of Medical History, DD-2807-1 must be included in the member's health record. Entries must be printed, in the examinees and examiner's own handwriting, using either ball-point pen or ink pen (black or dark blue). Pencils or felt-tip pens will not be used. Information in the numbered blocks on the form will be entered in the following manner:

      (a) Item 1: Last Name, First, Middle Name. BUNZEY, Michael D. Record the surname in all capital letters. Record the given name(s) in full, without abbreviation. If the individual's first or middle name consists only of an initial, enclose each initial within quotation marks. If the individual has no middle name, enter the letter "(n)" in parenthesis. Designations such as "Jr." or "II" will appear after the middle name or initial or after "(n)" if there is no middle name.

      (b) Item 2: Social Security Number. Enter SSN.

      (c) Item 3: Enter date format –year/month/day (ie 2001Sep04).

      (d) Item 4a: Home Address. Enter the evacuee's present residence and not the home of record.

      (e) Item 4b: Home Telephone. Enter home phone number.

      (f) Item 5: Examining Location and Address. For civilian or contract physician, enter the full name and address. For a Uniformed Services Military Treatment Facility (USMTF), enter only the facility name and the city and state in which located.

      (g) Item 6a: Service. Mark a box next to the appropriate service.

      (h) Item 6b: Component. Mark a box next to the appropriate component.

COMDTINST M6000.1E

(i) Item 6c: Purpose of Examination. Mark a box next to the appropriate purpose(s) of the examination. If not listed, mark "Other" and explain above the box such as: Diving Applicant; Biennial Aircrew; etc. For a medical board, indicate whether it is an IMB (Initial Medical Board)/DMB (Disposition Medical Board), etc. Do not use the incomplete terms "flight physical," "diving physical," or "aviation physical." Avoid nonstandard abbreviations. Differentiate between an applicant for a special program and a biennial physical for the same program.

(j) Item 7a: Position. Use official abbreviation of current grade or rate, branch of the Service, class and status; i.e., regular, reserve, or retired and if active or inactive. Example: HSCM, USCG; LTJG, USCGR; HSC, USCG (RET); HS3, USCG (TEMPRET). If not a Service member, enter "civilian."

(k) Item 7b: Usual Occupation. List current occupation.

(l) Item 8: Current Medications. List all current medications including over the counter meds.

(m) Item 9: Allergies. List any allergies to insect bites/stings, foods medicine or other substances.

(n) Item 10 to 28. Check appropriate box.

(o) Item 29: Explanation of "Yes" Answer(s). Describe all "yes" answers from section 10-28. Include date(s) of problems, name of doctor(s), and /or hospitals(s), treatment given and current medical status.

1. Append Item 29 to include: The statement to present health and a list of medications presently being taken by the examinee. For individuals receiving examinations more frequently, there is often little change in the medical history from year to year.

2. As an alternative to having the examinee complete Section 10-28 of the DD-2807-1 at a periodic examination, the following statement may be entered in Item 29 and initialed by the person undergoing the examination.
"I have reviewed my previous Report of Medical History and there have been no changes since my last medical examination, except as noted below." _____(initials).

(p) Item 30. Examiner's Summary and Elaboration of all Pertinent Data. Prior to performing the physical examination, the examiner

Chapter 4. B. Page 13

will review the completeness of the information furnished on the DD-2807-1. When this is done, summarize the medical history under (Item 30a. Comments) as outlined below and then sign the form. If additional space is needed, use Medical Record, SF-507.

(q) Do not use the term "usual childhood illnesses"; however, childhood illnesses (those occurring before age 12) may be grouped together enumerating each one. Incidents, other than those occurring in childhood, shall have the date recorded rather than the examinee's age. Do not use "NS" or "non-symptomatic" for items of history. Use "NCNS," "No Comp., No Seq." after items of recorded history where applicable. Elaborate on all items of history answered affirmatively except "Do you have vision in both eyes". The following specific questions shall also be asked on examination for initial entry into the CG, and for aviation and diving duty applicants:

1. "Is there a history of diabetes in your family (parent, sibling, or more than one grandparent)?"

2. "Is there a history of psychosis in your family (parent or sibling)?"

3. "Do you now or have you ever worn contact lenses?"

4. "Do you now or have you ever used or experimented with any drug, other than as prescribed by a physician (to include LSD, marijuana, hashish, narcotics, or other dangerous drugs as determined by the Attorney General of the United States)?"

5. "Have you ever required the use of an orthodontic appliance attached to your teeth or a retainer appliance? Month and year last worn? Are they still necessary?"

6. "Are there any other items of medical or surgical history that you have not mentioned?" All affirmative answers to the above questions shall be fully elaborated in Item 25. Negative replies to the above questions shall be summarized as follows: "Examinee denies history of psychosis, use of drugs, history of wearing of contact lenses, requirement for any orthodontic appliance, all other significant medical or surgical history; family history of diabetes." A rubber stamp or the overprinting of this information in Item 25 is recommended.

7. Distribution. Attach the original DD-2807-1 to the original DD-2808 and submit to reviewing authority. A copy of the DD-2807-1 and DD-2808 shall be kept on file at the unit

pending the return of the approved DD-2807-1 and DD-2808. After review and endorsement, the reviewing authority shall forward the original DD-2807-1 and DD-2808 to the member's parent command for insertion into the members health record.

12. <u>History and Report of OMSEP Examination, CG-5447.</u>

    a. <u>Introduction</u>. The CG-5447 is used to biennially update the Occupational Medical Surveillance and Evaluation Program. Demographic and identification information is vital to maintaining the database. CG-5447 will allow better tracking of personnel currently enrolled in OMSEP. Complete the form as follows:

      (1) Item 1: Last Name. Last Name - First Name - Middle Name. Record the surname in all capital letters. Record the given name(s) in full without abbreviation. If the individual's first or middle name consists only of an initial, enclose each initial in quotation marks (i.e., BRUNNER, Glen "W"). If the individual has no middle name, enter the letter "(n)" in parenthesis [i.e., COFIELD, Bernie (n)]. Designations, such as, "Jr." or "II" shall appear after the middle name or initial. In the absence of a middle name or initial, these designations shall appear after the "(n).

      (2) Item 2: Grade/Rate/Rank. Use official abbreviation of the current grade or rate, branch of service, class and status; i.e., regular, reserve, or retired, and if active or inactive. Example: HSCS, USCG; SN, USCG (TEMPRET); ETCM, USCG (RET). If not a service member, enter "civilian."

      (3) Item 3: SSN. Enter the Social Security Number.

      (4) Item 4: Date of Exam. Enter date in format e.g.04Sept03.

      (5) Item 5: Home Address. Enter home address in full (where examinee presently resides).

      (6) Item 6: Work/duty phone. Enter phone number beginning with area code. Include extension (if any), e.g., (xxx)-xxx-xxxx, ext xxxx.

      (7) Item 7: Unit Name and location. Enter unit, ship or station to where examinee is assigned.

      (8) Item 8: Home phone. Enter phone number beginning with area code. Include extension (if any), e.g., (xxx)-xxx-xxxx, ext xxxx.

      (9) Item 9: Unit Operating Facility (OPFAC)#. Enter OPFAC number of unit to which examinee is attached.

      (10) Item 10: Unit Zip Code: Enter unit's 5-digit zip code, e.g., 20593.

      (11) Item 11: Date of Birth & Age. Enter date followed by age in parentheses, e.g., 3Mar48 (54).

COMDTINST M6000.1E

(12) Item 12: Sex. Enter appropriate letter: (M) male or (F) female.

(13) Item 13: Race or Ethnicity. Enter a one character designator to identify the examinee's racial or ethnic group:

   (a) 1-Black.

   (b) 2-Hispanic (includes persons of Mexican, Puerto Rican, Cuban, Central and South American, or other Spanish origin or culture regardless of race).

   (c) 3-American Indian (including Alaskan Natives).

   (d) 4-Asian (including Pacific Islanders).

   (e) 5-All others (e.g., White/Caucasian, etc.).

(14) Item 14: Occupational or usual duties. Describe all primary duties, positions or billet assignments, (e.g. inspector, electrician, ASM).

(15) Item 15: Examining Facility Name & Location. For civilian or contract physician, enter the full name and address. For a USMTF, enter only the facility name and the city and state in which located.

(16) Item 16. Purpose of Examination. Mark appropriate box. If uncertain ask for assistance.

(17) Item 17. Years in Occupation. List number of years in present position or job title.

(18) Item 18-24. (Part 1-Section 1-Occupational History). Mark appropriate box Yes (Y) or No (N) as indicated.

(19) Item 25. (Part 1-Section 1-Occupational History). Explain all Yes (Y) answers to question 18-24 above.

(20) Item 26. (Part 1-Section II-Family History). Mark appropriate Yes (Y) or No (N) as indicated.

(21) Item 27. (Part 1-Section III-Social History). Mark appropriate box Yes (Y) or No (N) as indicated. Where indicated, please enter the number that best approximates the amount of tobacco products consumed/used by the examinee. If examinee does not consume tobacco products but is frequently exposed to second hand smoke (home; social group) please describe in Item 33 below.

(22) Item 28. (Part 1-Section III-Social History). Mark appropriate box Yes (Y) or No (N) as indicated. Where indicated, please enter the number that best approximates the amount of alcoholic beverages consumed/used by the examinee.

(23) Item 29. (Part 1-Section III-Social History). Mark appropriate box Yes (Y) or No (N) as indicated. Explain all YES answers.

COMDTINST M6000.1E

(24) Item 30. (Part 1-Section IV – Personal Health History). Mark appropriate box Yes (Y) or No (N) as indicated.

(25) Item 31. (Part 1-Section IV – Personal Health History). Mark the one box that best describes the examinees present health status.

(26) Item 32. (Part 1-Section IV – Personal Health History). Mark appropriate box Yes (Y) or No (N) as indicated.

(27) Item 33. (Part 1-Section IV – Personal Health History). Enter comments and explain all Yes (Y) responses to questions 27-32.

(28) Examinee must sign and date form.

(29) Item 34. (Part 1-Occupational Exposure History).

    (a) Column 1 - In chronological order list all known/documented exposures, including those occurring in prior employments.

    (b) Column 2 - Enter the date of the known exposure, e.g. year/day/month.

    (c) Column 3 - Enter the name of the place where exposure is known to have occurred.

    (d) Column 4 – List the type (if any) for protective equipment in use during the documented exposure.

(30) Examinee must sign and date form.

(31) Part 2 - Medical Officer Section.

    (a) Item 1-4. Same as Part 1 Items 1-4 first page. Provider must enter.

    (b) Item 5. Examining Facility Name & Location. For civilian or contract physician, enter the full name and address. For a USMTF, enter only the facility name and the city and state in which located.

    (c) Item 6. Enter the phone number of facility/medical provider performing the examination. Include area code and seven-digit number and extension, if indicated e.g. (xxx) xxx-xxxx extension xxx.

    (d) Item 7. Surveillance Protocols. Mark the indicated box for each of the examinee's documented exposure protocols for which an examination was performed. For a separation/termination examination, make sure to include ALL documented exposure protocols (past and present) for which surveillance was performed.

    (e) Item 8. Occupational related diagnosis. List ALL occupationally related diagnosis, e.g., asbestosis; leukemia, mesothelioma).

    (f) Item 9. Respirator Wear. Mark appropriate box.

    (g) Item 10. Conclusions. Mark appropriate box.

Chapter 4. B. Page 17

COMDTINST M6000.1E

- (h) Item 11. Next Occupational Medical Surveillance and Evaluation Program (OMSEP) Examination. For a regular schedule exam at the default time mark the space for"12 months". You may enter any specific time interval (of less than 12 months) under space marked "Other".

- (i) Item 12. Enter appropriate date when examinee was notified of examination results. This is a mandatory requirement.

- (j) Item 13. Provider should utilize this space to expand on all aforementioned diagnosis, to provide recommendations on follow-up care, and advice on future testing or procedures.

- (k) Medical provider must print name, sign and date form in space provided. Signature must include name, rank, and professional discipline.

13. Periodic History and Report of OMSEP Examination, CG-5447A.

   a. Introduction. The CG-5447A, Periodic History and Report of OMSEP Examination, is to be used for all scheduled periodic examinations. The member should review the last/previous OMSEP examination prior to completing this form.

   b. Items 1-10. Follow the same guidelines for part 1, CG-5447, Chapter 4 Section B 12.

   c. Item 11. Follow the same guidelines in Item 15 part 1, CG-5447, Chapter 4 Section B 12.

   d. Item 12. Last OMSEP Exam. Enter date of last OMSEP Initial/periodic or separation examination on record.

   e. Item 13. Present Exposure Protocols. Enter all documented exposure protocols for which examinations are scheduled.

   (1) Any changes since the last examination should be listed and describe in the "comments" area indicated for each of the particular sections. If no changes have occurred the member need only check the "no change " box, as indicated, for each of the particular sections.

   Section 1- Occupational History
   Section 2- Family History
   Section 3- Social History
   Section 4- Personal Health History
   Occupational Exposure

   (2) Health Care Provider Review. The Medical Officer is responsible for reviewing the completed CG-5447A and accompanying laboratory and radiological study results (if any), as well as making any final recommendations. The Medical Officer MUST enter all appropriate

comments in the "recommendations" space, including any additional studies, follow-up examinations or consultations. The medical provider MUST also initial the appropriate boxes indicating the review of any laboratory studies or radiological procedures performed as part of this examination.

    (3) The Medical Officer MUST provide name and signature (to include name, rank, and professional discipline) as well as date the CG-5447A (in the spaces provided) indicating the examinee was notified of any results and recommendations. When finalized the CG-5447A is to be placed into the member's medical record.

    (4) Note: If no changes have been reported by the examinee since the last examination and laboratory studies or radiological procedures (if any) are all within normal parameters, the designated health services technician (HST) may review and initial (sign and stamp) the completed CG-5447A after discussing the results with the cognizant Medical Officer and obtaining approval. The HST must make the following notation: "discussed and approved by Medical Officer" below the signature block. This allowance is intended primarily for situations where the cognizant Medical Officer is geographically separated and travel to/from the units negatively impacts unit operations.

14. <u>Medical Board Report Cover Sheet, CG-5684</u>.

    a. The CG-5684 is used in preparing a medical board. A copy of the CG-5684 and the complete medical board shall be inserted into the individual's health record.

    b. Detailed instructions for preparing and distributing this form are contained in Physical Disability Evaluation System, COMDTINST M1850.2 (series).

15. <u>Chronological Record of Medical Care, SF-600</u>.

    a. <u>General</u>.

    (1) This form provides a current, concise, and comprehensive record of a member's medical history. Properly maintained, the SF-600 should: aid in evaluating a patient's physical condition; greatly reduce correspondence to obtain medical records; eliminate unnecessary repetition of expensive diagnostic procedures; and serve as an invaluable permanent record of health care received. The SF-600 shall be continuous and include the following information as indicated: complaints; duration of illness or injury, physical findings, clinical course, results of special examinations; treatment; physical fitness at time of disposition; and disposition. The SF-600 also serves as the patient's prescription from which pharmacy services are provided.

(2) When a new SF-600 is initiated, complete the identification block with the name (last, first, middle initial), sex (M or F), year of birth, component (active duty or reserve), service (USCG, USN, USA, etc.), Social Security Number, and the member's grade/rate and organization at the time the form is completed.

(3) File SF-600's on the right side of the medical record with the most current SF-600 on top.

(4) Enter sick call entries on SF-600 in the following SOAP format:

SOAP METHOD OF SICK CALL WRITE UPS

S: (Subjective).

- cc: (Chief Complaint) sore throat, cough, diarrhea, etc.
- hpi: (History Present Illness) onset of symptoms, all problems, review of symptoms.
- pmh: (Past Medical History) any related problems in past that may be present with chief complaint.
- fh: (Family History) any diseases, chronic/acute, possibly related to present complaint.
- all: (Allergies) any known allergies to drugs/medications, etc.

O: (Objective).

First visual assessment/evaluation of the patient's general appearance: limping, bleeding doubled over, etc.

PE: All results of physical exam, vital signs, lab, x-ray, and any other study results.

A: (Assessment).

Imp: (Impression, Diagnosis) includes R/0 (rule out)

NOTE: THIS IS TO INCLUDE, AFTER IMPRESSION, WHAT YOU ARE GOING TO DO NOW AND WHY--SUCH AS, SUTURING, TOURNIQUET, ETC.

P: (Plan).

List of medications given, lab, x-ray, special studies ordered, duty status, return appointments, referrals, etc.

(5) The entries for all treatments shall be complete with regard to place, date, problem number (if appropriate), number of sick days, diagnosis of all conditions for which treated and signature of individual

furnishing treatment. Note all facts concerning the origin of the disease, pregnancy status, symptoms, course, treatment, and if a conflicting opinion is expressed subsequently by the same, or another Medical Officer, fully state the reason for such change. The record need not be voluminous, but it shall be thorough, concise, clearly phrased, and complete in each case. All entries, including signatures, must be legible.

(6) When a member is injured or contracts a disease while on leave, or when for any other reason the facts concerning an injury or sickness have not been entered in the individual's health record, the record custodian shall ascertain the facts in the case and make the necessary entries on SF-600. Discuss and document the instructions given to the patient. Include the intended treatment and, as appropriate, possible alternative treatments, possible complications, and long term prognosis. Information regarding previous treatments should be entered giving the following: date, place, and full details of treatment; laboratory reports; x-ray results; etc. The following shall also be entered:

   (a) "Date.

   (b) "Transcribed From Official Records.

   (c) Signature/Rate.

   (d) Duty Station of Transcriber.

(7) When an individual is required to carry the PHS-731, enter a statement of acknowledgment on the SF-600.

(8) When an individual is diagnosed as having a Sexually Transmitted Infection (STI) make an entry to record that an interview was conducted and that the following was discussed with the patient:

   (a) Symptoms.

   (b) Complications.

   (c) Treatments and contacts.

   (d) Treatment at Other Than Unit Assigned. When an activity furnishes sick call treatment to an individual whose health record is not available, an entry shall be made on a new SF-600, placed in a sealed envelope labeled "Sensitive Medical Information – Confidential," and forwarded to the individual's duty station for inclusion in the health record.

16. Emergency Care and Treatment, SF-558. This form provides a comprehensive yet concise record of emergency health care. It shall be used whenever an individual receives emergency treatment. Detailed instructions for completing the form are as follows:

COMDTINST M6000.1E

a. Patient's Home Address or Duty Station. Complete all blocks in this section.

b. Arrival. Record the date and time the patient arrived at the clinic or emergency room for care.

c. Transportation to Facility. Record the name of the ambulance company or unit that transported the patient for care, if appropriate. If patient was not transported by ambulance or other emergency vehicle, enter "N/A'.

d. Third Party Insurance. List detailed insurance if known by patient. If potential third party liability exists, forward a copy of SF-558 to Commandant (CG-1012). Note: Disregard DD-2568 in chart, enter N/A.

e. Current Medications. List all medications patient is presently taking.

f. Allergies. Record any substance or drug to which the patient has a known or suspected allergy. If none, enter "NKA" (No Known Allergy).

g. Injury or Occupational Illness. Most fields. When, refers to date injury was sustained. Where, refers to location injury occurred. How, refers to what happened (briefly).

h. Emergency Room Visit. Self-Explanatory.

i. Date of Last Tetanus Shot. Self-Explanatory.

j. Chief Complaint. Record a brief description of why the patient is seeking health care.

k. Category of Treatment. If Condition is Result of Accident/Injury. Check the block that best describes the patients' condition upon arrival.

   (1) Emergent. A condition which requires immediate medical attention and for which delay is harmful to the patient; such a disorder is acute and potentially threatens life or function.

   (2) Urgent. A condition which requires medical attention within a few hours or danger can ensue; such a disorder is acute but not necessarily severe.

   (3) Non-Urgent. A condition which does not require the immediate resources of an emergency medical services system; such a disorder is minor or non-acute.

l. Vital Signs. Take and record all vital signs. Indicate the time vitals were taken. Use 24-hour clock annotation i.e. 0215.

m. Lab Orders and X-Ray Orders. Self-Explanatory, check appropriate box.

n. Orders. List orders given by provider. Record all medications, appointments made. Or any other follow-up plans.

o. Disposition. Check appropriate box. Ensure patient understands this section.

COMDTINST M6000.1E

p. <u>Patient/Discharge Instructions</u>. Be specific. Ensure patient understands instructions given.

q. <u>Patients Signature and Date</u>. Have the patient or person accompanying the patient sign the form. This signature only acknowledges that instructions were given to the patient.

r. <u>Time Seen by Provider</u>. Record the time when the patient received treatment. Use 24-hour clock annotation i.e. 0215.

s. <u>Test Results</u>. Record results of tests ordered on patient.

t. <u>Provider History/Physical</u>. Self-explanatory, use standard S.O.A.P. format.

u. <u>Consult With</u>. List all individuals that on-scene provider received medical advice from. Example Dr. Richard Smith.

v. <u>Diagnosis</u>. Record patient diagnosis.

w. <u>Providers Signature and Date</u>. The Medical Officer or other health care provider shall sign and date the form. The signature shall include name, rank, and professional discipline.

x. <u>Codes</u>. List all ICD-9 codes applicable to the patient.

y. <u>Patients' Identification</u>. Ensure all patient identification information is entered.

17. <u>Emergency Medical Treatment Report, CG-5214</u>.

    a. <u>Purpose</u>. CG-5214 provides a multiple copy record of all emergency medical care rendered by CG personnel outside of a clinic or sickbay. All care rendered by crews of CG emergency vehicles must be documented with a CG-5214. (Alternatively, compatible state-approved forms may be used in lieu of the CG-5214).

        (1) Part 1, Copy to Patient. This copy shall be placed in the patients' health record in Section II behind the SF 558.

        (2) Part 2, Copy to Receiving Unit. This copy shall be given to the hospital, clinic, or Emergency Medical Services (EMS) crew assuming responsibility for patient care.

        (3) Part 3, Copy to Triage Officer. In multi-casualty incidents, this copy shall be given to the triage officer to account for the patients' treatment priority and status. Otherwise, this copy shall be kept on file at the clinic or sickbay.

    b. <u>Preparation and Submission of CG-5214</u>. The form provides an accurate account of the patient's injury or illness, and a detailed report of all treatments rendered en route to a receiving facility. If possible, the report should be completed during the transport phase. Detailed instructions for completing the CG-5214 are as follows:

(1) Victim Identification.

   (a) Item 1: Name. Enter last, first, and middle initial.

   (b) Item 2: Sex. Check one.

   (c) Item 3: Estimated Age. Enter in years or months.

(2) Description of Incident.

   (a) Item 4: Date. Enter date incident occurred.

   (b) Item 5: Type of Incident. Check one and give pertinent details under "Nature of Emergency/Mechanism of Injury".

   (c) Item 6: Time on Scene. Enter (using 24 hour clock).

   (d) Item 7: Time of Incident. Enter (using 24 hour clock).

   (e) Item 8: Location. Enter exact geographical area.

(3) Observation of Victim. Stick-Man figure: Place applicable injury letter code over injured area.

(4) Skin. Circle applicable number.

(5) Vital Signs. Note time observed (24 hour clock).

(6) Level of Consciousness. Check only one per time observed.

(7) Pupils. Check only one per time observed.

(8) Pulse. Place numerical value under rate and check appropriate space for quality.

(9) Breathing. Place numerical value under rate and check appropriate space for quality.

(10) Blood Pressure. Enter systolic and diastolic values under applicable time.

(11) Temperature. Circle either oral or rectal and enter in numerical value.

(12) Mast. Beside "Mast BP" enter blood pressure values. Circle applicable compartments inflated.

(13) Triage Information. Circle one of the following:

   (a) Priority I: Patients with airway and/or breathing problems, cardiac arrest, uncontrolled bleeding or controlled bleeding with symptoms of shock, severe head or abdominal injuries, and severe medical problems to include possible heart attack, severe burns, and severe poisonings.

   (b) Priority II: Patients with less serious burns, multiple fractures, potential C-Spine injuries without shock, or medical conditions of a less serious note.

(c) Priority III: Patients with obvious minor injuries or patients who are obviously dead or mortally wounded.

(14) Medications. List any medications the patient is currently taking.

(15) Allergies. List any known allergies for the patient.

(16) Medications Administered. Note the time, dosage, and route of administration for any medications administered to the patient.

(17) Rescuer Information.

  (a) Item 10: Name. Enter last, first, and middle initial.

  (b) Item 11: Level. Circle appropriate certification level.

  (c) Item 12: Unit. Rescuer's assigned unit.

  (d) Item 13: OPFAC#. Enter.

  (e) Item 14: Rescue vehicle. Identity of the responding vehicle, vessel, or aircraft.

  (f) Item 15: Receiving unit. Hospital, EMS vehicle, or clinic assuming responsibility for patient care.

  (g) Time patient transferred. Enter (24 hour clock).

18. <u>Radiographic Reports, SF-519</u>.

   a. This is a display form for mounting Radiographic Reports (SF-519-A). Attach the SF-519-A to the indicated spaces, with the most recent report on top.

   b. Use SF-519-A to request x-ray examinations. All patient data must be completed as indicated. Ensure that examinations requested are in standard terms or abbreviations. ALL pertinent clinical history, operations, physical findings, pregnancy status, and provisional diagnoses must be recorded in the appropriate space. This information is needed by the radiologist in order to render a proper interpretation of the film.

   c. Complete the required patient's identification information.

19. <u>Laboratory Reports</u>. Attach the laboratory reports to the indicated spaces with the most recent on top.

20. <u>Eyewear Prescription, DD-771</u>. Type DD-771 for clarity and to avoid errors in interpretation, using the following format:

   a. <u>Date</u>. Enter as follows, 22 JAN 87, etc.

   b. <u>Order Number</u>. Enter unit identifying number, issued by the Naval Ophthalmic Support & Training Activity (NOSTRA), above the order number block. Complete order number block if desired.

COMDTINST M6000.1E

c. To. Appropriate fabricating facility.

d. From. Enter complete unit address of unit ordering the eyewear.

e. Name, Service Number/Social Security Number. Enter as HINSON, Frank W. HSC 123-45-6789.

f. Age. Self-explanatory.

g. Unit and Address. Enter complete mailing address of unit to which individual is attached. If retiree, use the individual's home or mailing address.

h. Active Duty, etc. Check appropriate block.

i. USA, USN, etc. Check appropriate block.

j. Spectacles. Check appropriate block.

k. Aviation Spectacles. Use this block only when ordering aviation frames. Check as appropriate:

   (1) N-15 tinted lenses;

   (2) Coated lenses (coated with an anti-glare compound) are not authorized for Coast Guard personnel.

l. Other. Leave blank.

m. Interpupillary Distance. Copy directly from patient's Prescription, previous DD-771, or SF-600.

n. Eye Size. As above. (Not required for aviation goggles).

o. Bridge Size. As above. (Not required for aviation goggles).

p. Temple Length and Style. As above. (Not required for aviation goggles).

q. Number of Pairs. Enter the number of pairs requested.

r. Case. Enter the number of cases requested.

s. Single Vision.

   (1) Sphere. Copy directly from individual's prescription, previous DD-771, or SF-600 (+1.00, -1.25, etc.). Prescriptions are filled in multiples of 0.25 diopters only.

   (2) Cylinder. As above, except that prescriptions or multi-vision lenses must be in "minus cylinder" form, (-0.50, -0.75, etc.).

   (3) Axis. Copy directly from individual's prescription, previous DD-771, or SF-600. The axis must contain three (3) digits such as: 180, 090, 005, etc.

   (4) Decentration. Need not be completed unless specified as a part of prescription.

Chapter 4. B. Page 26

(5) Prism. As indicated on individual's prescription, previous DD-771, or SF-600.

(6) Base. As above.

t. Multivision. If the individual needs multivision lenses (bifocals, trifocals, etc.) then the prescription must be in minus cylinder form.

u. Special Lenses or Frames. This block is used for special instructions or justification for aviation spectacles, or nonstandard lenses, and frames, etc.

(1) When replacement eyewear is ordered from a prescription extracted from the health record, enter the following entry in this block: "REPLACEMENT ORDER: PRESCRIPTION FROM REFRACTION PERFORMED ON DATE."

(2) When eyewear is ordered for recruits, enter the following entry in this block: "RECRUIT - PLEASE EXPEDITE."

(3) When tinted lenses are ordered for non-aviation personnel, enter a written justification in this block. "Tinted lenses STATE JUSTIFICATION."

(4) When nonstandard temples or frames are ordered, enter type frame or temple requested, and justification:

(a) Riding Bow Cables, (Justification).

(b) Adjustable Nose Pads, (Justification).

(5) When an individual's pupillary distance is less than 60 mm it must be verified and an entry placed in this block: "PD of ____ verified and correct."

v. Signature of Approving Authority. Shall be signed by the Senior Medical Executive, designated representative, or the Commanding Officer where no Medical Officer is present.

w. Signature of the Prescribing Officer. Shall be signed by the Medical Officer or person performing the refraction. When this is not possible, i.e., examination obtained from a civilian source, transcribed from the health record, etc., the person transcribing the information shall sign as prescribing officer. Flight Surgeons may sign prescriptions as both the prescribing and approving authority.

21. Syphilis Record, SF-602.

a. Purpose. This form shall be prepared and inserted in the health record for each person for whom a confirmed diagnosis of syphilis or any of its complications or sequela has been established.

b. Providers and patients responsibilities. The Medical Officer shall carefully and thoroughly explain to the patient the nature of the infection and the reasons why treatment, prolonged observation and the repeated performance of certain prescribed tests are necessary. The patient shall then be requested to sign the statement in Section II of SF-602.

22. Authorization for Anesthesia, Operations, etc., OF-522. Complete a OF-522 describing the general nature of the procedure and have the patient sign prior to administering anesthesia (local or general). except for dental anesthesia. An SF- 522 is required for dental surgical procedures such as exodontia, root canal therapy, and periodontal surgery; a OF-522 is not required for routine dental anesthesia. File the OF-522 for dental procedures in Section VI of the Medical Record in chronological order behind the SF-603.

23. Record of Occupational Exposure to Ionizing Radiation, DD-1141.

    a. Requirements. The custodian of the medical records shall prepare and maintain as DD-1141 for each person occupationally exposed to ionizing radiation. Enter all exposures in rems.

    b. Recording Procedures.

        (1) Initial Determination of Accumulated Dose.

            (a) In the initial preparation of DD-1141, obtain complete reports of previous exposure. For each period in which the individual was engaged in activities where occupational exposure was probable, and no record, or only an incomplete record of exposure during the period can be obtained, assume that an occupational exposure of 1.25 rems was incurred per quarter of each calendar year or fraction thereof.

            (b) In cases where the nature of the radiation is unknown, assume gamma radiation.

            (c) If an individual was exposed at more than one facility, calculate the cumulative exposures and record them in Items 7 through 12 as appropriate. Enter the sum of the whole body exposure in Item 13, and a statement regarding the sources of that information in Item 16, REMARKS.

        (2) Current Record.

            (a) Quarterly, make appropriate entries on each individual's DD-1141 from the exposure records received from the Public Health Service Contractor.

            (b) Maintain separate DD-1141 to record exposures other than whole body, with appropriate descriptions under Item 16, REMARKS.

    c. Completion Instructions.

(1) Item 1. Leave blank.

(2) Item: 2. Enter last name, first name, and middle initial. If the combination of last name and first name exceed 19 spaces, enter last name and initials only.

(3) Item 3. Enter SSN.

(4) Item: 4. Enter in not more than 10 spaces, rate, grade, title or position the individual is currently holding. Use standard service abbreviations (i.e., CAPT, HSCS, HSl, etc.). Abbreviate civilian occupation titles as needed (i.e., Radiological Physicist to Rad Physic, Radiation Physiologist to Rd Physiol, Electrical Welder to Elec Wldr, etc.).

(5) Item 5. Enter date of birth: i.e., 4 SEP 87.

(6) Item 6. Enter name of activity or unit.

(7) Items 7 & 8. "Period of Exposure." Enter the day, month, and year: i.e., 1 MAR 87.

(8) Items 9-12. "Dose This Period." Enter radiation dose received this period to three decimal places: i.e., 02.345rem. Use five digits including zeros as necessary for all entries.

   (a) Item 9. Enter skin dose (soft) which includes low energy gamma and x-ray of less than 20 kilovolts peak (kVp) effective energy and beta radiation. Total skin dose is the addition of columns 9 and 12.

   (b) Item 10. Enter gamma and x-ray dose greater than 20 KVE effective energy in REM.

   (c) Item 11. Enter neutron dose in REM.

   (d) Item 12. Enter sum of items 10 and 11.

(9) Item 13. Add item 12 to previous item 13; enter total in item 13.

(10) Item 14. Enter permissible dose calculated from the age formula $5(N-18)$ REM, where N equals the present age in years.

(11) Item 15. Recorder certifies entries by initial.

(12) Item 16. Enter other pertinent information such as known exposure from internally deposited radioactive material or from any external radioactive sources. Describe briefly any activity or assignment bearing a potential for exposure and estimate dose-time relationships, if feasible. If this form is used for other than whole body and skin of whole body, specify the use; i.e., hands and forearms, feet and ankles, thyroid, etc. When recorded dose is not obtained from film badge readings, specify whether estimates were obtained from pocket dosimeters, area or air monitoring, bioassay, etc.

24. <u>Audiogram Results</u>. The Microprocessor will generate a legal archival test result strip which shall filed chronologically in the health records.

25. Reference Audiogram, DD-2215. Place form in section V of the Health Record.

26. Hearing Conservation Data, DD-2216. Place form in section V of the Health Record.

27. Chronological Record of Service, CG-4057.

    a. Purpose. Use this form:
       (1) As a statement of agreement or disagreement with the assumption of fitness for duty upon separation from the CG.
       (2) To terminate the health record.

    b. Agreement or disagreement with the assumption of fit for duty at the time of separation. Members not already in the physical disability evaluation system, who disagree with the assumption of fitness for duty at separation, shall indicate on the reverse of the Chronological Record of Service, CG-4057. They shall then proceed as indicated in paragraph Chapter 3 Section B 5 of this Manual. Members who agree with the assumption shall check the box indicating agreement. This is a health services department responsibility when there is a health services department representative attached; otherwise it becomes a personnel action.

    c. Terminating the health record. The reverse side of the form is also used to terminate a member's health record upon definite separation from active service. The date of termination is the effective date of separation. Make appropriate entries giving the reason for termination, the date of termination and the grade and signature of the responsible commissioned officer in the bottom portion of the form. Additionally, an entry, signed by the member whose health record is being terminated, acknowledging the receipt of a copy all available NAVMED 6150/2's, a copy of separation examination if done (either DD-2808 or SF-600 entry), a signed copy of the Chronological Record of Service, CG-4057, and the PHS-731 (if available) shall be made in the Remarks section of the Chronological Record of Service, CG-4057.

    d. Notification of benefits. This form is also used to notify the individual of the possibility of certain disability benefit entitlements from the Department of Veterans Affairs after separation.

    e. Chronological Record of Service, CG-4057 is filled. If either side of the Chronological Record of Service, CG-4057 is filled, the reverse side shall have a line drawn diagonally through it in red and a second Chronological Record of Service, CG-4057, marked "Supplement started this date" at the top.

28. Authorization for Disclosure of Medical or Dental Information, DD-2870. In order to use or disclose patient health information for purposes beyond the treatment, payment and health care operations and other purposes described in the MHS Notice of Privacy Practices, written authorization from the patient must be obtained on form DD-2870.

29. Request to Restrict Medical or Dental Information, DD-2871. Individuals have the right to request restrictions on the use or disclosure of their health information. Requests must be made in writing on form DD-2871. Requests for restriction may be denied upon review by the clinic HIPAA Privacy/Security Official, or the CG HIPAA Privacy/Security Official.

30. International Certificate of Vaccination, PHS-731.

    a. General.

        (1) When required, prepare PHS-731 for each member of the CG (for reserve personnel when ordered to Active Duty for Training). This form shall be carried only when required for performing international travel.

        (2) A reservist not on extended active duty who plans international travel either under official orders or privately, may request that the appropriate district commander (r) furnish a PHS-731 for this purpose. The reservist shall return the PHS-731 to the district commander (r) when travel is completed.

        (3) When properly completed and authenticated, the PHS-731 contains a valid certificate of immunization for international travel and quarantine purposes in accordance with World Health Organization Sanitary Regulations.

        (4) All military and nonmilitary personnel performing international travel under CG cognizance shall be immunized in accordance with Commandant Instruction 6230.4 (series) and shall have in their possession a properly completed and authenticated PHS-731, if required by the host country.

    b. Detailed Instructions.

        (1) Stamp or type the following address on the front of PHS-731:

            COMMANDANT (CG-11)
            ATTN HEALTH SAFETY AND WORKLIFE
            US COAST GUARD
            2100 2ND ST SW STOP 7902
            WASHINGTON DC 20593-7902

        (2) Enter data by hand, rubber stamp, or typewriter.

        (3) Enter the day, month, and year in the order named (i.e., 4 SEP 87).

        (4) Record the origin and batch number for yellow fever vaccine.

        (5) Entries for cholera and yellow fever must be authenticated by the Department of Defense Immunization Stamp and the actual signature of the Medical Officer. Other immunizations may be authenticated by

COMDTINST M6000.1E

initialing. Entries based on prior official records shall have the following statement added: "Transcribed from Official Records."

c. <u>International Certificate of Vaccination, PHS-731</u>. Remove the PHS-731 from the health record and give it to the individual upon separation from the Service.

31. <u>Tissue Examination, SF-515.</u>

a. Prepare a SF-515 or use the contract lab form whenever a tissue specimen is forwarded to a laboratory for examination.

b. Ensure patient's identification information is completed.

32. <u>Request for Medical/Dental Records or Information, DD-877.</u>

a. <u>Purpose</u>. The Request for Medical/Dental Records or Information, DD-877 is a form used to track health records between clinics and units as well as to request records from clinics, units, or MTFs.

b. <u>General</u>. This form shall be initiated and included with health and clinical records as directed in Chapter 4 Section A 5 c (2) (a) 3. and Chapter 4 Section D 7 of this Manual.

c. <u>Detailed Instruction</u>.

(1) Each DD-877 must have all boxes completed.

(2) In all instances when a DD-877 is initiated, remarks concerning the reason for sending the record, the name of the gaining unit for the member/ sponsor and a request for action will be included on the form. When preparing a DD-877 for a record to be forwarded, place the following in section 9, REMARKS: "Health {clinical} record for this member (family member) is forwarded to you for appropriate filing. Member (sponsor) assigned to (insert gaining unit name)."

(3) For members entering the Individual Ready Reserve, (IRR) follow the instructions given by the Servicing Personnel Office as per the Military Personnel Data Records (PDR) System, COMDTINST M1080.10 (series).

(4) A copy of the DD877 will be retained at the unit sending the record for 6 months after the record is mailed, and then may be discarded.

33. <u>Modified Screening For: Overseas Assignment and/or Sea Duty Health Screening, CG-6100.</u>

a. <u>General</u>. Refer to Chapter 3 of this manual for the completion of this form.

34. <u>Bloodborne Pathogens Exposure Guidelines, CG-6201</u>.

a. General. Refer to Chapter 13 of this manual for the completion of this form.

35. Examination Protocol for Exposure to: CHROMIUM COMPOUNDS, CG-6202.

    a. General. Refer to Chapter 12 of this manual for the completion of this form.

36. Examination Protocol for Exposure to: ASBESTOS, CG-6203.

    a. General. Refer to Chapter 12 of this manual for the completion of this form.

37. Examination Protocol for Exposure to: BENZENE, CG-6204.

    a. General. Refer to Chapter 12 of this manual for the completion of this form.

38. Examination Protocol for Exposure to: NOISE, CG-6205.

    a. General. Refer to Chapter 12 of this manual for the completion of this form.

39. Examination Protocol for Exposure to: HAZARDOUS WASTE, CG-6202.

    a. General. Refer to Chapter 12 of this manual for the completion of this form.

40. Examination Protocol for Exposure to: LEAD, CG-6207.

    a. General. Refer to Chapter 12 of this manual for the completion of this form.

41. Examination Protocol for Exposure to: RESPIRATOR WEAR, CG-6208.

    a. General. Refer to Chapter 12 of this manual for the completion of this form.

42. Examination Protocol for Exposure to: PESTICIDES, CG-6209.

    a. General. Refer to Chapter 12 of this manual for the completion of this form.

43. Examination Protocol for Exposure to: RESPIRATORY SENSITIZERS, CG-6210.

    a. General. Refer to Chapter 12 of this manual for the completion of this form.

44. Examination Protocol for Exposure to: BLOODBORNE PATHOGENS, CG-6211.

COMDTINST M6000.1E

a. <u>General</u>. Refer to Chapter 12 of this manual for the completion of this form.

45. Examination Protocol for Exposure to: TUBERCULOSIS, CG-6212.

    a. <u>General</u>. Refer to Chapter 12 of this manual for the completion of this form.

46. Examination Protocol for Exposure to: SOLVENTS, CG-6213.

    a. <u>General</u>. Refer to Chapter 12 of this manual for the completion of this form.

47. Examination Protocol for Exposure to: RADIATION, CG-6214.

    a. <u>General</u>. Refer to Chapter 12 of this manual for the completion of this form.

48. How to Calculate a Significant Threshold Shift, CG-6215.

    a. <u>General</u>. Refer to Chapter 12 of this manual for the completion of this form.

Section C. Dental Records Forms, Classification, and Treatment Priority.

    FORM   TITLE

1. Dental Record Cover, CG-3443-2. 1
2. Dental Health Questionnaire, NAVMED 6600/3. 2
3. Dental Record, SF-603. 2
4. Dental Continuation, SF-603-A. 14
5. Consultation Sheet, SF-513. 14
6. Lost Dental Records...14
7. Special Dental Records Entries..14
8. Dental Examination Requirements. 14
9. Recording of Dental Treatments on Chronological Record of Care, SF-600.........15

This page intentionally left blank.

C. Dental Record Forms, Classification, and Treatment Priority.

1. Dental Record Cover, CG-3443-2.

   a. Open a Dental Record Cover, CG-3443-2 for each individual upon arrival at a training center or initial entry into the CG or CG Reserve. When an individual on the retired list returns to active duty, submit a request for a copy of the closed out dental record to Commandant (G-PIM). Whenever the original record is lost or destroyed, a new dental record shall be opened immediately. The dental record shall be kept in the Health Record Cover, CG-3443 of each individual.

   b. All dental forms and radiographs will be contained in the Dental Record.

   c. Detailed Instructions.

      (1) Surname. Record the surname in all capital letters.

      DOE

      SURNAME

      (2) Given name(s). Record in full without abbreviation. If the individual has no middle name or initial then record the lower case letter "n" in parentheses (n). If the individual has only a middle initial(s), record each initial in quotation marks. When "Jr." or "II" or other similar designations are used, they shall appear after the middle name or initial.

      DOE   JANE   ANN

      SURNAME   First Name   Middle Name

      (3) Social Security Number (SSN). Enter Social Security Number.

      (4) Date of Birth. Enter day, month (abbreviated JAN, FEB, MAR, etc.), and the year: i.e., 4 SEP 49.

      (5) Change in Grade or Rate. Enter as they occur.

      (6) Blood Type. Enter the individual's blood type in the appropriate box. If not known, perform a blood type test.

      (7) RH Factor. Enter the individual's RH factor in the appropriate box. If not known, perform an RH factor test.

      (8) Drug Sensitivity Sticker. When required, affix the Drug Sensitivity Sticker, CG-5266 to the lower left corner of the front of the Dental Record Cover. Do not cover other identification data.

      (9) Dental Radiographs. Dental Bitewing Radiograph Storage. Bitewing radiographs shall be stored in the standard stock 5-year x-ray card (FSC# 6525-00-142-8732). This shall replace the single bitewing x-ray card (FSC# 6525-00-817-2364). X-ray film is mounted in the x-ray card with the raised dot side of the film on the **front** side of the card.

2. Dental Health Questionnaire, NAVMED 6600/3.

   a. General. The Dental Health Questionnaire, NAVMED 6600/3 will help the Dental Officer detect any present or past health problem (i.e., positive Human Immunodeficiency Virus (HIV)) that might interfere with definitive dental treatment. All positive answers from the health history section must be followed up by the Dental Officer for impact on health care and so annotated on the Dental Health Questionnaire, NAVMED 6600/3 and the Dental Continuation, SF-603-A.

   b. Detailed Instructions. Insert the Dental Health Questionnaire as the first page of the dental record. Patients shall fill out a new Dental Health Questionnaire at least annually, or when information changes. Maintain the two most recent forms in the dental record with the current Dental Health Questionnaire, NAVMED 6600/3 on top.

      (1) Chief Complaint. Have the patient enter the problem they are presently having.

      (2) Check and Sign. Have the patient enter yes/no in each box of the history. The signature indicates the authenticity of the history.

      (3) Summary of Pertinent Findings. Include baseline BP reading.

3. Dental Record, SF-603.

   a. General. The Dental Record is a continuous history and must contain accurate and complete entries of dental examinations and treatments. Each entry shall clearly indicate the name of the Dental Officer conducting the examination and/or rendering the treatment. Dental Hygienists or other auxiliary personnel providing care shall also follow this requirement. Each dental officer is personally responsible for ensuring that all entries are properly recorded.

   b. Numerical Classification for Record Purposes. Chart markings have been standardized so that dental conditions, treatments needed, and treatments completed may be readily identified. This facilitates efficient continuity of treatments and may establish identification in certain circumstances.

      (1) Use the following numbering system for permanent dentition starting with the maxillary right third permanent molar as tooth #1:

1	2	3	4	5	6	7	8	9	10	11	12	13	14	15	16
32	31	30	29	28	27	26	25	24	23	22	21	20	19	18	17

(2) Use the following numbering system for deciduous dentition starting with the maxillary right second deciduous molar as tooth A:

A	B	C	D	E	F	G	H	I	J
T	S	R	Q	P	O	N	M	L	K

(3) Indicate a supernumerary tooth by placing "s" in the location of the supernumerary tooth and in the remarks section enter a statement that the examinee has a supernumerary tooth.

(4) Indicate deciduous and supernumerary teeth on the SF-603 in SECTION I, Part 5 (Diseases, Abnormalities, and Radiographs) and enter a statement in the remarks section of Section 5.

c. Detailed Instructions. SECTION 1. DENTAL EXAMINATION

(1) Purpose of Examination. To assess the oral health status of cadets, officer candidates and enlisted recruits upon initial entry into the CG, and to provide periodic (but at least annual) examinations of active duty personnel. Enter an "X" in the appropriate box. Mark the "Initial" box for the dental examination made upon entrance into the CG. All other examinations fall under the "Other" category and shall be identified: i.e., "Academy", "Reenlistment", etc.

(2) Type of Examination. Enter an "X" in the proper box of item 2, "Type of Exam."

(a) Type 1, Comprehensive Examination. Comprehensive hard and soft tissue examination, shall include: oral cancer screening examination; mouth-mirror, explorer, and periodontal probe examination; adequate natural or artificial illumination; panoramic or full-mouth periapical, and posterior bitewing radiographs as required; blood pressure recording; and when indicated, percussive, thermal, and electrical tests, transillumination, and study models. Included are lengthy clinical evaluations required to establish a complex total treatment plan. For example, treatment planning for full mouth reconstruction, determining differential diagnosis of a patient's chief complaint, or lengthy history taking relative to determining a diagnosis. Use S.O.A.P. format to record the results of a Type 1 examination.

(b) Type 2, Oral Examination (annual or periodic). Shall include hard and soft tissue examination, which shall include: oral cancer screening examination; mouth mirror and explorer examination include Periodontal Screening and Recording™ (PSR) with sextant scores; appropriate panoramic or intraoral radiographs as indicated by the clinical examination; and blood pressure recording. An appropriate treatment plan shall be recorded. This type is the routine examination, which is normally performed one time per treatment regimen per patient, unless circumstances warrant another complete examination. Use S.O.A.P. format to record the results of Type 2 examination.

(c) Type 3, Other Examination. Diagnostic procedure as appropriate for: consultations between staff; observation where no formal consult is prepared; certain categories of physical examination; and emergency oral examination for evaluation of pain, infection, trauma, or defective restorations and follow-up exams for previously rendered treatment.

(d) Type 4, Screening Evaluation. Mouth mirror and explorer or tongue depressor examination with available illumination. This includes the initial dental processing of candidates without necessarily being examined by a dentist, or other dental screening procedures.

(e) If not specified by this Manual, it shall be the professional responsibility of the Dental Officer to determine the type of examination which is appropriate for each patient. However, Type 3 and Type 4 examinations are not adequate to definitively evaluate the oral health status of patients. When the Dental Officer determines that a comprehensive periodontal examination is to be accomplished, use the Navy Periodontal Chart, NAVMED 6600/2 (3-90).

(3) Dental Classification of Individuals. Dental classifications are used to designate the health status and the urgency or priority of treatment needs for active duty personnel. Use the following guidelines and criteria for the classification of patients. When a criterion for a specific condition is not listed, the dental officer shall evaluate the prognosis for a dental emergency and assign the appropriate classification.

(a) Class 1 (Oral Health). Patients with a current dental examination, who do not require dental treatment or reevaluation. Class 1 patients are worldwide deployable.

(b) Class 2. Patients with a current dental examination, who require non-urgent dental treatment or reevaluation for oral conditions, which are unlikely to result in dental emergencies within 12 months. Class 2 are worldwide deployable. Patients in dental class 2 may exhibit the following:

1. Treatment or follow-up indicated for dental caries or minor defective restorations that can be maintained by the patient.

2. Interim restorations or prostheses that can be maintained for a 12-month period. This includes teeth that have been restored with permanent restorative materials for which protective cuspal coverage is indicated.

3. Edentulous areas requiring prostheses but not on an immediate basis.

4. Periodontium that:

   a. Requires oral prophylaxis.

b. Requires maintenance therapy.

  c. Requires treatment for slight to moderate periodontitis and stable cases of more advanced periodontitis.

  d. Requires removal of supragingival or mild to moderate sub-gingival calculus.

 5. Unerupted, partially erupted, or malposed teeth that are without historical, clinical, or radiographic signs or symptoms of pathosis, but which are recommended for prophylactic removal.

 6. Active orthodontic treatment. The provider should consider placing the patient in passive appliances for deployment up to six months. For longer periods of deployment, the provider should consider removing active appliances and placing the patient in passive retention.

 7. Temporomandibular disorder patients in remission. The provider anticipates patient can perform duties while deployed without ongoing care and any medications or appliances required for maintenance will not interfere with duties.

(c) <u>Class 3</u>. Patients who require urgent or emergent dental treatment. Class 3 patients normally are not considered to be worldwide deployable.

 1. Treatment or follow-up indicated for dental caries, symptomatic tooth fracture or defective restorations that cannot be maintained by the patient.

 2. Interim restorations or prostheses that cannot be maintained for a 12-month period.

 3. Patients requiring treatment for the following periodontal conditions that may result in dental emergencies within the next 12 months.

  a. Acute gingivitis or pericoronitis.

  b. Active progressive moderate or advanced periodontitis.

  c. Periodontal abscess.

  d. Progressive mucogingival condition.

  e. Periodontal manifestations of systemic disease or hormonal disturbances.

  f. Heavy subgingival calculus.

4. Edentulous areas or teeth requiring immediate prosthodontic treatment for adequate mastication or communication, or acceptable esthetics.

5. Unerupted, partially erupted, or malposed teeth with historical, clinical or radiographic signs or symptoms of pathosis that are recommended for removal.

6. Chronic oral infections or other pathologic lesions.

7. Pulpal, periapical, or resorptive pathology requiring treatment.

8. Lesions requiring biopsy or awaiting biopsy report.

9. Emergency situations requiring therapy to relive pain, treat trauma, treat acute oral infections, or provide timely follow-up care (e.g., drain or suture removal) until resolved.

10. Acute Temporomandibular disorders requiring active treatment that may interfere with duties.

(d) Class 4: Patients who require periodic dental examinations or patients with unknown dental classifications. Class 4 patients normally are not considered to be worldwide deployable.

(4) Priority of Dental Treatment. To further indicate priority of treatment within a class, the following groupings shall be used when necessary (listed in order of decreasing priority).

(a) Group 1. CG active duty personnel in receipt of orders to sea, overseas, or combat duty.

(b) Group 2. CG active duty personnel upon return from sea, overseas, or combat duty.

(c) Group 3. Other CG personnel.

(d) Group 4. Active duty personnel of other Services assigned to duty with the CG.

(e) Group 5. Active duty personnel of other Services.

(5) Missing Teeth and Existing Restorations.

(a) Markings shall be made on examination chart as follows:

1. Missing Teeth. Draw a large "X" on the root(s) of each tooth that is not visible in the mouth.

2. Edentulous Mouth. Inscribe crossing lines, one extending from the maxillary right third molar to the mandibular left third molar and the other from the maxillary left third molar to the mandibular right third molar.

3. <u>Edentulous Arch</u>. Make crossing lines, each running from the uppermost aspect of one third molar to the lowest aspect of the third molar on the opposite side.

4. <u>Amalgam Restorations</u>. In the diagram of the tooth, draw an outline of the restoration showing size, location, and shape, and block solidly.

5. <u>Nonmetallic Permanent Restorations (includes ceramics and resins)</u>. In the diagram of the tooth, draw an outline of the restoration showing size, location, and shape.

6. <u>Gold Restorations</u>. Outline and inscribe horizontal lines within the outline.

7. <u>Combination Restorations</u>. Outline showing overall size, location, and shape; partition and junction materials used and indicate each, as in "4." above.

8. <u>Porcelain and Acrylic Post Crowns</u>. Outline the crown and approximate size and position of the post(s).

9. <u>Porcelain Veneers</u>. Outline each aspect.

10. <u>Acrylic Resin Jacket Crowns</u>. Outline each aspect.

11. <u>Fixed Bridges</u>. Outline each, showing overall size, location, teeth involved and shape by the inscription of diagonal lines in abutments and pontics.

12. <u>Removable Appliances</u>. Place an "X" through the missing tooth, place a line over replaced teeth and describe briefly in "Remarks."

13. <u>Root Canal Fillings</u>. Outline canal filled and black in solidly.

14. <u>Apicoectomy</u>. Draw a small triangle apex of the root of the tooth involved, the base line to show the approximate level of root amputation.

15. <u>Drifted Teeth</u>. Draw an arrow from the designating number of the tooth that has moved; the point of the arrow to indicate the approximate position to which it has drifted. Under "Remarks" note the relationship to the drifted tooth in respect to occlusion.

(b) If an individual is appointed or enlisted with dental defects which have been waived, the defects shall be described fully in the dental record under "Remarks" (Section I).

(c) The examining Dental Officer shall sign, date, and record the place of examination where indicated.

(6) <u>Diseases, Abnormalities, and Radiographs</u>.

(a) Markings on the examination chart of Diseases, Abnormalities, and Radiographs shall be made as follows:

1. <u>Caries</u>. In the diagram of the tooth affected, draw an outline of the carious portion, showing size, location and shape, and block in solidly.

2. <u>Defective Restoration</u>. Outline and block in solidly the restoration involved.

3. <u>Impacted Teeth</u>. Outline all aspects of each impacted tooth with a single oval. Indicate the axis of the tooth by an arrow pointing in the direction of the crown.

4. <u>Abscess</u>. Outline approximate size, form, and location.

5. <u>Cyst</u>. Outline the approximate form and size in relative position of the dental chart.

6. <u>Periodontal Disease</u>. Inscribe a horizontal continuous line on the external aspect of root(s) involved in a position approximating the extent of gingival recession or the clinical depth of the pocket. If known, indicate the position of the alveolar crest by a second continuous line in relative position to the line indicating the gingival tissue level.

7. <u>Extraction Needed</u>. Draw two parallel vertical lines through all aspects of the tooth involved.

8. <u>Fractured Tooth Root</u>. Indicate fracture with a zigzag line on outline of tooth root.

(b) A statement regarding hypersensitivity to any other drug known to the person for whom a Dental Record is prepared shall be entered under "Remarks." (Example: HYPERSENSITIVITY TO PROCAINE).

(c) Complete items A through E.

(d) The examining Dental Officer shall sign, date, and record the place of examination where indicated.

(e) NOTE: Section I, Subsections 4 and 5 of SF 603 are used to record findings of initial and replacement examinations. These charts shall not be altered thereafter.

(7) <u>SECTION 2. PATIENT DATA</u>. Complete items 6 through 14 as indicated.

COMDTINST M6000.1E

(8) <u>SECTION 3. ATTENDANCE RECORD</u>. Restorations and Treatments (Completed during service) (Item 15).

   (a) Record restorations or treatments provided a patient after the initiation of a Dental Record on the chart "Restorations and Treatments" of Section III, in accordance with the following:

   1. Carious Teeth Restored. In the diagram of the tooth involved, draw an outline of the restoration showing size, location and shape, and indicate the material used. Amalgam restorations would be outlined and blocked in, composite resin restorations outlined only, etc.

   2. Extractions. Draw a large "X" on the root(s) of each tooth extracted.

   3. Root Canal Fillings. Outline each canal filled on the diagram of the root(s) of the tooth involved and block it in solidly.

   4. Apicoectomy. Draw a small triangle on the root of the tooth involved, apex away from the crown, the base line to show the approximate level of tooth amputation.

   5. Bridge and Crowns. Outline and fill in as specified above.

   6. Removable Appliances. Place a line over numbers of replaced teeth and give a brief description under "Remarks".

   7. Unrecorded Operations and Conditions. Operations performed by other than CG Dental Officers subsequent to the original examination will be indicated by the Dental Officer discovering the condition just as if they had been done by a CG Dental Officer. Make appropriate entries indicating the nature of the treatment and adding the abbreviation "CIV" or other abbreviation as the case may be. The date entered will be the date of the discovery.

   8. Other. Similarly, note operations known to have been performed by CG Dental Officers whose identity is not recorded, except use the abbreviation "CGDO." The date entered shall be the date the operation is discovered. Account for teeth which are shown as missing in the chart, Missing Teeth and Existing Restorations, and which have erupted subsequently, by an entry in the following manner: "1 and 32," eruption noted, date, and signature of Dental Officer making the notation. Record other conditions of comparable importance in a similar manner.

   (b) Record a series of treatments for a specific condition not producing lasting changes in dental characteristics by entering of initial and final treatment dates (i.e., POT daily 1 AUG 87 thru 5 AUG 87 or Vin Tr. twice daily 1 AUG 87 thru 10 AUG 87).

Chapter 4. C. Page 9

COMDTINST M6000.1E

(c) Authenticate each entry in this record by a written entry in the spaces provided under "Services Rendered".

(9) <u>Subsequent Disease and Abnormalities (Item 16)</u>. Chart subsequent conditions, in pencil only, using the instructions in Chapter 4-C.3.(6). Once treatment is completed and documented in item 17, erase pencil entry in item 16 and permanently transfer in ink to item 15 (Restorations and Treatments).

(10) <u>Services Rendered (Item 17)</u>. The accuracy and thoroughness in recording patient histories and treatment progress notes are essential elements in the diagnosis and treatment of the dental patient. In addition to the conventional listing of the tooth number and procedure, all dental materials used intraorally shall be identified. Use trade names where possible. This includes, but is not limited to; bases and liners, metallic and nonmetallic restorative materials, denture frameworks and bases, impression materials, medicaments, and anesthesia. Record prescribed medications.

(a) Standard Subjective. Objective. Assessment. Plan. (S.O.A.P.) format. The S.O.A.P. format shall be used to document all sickcall and emergency dental treatments, to document Type 1 and Type 2 examinations, and to record the results of the examination of patients in preparation for comprehensive treatment planning. S.O.A.P. format is not required to document ongoing delivery of treatment, which has been previously planned. All entries are to be on the SF-603/603-A, item 17. The S.O.A.P. format uses a problem-oriented record as a tool in management of patient care. The acronym is derived from the first letter of the first four record statements as follows:

1. "S" Subjective data. This data includes the reason for the visit to the dental clinic, and if appropriate, a statement of the problem (chief complaint "in the words of the patient") and the qualitative and quantitative description of the symptoms appropriate to the problem.

2. "O" Objective data. A record of the type of examination and the diagnostic aids, including the ordering of radiographs, and the actual clinical findings, x-ray results, or laboratory findings appropriate to the problem. This is to include all the provider's findings such as carious teeth, inflammation, periodontal status, pocket depths, blood pressure measurement, etc.

3. "A" Assessment. This portion is the assessment of the subjective data, objective data, and the problem statement which leads the provider to a diagnosis, e.g.,"needs" (existing conditions or pathoses).

4. "P" Plan. This is the plan of treatment to correct or alleviate the stated problems or needs, irrespective of the treatment capability of the dental treatment facility. Include recommended treatment and, as appropriate, possible complications, alternative treatment, and prognosis with and without intervention. Include consultations, a record of the specific treatment performed, pre- and postoperative instructions, prescriptions, and any deviations from the original treatment plan.

(b) The following classification of tooth surfaces are listed in order of precedence and shall be used in connection with recording restorations of defective teeth:

Surface	Designation
Facial (Labial) (Anterior teeth)	F
Buccal (Posterior teeth)	B
Lingual	L
Occlusal (Posterior teeth)	O
Mesial	M
Distal	D
Incisal (Anterior teeth)	I

(c) Use combinations of designators to identify and locate caries, operations, or restorations in the teeth involved; for example, 8-MID would refer to the mesial, incisal, and distal aspects of the left mandibular cuspid; 30-MODF, the mesial, occlusal, distal, and facial aspects of a right mandibular first molar.

Surface	Designation
Mesial-Occlusal	MO
Distal-Occlusal	DO
Mesial-Incisal	MI
Distal-Incisal	DI
Occlusal-Facial	OF
Occlusal-Lingual	OL
Incisal-Facial	IF
Incisal-Lingual	IL
Mesial-Occlusal-Distal	MOD
Mesial-Occlusal-Facial	MOF
Mesial-Occlusal-Lingual	MOL

Mesial-Incisal-Distal	MID
Mesial-Incisal-Facial	MIF
Mesial-Incisal-Lingual	MIL
Distal-Occlusal-Facial	DOF
Distal-Occlusal-Lingual	DOL
Mesial-Occlusal-Distal-Facial	MODF
Mesial-Incisal-Distal-Facial	MIDF
Mesial-Occlusal-Distal-Facial-Lingual	MODFL
Mesial-Incisal-Distal-Facial-Lingual	MIDFL

(d) The use of abbreviations is not mandatory but is desirable for purposes of brevity in view of the limited space available in the dental record for recording services rendered. Whenever there is a possibility of misinterpretation due to the use of abbreviations, dental operations shall be written in full. When abbreviations are used, they shall conform to the following:

Operation, Condition, or Treatment	**Abbreviation**
Abrasion	Abr.
Abscess	Abs.
Acrylic	Acr.
Adjust (ed)(ment)	Adj.
Amalgam	Am.
Anesthesia	Anes.
Apicectomy	Apico.
Bridge (denotes fixed unless otherwise noted)	Br.
Calcium Hydroxide	CaOH
Calculus	Calc.
Cavity Varnish	C.Var.
Cement	Cem.
Complete Denture (full unless otherwise noted)	CD.
Composite Resins	Comp. Res.
Crown	Cr.

Deciduous	Decid.
Defective	Def.
Drain.	Drn.
Equilibrate (action)	Equil.
Eugenol	Eug.
Extraction	Ext.
Fluoride	Fl.
Fracture(s)	Frac.
General	Gen.
Gingival (itis) (state type in parenthesis)	Ging.
Gutta percha	G.P.
Impacted (ion)	Imp.
Impression	Impr.
Maxillary	Max.
Mandibular	Mand.
Periapical	PA.
Pericoronitis	P-Cor.
Periodontitis	Perio.
Porcelain	Porc.
Post Operative Instructions Given	POIG.
Post Operative Treatment	POT.
Prepared (ation)	Prep.
Prophylaxis	Prophy.
Reappoint (ment)	Reappt.
Recement (ed)	Recem.
Reduce (d)	Red.
Removable Partial Denture	RPD.
Sedative (ation)	Sed.
Sequestrum	Seq.
Surgical	Surg.
Suture (s)(d)	Su.
Treatment (ed)	Tx.
Zinc Chloride	ZnCl.

COMDTINST M6000.1E

(11) Space is provided in the lower right margin under Section III for the patient's name which is for convenience in filing in the dental record. Record the last name in capital letters. Do not abbreviate any part of the name.

4. Dental Continuation, SF-603-A.

   a. General. Use a Dental Continuation, SF-603-A whenever the original Dental Record, SF-603 becomes filled or when the record cannot be satisfactorily brought up-to-date by entries on the appropriate chart.

   b. Detailed Instructions.

      (1) Enter individual's name and SSN in the space provided on the right margin of both the front and backside of the form.

      (2) Number the continuation sheet in the upper right corner following the phrase "DENTAL-Continuation." Thus, the earliest Dental Continuation, SF-603-A is labeled "DENTAL-Continuation #1" and subsequent sheets are labeled "DENTAL-Continuation #2", "DENTAL-Continuation #3", etc.

      (3) File the Dental Continuation, SF-603-A forms on top of the Dental Record, SF-603 form in reverse chronological order, i.e., the most recent on top.

5. Consultation Sheet, SF-513.

   a. Purpose. The Consultation Sheet, SF-513 shall be used whenever a patient is referred to another facility for evaluation or treatment.

   b. Detailed Instructions. Complete the form as detailed in paragraph 4-B-14.b.

6. Lost Dental Records.

   a. Forward "stray" dental records, disposition of which cannot be determined, to Commander PSC-adm-3 with a letter of explanation.

   b. When a Dental Record is missing, prepare a new record. Prominently mark the Dental Record Cover, CG-3443-2 and the Dental Record, SF-603 "REPLACEMENT." Request the old Dental Record from the individual's last unit or Commander PSC-adm-3.

   c. In case a lost Dental Record is recovered, incorporate the replacement record into the original record.

7. Special Dental Records Entries. When dental treatment is refused, make an appropriate entry on the Dental Record, SF-603 or Dental Continuation, SF-603-A, signed by both the Dental Officer and patient.

8. Dental Examination Requirements.

   a. Any peculiarities or deviations from normal are particularly valuable for identification purposes and shall be recorded on Dental Record, SF-603 under "Remarks." Abnormalities such as erosion, mottled enamel, hypoplasia, rotation, irregularity of alignment and malocclusion of teeth, presence of supernumerary teeth, denticles, Hutchinson's incisors, fractures of enamel or teeth, abnormal interdental spaces, mucosal pigmentation, leukoplakia, diastema, hypertrophied frenum labium, torus palantinus and torus mandibularis, tattoos, piercings, embedded foreign bodies and descriptions of unusual restorations or appliances are, when noted, especially useful in this connection. Malocclusion shall be simply and clearly described. Dentures and other removable dental appliances shall also be described under "Remarks".

b. When all teeth are present, and free of caries or restorations, take special effort to discover and record any abnormalities, however slight. If no caries, restorations, or abnormalities are found, make an entry to that effect on Dental Record, SF-603 under "Remarks."

c. Inquire about the patients' tobacco use during routine dental examinations and document. Advise users of the health risks associated with tobacco use, the benefits of stopping, and where to obtain assistance in stopping if available. Advise all pregnant tobacco users of the health risks to the fetus.

d. Oral hygiene and periodontal status at time of examination shall be recorded. Upon initial examination, complete items 5A-5C, Dental Record SF-603, with additional comments placed in "Remarks" if needed. For all subsequent examinations, describe oral hygiene level and periodontal status in item 17 of Dental Record SF-603/Dental Continuation SF-603-A, including PSR scores.

e. For all patients 16 years of age or older, blood pressure readings shall be taken and recorded on the Dental Health Questionnaire CG-5605 and the Dental Record SF-603/Dental Continuation SF-603-A at initial and subsequent dental examinations.

9. Recording of Dental Treatments on a Chronological Record of Care, SF-600. Make entries of dental treatment on the Chronological Record of Care, SF-600 when the patient is on the sick list and when treatment is related to the condition for which the patient is admitted. Such entries shall be made and signed by the dental officer. Notes concerning conditions of unusual interest and of medical or dental significance may be made when appropriate.

This page intentionally left blank.

Section D. Clinical Records (Dependent/Retiree).

1. Purpose and Background 1
2. Contents of Clinical Records 2
3. Extraneous Attachments 3
4. Opening Clinical Records 3
5. Terminating Clinical Records 4
6. Custody of Clinical Records 4
7. Safekeeping of Clinical Records 4
8. Transfer of Clinic Records 4
9. Lost, Damaged, or Destroyed Clinical Records 5

COMDTINST M6000.1E

This page intentionally left blank.

D. Clinical Records (Dependent/Retiree).

1. Purpose and Background. The Clinical Record, CG-3443-1 is the chronological medical and dental record of a non-active duty beneficiary (dependent or retiree) eligible for health care at a CG facility. The Clinical Record Cover is used whenever a Clinical Record is opened on dependents or retirees. The primary reasons for compiling a clinical record are:

    a. Purpose. To develop records to facilitate and document the health condition in order to provide health care and to provide a complete account of such care rendered, including diagnosis, treatment, and end result. CG clinics are Primary Care Managers (PCM) for active duty members only. The family member may be given a copy of the clinical record contents to carry with them when the family will no longer receive care at the CG clinic. Inactive health records of dependents will be forwarded to the National Personnel Records Center in St. Louis, MO.

    b. Uses. To protect the Government, the individual concerned, and the individual's dependents: It may be used:

        (1) To provide, plan and coordinate health care.

        (2) To aid in preventive health and communicable disease control programs; in reporting medical conditions required by law to Federal, state, and local agencies.

        (3) To compile statistical data; for research; to teach health services personnel.

        (4) To determine suitability of persons for service or assignments.

        (5) To adjudicate claims and determine benefits; for law enforcement or litigation.

        (6) To evaluate care provided.

        (7) To evaluate personnel and facilities for professional certification and accreditation.

        (8) To facilitate communication among health care providers, utilization managers, quality assurance and medical records personnel.

    c. To aid in identifying deceased persons when other means may be inadequate.

    d. Detailed Instructions.

        (1) Last Name. Record the last name in all capital letters.

            SMITH

        (2) Given Name(s). Record given name(s) in full without abbreviation. If the individual has no middle name or initial, use the lower case letter "n" in parentheses (n). If the individual has only a middle initial(s), record each initial in quotation marks. When "Jr." or "II" or other similar designations are use, they shall appear after the middle name or initial.

            SMITH,   Helen   (n)

Last Name   First Name   Middle Name

    (3) Date of Birth. Enter day, month (abbreviated JAN, FEB, MAR, etc.) and the year; i.e., 3 FEB 77.

    (4) Social Security Number. Enter sponsor's SSN.

    (5) Status. Check the appropriate block; i.e., Retiree USCG, Dependent USPHS, etc.

    (6) Other. Use this block to indicate special status or other information useful for either proper monitoring of the patient or for aid in identifying the patient or record.

    (7) Occupational Monitoring. Indicate the reason for occupational monitoring if monitoring is required.

    (8) Med-Alert. Check this block to indicate that the patient has a medical problem that must be considered in rendering treatment; i.e., allergy, diabetes, cardiac problems, etc. Describe the specific medical problem within the medical record on Adult Preventive and Chronic Care Flowsheet, DD-2766.

2. <u>Contents of Clinical Records</u>.

    a. <u>Contents</u>. Each clinical record shall consist of CG-3443-1 with dental and medical records arranged in the following bottom to top sequence: (Notes * when required)

        (1) Right Side - Dental: CG-3443-2 Dental Record Cover* with Drug Sensitivity Sticker, CG-5266*, containing the following:

FORM	TITLE
(a) OF-522	Authorization for Administration of Anesthesia and for Performance of Operations and Other Procedures*.
(b) SF-513	Consultation Sheet.
(c) SF-603	Dental Record *.
(d) SF-603A	Dental Record – Continuation*.
(e) CG-5605	Dental Health Questionnaire*.

        (2) Right Side - Medical:

            (a) PHS-731   International Certificate of Vaccination* (Attached to the lower right corner of the inside of the Clinical Record Cover.)

            (b) DD-1141   Record of Occupational Exposure to Ionizing Radiation.*

            (c) SF-507   Medical Record.*

            (d) SF-602   Syphilis Record.*

(e) SF-601   Immunization Record.*

(f) DD-771   Spectacle Order Form.*

(g) Electrocardiographic Report.*

(h) SF-519   Radiographic Reports.

(i) Laboratory Reports.

(j) SF-541   Gynecologic Cytology.*

(k) SF-515   Tissue Examination.*

(l) OF-522   Authorization For Administration of Anesthesia and for Performance of Operations and Other Procedures.*

(m) SF-513   Consultation Sheet.*

(n) SF-507   Medical Record*

(o) CG-5447   Occupational Medical Surveillance and Evaluation Program.*

(p) DD-2807-1   Report of Medical History.*

(q) DD-2808   Report of Medical Examination.*

(r) SF-558   Emergency Care and Treatment.

(s) SF-600   Chronological Record of Medical Care.

(t) DD-2766   Adult Preventive and Chronic Care Flowsheet Form.

(u) CG-5266   Drug Sensitivity Sticker.*

(v) DD-2870   Authorization for Disclosure.

(w) DD-2871   Request for Restriction of Information.

* Annotates when required

b. <u>Filing system</u>. File forms of the same number in their assigned sequence, with the most recent placed on top of each previous form, i.e., file Chronological Record of Care, SF-600 dated 3 AUG 89 on top of Chronological Record of Care, SF-600 dated 20 MAY 86.

c. <u>Dates</u>. Enter all dates on Clinical Record forms, including the Clinical Record Cover, in the following sequence: day (numeral), month (in capitals abbreviated to the first three letters), and year (numeral); i.e., 30 AUG 86.

3. <u>Extraneous Attachments</u>. In order to ensure that the clinical record is an accurate, properly documented, concise and dependable record of the medical and dental history of the individual, keep extraneous attachments to a minimum. When they are necessary, file them beneath all other forms.

4. <u>Opening Clinical Records</u>. Open a Clinical Record when an eligible non-active duty beneficiary initially reports to a CG health care facility for treatment.

5. Terminating Clinical Records. The Clinical Record shall be terminated four years after the last record entry. Make an entry on SF-600 explaining the circumstances under which the record was terminated. Forward the record, placed in a sealed envelope labeled "Sensitive Medical Information – Confidential," to:

Dependant/Retirees:	Military Records:
NPRC-ANNEX	VA RECORDS MANAGEMENT CENTER
1411 BOULDER BLVD	4300 GOODFELLOW BLVD BLDG 104
VALMEYER, IL 62295	ST LOUIS MO 63115-1703

6. Custody of Clinical Records.

    a. Custody. Clinical Records shall be retained in the custody of the Senior Health Services Officer of the unit providing care. At times when there is no medical or dental officer, the clinical record will become the responsibility of the senior health services department representative.

    b. Entries. The name, grade, or rate of the health care provider making entries in clinical records shall be typed, stamped, or printed under their official signatures. Do not use facsimile signature stamps.

    c. Erroneous entry. The author of the entry shall draw a diagonal line through the complete entry, make an additional entry showing wherein and to what extent the original entry is in error, and initial clearly next to the correction.

    d. Completeness. Each health care provider is responsible for the completeness of the entries they make on any medical or dental form in the Clinical Record.

    e. Removal of material. Nothing shall be removed from the Clinical Record except under conditions specified in this Manual.

7. Safekeeping of Clinical Records. Clinical Records are the property of the Federal government and must be handled in accordance with the provisions of the Privacy Act of 1974 and the Freedom of Information Act. Guidance in this area is contained in The Coast Guard Freedom of Information and Privacy Acts Manual, COMDTINST M5260.3 (series).

    a. Security class. Since Clinical Records contain personal information of an extremely critical or sensitive nature, they are For Official Use Only requiring maximum security (high security locked cabinets or areas).

    b. Disclosure. Except as contained in The Coast Guard Freedom of Information and Privacy Acts Manual, COMDTINST M5260.3 (series), the information contained in Clinical Records shall not be disclosed by any means of communication to any person or to any agency, unless requested in writing by or with the prior consent of the individual to whom the record pertains. It is the requestor's responsibility to obtain the consent.

8. Transfer of Clinical Records.

    a. Dependents. When dependents of active duty personnel accompany their sponsor to a new duty station, the Senior Health Services Officer, his designee, the Executive Officer, or the senior health services department representative shall ensure that the "TRANSFERRED TO" line of the Health Record Receipt Form, NAVMED 6150/7, is completed in accordance with Chapter 4 Section A of this Manual.

b. <u>Request For Medical/Dental Records or Information, DD-877</u>. A DD-877, Request For Medical/Dental Records or Information shall be initiated for each record transferred. Send records via traceable means (e.g. DHS authorized Commercial Carriers FedEx or UPS); US Postal Service (USPS): 1) Express Mail or 2) Proof of Delivery using Extra Services which are either Certified, Delivery Confirmation, or Signature Confirmation. In instances where the family member will not be located near a CG Clinic, the record may be mailed to the appropriate MTF.

c. <u>CG Clinics are Primary Care Managers for Active Duty Members Only</u>. The family member may be given a copy of the clinical record contents to carry with them when the family will no longer receive care at the CG clinic. Inactive health records of dependents will be forwarded to the National Personnel Records Center in St. Louis, MO.

d. <u>Request for copies</u>. Clinics will give family members written information containing address and POC information to facilitate requests for record copies after transfer. All requests for clinical record copies must be in writing. The family member may request that a copy of the record be forwarded to their new care provider once they arrive at the new location, or they may request that the original record be forwarded to their new military primary care manager once they arrive at the new location. In these cases, the clinic shall send a copy of the clinical record contents to the care provider within 10 working days of receipt of the written request. If the clinic cannot comply with this requirement for some reason, the family member will be notified within 10 working days of the request of a projected date when the record copy will be available.

e. <u>Concern about potential loss</u>. In any instance where there is concern about potential loss of the clinical record, or that its contents may become unavailable to the treating clinic or its provider, the Clinic Administrator or the Senior Health Services Officer shall direct that copies of parts or all of the clinical record shall be made and retained at the clinic.

f. <u>Originals and copies</u>. Originals and copies of clinical records shall be retained and subsequently archived in accordance with directions contained in the Information and Life Cycle Management Manual, COMDTINST M5212.12 (series).

9. <u>Lost, Damaged, or Destroyed Clinical Records</u>.

a. <u>Lost or destroyed</u>. If a Clinical Record is lost or destroyed, the unit which held the record shall open a new record. The designation "REPLACEMENT" shall be stamped or marked on the cover. If the missing Clinical Record is recovered, insert in it any additional information or entries from the replacement record, then destroy the replacement record cover.

b. <u>Illegible</u>. Clinical Records which become illegible, thus destroying their value as permanent records, shall be duplicated. The duplicate shall, as nearly as possible, be an exact copy of the original record before such record became illegible. The new record shall be stamped or marked "DUPLICATE" on the cover. The circumstances necessitating the duplication shall be explained on the SF-600. Forward Clinical Records replaced by duplicate records to the National Personnel Records Center.

Section E. Employee Medical Folders.

1. Purpose and Background 1
2. Custody of Employee Medical Folders (EMF's)..1
3. Contents of the Employee Medical Folders...2
4. Accountability of Disclosures...3
5. Opening Employee Medical Folder..3
6. Terminating Employee Medical Folders 3
7. Transferring to Other Government Agencies 4
8. Lost, Damaged, or Destroyed Employee Medical Folders 4
9. Employee Medical Folder, SF-66 D 4

This page intentionally left blank.

E. Employee Medical Folders.

1. Purpose and Background. The Employee Medical Folder (EMF), SF-66 D is the chronological medical record of Federal employees eligible for health care at CG facilities. These are the primary reasons for compiling an EMF.

    a. Documentation. Develop records to facilitate and document the health condition in order to provide health care and to provide a complete account of care rendered, including diagnosis, treatment, and end result.

    b. To protect the Government and the individual concerned.

    c. Provide quality health care. The information in the EMF is routinely used: to provide, plan and coordinate health care; to aid in preventive health and communicable disease control programs; in reporting medical conditions required by law to Federal, state, and local agencies; to compile statistical data; for research; to teach health services personnel; to determine suitability of persons for service or assignments; to adjudicate claims and determine benefits; for law enforcement or litigation; to evaluate care provided; and to evaluate personnel and facilities for professional certification and accreditation.

2. Custody of Employee Medical Folders (EMF's).

    a. Privacy. EMF's are the property of the Federal government handled in accordance with the provisions of the Privacy Act of 1974 and the Freedom of Information Act. Guidance in this area is contained in the Coast Guard Freedom of Information and Privacy Acts Manual, COMDTINST M5260.3 (series).

        (1) Since EMF's contain personal information of extremely critical or sensitive nature, they are considered "For Official Use Only" records according to the CG Freedom of Information and Privacy Acts Manual, COMDTINST M5260.3 (series), requiring maximum security (high security locked cabinets or areas).Except as contained in the Coast Guard Freedom of Information and Privacy Acts Manual, COMDTINST M5260.3 (series), the information contained in the EMF shall not be disclosed by any means of communication to any person or to any agency, unless requested in writing by or with the prior consent of the individual to whom the record pertains. It is the responsibility of the requester to obtain the consent.

    b. Custody. EMF's shall be retained in the custody of the Medical Officer of the unit at which the individual is employed. At no time shall individual employees keep or maintain their own records.

    c. Individual's rights. Individuals may examine their EMF in the presence of a health services department representative, providing it does not interrupt the scheduled mission of the unit and there is no information contained therein which would be detrimental to the individual's mental well-being.

COMDTINST M6000.1E

    d.   <u>Entries</u>. Health services personnel making entries in EMF shall ensure that all entries, including signatures, are neat and legible. Signature information shall include the name and grade or rate. Do not use facsimile signature stamps.

    e.   <u>Erroneous entry</u>. If an erroneous entry is made in an EMF, draw a diagonal line through the complete entry. Make an additional entry showing wherein and to what extent the original entry is in error.

    f.   <u>Completeness</u>. Health services personnel are responsible for the completeness of the entries made on any form while the EMF is in their custody. No sheet shall be removed from the EMF except under conditions specified in this Manual.

    g.   <u>Storage</u>. Health services personnel shall ensure that, if EMF's are located in the same office as the Official Personnel Folder (OPF), the records are maintained physically apart from each other.

3.   <u>Contents of the Employee Medical Folders</u>.

    a.   Employee Medical Folder. Each medical folder shall consist of Employee Medical Folder (EMF), SF-66 D with medical records arranged in the following bottom to top sequence:

        (1)   Left Side Dental: Leave blank.

        (2)   Right Side - Medical:

	FORM	TITLE
(a)	PHS-731	International Certificate of Vaccination* (Attached to the lower right corner of the inside of the EMF. This form is optional.)
(b)	DD-1141	Record of Occupational Exposure to Ionizing Radiation*
(c)	SF-507	Medical Record**
(d)	CG-5447	Occupational Medical Surveillance and Evaluation Program*
(e)	SF-602	Syphilis Record*
(f)	SF-601	Immunization Record*
(g)	DD-771	Spectacle Order Form*
(h)		Electrocardiographic Report*
(i)	SF-519	Radiographic Reports
(j)		Laboratory Reports
(k)	SF-541	Gynecologic Cytology*
(l)	SF-515	Tissue Examination*

Chapter 4. E. Page 2

(m) OF-522   Authorization For Administration of Anesthesia and for Performance of Operations and Other Procedures*

(n) SF-513   Consultation Sheet*

(o) DD-2807-1   Report of Medical History*

(p) DD-2808   Report of Medical Examination*

(q) SF-558   Emergency Care and Treatment*

(r) SF-600   Chronological Record of Medical Care

(s) DD-2766   Adult Preventive and Chronic Care Flowsheet

(t) CG-5266   Drug Sensitivity Sticker*

(u) DD-2870   Authorization for Disclosure

(v) DD-2871   Request for Restriction of Information

  * Annotates when required

  ** Medical Record, SF-507 are attached to and filed after the form is continued.

b. <u>Sequence</u>. File forms of the same number in their assigned sequence, with the most recent placed on top of each previous form, i.e., file Chronological Record of Care, SF-600 dated 3 AUG 87 on top of the Chronological Record of Care, SF-600 dated 20 MAY 86.

c. <u>Dates</u>. Enter all dates in the following sequence: day (numeral), month (in capitals abbreviated to the first three letters), and year (numeral); i.e., 30 AUG 86.

4. <u>Accountability of Disclosures</u>. The accountability of disclosure of records, as required by the HIPAA Privacy Regulation and the Privacy Act of 1974, will be maintained in accordance with Chapter 8, of The Coast Guard Freedom of Information (FOIA) and Privacy Acts Manual, COMDTINST M5260.3 (series), in the Protected Health Information Management Tool (PHIMT); see Chapter 14 Section B.2.e of this Manual. The information will be retained for six years after the last disclosure or for the life of the record, whichever is longer.

5. <u>Opening Employee Medical Folder</u>. Open an EMF when an eligible Federal employee initially reports for treatment.

6. <u>Terminating Employee Medical Folders</u>. Terminate the EMF in accordance with the Information and Life Cycle Management Manual, COMDTINST 5212.12 (series). Make an entry on the Chronological Record of Care, SF-600 explaining the circumstances under which the folder was terminated.

7. <u>Transferring to Other Government Agencies</u>. When transferring an EMF to other agencies, complete a Request for Medical/Dental Records or Other Information, DD-877.

8. <u>Lost, Damaged, or Destroyed Employee Medical Folders</u>.

a. Lost or destroyed. If an EMF is lost or destroyed, the unit which held the record shall open a complete new Employee Medical Folder. Stamp or mark "REPLACEMENT" on the cover. If the missing folder is recovered, insert in it any additional information or entries from the replacement folder, then destroy the replacement folder.

b. Illegible. EMF's which become illegible, thus destroying their value as permanent records, will be duplicated. The duplicate shall, as nearly as possible, be an exact copy of the original record before such record becomes illegible. Stamp or mark "DUPLICATE" on the new record cover. Document the circumstances necessitating the duplication on a Chronological Record of Care, SF-600. Forward EMF's replaced by duplicate records to the National Personnel Records Center.

9. Employee Medical Folder, SF-66 D.

   a. Last Name. Record the last name in all capital letters.

   BROOKS

   b. Given Name(s). Record given name(s) in full without abbreviation. If the individual has no middle name or initial, use the lower case letter "n" in parentheses (n). If the individual has only a middle initial(s), record each initial in quotation marks. When "Jr." or "II" or other similar designations are use, they shall appear after the middle name or initial.

BROOKS	Cecilia	(n)
Last Name	First Name	Middle Name

   c. Date of Birth. Enter day, month (abbreviated JAN, FEB, MAR, etc.) and the year; i.e., 8 JUN 62.

   d. Social Security Number. Enter SSN.

Section F. Inpatient Medical Records

1. Purpose and Background. 1
2. Maintenance and Storage. 2
3. Disposition of IMRs...3
4. Inpatient Medical Record Forms and Required Entries.......................................4

This page intentionally left blank.

F. Inpatient Medical Records.

1. Purpose and Background.

   a. Overnight care. Certain CG health care facilities have the capability and staffing to provide overnight care. Overnight care is defined as any period lasting more than four hours during which a beneficiary remains in the facility under the care or observation of a provider. By definition, overnight care may last less than 24 hours or it may last several days. Overnight care is utilized when a patient's condition or status requires observation, nursing care, frequent assessment, or other monitoring.

   b. Inpatient Medical Records (IMRs). Facilities providing overnight care shall create an Inpatient Medical Record (IMR) separate from the health record for the purpose of recording and preserving information related to the overnight care. The IMR shall be assembled as soon as a person is identified as needing overnight care. The IMR shall contain the following forms in a TOP TO BOTTOM sequence:

      (1) Inpatient Medical Record Cover Sheet and Privacy Act Statement.

      (2) Doctor's Orders, SF-508 (most recent on top).

      (3) Clinical Record/Physical Exam, SF-506.

      (4) Medical Record, SF-507.

      (5) Doctor's Progress Notes, SF-509 (most recent on top).

      (6) Vital Signs Record, SF-511.

      (7) Laboratory Report Display.

      (8) Radiologic Reports, SF-519.

      (9) Patient Care Kardex.

      (10) Medication Kardex.

      (11) Consultation Sheet, SF-513.

      (12) Miscellaneous forms (e.g., audiograms).

   c. Abbreviated Inpatient Medical Records (AIMRs). For patients who receive overnight care lasting 24 hours or less, an Abbreviated Inpatient Medical Record (AIMR) shall be created. The AIMR shall consist of at least an Inpatient Medical Record Cover Sheet, Privacy Act Statement, an Abbreviated Medical Record, DD-2770, Radiologic Consultation Reports SF-519, Kardexes, and other forms may be included at the discretion of the clinic. The AIMR shall be maintained while in use, completed, stored, and retired following the same requirements as listed for IMRs below.

   d. Organizing the IMR. During the time that the patient is receiving care, the IMR may be maintained in a loose-leaf binder, clipboard, or other convenient device, at the facility's discretion. Devices should be chosen and maintained so that the privacy, confidentiality and security of the patient information contained therein is protected at all times. Keeping or storing the record at the patient's bedside is discouraged for privacy reasons.

    e. <u>Patients release</u>. Once the patient is released from overnight care, providers shall have 48 hours to complete their notations in the record (excluding dictated entries). All laboratory, radiology and consultation forms shall also be included in the IMR within 48 hours of the patient's release from overnight care.

    f. <u>Dictated entries</u>. Dictated entries shall be entered in the medical record within 7 days of discharge. The record may be held in medical records and flagged as needing a dictated entry.

    g. <u>Storage</u>. After all notations, lab reports, radiology reports and consultations have been entered into the IMR, the IMR forms shall be placed in a bifold Clinical Record, CG-3443-1, and secured via a two prong device. The medical records staff is responsible for ensuring that the documents are in the correct order and are stored properly.

2. <u>Maintenance and Storage</u>. IMRs are the property of the Federal Government and must be handled in accordance with the provisions of the HIPAA Regulations, the Privacy Act of 1974 and the Freedom of Information Act. Guidance concerning these acts is contained in the CG Freedom of Information and Privacy Acts Manual, COMDTINST M5260.3 (series). All requirements and directions for handling and storing IMRs also apply to AIMRs.

    a. <u>Security</u>. Since IMRs contain personal information of an extremely critical or sensitive nature, they are considered "For Official Use Only" records requiring maximum security (high security locked cabinets or areas). IMRs shall be stored in well ventilated and sprinklered areas. Fire-resistant cabinets or containers shall be used for storage whenever possible.

    b. <u>IMRs shall be retained at the health care facility which created the record</u>. IMRs will not be transferred with personnel who change duty stations. Copies of the IMR may be given to the individual if such a request is made in writing, or may be released to other persons, e.g., physicians or hospitals, if the patient requests or authorizes such release in writing. All release requests and authorizations will be inserted into the IMR cover.

    c. <u>Retention of records</u>. IMRs will be retained at the creating health care facility for six (6) years after the date the patient is released from overnight care.

3. <u>Disposition of IMRs</u>. The IMR will be forwarded to the National Personnel Records Center (NPRC) as described in Information and Life Cycle Management Manual, COMDTINST M5212.12 (series), six years after the date the patient was released from inpatient care. The NPRC requirements must be met in order for the NPRC to accept the records.

   a. <u>Records must be sent in prescribed standard cubic foot cartons</u>. Cartons are available from the General Services Administration Federal Supply Service (FSS). The FSS stock number is NSN 8115-00-117-8344. All non-standard cartons will be returned at the expense of the originating organization.

   b. <u>NPRC does not accept accessions of less than one cubic foot</u>. Small amounts shall be held until a volume of one cubic foot or more is reached.

   c. <u>Accession number</u>. Print the accession number on each box, starting in the upper left hand corner. Mark the front of the box only. The accession number consists of the RG, which is always 26 for the CG, the current FY in which the records are being shipped, and a four digit number assigned by NPRC (see 4-F-3.j. for SF-135 preparation). Mark the front of the box only. Ensure that the information printed on the box is not obscured in any way, and that removal of tape or other sealing materials will not remove vital information.

   d. <u>Number each box consecutively</u>, e.g., 1 of 8, 2 of 8, 3 of 8,.8 of 8; or 1/8, 2/8, 3/8...8/8, in the upper right hand corner.

   e. <u>Records shall be arranged in each storage box either alphabetically or numerically</u>. Print the identifier of the first and last record/folder that is contained in the box on the center front of each box.

   f. <u>Enclose in the first box of each accession one copy of the SF-135</u> and any alphabetical or numerical listing needed to reference the records.

   g. <u>Ship records together so they arrive at the NPRC at the same time</u>. Shipments of 10 cubic feet or more shall be palletized.

   h. <u>Records must be shipped within 90 days of being assigned</u> an accession number. Failure to ship within 90 days will void the accession number.

   i. <u>Each clinic that transfers IMRs to NPRC must keep a master list (hard copy) of the records sent</u>. The master list must be retained at the clinic for a period of 50 years.

   j. <u>All shipments to NPRC must be accompanied by SF-135</u>, Records Transmittal and Receipt form. The transmittal form must include the name on the record and the individual's social security number. The accession number elements include the RG which is always 26 for the CG, the current

FY during which the record is shipped, and the 4 digit sequential number assigned by NPRC. Also include the date sent. Complete SF-135 preparation and submission instructions are contained in the Information and Life Cycle Management Manual, COMDTINST M5212.12 (series).

4. Inpatient Medical Record Forms and Required Entries.

   a. Doctor's Orders, SF-508.

      (1) Purpose. Doctor's Orders, SF-508 is used to record written and verbal orders of the medical or dental staff; record that nurses have noted orders; record automatic stop dates for medications and time limited treatments; and record the RN review of orders which shall be performed every 24 hours.

      (2) Preparation.

         (a) When Prepared. Doctor's Orders, SF-508 shall be used to communicate doctor's orders for all persons admitted to the medical facility inpatient area.

            1. Required Entries.
            2. Patient identification information may be written in or overprinted using a patient identification card.
            3. The date and time at which the order is written by the provider will be listed under the start column. If a verbal order is received, the date and time at which the order was received will be noted by the person who received the order in the start column. All verbal orders must be countersigned by the admitting provider on the next working day.
            4. Certain orders may be defined as time limited, e.g., complete bed rest for 24 hours, tilts q 8 hours X 3, etc. In addition, the facility shall define the length of time between renewal of orders for medications, treatments, etc. For orders which are time limited, the date and time when the order expires shall be noted under the stop column.
            5. All doctor's orders shall be listed on the form under drug orders. Orders shall be printed clearly in black ink. Only approved abbreviations shall be used. Nursing staff and/or health services technicians are required to contact the provider who wrote the order if there are any questions or difficulty encountered in reading the written order.

b. Clinical Record/Physical Exam, SF-506.

   (1) Purpose. The Clinical Record/Physical Exam, SF-506 is part of the inpatient medical record. It is used to record information obtained from physical examinations.

   (2) Preparation. When Prepared. SF-506 shall be prepared when a patient is admitted to the medical facility.

      (a) Required Entries.

         1. Patient identification information may be written in or printed using a patient identification card.

         2. Fill in the date that the exam is conducted in the upper left corner. The patient's self reported height may be used. Patients shall be weighed accurately on the day of admission and the weight entered as present weight. Vital signs to include temperature, pulse and blood pressure are recorded in the appropriate boxes. Rectal temperatures shall be identified by an "R" after the temperature reading. Axillary temperatures in adults are unreliable and will not be used.

         3. A physical examination must be thorough, recorded accurately, and contain sufficient information to substantiate the treatment plan and interventions. Examination notations may be continued on the reverse of the form. If the back of the form is used, this must be indicated on the front of the form. The examiner will sign the form at the end of his/her notations and use a printed ink stamp to clearly mark name, rank, and SSN.

c. Progress Notes, SF-509.

   (1) Purpose. The Progress Notes, SF-509 is part of the inpatient medical record. It is used to record the progress of the patient's condition, therapy or other treatment(s), as well as any other information relevant to the patient's condition or treatment such as laboratory tests and results.

   (2) Preparation.

      (a) When Prepared. The Progress Note, SF-509 shall be prepared when a patient is admitted to the medical facility inpatient area.

      (b) Required Entries.

         1. Patient identification information may be written in or overprinted using a patient identification card.

         2. Fill in the left column with the date and time at which the entry is being created. Begin writing to the right of the solid brown line. Notes will be written in SOAP format (see 4-B-

COMDTINST M6000.1E

5.a.(4)). The person creating the note will sign the form at the end of his/her notations and use a printed ink stamp to clearly mark name, rank, and SSN.

d. Vital Signs Record, SF-511.

(1) Purpose. Vital Signs Record, SF-511 shall be used to document vital sign measurements, height, weight, hospital day and, if appropriate, postoperative day for patients admitted to the medical facility inpatient area.

(2) Preparation.

(a) When Prepared. Vital Signs Record, SF-511 shall be prepared when a patient is admitted to the medical facility inpatient area.

(b) Required Entries.

1. Patient identification information may be written in or overprinted using a patient identification card.

2. Hospital day one shall be the day of admission. If the patient undergoes an invasive procedure, "op" shall be written after the word post in the left column. The day of surgery shall be noted by writing "DOS" in the appropriate column. The day following the day of surgery is post-op day one. Post-op days shall be numbered consecutively thereafter.

3. The month in which the patient is admitted shall be written on the fifth line, first column. The year shall be completed by writing in the correct numerals after "19" on the fifth line.

4. The calendar date on which the patient is admitted shall be written in on the line next to the word day, e.g., if the patient is admitted on 3 June, the hospital day is one, and a "3" is written on the line next to the word day.

5. The hour at which the vital sign measurements are to be made are noted in the spaces next to the word hour. Use 24 hour clock notations, e.g., 11 p.m. is 2300, etc.

6. Once vital signs have been measured, they shall be recorded on the form using the symbols for pulse and temperature. Symbols are placed in the columns, not on the brown dotted lines.

7. Blood pressure measurements are written in the spaces to the right of the words "blood pressure". The first measurement made after midnight is written in the top left column, the second is written below it. The first measurement made after noon is written in the top box in the right side column, the second below that, etc. Blood pressure may also be represented by x marks placed at the systolic and diastolic

Chapter 4. F. Page 6

measurements corresponding to the scale for pulse measurements.

8. Other vital signs measurements or intake and output measurements may be written in the spaces on the lower part of the form, or a local overprint/stamp may be used.

9. Both sides of the form will be used. If the second side of the form is used, the word "continued" will be clearly written on the bottom of the first page.

e. Laboratory Reports. Laboratory Reports are part of the inpatient medical record.

f. Radiologic Consultation Reports, SF-519 (no longer used).

(1) Purpose. Radiologic Consultation Reports, SF-519 is part of the inpatient medical record.

g. Abbreviated Medical Record, DD-2770 (replaces SF 539).

(1) Purpose. Abbreviated Medical Record, DD-2770 is used to record history, exam findings, patient progress, doctor's orders, vital signs, output, medications and nurse's notes for patients requiring overnight care who remain 24 hours or less.

(2) Preparation.

(a) When prepared, Abbreviated Medical Record, DD-2770 may be used for any overnight care patient for whom total stay is anticipated to be 24 hours or less. If length of stay exceeds 24 hours, a full IMR must be initiated to provide proper documentation of the patient's stay. The Abbreviated Medical Record, DD-2770 shall be prepared when a short stay patient is admitted to the inpatient medical area.

(b) Required Entries.

1. Patient identification information may by written in or overprinted using a patient identification card.

2. History, chief complaint, and condition on admission must be documented in the top box on page one. Date of admission shall be noted here also.

3. Physical examinations findings shall be noted in the center box on page one. Physical exam findings shall be completely noted and appropriate to the condition. Deferred exams, such as rectal exams, shall be noted as such.

4. The patient's progress over the 24 hour period between admission and discharge will be noted by the Medical Officer

in the third box on page one. Date of discharge and final diagnosis shall be noted here also.

5. The physician shall sign the form in the box provided and use a printed ink stamp to clearly mark his/her name, rank, and SSN. The date the form is signed shall be written in the box provided next to the signature.

6. The location of the clinic or dispensary, for example, Dispensary TRACEN Cape May, shall be written or stamped in the box marked organization.

7. Doctor's orders shall be written only in the space provided on page two. Each order group written shall be dated and signed. A printed ink stamp shall be used by Medical Officers to mark name, rank, and SSN. All medical and dental orders given during the patient's stay must be recorded. A second page should be started if the number of orders exceeds space available on one page.

8. Vital sign measurements shall be recorded in the spaces provided with the date and time of each notation. Bowel movements and urine output are noted in the columns marked stools and weight.

9. Medications administered and brief notes regarding the patient's condition shall be made in the nurse's notes area. Medication name, dose, route, and time given shall be recorded for each dose of medication administered. Each notation shall be signed with the name, military rank, or title for civilians, e.g., RN or LPN, of the person making the note.

Section G. Mental Health Records.

1. Active Duty...1
2. Non-active Duty...1
3. Psychiatric Evaluation Format...1
4. Custody of Mental Health Records..1

This page intentionally left blank.

G. Mental Health Records.

1. Active Duty. Complete mental health assessments and visits will be done in an IMB, DMB, or traditional psychiatric evaluation format and recorded on a Chronological Record of Care, SF-600, Consultation Sheet, SF-513, IMB, DMB, or typed psychiatric evaluation forms as appropriate. Active duty episodic visits and routine appointments will be recorded on a Chronological Record of Care, SF-600 in SOAP format. The Objective ("O") section shall include mental status observations and any other pertinent findings. Records of active duty mental health assessments and visits will be kept in the CG Health Record, CG-3443. An additional separate mental health record may be created and maintained in a system of records approved by the local QI Committee and kept secure in the mental health practitioner's office. New patients shall be evaluated in accordance with traditional psychiatric evaluation processes.

2. Non-Active duty. Separate records of mental health care may be created and maintained in a system of records approved by the local QI Committee and kept secure in the mental health practitioner's office. Alternatively, the mental health practitioner may elect to keep records of visits in the dependent's or retiree's primary Clinical Record, CG-3443-1. Should the practitioner elect to maintain a separate office based record for non-active duty patients, the primary record must include at a minimum, the diagnosis on the problem summary list, current psychiatric medications on a Chronological Record of Care, SF-600, and laboratory analysis ordered by the mental health care provider. New patients shall be evaluated in accordance with traditional psychiatric evaluation processes. Episodic and follow-up visits shall be recorded in SOAP format.

3. Psychiatric evaluation format. The psychiatric evaluation shall include at a minimum, patient information, chief complaint, history of present illness, past history (psychiatric symptoms, diagnoses, chronic illnesses, surgical procedures, current medications, allergies, and alcohol and drug history), personal history, family history, mental status exam, assessment (DSM-IV), prognosis, and plan. Included in all assessments and other visits, as appropriate, an estimation of potential harm to self or others. In addition, notes should contain sufficient information to establish that the criteria for any new DSM based diagnosis are met.

4. Custody of Mental Health Records. Records kept in the mental health practitioner's office are property of the USCG and copies should be made available to other practitioner's or agencies at the patient's request. These records should also be made available to other CG providers as part of an official records review process and as directed by Chapter 4, Section A.3 of this Manual.

This page intentionally left blank.

COMDTINST M6000.1E

CHAPTER 5

DEATHS AND PSYCHIATRIC CONDITIONS

Section A. Deaths.

1. General 1
2. Duties of health services department 1
3. Determining Cause of Death..1
4. Death Certificates for Deaths Occurring Away From Command or in Foreign Ports.........1
5. Relations with Civilian Authorities 2
6. Reporting Deaths to Civilian Authorities 2
7. Death Forms for Civilian Agencies and Individuals..2
8. Identification of Remains...2

Section B. Psychiatric Conditions.

1. General 1
2. Personality Disorders 1
3. Adjustment Disorders 2
4. Organic Mental Disorders...2
5. Psychoactive Substance Use Disorders 3
6. Schizophrenia..3
7. Psychotic Disorders Not Elsewhere Classified 4
8. Delusional (Paranoid) Disorder 4
9. Neurotic Disorders 4
10. Mood Disorders 4
11. Anxiety Disorders (or Anxiety and Phobic Neuroses) 5
12. Somatoform Disorders 5
13. Dissociative Disorders (or Hysterical Neuroses, Dissociative Type)..................................5
14. Sexual Disorders 6
15. Sexual Dysfunctions 6
16. Factitious Disorders 7
17. Disorders of Impulse Control Not Elsewhere Classified 7
18. Disorders Usually First Evident in Infancy, Childhood, or Adolescence...........................7
19. Psychological Factors Affecting Physical Condition 9
20. V Codes for Conditions Not Attributable to a Mental Disorder that are a Focus of Attention or Treatment...9
21. Additional Codes 10

Section C. Command directed Mental Health Evaluation of Coast Guard Service members.

1. Active Duty Mental Health Evaluation Protection 1
2. Emergency Evaluations 1
3. Non-emergent Mental Health Evaluation 1
4. Service Member's Rights..2

5. Things Not To Do 2
6. Evaluations NOT covered 3
7. Memorandum Requesting a Mental Health Evaluation 3

Section A. Deaths.

1. General 1
2. Duties of health services department 1
3. Determining Cause of Death..1
4. Death Certificates for Deaths Occurring Away From Command or in Foreign Ports 1
5. Relations with Civilian Authorities 2
6. Reporting Deaths to Civilian Authorities 2
7. Death Forms for Civilian Agencies and Individuals 2
8. Identification of Remains...2

This page intentionally left blank.

CHAPTER FIVE – DEATHS AND PSYCHIATRIC CONDITIONS

Section A. Deaths.

1. General. Chapter 11 of the Personnel Manual, COMDTINST M1000.6 (series) contains further guidance concerning casualties and decedent affairs. Chapter 2 of the Administrative Investigations Manual, COMDTINST M5830.1 (series) contains guidance for notifying CGIS about incidents of death or injury to CG military and civilian members.

2. Duties of Health Services Department. In the event of a death at a CG unit the Medical Officer or Health Services Department Representative shall report immediately to the scene and:

    a. Make contact with on-scene law enforcement (e.g., CGIS, other state, local or Federal law enforcement) and advise them of identifying information needed regarding the deceased.

    b. Advise the Commanding Officer of the name, grade or rate, and social security number of the deceased.

    c. Advise the Commanding Officer of the time and place of death.

    d. Advise the Commanding Officer, insofar as possible, as to the cause of death.

    e. Ensure notification of the Quarantine Officer or Coroner if required.

    f. Arrange with local civilian authorities for issuing a death certificate.

3. Determining Cause of Death. When an active duty CG member dies aboard a CG vessel or station under unnatural or suspicious circumstances, or when the cause of death is unknown, an administrative investigation shall immediately be convened in accordance with Section 11-A-3 of the Personnel Manual, COMDTINST M1000.6 (series) and Chapter 7 of the Administrative Investigations Manual, COMDTINST M5830.1 (series).

4. Death Certificates for Deaths Occurring Away From Command or in Foreign Ports.
    a. Active duty member dies while away from his/her duty station. When an active duty member dies while away from his/her duty station, the Commanding Officer or designated representative shall obtain a death certificate from civilian authorities. CGIS may be able to assist, if necessary. If the civilian death certificate does not furnish all necessary information, the district commander of the district in which the death occurred shall request additional information.

    b. If death occurs abroad, request the nearest United States Consular Office to obtain a death certificate from civilian authorities.

    c. Missing status. When an active duty member, or a reserve performing inactive duty for training, is in a missing status because of events in international waters and no identifiable remains can be recovered, and no civilian death certificate is issued, a report (including recommendations) shall be made as per Section 11-A of the Personnel Manual, COMDTINST M1000.6 (series).

5. Relations with Civilian Authorities. As appropriate, CGIS will be the liaison between commands and civilian authorities. When a CG member dies outside the limits of a CG reservation, the body shall not be moved until permission has been obtained from CGIS and/or civilian authorities (e.g., Coroner's office and/or Medical Examiner). In order that there may be full understanding and accord between the CG and civilian authorities, appropriate procedures will be developed for each command area, in consultation with CGIS and the civilian authorities, covering deaths of personnel within and outside the limits of CG commands. In general, and except where the state has retained concurrent jurisdiction with the United States, civilian authorities have no jurisdiction over deaths occurring on Coast Guard reservations. A transit or burial permit, however, issued by civilian authorities is required for removal of a body from a Coast Guard reservation for shipment or burial.

6. Reporting Deaths. In conjunction with the action required in Ch. 4-A-6.j of the Manual, verbal briefs are provided to those on a need to know basis (i.e. Commandant (CG-112), HSWL, etc.). CG Investigative Service (CGIS) may also inquire and request to review the health record. The health record shall be forwarded to the HSWL SC for a Quality Improvement (QI) review upon conclusion of local review(s). Findings of the review are forwarded to Commandant (CG-11) via Commandant (CG-112) to determine if additional investigation, process improvement, or adverse privileging action is warranted. The HSWL SC shall forward the original health record to Commander (PSC-mr).

7. Reporting Deaths to Civilian Authorities. When a death occurs at a CG activity in any state, territory, or insular possession of the United States, the death must be reported promptly to CGIS and civilian authorities. Local agreements concerning reporting and preparing death certificates shall be made between the Commanding Officer, or designated representative, and the civilian authorities.

8. Death Forms for Civilian Agencies and Individuals. Forward all requests for completing blank forms concerning death of CG personnel to Commander PSC (PSD-fs) for action.

9. Identification of Remains. Identification of remains may be established by DNA, marks and scars, dental records, fingerprints, and personal recognition. In questionable cases, a Dental Officer shall examine the remains and record observations on a SF-603, Dental Record for comparison with other available records.

Section B. Psychiatric Conditions.

1. General 1
2. Personality Disorders 1
3. Adjustment Disorders 2
4. Organic Mental Disorders 2
5. Psychoactive Substance Use Disorders 3
6. Schizophrenia 3
7. Psychotic Disorders Not Elsewhere Classified 4
8. Delusional (Paranoid) Disorder 4
9. Neurotic Disorders 4
10. Mood Disorders 4
11. Anxiety Disorders (or Anxiety and Phobic Neuroses) 5
12. Somatoform Disorders 5
13. Dissociative Disorders (or Hysterical Neuroses, Dissociative Type) 5
14. Sexual Disorders 6
15. Sexual Dysfunctions 6
16. Factitious Disorders 7
17. Disorders of Impulse Control Not Elsewhere Classified 7
18. Disorders Usually First Evident in Infancy, Childhood, or Adolescence 7
19. Psychological Factors Affecting Physical Condition 9
20. V Codes for Conditions Not Attributable to a Mental Disorder that are a Focus of
    Attention or Treatment 9
21. Additional Codes 10

This page intentionally left blank.

B. Psychiatric Conditions (including personality disorders).

1. General.

    a. Initial assessment. The following diagnostic categories conform to Diagnostic and Statistical Manual (DSM) IV-R and indicate the appropriate reference for disposition. In determining qualification for appointment, enlistment, and induction, or appropriate disposition (when the condition has been determined to be disqualifying for retention in accordance with paragraph 3-F-16 of this Manual), the diagnosis appears under DSM IV Axis I or Axis II. Conditions generally considered treatable and not grounds for immediate separation, mental health treatment may be authorized for members when medically necessary to relieve suffering and/or maintain fitness for unrestricted duty. The decision to provide treatment for mental health conditions will be based on a review of all factors, including the opinion of experts, probability of a successful outcome, and the presence of other physical or mental conditions. If a successful outcome (availability for worldwide assignment) is not realized within six months of the initiation of therapy, the patient's condition must be reassessed. If the reassessment indicates that the prognosis for a successful outcome is poor, the member shall be processed for discharge pursuant to Chapter 12 of the Personnel Manual, COMDTINST M1000.6 (series), or through the Physical Disability Evaluation System, COMDTINST M1850.2 (series).

    b. PDES Determination. Examination for purposes of PDES determination shall include a mental health evaluation performed by a military or VA mental health care provider. A military or VA mental health care provider is a psychiatrist, a doctoral level clinical psychologist, or doctoral level clinical social worker with necessary and appropriate professional credentials who is privileged to conduct mental health evaluations for the DoD, VA or the CG.

2. Personality Disorders. These disorders are disqualifying for appointment, enlistment, and induction under Section 3-D of this Manual and if identified on active duty shall be processed in accordance with Chapter 12-B-16, Personnel Manual, COMDTINST M1000.6 (series). These are coded on Axis II.

    a. 301.00 Paranoid.

    b. 301.20 Schizoid.

    c. 301.22 Schizotypal.

    d. 301.4 Obsessive compulsive.

    e. 301.50 Histrionic.

    f. 301.6 Dependent.

    g. 301.7 Antisocial.

h. 301.81 Narcissistic.

  i. 301.82 Avoidant.

  j. 301.83 Borderline.

  k. 301.9 Personality disorder NOS (includes Passive-aggressive).

  l. Personality trait(s) considered unfitting per paragraph 3-F-16.c.

3. Adjustment Disorders. These disorders are generally treatable and not usually grounds for separation. However, when these conditions persist or treatment is likely to be prolonged or non-curative, (e.g., inability to adjust to military life/sea duty, separation from family/friends) process in accordance with Chapter 12, Personnel Manual, COMDTINST M1000.6 (series) is necessary.

  a. 309.0 With depressed mood.

  b. 309.24 With anxiety.

  c. 309.28 With mixed anxiety and depressed moods.

  d. 309.3 With disturbance of conduct.

  e. 309.4 With mixed disturbance of emotions and conduct.

  f. 309.90 Adjustment disorder unspecified.

4. Organic Mental Disorders. These disorders are either disqualifying for appointment, enlistment, and induction under Section 3-D-29 of this Manual or if identified on active duty shall be processed in accordance with Physical Disability Evaluation System, COMDTINST M1850.2 (series).

  a. Dementias arising in the senium and presenium.

    (1) Dementia of the Alzheimer type, with early onset.

      (a) 290.00 Uncomplicated.

      (b) 290.11 With delirium.

      (c) 290.12 With delusions.

      (d) 290.13 With depressed mood.

    (2) 290.4 Vascular Dementia (various subtypes).

    (3) 294.x Dementia due to other medical conditions (various subtypes).

    (4) 294.8 Dementia NOS.

  b. Other Organic Mental Disorders associated with Axis III physical disorders or conditions, or etiology is unknown, including but not limited to the following:

    (1) 293.0 Delirium due to general medical condition.

(2) 293.81 Psychotic disorder with delusions due to a general medical condition.

(3) 293.82 Psychotic disorder with hallucinosis due to a general medical condition.

(4) 293.83 Mood disorder due to a general medical condition.

(5) 294.00 Amnestic disorder due to general medical condition.

(6) 310.1 Personality change due to a general medical condition.

5. <u>Psychoactive Substance Use Disorders</u>. These disorders are disqualifying for appointment, enlistment, or induction under Section 3-D-32 of this Manual or if identified on active duty shall be processed in accordance with Chapter 20, Personnel Manual, COMDTINST M1000.6 (series).

   a. 303.90 Alcohol dependence (alcoholism).

   b. 304.00 Opioid dependence.

   c. 304.10 Sedative, hypnotic, or anxiolytic dependence.

   d. 304.20 Cocaine dependence.

   e. 304.30 Cannabis dependence.

   f. 304.40 Amphetamine dependence.

   g. 304.50 Hallucinogen dependence.

   h. 304.60 Inhalant dependence.

   i. 304.90 Other (or unknown) substance, including PCP dependence.

   j. 305.00 Alcohol abuse.

   k. 305.20 Cannabis abuse.

   l. 305.30 Hallucinogen abuse.

   m. 305.40 Sedative, hypnotic, or anxiolytic abuse.

   n. 305.50 Opioid abuse.

   o. 305.60 Cocaine abuse.

   p. 305.70 Amphetamine abuse.

   q. 305.90 Other (or unknown) Substance abuse, including inhalant and PCP abuse.

6. <u>Schizophrenia</u>. These disorders are disqualifying under Section 3-D-30 of this Manual or if identified on active duty shall be processed in accordance with Physical Disability Evaluation System, COMDTINST M1850.2 (series).

   a. 295.10 Disorganized type.

   b. 295.20 Catatonic type.

c. 295.30 Paranoid type.

d. 295.60 Residual type.

e. 295.90 Undifferentiated type.

7. <u>Psychotic Disorders Not Elsewhere Classified</u>. These disorders are disqualifying under Section 3-D-30 of this manual or if identified on active duty shall be processed in accordance with Physical Disability Evaluation System, COMDTINST M1850.2 (series).

    a. 295.40 Schizophreniform disorder.

    b. 295.70 Schizoaffective disorder.

    c. 297.30 Induced psychotic disorder.

    d. 298.80 Brief psychotic disorder.

    e. 298.90 Psychotic disorder NOS.

8. <u>Delusional (Paranoid) Disorder</u>. 297.1, Delusional (Paranoid) Disorder, is disqualifying under Section 3-D of this Manual or shall be processed in accordance with Physical Disability Evaluation System, COMDTINST M1850.2 (series).

9. <u>Neurotic Disorders</u>. These disorders are now included in Anxiety, Somatoform, Dissociative, and Sexual Disorders.

10. <u>Mood Disorders</u>. These disorders are disqualifying for enlistment under Chapter 3 Section D of this Manual or if identified on active duty shall be processed in accordance with Physical Disability Evaluation System, COMDTINST M1850.2 (series). These disorders may be disqualifying for retention under Chapter 3 Section F of this Manual.

    a. <u>Bipolar I Disorders</u>.

        (1) 296.0X Bipolar I disorder, single manic episode (various subtypes).

        (2) 296.40 Bipolar I disorder, most recent episode hypomanic.

        (3) 296.4X Bipolar I disorder, most recent episode manic (various sub-types).

        (4) 296.5X Bipolar I disorder, most recent depressed (various sub-types).

        (5) 296.6X Bipolar I disorder, most recent episode mixed, (various sub-types).

        (6) 296.7 Bipolar I disorder, most recent episode unspecified.

        (7) 296.89 Bipolar II disorder.

        (8) 301.13 Cyclothymia.

    b. <u>Depressive Disorders</u>.

        (1) 296.XX Major depressive disorder (various sub-types).

(2) 300.4 Dysthymic disorder (or depressive neurosis).

(3) 311 Depressive disorder NOS.

11. Anxiety Disorders (or Anxiety and Phobic Neuroses). These disorders are disqualifying for appointment, enlistment, or induction under Chapter 3 Section D of this Manual or if identified on active duty shall be processed in accordance with Physical Disability Evaluation System, COMDTINST M1850.2 (series), except as noted on (5) below. These disorders may be disqualifying for retention under Chapter 3 Section F of this Manual.

   a. Panic Disorders.

      (1) 300.01 Without agoraphobia.

      (2) 300.21 With agoraphobia.

      (3) 300.22 Agoraphobia without history of panic disorder.

      (4) 300.23 Social phobia.

      (5) 300.29 Specific phobia. [Chapter 12, Personnel Manual, COMDTINST M1000.6 (series).]

   b. Other Anxiety disorders.

      (1) 300.00 Anxiety disorder NOS.

      (2) 300.02 Generalized anxiety disorder.

      (3) 300.3 Obsessive-compulsive disorder (or obsessive compulsive neurosis).

      (4) 309.81 Post-traumatic stress disorder.

12. Somatoform Disorders. These disorders are disqualifying for appointment, enlistment, or induction under Chapter 3 Section D of this Manual or if identified on active duty shall be processed in accordance with Physical Disability Evaluation System, COMDTINST M1850.2 (series). These disorders may be disqualifying for retention under Chapter 3 Section F of this Manual.

   a. 300.11 Conversion disorder.

   b. 300.70 Hypochondriasis (or hypochondrical neurosis). Body Dysmorphic disorder. Somatoform disorder NOS.

   c. 300.81 Somatization disorder or undifferentiated somatoform disorder.

   d. 307.80 Pain disorder associated with psychological factors.

13. Dissociative Disorders (or Hysterical Neuroses, Dissociative Type). These disorders are disqualifying for appointment, enlistment, or enlistment under Section 3-D of this Manual or if identified on active duty shall may be processed in accordance with Physical Disability Evaluation System, COMDTINST M1850.2 (series).

   a. 300.12 Dissociative amnesia.

b. 300.13 Dissociative fugue.

c. 300.14 Dissociative identity disorder.

d. 300.15 Dissociative disorder NOS.

e. 300.6 Depersonalization disorder.

14. <u>Sexual Disorders</u>. These disorders are processed in accordance with Chapter 12 of the Personnel Manual, COMDTINST M1000.6 (series).

    a. <u>Gender Identity Disorders</u>.

        (1) 302.6 Gender identity disorder in children (history of) or NOS.

        (2) 302.85 Gender identity disorder in adolescents or adults.

    b. <u>Paraphilias</u>.

        (1) 302.2 Pedophilia.

        (2) 302.3 Transvestic fetishism.

        (3) 302.4 Exhibitionism.

        (4) 302.81 Fetishism.

        (5) 302.82 Voyeurism.

        (6) 302.83 Sexual masochism.

        (7) 302.84 Sexual sadism.

        (8) 302.89 Frotteurism.

        (9) 302.9 Paraphilia NOS (includes Zoophilia).

15. <u>Sexual Dysfunctions</u>. These are not grounds for action as they have no direct bearing upon fitness for duty.

    a. 302.70 Sexual dysfunction NOS.

    b. 302.71 Hypoactive sexual desire.

    c. 302.72 Female arousal disorder. Male erectile disorder.

    d. 302.73 Female orgasmic disorder.

    e. 302.74 Male orgasmic disorder.

    f. 302.75 Premature ejaculation.

    g. 302.76 Dyspareunia.

    h. 302.79 Sexual aversion disorder.

    i. 302.9 Sexual Disorder NOS.

    j. 306.51 Vaginismus.

16. <u>Factitious Disorders</u>. These disorders are disqualifying for appointment, enlistment, or induction under Section 3-D-29 of this Manual or if identified on

active duty shall be processed in accordance with Chapter 12 of the Personnel Manual, COMDTINST M1000.6 (series).

   a. 300.16 With predominantly psychological symptoms.

   b. 300.19 Factitious disorder NOS.

   c. 301.51 With predominantly physical symptoms, or combined.

17. Disorders of Impulse Control Not Elsewhere Classified. These disorders are disqualifying for enlistment under Section 3-D-30 of this Manual or if identified on active duty shall be processed in accordance with Chapter 12 of the Personnel Manual, COMDTINST M1000.6 (series).

   a. 312.30 Impulse control disorder NOS.

   b. 312.31 Pathological gambling.

   c. 312.32 Kleptomania.

   d. 312.33 Pyromania.

   e. 312.34 Intermittent explosive disorder.

   f. 312.39 Trichotillomania.

18. Disorders Usually First Evident in Infancy, Childhood, or Adolescence. Except as indicated in parentheses, these disorders are disqualifying for appointment, enlistment, or induction under Section 3-D-30 of this manual, or if identified on active duty shall be processed in accordance with Chapter 12 of the Personnel Manual, COMDTINST M1000.6 (series), if the condition significantly impacts, or has the potential to significantly impact performance of duties (health, mission, and safety).

   a. Mental Retardation (Note: these are coded on Axis II).

      (1) 317 Mild mental retardation, IQ 50-70.

      (2) 318.X Moderate, severe, or profound mental retardation, IQ 35-49.

      (3) 319 Mental retardation, severity unspecified.

   b. Disruptive Behavior Disorders.

      (1) 314.0X Attention deficit hyperactivity disorder (various types).

      (2) 312.8 Conduct disorder.

      (3) 312.9 Disruptive behavior disorder or attention deficit disorder, NOS.

      (4) 313.81 Oppositional defiant disorder.

   c. Other Disorders of Infancy, Childhood, or Adolescence.

      (1) 307.30 Stereotypic movement disorder.

      (2) 309.21 Separation anxiety disorder.

      (3) 313.23 Selective mutism.

(4) 313.82 Identity problem.

(5) 313.89 Reactive attachment disorder of infancy or early childhood.

d. Eating Disorders. Eating disorders have a potential to affect fitness for duty, but the diagnosis of an eating disorder does not automatically mean the member is unsuitable for continued service. Individuals suspected of having an eating disorder shall be referred for evaluation by an Armed Forces psychiatrist or Armed Forces clinical psychologist. Treatment may be authorized in accordance with the same criteria as other mental conditions. See paragraph 5.B.1 of this Manual.

(1) 307.1 Anorexia nervosa. (Shall be processed through Physical Disability Evaluation System, COMDTINST M1850.2 (series)).

(2) 307.50 Eating disorder NOS. Shall be processed in accordance with Chapter 12.B.12 or 12.A.15.h (as applicable) of the Personnel Manual, COMDTINST M1000.6 (series), if the condition significantly impacts or has the potential to significantly impact performance of duties (health, mission, and safety).

(3) 307.51 Bulimia nervosa. (Shall be processed through Physical Disability Evaluation System, COMDTINST M1850.2 (series)).

(4) 307.52 Pica.

(5) 307.53 Rumination disorder.

e. Tic Disorders.

(1) 307.20 Tic disorder NOS.

(2) 307.21 Transient tic disorder.

(3) 307.22 Chronic motor or vocal tic disorder.

(4) 307.23 Tourette's disorder.

f. Communication Disorder.

(1) 307.0 Stuttering.

(2) 315.31 Expressive or mixed (expressive-receptive) language disorder.

(3) 315.39 Phonological disorder.

g. Elimination Disorders.

(1) 307.46 Sleepwalking disorder.

(2) 307.46 Sleep terror disorder.

(3) 327.4 Parasomnia

(4) 307.6 Enuresis (not due to a general medical condition).

(5) 307.7 Encopresis (without constipation and overflow incontinence.)

h. Pervasive Developmental Disorder.

(1) 299.00 Autistic disorder.

(2) 299.80 Pervasive developmental disorder NOS.

i. <u>Specific Learning Developmental Disorders</u> - (Note: These Are Coded on Axis II).

(1) 315.00 Reading disorder.

(2) 315.1 Mathematics disorder.

(3) 315.2 Disorder of written expression.

(4) 315.4 Developmental coordination disorder.

(5) 315.9 Learning disorder NOS.

19. <u>Psychological Factors Affecting Physical Condition</u>. Psychological factors affecting physical conditions (316.00). This disorder is not generally grounds for action alone. The physical condition must be specified on Axis III and will determine fitness.

20. <u>V Codes for Conditions Not Attributable to a Mental Disorder that are a Focus of Attention or Treatment</u>. These disorders are generally not of such severity as to lead to disqualification for enlistment or to separation. Where separation is indicated, process in accordance with Chapter 12 of the Personnel Manual, COMDTINST M1000.6 (series).

a. V15.81 Noncompliance with medical treatment.

b. V61.1 Partner relational problem.

c. V61.20 Parent-child relational problem.

d. V61.8 Sibling relational problem.

e. V62.2 Occupational problem.

f. V62.3 Academic problem.

g. V62.81 Relational problem NOS.

h. V62.82 Bereavement.

i. V62.89 Borderline intellectual functioning.

j. V62.89 Phase of life problem or religious or spiritual problem.

k. V65.2 Malingering. (May be grounds for legal, administrative, or medical board proceedings in accordance with Section 2-A-4 of this manual depending on the circumstances)

l. V71.01 Adult antisocial behavior.

m. V71.02 Child or adolescent antisocial behavior.

21. <u>Additional Codes</u>.
These are non-diagnostic codes for administrative use and require no action.

a. V71.09 No diagnosis or condition on Axis I.

b. V71.09 No diagnosis on Axis II.

c. 300.9 Unspecified mental disorder (nonpsychotic).

d. 799.9 Diagnosis or condition deferred on Axis I.

e. 799.9 Diagnosis deferred on Axis II.

Section C. Command directed Mental Health Evaluation of Coast Guard Service members.

1. Active Duty Mental Health Evaluation Protection 1
2. Emergency Evaluations 1
3. Non-emergent Mental Health Evaluation 1
4. Service Member's Rights..2
5. Things Not To Do 2
6. Evaluations NOT covered..3
7. Memorandum Requesting a Mental Health Evaluation...3

This page intentionally left blank.

C. Command Directed Mental Health Evaluation of CG Members.

1. Active Duty Mental Health Evaluation Protection. Active Duty Mental Health Conditions and Emergencies, COMDTPUB P6520.1 refers to Public Law 102-484, Section 546, also known as the "Boxer Amendment". The CG is not included and therefore not subject to the Boxer Amendment. The restrictions in this Amendment are intended to prevent unwarranted involuntary mental health evaluations or involuntary hospitalization as a form of harassment or retaliation. Accordingly, the following instructions meet many of the criteria of PL 102-484, Section 546.

2. Emergency Evaluations.
    a. When to make the mental health referral. A CO should consider making an emergency mental health referral for any member who indicates intent to cause harm to themselves or others and who appears to have a severe mental disorder.

    b. Communicate with provider. The CO should make every effort to consult with a mental health care provider (MHCP) at the location of the desired evaluation, prior to transporting a Service Member for a mental health evaluation. If this is not possible, the CO must consult with a MHCP, or other health care provider if a MHCP is not available, at the MTF or location of the evaluation, as soon as possible after transporting the Service Member for an emergency evaluation. The purpose of this consultation is to communicate the observations and circumstances which led the CO to believe that an emergency referral was required. The CO will then forward to the MHCP consulted, a memorandum documenting the information discussed.

3. Non-emergent Mental Health Evaluation. Signs of mental illness can include changes in behavior, mood, or thinking that interfere with normal functioning. When a CO believes a Service Member has a mental illness that requires a Command Directed Mental Health Evaluation they will:
    a. Contact the servicing CG Clinic. The CO should speak directly with a health care provider to discuss the request for a Command Directed Mental Health Evaluation. The CO should clearly state the Service Member's actions and behaviors that led to the request for a Command Directed Mental Health Evaluation. The health care provider will clarify the request, urgency of the referral, and schedule an appointment.

    b. Provide a memorandum. The CO must provide a memorandum to the Senior Health Services Officer (SHSO), or DoD MTF clinic CO, documenting this request for a Command Directed Mental Health Evaluation. The subject line of the memorandum shall read, Subject: Command Referral for Mental Health Evaluation of (Service Member Rank, Name, Branch of Service and SSN. (Sample letter Figure 1).

    c. Counsel the Service Member. Along with counseling the Service Member regarding the reasons for the Command Directed Mental Health Evaluation, the CO will ensure that the Service Member is provided written notice of the referral. The notice, Subject: Notification of Commanding Officer Referral for Mental Health Evaluation (Non-Emergency), will include the following: (Sample letter Figure 2)

(1) Date and time the mental-health evaluation is scheduled.

(2) A brief, factual description of the Service Member's behavior and/or statements that indicate a mental-health evaluation is necessary.

(3) Names of mental-health professionals the commander has consulted before making the referral. If prior consultation with a MHCP is not possible, commanders must include the reasons in the notice.

d. Request the Service Member sign the notice to report for a mental health evaluation. If the Service Member refuses to sign, the CO will note this response in the notice.

e. Provide an escort for Service Member referred for a mental health evaluation.

4. Service Members Rights. COs shall provide a copy of the following rights to Service Members who are referred: (Sample letter Figure 2)

a. Second opinion. A Service Member has the right to obtain a second opinion at his/her own expense. The evaluation should be conducted within a reasonable period of time, usually within 10 days, and will not delay nor substitute for an evaluation performed by a DoD mental health care provider.

b. Free communication. No person may restrict the Service Member from communicating with an Attorney, IG, Chaplain, Member of Congress, or other appropriate party about the member's referral.

c. Two workdays before appointment. Other than emergencies, the Service Member will have at least 2 workdays before a scheduled mental health evaluation to meet with an Attorney, Chaplain, IG, or other appropriate party. If a CO has reason to believe the condition of the Service Member requires an immediate mental health evaluation, the CO will state the reasons in writing as part of the request for evaluation.

d. If military duties prevent the Service Member from complying with this policy, the CO seeking the referral will state the reasons in a memorandum.

5. Things Not To Do.

a. Use Command Directed Mental Health Evaluations as a Reprisal. No one will refer a Service Member for a mental health evaluation as a reprisal for making or preparing a lawful communication to a Member of Congress, an authority in the Service Member's chain of command, an IG, or a member of a DoD audit, inspection, investigation, or law enforcement organization.

b. **Withhold communication.** A Service Member will NOT be restricted from lawfully communicating with an IG, Attorney, Member of Congress, or others about the Service Member's referral for a mental health evaluation.

c. **CO's authority to refer Service Members.** These policies are not designed to limit the CO's authority to refer Service Members for emergency mental health evaluations and treatment when circumstances suggest the need for such action.

6. **Evaluations NOT covered.** The specific procedures required by these regulations apply to mental health evaluations directed by a Service Member's CO as an exercise of the CO's discretionary authority. Evaluations NOT covered by these procedures include:

   a. Voluntary self-referrals.

   b. Criminal responsibility and competency inquiries conducted under Rule for Court-Martial 706 of the Manual for Courts-Martial.

   c. Interviews conducted according to the Family Advocacy Program.

   d. Referrals to the Alcohol and Drug Abuse Prevention and Control Program.

   e. Security clearances.

   f. Diagnostic referrals from other health care providers not part of the Service Member's chain of command when the Service Member consents to the evaluation.

   g. Referrals for evaluations expressly required by regulation, without any discretion by the Service Member's CO, such as enlisted administrative separations.

7. **Memorandum Requesting a Mental Health Evaluation.** Procedures for using the memorandum requesting a mental health evaluation in emergency situations, COs will:

   a. Complete the memorandum including as many details as possible.

   b. Make one copy to give to the Service Member.

   c. Escort hand carries the memorandum. Ensure that the Service Member's escort hand carries the memorandum to the treatment facility. The memorandum will not be hand carried by the Service Member being referred. This memorandum will not be sent through distribution channels, nor will it become part of the Service Member's health record. The memorandum will be filed in the Department of Psychiatry of the medical treatment facility where the Service Member was evaluated.

COMDTINST M6000.1E

FIGURE 1

SAMPLE COMMAND REFERRAL FOR MENTAL HEALTH EVALUATION

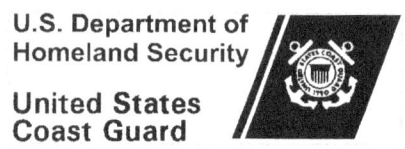

U.S. Department of
Homeland Security

United States
Coast Guard

Commanding Officer
United States Coast Guard

xxxxxxxxxxxxxxx
xxxxxxxxxxxxxxx
Staff Symbol: xxx
Phone: (xxx) xxx-xxxx
Fax: (xxx) xxx-xxxx
Email:

MEMORANDUM

SSIC

Date 3 Jan 2005

From: Commanding Officer, (Name of Command)   Reply to
                                                  Attn of:

To: Commanding Officer, (Name of Medical Treatment Facility (MTF) or Clinic)

Thru:

Subj: COMMAND REFERRAL FOR MENTAL HEALTH EVALUATION OF (Service Member Rank, Name, Branch of Service and SSN)

Ref: (a) CG Medical Manual, COMDTINST M6000.1 (series)
        (b) Active Duty Mental Health Conditions and Emergencies, COMDTPUB P6520.1

1. In accordance with references (a. b.), I request a formal mental health evaluation of (rank and name of service member).

2. On _____ (date) I consulted with _____ (name and rank of mental health care provider consulted) or I was unable to consult with a mental health care provider because _____.

3. (Name and rank of Service Member) has ___ (years) and ___ (months) active duty service and has been assigned to my command since ____ (date). Armed Services Vocational Aptitude Battery (ASVAB) scores upon enlistment were: ____ (list scores). Past average performance marks have ranged from _____ to _____ (give numerical scores). Legal action is/is not currently pending against the service member. (If charges are pending, list dates and UCMJ articles.) Past legal actions include: _____ (List dates, charges, non-judicial punishments (NJPs) and/or findings of Courts Martial.)

4. I have given the service member a memorandum that advises _____ (rank and name of Service Member) of his/her rights, and explains my reasons for the referral. I have also informed the Service Member of the name of the mental health care provider(s) with whom I consulted, and the names and telephone numbers of persons who

COMDTINST M6000.1E

may advise the Service Member. A copy of this memorandum is attached for your review.

5. I directed _____ (Service Member's rank and name) to meet with _____ (name and rank of mental health care provider) at _____ (MTF or clinic) on _____ (date) at _____ (hours).

6. Should you wish additional information, you may contact me or _____ (POC name and rank) at _____ (telephone number).

7. Please provide a summary of your findings and recommendations as soon as they are available to _____.

#

Enclosures:

Dist:

Copy:

COMDTINST M6000.1E

FIGURE 2

SAMPLE SERVICE MEMBER NOTIFICATION OF COMMANDING OFFICER REFERRAL FOR MENTAL HEALTH EVALUATION.

U.S. Department of
Homeland Security

United States
Coast Guard

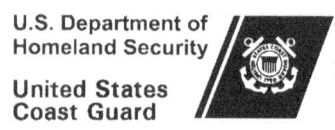

Commanding Officer
United States Coast Guard

xxxxxxxxxxxxx
xxxxxxxxxxxxx
Staff Symbol: xxxxx
Phone: (xxx) xxx-xxxx
Fax: (xxx) xxx-xxxx
Email:

MEMORANDUM

SSIC

Date 3 Jan 2005

From: Commanding Officer, (Name of Command)   Reply to
Attn of:

To: (Service Member being directed for mental health evaluation)

Thru:

Subj: NOTIFICATION OF COMMANDING OFFICER REFERRAL FOR MENTAL HEALTH EVALUATION (NON EMERGENCY) (Service Member Rank, Name, Branch of Service and SSN)

Ref: (a) CG Medical Manual, COMDTINST M6000.1(series)
(b) Active Duty Mental Health Conditions and Emergencies, COMDTPUB P6520.1

1. In accordance with references (a) and (b), this memorandum is to inform you that I am referring you to a mental health provider for a mental health evaluation.

2. I direct you to meet with _____ (name & rank of mental health care provider(s)) at _____ (MTF or clinic) on _____ (date) at _____ (hours).

3. I am referring you for a mental health evaluation because of your behavior and/or statements on _____ (date(s)). On the stated date(s), you (brief description of behaviors and statements): _____
_____.

4. In accordance with reference (a), before the referral, on _____ (date) I consulted with _____ (name, rank, and branch of each medical or mental health care provider consulted) from the _____ (MTF or clinic) about your recent behavior and/or statements and _____ (name and rank of each mental health or medical provider) (did) (did not) concur(s) that a mental health evaluation is necessary.

OR

5. Consultation with a mental healthcare provider prior to this referral is (was) not possible because _____ (give reason; e.g., geographic isolation from available mental healthcare provider, etc.)

Per references (a) and (b), you are entitled to the following rights:

6. The right to speak to a civilian attorney of your own choosing and expense, for advice on how to rebut this referral if you believe it is improper.

7. The right to submit to the USCG or the IG a complaint that your mental health evaluation referral was a reprisal for making or preparing a protected communication to a statutory recipient. Statutory recipients include members of Congress, an IG, and personnel within USCG or DoD audit, inspection, investigation, or law enforcement organizations. Statutory recipients also include any appropriate authority in your chain of command, and any person designated by regulation or other administrative procedures to receive your protected communication.

8. The right to be evaluated by a mental health care provider (MHCP) of your own choosing, at your own expense, provided the MHCP is reasonably available. Such an evaluation by an independent mental healthcare provider shall be conducted within a reasonable period of time, usually within 10 business days. The evaluation performed by your MHCP will not delay or substitute for an evaluation performed by a DoD mental healthcare provider.

9. The right to communicate, provided the communication is lawful, with an IG, Attorney, Member of Congress, or others about your referral for a mental health evaluation.

10. The right, except in emergencies, to have at least two business days before the scheduled mental health evaluation to meet with an Attorney, IG, Chaplain, friend, or family member. If I believe your situation constitutes an emergency or that your condition appears potentially harmful to your well being and I judge that it is not in your best interest to delay your mental health evaluation for two business days, I shall state my reasons in writing as part of the request for the mental health evaluation.

11. If applicable: Since you are _____ (deployed) (in a geographically isolated area) because of circumstances related to military duties, compliance with the following procedures _____ are impractical for the following reasons _____.

12. You may seek assistance from the chaplain located in building number _____, Monday through Friday from ___ hours to ____ hours.

#

I have read the memorandum above and have been provided a copy.

Service Member's signature:_____ Date:_____

IF SERVICE MEMBER REFUSES TO SIGN

The Service Member declined to sign this memorandum containing the notice of referral and notice of Service Member's rights because _____ (gave no reason or give reason and/or quote Service Member).

Witness signature:_____ Date:_____
Witness rank and name:_____ Date:_____

After the witness signed this memorandum, I provided a copy of this memorandum to the Service Member.

CHAPTER 6

MEDICAL READINESS/DEPLOYMENT HEALTH

Section A. Overview.

1. Purpose..1
2. Responsibilities..1
3. Individual Medical Readiness..1
4. Standard Definitions and Scoring..1
5. Medically Ready...3
6. Deployment Definitions...3

Section B. Expeditionary Deployment.

1. Electronic Deployment Health Assessment (EDHA)..1
2. Responsibility and timeline for the EDHA..1
3. EDHA Overview..1
4. EDHA Healthcare Provider Review Process..1
5. Pre-Deployment Requirements..2
6. Deployment..3
7. Post-Deployment..3
8. DD-2900, Post-Deployment Health Reassessment via the EDHA (see above) 4
9. Compliance Program 4

Section C. Routine Deployment.

1. Pre Deployment Requirements..1
2. Deployment..1
3. Post-Deployment..1
4. Additional References...2

COMDTINST M6000.1E

This page intentionally left blank

Chapter 6 Contents

Section A. Overview

1. Purpose...1
2. Responsibilities..1
3. Individual Medical Readiness...1
4. Standard Definitions and Scoring...1
5. Medically Ready..3
6. Deployment Definitions..3

This page intentionally left blank.

CHAPTER SIX – MEDICAL READINESS/DEPLOYMENT HEALTH

Section A. Overview.

1. Purpose. This chapter describes procedures for, and directs implementation of medical readiness and deployment health requirements for all CG expeditionary and routine deployments. The goal of this program is for all active duty and reserve CG members to meet medical readiness requirements in order to deploy in support of CG missions. For the purpose of this Chapter, medical readiness includes dental readiness. Also, for the purpose of this Chapter, reserve refers to selected reserves.

2. Responsibilities. Medical readiness and deployment health are Commandant programs, and Commanding Officers/Officers-in-Charge are responsible for full compliance. These program requirements are mandated by DoD Instruction 6025.19 – Individual Medical Readiness, which applies to the CG and meet the requirements of the National Defense Authorization Act of 2005 (NDAA 05), Public Law 108-375. It is the personal responsibility of each CG active duty and reserve member to maintain their medical readiness levels at all times.

3. Individual Medical Readiness. Individual Medical Readiness (IMR) is the extent to which an individual active duty or reserve member is free from health related conditions that could limit their ability to fully participate in CG operations (i.e. fit for full duty-FFFD). All active duty and reserve CG members are required to be medically ready for deployment. All IMR requirements, as delineated in the Coast Guard Periodic Health Assessment (PHA), COMDTINST M6150.3, are required to be met by CG AD and SELRES members (to include Direct Commission Officers and those at various points of accession). The CG clinic affiliated with the point of accession is responsible for inputting the IMR data into the applicable medical information system (MIS) database (i.e. Medical Readiness Reporting System (MRRS), etc.). Refer to Chapter 2 Section A 1.c. for the CO's and the medical department's responsibilities in relation to medical readiness documentation.

4. Standard Definitions and Scoring. DODI 6025.19 has established the following standard definitions for six Individual Medical Readiness (IMR) elements for all Armed Forces:

    a. Periodic Health Assessment (PHA). Each active duty and reserve member must have an annual Periodic Health Assessment (PHA) to closely monitor their health. The PHA will consolidate periodic clinical preventive examinations, individual medical readiness, occupational health and risk screening services, medical record review, preventive counseling and risk communication. The PHA will replace the routine periodic physical examination.

    b. Dental. To meet IMR standards service members must be rated as either Class 1 or Class 2. Service members who are categorized as Class 3 or Class 4 will not meet IMR standards. All active duty and reserve members must have an annual dental screening.

Dental Classification	Definition
Class 1	A service member who does not require dental treatment or revaluation within 12 months.
Class 2	A service member who has an oral condition that, if not treated or followed up, has the potential to, but is not expected to, result in emergencies within 12 months.
Class 3	A service member who has an oral condition that if not treated is expected to result in a dental emergency within 12 months.
Class 4	Patients who require periodic dental examinations or patients with unknown dental classifications. Class 4 patients normally are not considered to be worldwide deployable

Table 6-A-1

c. *Immunizations*. All active duty and reserve members shall be current on the following readiness immunizations – (1) Hepatitis A (or Twinrix), (2) Hepatitis B (or Twinrix), (3) Influenza, (4) Measles, Mumps and Rubella (MMR), (5) Inactivated Poliovirus, (IPV), and (6) Tetanus Diphtheria (or Tetanus Diphtheria acellular Pertussis). Additional immunizations may be required prior to specific deployment or assignment. See the CG's current immunization policies, Immunization and Chemoprophylaxis COMDTINST M6230.4 (series), the Coast Guard Anthrax Vaccine Immunization Program (CG AVIP), COMDTINST M6230.3 (series), and the CG Smallpox Vaccine Program COMDTINST M6230.10 for additional immunization requirements.

d. *Individual Medical Equipment (IME)*. Service members who are in the process of being deployed on an expeditionary deployment (e.g. CENTCOM AOR) and Deployable Operational Group units shall have the following IME – (1) Ballistic Protection Optical Inserts, (2) Protective (Gas) Mask Inserts, and (3) Medical Warning Tags. Members requiring eye-wear must possess two pairs of eyeglasses. Contact lenses are time consuming to take care of and have been identified during Central Command (CENTCOM) deployments as an operational safety issue. Personnel deploying must contend with field conditions that may not allow for proper contact lens hygiene, and poor hygiene leads to an increase in eye abrasions, infections and ulcers. This should be taken into account by personnel desiring to deploy with contact lenses in addition to their spectacles.

e. <u>Medical Readiness Labs</u>. The basic laboratory studies include – (1) blood type and Rh factor, G6PD status, deoxyribonucleic acid (DNA) specimen, a baseline Tuberculin Skin Test, and a current HIV antibody test. A negative pregnancy test for women of child bearing age should be determined prior to deployment

f. <u>Deployment Limiting Conditions</u>. Service members who are in the process of deploying (on an expeditionary deployment) must not have any deployment limiting conditions (DLC). DLC includes – (1) pregnancy and 6 weeks post-partum, (2) injuries or illnesses that require a 6 month or greater Temporary Limited Duty (TLD) assignment, and Dental Class III or IV.

5. <u>Medically Ready</u>. To be fully medically ready, an individual must meet all six of the criteria. Medical readiness does not mean deployability. Deployability includes other factors determined by the CO such as core competencies in job skills. All medically ready individuals are deployable from a medical standpoint. It is the CO's decision whether to deploy members who do not meet CG medical readiness criteria.

6. <u>Deployment Definitions</u>.

   a. <u>Expeditionary Deployment</u>. Expeditionary deployments include active duty and reserve CG members supporting DoD troop movements resulting from a Joint Chiefs of Staff/Combatant Command deployment for 30 continuous days or more to a location outside the United States where there is not a fixed U.S. military medical treatment facility (MTF). Operation Iraqi Freedom (OIF) and Operation Enduring Freedom (OEF) are examples of expeditionary deployments.

   b. <u>Routine Deployment</u>. Routine deployment include active duty and reserve CG personnel involved in CG patrols and deployments outside the US, its territories or possessions, in support of CG missions. This includes joint DoD deployments not associated with expeditionary deployments. This also includes special named operations/contingencies as designated by Commandant (CG-11) (e.g. deployments to identified domestic disaster relief (i.e. hurricane) operations).

This page intentionally left blank.

Section B. Expeditionary Deployment

1. Electronic Deployment Health Assessments (EDHA). 1
2. Responsibility and timeline for the EDHA. 1
3. EDHA Overview. 1
4. EDHA healthcare provider review process: 1
5. Pre-Deployment Requirements. 2
6. Deployment. 3
7. Post-Deployment. 3
8. DD-2900, Post-Deployment Health Reassessment via the EDHA (see above). 4
9. Compliance Program. 4

This page intentionally left blank.

B. Expeditionary Deployment.

1. Electronic Deployment Health Assessments (EDHA). All Active Duty and Selected Reserve CG personnel who are on an expeditionary deployment for at least thirty (30) consecutive days must complete pre and post deployment health assessments electronically. The Armed Forces Health Surveillance Center (AFHSC) will no longer accept submission of paper based deployment health forms.

2. Responsibility and timeline for the EDHA. It is the member's responsibility to complete the deployment health assessments within the appropriate time lines as follows:

    a. DD-2795, Pre-Deployment Health Assessment. Within 30 days prior to deployment,

    b. DD-2796, Post Deployment Health Assessment. No earlier than 7 days before returning and no later than 30 days after returning to the home stations, and

    c. DD-2900, Post Deployment Health Reassessment (PDHRA). During the 3 month to 6 month time period after returning from deployment. After members have completed the form, a healthcare provider will discuss with the service member any health concerns which they have indicated on the form, and will make referrals to appropriate healthcare or community-based services if further evaluation or treatment is needed. CG Active Duty and Reserve Members who are not located near a CG clinic or a Navy Military Treatment Facility must call the PDHRA Call Center at 1-888-PDHRA-99 (press Option 3) to complete their PDHRA with a DoD contracted healthcare provider via the telephone. The DoD contracted healthcare providers have access to the EDHA and will complete the PDHRA electronically.

3. EDHA Overview. All deploying members will access the Navy Electronic Deployment Health Assessment (EDHA) located at https://www-nehc.med.navy.mil/edha. Members must select "New User" and enter "Coastie1234$" as the pass phrase. Members must enter the required information and then select "Register". After registering, members must select "Create a New Survey" and select the required deployment health survey (i.e. DD-2795, Pre-Deployment Health Assessment, DD-2796, Post Deployment Health Assessment, or the DD-2900, Post Deployment Health Reassessment). After completing the survey, members must select "Save" and exit out of the program. For subsequent access to the EHDA, the member must enter his or her social security number as the login ID and enter his or her newly created password. If a member has forgotten his or her password or the pass phrase, he or she should contact Commandant (CG-1121) for assistance.

4. EDHA healthcare provider review process.

    a. DD-2795, Pre-Deployment Health Assessment. The DD-2795, Pre-Deployment Health Assessment must be reviewed by a healthcare provider. The healthcare provider can be a health services technician (HS), and independent duty health services technician (IDHS), or a Medical Officer. Medical appointment or follow-up with a IDHS or Medical Officer is only necessary for the DD-2795, Pre-Deployment Health Assessment if the member responded positively to questions 2-4 or 7-8.

    b. DD-2796, Post Deployment Health Assessment. For the DD-2796, Post Deployment Health Assessment members must schedule a medical appointment with an IDHS or

COMDTINST M6000.1E

   Medical Officer as soon as possible, after completing the DD-2796, Post Deployment Health Assessment.

   c. <u>DD-2900, Post Deployment Health Reassessment</u>. For the PDHRA, members must either schedule a medical appointment with an IDHS or Medical Officer at a CG or Navy Medical Treatment Facility or call the PDHRA Call Center after completing the DD-2900, Post Deployment Health Reassessment.

   d. <u>Healthcare providers Responsibility</u>. Healthcare providers will review the member's deployment health assessment forms via the EDHA. All healthcare providers who perform deployment health screenings (for expeditionary deployments) must contact Commandant (CG-1121) via phone or email for their login ID and password. After logging into the EDHA, the provider must review the member's survey, complete the remainder of the survey and select "Save" to finish. Providers should print the member's signed deployment health survey (using the print icon) and exit out of the EDHA. The provider must place the signed original assessment in the ember's medical record. When the assessments are completed and saved, they are electronically submitted to AFHSC.

5. <u>Pre-Deployment Requirements</u>. The following pre-deployment health activities are required for all expeditionary deployments:

   a. Completion of the DD-2795, Pre-Deployment Health Assessment via the EDHA (see above).

   b. Administer deployment specific immunizations, prophylaxis, and other countermeasures (see Chapter 6, Section A).

   c. Ensure all IMR requirements have been met (see Chapter 6, section A).

   d. Medications. Ensure members have a sufficient supply of medications for duration of orders (at least a 90-day supply).

   e. Allergies. Review member's allergies and ensure documentation on the DD-2766, Adult Preventive and Chronic Care Flowsheet.

   f. Review and update the DD-2766, Adult Preventive and Chronic Care Flowsheet. The original DD-2766, Adult Preventive and Chronic Care Flowsheet should be taken with the member during the deployment rather than filed in the member's health record.

   g. <u>Countermeasures</u>. Ensure deploying personnel have access to appropriate Force Health Protection Prescription Products (FHPPP) which include malaria prophylaxis, atropine/2-Pam chloride autoinjectors, pyridostigmine bromide (PB) tablets, and CANA. Document any FHPPP dispensed/prescribed in the comments section of the DD-2795, Pre-Deployment Health Assessment. Ensure all FHPPP are issued in accordance with ASD(HA) Memorandum, Policy for Use of Force Health Protection Prescription Products (24 Apr 03) - http://www.ha.osd.mil/policies/2003/03-007.pdf.

   h. <u>Medical Threat Briefing</u>. Provide specific medical threat briefing and recommend appropriate countermeasures before each deploying member. This briefing should summarize any preventive medicine threats at the deployment location. Information on medical threats can be found at: Armed Forces Medical Intelligence Center (AFMIC) website http://www.afmic.detrick.army.mil/ (must register for an account); U.S. Army Center for Health Promotion and Preventive Medicine http://chppm-www.apgea.army.mil/

and the Deployment Health Clinical Center http://www.pdhealth.mil/dcs/pre_deploy.asp. HSWL SC or Commandant (CG-1121) will provide a list of any additional required immunizations or chemoprophylaxis for each deployment based on medical threat assessment. The recommendations, to include all medically related personal protective measures, will be communicated to all deploying personnel during the pre-deployment medical threat brief and/or via message. When possible, Commandant (CG-1121) or HSWL SC will contact the agency that will serve as the CG supporting medical unit in joint DoD operations, and the medical threat brief will be obtained to provide to CG deploying units. If not involved in joint operations, medical threat brief and recommended countermeasures will be provided by HSWL SC, Commandant (CG-1121) and Commandant (CG-1133) based on the deployment requirements.

i. Health Record Review. Review each member's health record for accuracy. Enter and verify all required data into MRRS.

j. Pre-Deployment Serum Sample. Verify that a serum sample has been provided within one year prior to deployment. The HIV test will serve as pre-deployment serum sample provided the HIV test was completed within one year prior to deployment. If more than one year, a new HIV test will be drawn and must be processed through the VIROMED contract. Members who refuse the blood draw will have an SF-600, Chronological Record of Care entry to that effect placed in their health record. No further legal or medical action will be required

6. Deployment.

   a. <u>Disease Non-Battle Injury (DNBI) Reports</u>. Weekly DNBI reports will be used to assess operational readiness at the unit level. The unit corpsman will review DNBI rates for trends. Weekly reports will be provided to Commandant (CG-1121). Blank DNBI reports are available for download on Commandant (CG-1121) Operational Medicine website http://www.uscg.mil/hq/cg1/cg11/ (Preventive Medicine section).

   b. <u>Other Deployment Requirements</u>. All other deployment surveillance requirements will be fulfilled in conjunction with the supporting medical unit as designated by Commandant (CG-1121).

7. <u>Post-Deployment</u>. After the member completes the DD-2796, Post Deployment Health Assessment via the EDHA, (this must be completed no earlier than 7 days before returning and no later than 30 days after returning to the home station) they must set up an appointment with a healthcare provider (IDHS or Medical Officer). This is required for all expeditionary deployments. The following are special requirements for reserve personnel:

   a. Reserve members requiring a more detailed medical evaluation or treatment shall, with the member's consent, be retained on active duty until the member is determined fit for full duty, or until the resulting incapacitation cannot be materially improved by further hospitalization or treatment and the case has been processed and finalized through physical disability evaluation system (PDES).

   b. Reserve members no longer on active duty, who have deployment health concerns should initiate contact with their reserve activity or a Department of Veterans Affairs (VA) medical facility. Combat veterans are eligible for care two years post discharge in the VA

COMDTINST M6000.1E

  health system for any illness, even if there is insufficient medical evidence to conclude that their illness is attributable to their military service.

 c. Members who refuse to complete the DD-2796, Post-Deployment Health Assessment will have an SF-600, Chronological Record of Care entry to that effect placed in their health record. No further legal or medical action will be required. A member can request to complete a DD-2796, Post-Deployment Health Assessment for any reason and at any time (even if the member was not on an expeditionary deployment).

8. DD-2900, Post-Deployment Health Reassessment (PDHRA) via the EDHA (see above). Complete the PDHRA over the next few months after returning from deployment via the EDHA. Other post deployment requirements include the following:

 a. Review and update the DD-2766, Adult Preventive and Chronic Care Flow Sheet and place it in the member's health record.

 b. Countermeasures. Assess the need for specific post deployment requirements such as tuberculosis screening and malaria terminal chemoprophylaxis and ensure members are scheduled to meet these requirements.

 c. Medical Threat Debriefing. Provide a medical threat debriefing on all significant health events, exposures and concerns within 5 days (ideally) of return to home station. Additional information can be found at the Deployment Clinical Care Center - http://www.pdhealth.mil/dcs/.

 d. Health Record Review. Review and update the member's health record regarding theater medical encounters, adverse events related to taking FHPPP.

 e. Post-Deployment Serum Sample. Verify that redeploying members have had a blood sample drawn for submission to the DoD serum repository within 30 days of return to home station or demobilization site. All blood samples will be submitted to the CG HIV Contractor per Coast Guard Human Immunodeficiency Virus (HIV) Program, COMDTINST M6230.9 (series). Utilizing the CG HIV Contractor ensures that a serum sample is sent to the repository and that the member has a current HIV test. The date of the HIV test will be entered into MRRS. Members who refuse the blood draw will have an SF-600, Chronological Record of Care entry to that effect placed in their health record. No further legal or medical action will be required.

 f. Physical examination. A physical examination is required for a member being released from an active duty assignment of 30 days or greater, if the member has not had a physical examination within the previous 12 months. A member being released from active duty can request a physical examination at any time, even if the member had a physical examination within the previous 12 months. A health care provider can recommend a member undergo a physical examination based on the results of the member's post deployment health assessment.

9. Compliance Program. Commanding Officers will implement a quality improvement program to ensure their compliance with guidelines as outlined in this Chapter. This requirement is primarily focused on completeness of execution and includes the ability to answer the following questions:

TASK	YES	NO
Did all those covered by the policy get screened?		
Is a copy of the completed deployment health forms in the permanent medical record?		
Was a copy of the deployment health forms electronically sent to AFHSC?		
Was a blood sample collected and sent through CG HIV Contractor for the serum repository?		
Were recommended referrals/consultations completed?		

Table 6-B-1

At a minimum, report the following data to MLC (k):

The number of personnel requiring screening?	
The number of personnel screened (e.g. completion of a the deployment health forms	
Confirmation that a blood sample was sent to CG HIV Contractor	
Tracking of clinical follow-up for those indicated on the deployment health forms is being accomplished.	

Table 6-B-2

This page intentionally left blank.

Section C. Routine Deployment

1. Pre-Deployment Requirements 1
2. Deployment 1
3. Post-Deployment 1
4. Additional references 2

This page intentionally left blank.

C. Routine Deployment.

1. Pre-Deployment Requirements.

    a. Individual Medical Readiness (IMR) Review. Perform an IMR review on all deploying personnel per Chapter 6, Section A.

    b. Medical Threat Briefing. Provide specific medical threat briefing and recommend appropriate countermeasures fore each deploying member. This briefing should summarize any preventive medicine threats at the deployment location. Information on medical threats can be found at the National Center for Medical Intelligence website at http://www.intelink.gov/ncmi/index.php, U.S. Army Center for Health Promotion and Preventive Medicine at http://chppm-www.apgea.army.mil and the Deployment Health Clinical Center at http://www.pdhealth.mil/dcs/pre_deploy.asp. HSWL SC or Commandant (CG-1121) will provide a list of any additional required immunizations or chemoprophylaxis for each deployment based on medical threat assessment.

    c. Health Record Review. Review each member's health record for accuracy. Enter and verify all required data into MRRS.

2. Deployment.

    a. Sick logs. Complete and tabulate daily logs for sick call to determine any trends of illness while deployed. This will facilitate identification and development of preventive measures that can be taken for future deployments.

    b. Occupational Medical Surveillance and Evaluation Program (OMSEP). Enroll members with occupational exposures into the OMSEP if they meet the program requirements.

    c. Medical Event Reports (MERs). Complete MERs per Chapter 7 for illnesses that occur during deployment. MERs should be entered into the Naval Disease Reporting System Internet (NDRSi) system. Critical conditions should be reported to HSWL SC or Commandant (CG-1121) as required per Chapter 7.

3. Post-Deployment.

    a. Countermeasures. Assess the need for specific post deployment requirements such as tuberculosis screening and malaria terminal chemoprophylaxis and ensure members are scheduled to meet these requirements.

    b. Medical Threat Debriefing. Provide a medical threat debriefing on all significant health events, exposures and concerns within 5 days (ideally) of return to home station. Additional information can be found at the Deployment Clinical Care Center - http://www.pdhealth.mil/dcs/.

c. <u>Health Record Review</u>. Review and update the member's health record regarding medical encounters during the deployment.

4. <u>Additional references</u>. The following Websites have information that may be helpful pre-, during and post-deployment:

Source	Website
Center for Health Promotion and Preventive Medicine	http://chppm-www.apgea.army.mil/
Centers for Disease Control Travel Page	http://www.cdc.gov/travel/
Headquarters Operational Medicine Division	http://www.uscg.mil/hq/cg1/cg112/cg1121/default.asp
HSWL SC	http://www.uscg.mil/mlclant/KDiv/kseHomePage.htm http://www.uscg.mil/mlcpac/mlcp/

Table 6-C-1

CHAPTER 7

PREVENTIVE MEDICINE

Section A. General.

1. Scope 1
2. Responsibilities 1

Section B. Communicable Disease Control.

1. General 1
2. Disease Outbreak 1
3. Medical Event Reporting 1
4. Figure 7-B-1 Medical Event Reporting Chart Within 24 Hours 3
5. Figure 7-B-2 Medical Event Reporting Chart Within 7 Days 4
6. Sexually Transmitted Infection (STI) Program 5
7. STI Treatment 7
8. STI Drug Prophylaxis 7
9. STI Immunizations 7
10. STI Reporting 7

Section C. Immunizations and Allergy Immunotherapy (AIT)

1. General 1
2. Unit Responsibilities 1
3. Equipment and Certification Requirement 1
4. Immunization Site Responsibilities 1
5. Immunization on Reporting for Active Duty for Training 4
6. Specific Vaccination Information 4

COMDTINST M6000.1E

This page intentionally left blank

Chapter 7 Contents

Section A. General

1. Scope..1
2. Responsibilities..1

This page intentionally left blank.

CHAPTER SEVEN – PREVENTIVE MEDICINE

Section A. General.

1. Scope. The scope of preventive medicine involves all activities that prevent illness and disease, including immunizations; communicable disease control; and epidemiology.

2. Responsibilities.

    a. The unit Medical Officer (MO) is responsible to the Commanding Officer for implementing all directives issued by the Commandant which relate to the health of members of the command. The MO shall:

        (1) Evaluate the command's health care capabilities to fulfill Occupational Medical Surveillance and Evaluation Program (OMSEP) requirements.

        (2) Develop and supervise an environmental health program to prevent disease and maintain the Commandant's established sanitation standards.

        (3) Monitor the incidence of disease or disability in personnel and, when indicated, in adjacent communities.

        (4) Use epidemiological methods to determine the cause of disease patterns, if there is an increase in incidence.

    b. Preventive Medicine Technicians (PMTs) are individuals who are highly proficient in all aspects of preventive medicine. If assigned or available to a unit, the unit shall gainfully employ their services.

    c. The Preventive Medicine (PM) physician at Commandant (CG-1121) will provide policy recommendations and other consultation as needed to Commandant (CG-11), the HSWL SC, and individual health care providers. The PM Physician will develop evidence-based policies for the control of disease of public health importance and will maintain liaison with civilian and public health (local, State, Federal) and military medical authorities to coordinate appropriate response to public health threats. The PM physician will also serve as the Public Health Emergency Officer (PHEO) for the CG.

This page intentionally left blank.

Section B. Communicable Disease Control.

1. General 1
2. Disease Outbreak 1
3. Medical Event Reporting 1
4. Figure 7-B-1 Medical Event Reporting Chart Within 24 Hours 3
5. Figure 7-B-2 Medical Event Reporting Chart Within 7 Days 4
6. Sexually Transmitted Infection (STI) Program 5
7. STI Treatment 7
8. STI Drug Prophylaxis 7
9. STI Immunizations 7
10. STI Reporting 7

This page intentionally left blank.

B. Communicable Disease Control.

1. General. The health services department representative is responsible for complying with Federal, State, and CG communicable disease reporting requirements. In order to have an effective communicable disease control program, health services department representatives should:

    a. Recognize communicable diseases (see Figures 7-B-1 & 7-B-2).

    b. Recommend preventive and control measures to the Commanding Officer.

    c. Submit required reports.

    d. Comply with state and local health department reporting requirements.

2. Disease Outbreak.

    a. Definition. An outbreak is defined as two or more linked cases with clinically compatible signs and symptoms of an infection in a given period of time in a specified location or two or more laboratory confirmed cases in a specified location within a given period of time or whatever is above normal in the population specified during a period of time.

    b. Each clinic and sickbay must have at least one designated staff member responsible for submitting medical event reports (MERs).

    c. The designated health services department representative shall:

        (1) Recognize outbreaks and establish a case definition.

        (2) Investigate the source of the agent and how it spread.

        (3) Recommend to Commanding Officer appropriate initial control/preventive measures.

        (4) Complete a Medical Event Report using the Naval Disease Reporting System Internet (NDRSi). The Tri-Service Reportable Events document provides detailed definitions of the reportable medical events. The Tri-Service Reportable Events document is located on the Commandant (CG-1121) web page.

        (5) Contact Commandant (CG-1121) if assistance is needed at any of the aforementioned steps.

        (6) Follow communicable disease policy guidance disseminated by the HSWL SC and/or Commandant (CG-11) in the event of a bioterrorist threat or a natural or manmade communicable disease threat.

3. Medical Event Reporting.

    a. Circumstances requiring reports.

        (1) Any outbreak,

(2) Any person diagnosed with any disease listed in Figures 7-B-1 and 7-B-2,

(3) Any epizootic (e.g. animal epidemic) transmissible from animals to man,

(4) Any quarantined CG vessel or aircraft (at a foreign port),

(5) Any medical condition deemed worthy of reporting by health services department personnel, or

(6) Any reportable medical condition as mandated by the local/state health department.

b. Reporting Process. CG health services personnel will no longer report Disease Alert Reports (DAR) using the DAR form. Additionally, CG health services personnel will no longer email DARS to the HQS-DG-Disease Alert Report email group. CG health services personnel must use the NDRSi system for all MERS.

(1) The NDRSi can be accessed at https://www-nehc.med.navy.mil/ndrsi/.

(2) For initial access to the NDRSi, the cognizant health services personnel must print out the DD-2875, System Authorization Access Request and complete part I of the form and initial block 27. Health services personnel must have completed the annual mandatory CG Information Systems Security (ISS) Training (which is the CG equivalent to the DoD Annual Information Awareness Training) in order to have NDRSi access approved. Part II of the form must be compelted by the Senior Health Services Officer (SHSO) or the cognizant Designated Medical Officer Advisor (DMOA). Additional directions for completing and submitting the form can be found on the NDRSi website.

(3) After completing, the SHSO or DMOA must submit the DD-2875, System Authorization Access Request in hard copy or electronic form to the Navy and Marine Corps Public Health Center (NMCPHC). NMCPHC will contact the individual listed in Part II of the form to verify the request and activate the NDRSi user account. NMCPHC will send a Login ID and Password to the user once they obtain the CHSD or DMOA approval.

(4) After obtaining a Login ID and password, health services personnel must login to the NDRSi. After logging in, directions on how to enter MERs into NDRSi can be found by clicking on the "Help" icon. The "Frequently Asked Questions" FAQ link on the Login page also has helpful information.

(5) CG units are listed in NDRSi by their OPFAC.

(6) For any critical conditions listed in Figure 7-B-1, health services personnel must contact Commandant (CG-1121) within 24 hours. Upon final confirmed diagnosis, the health services personnel must enter the medical event report into NDRSi. Commandant (CG-1121) will review the information in NDRSi and will contact the HSWL SC for all critical conditions.

Figure 7-B-1   COMDTINST M6000.1E

Medical Event Reporting Chart Within 24 Hours

PHONE COMMANDANT(CG-1121) WITHIN <u>24</u> HOURS & COMPLETE A MEDICAL EVENT REPORT IN NDRSI[1]

🌀 Potential agent of Bioterrorism

Animal Bites	Diphtheria	Influenza (HPAI / PI)[4]	Severe Acute Respiratory Syndrome (SARS)
Anthrax 🌀	*E. coli* O157:H7	Malaria	Smallpox 🌀
Arboviral Infection	Foodborne Outbreak	Measles	Syphilis
Botulism 🌀	*Haemophilus influezae*	Meningococcal Disease	Tuberculosis 🌀
Brucellosis 🌀	Hantavirus Infection	Pertussis	Tularemia
Carbon Monoxide Poisoning	Heat Related Injuries[3]	Plague 🌀	Yellow Fever
Chemical Agent Exposure	Hemorrhagic Fever 🌀	Poliomyelitis	UNUSUAL Disease/Cluster
Cholera	Hepatitis A (acute)	Q Fever 🌀	
Cold Weather Injuries[2]	Hemolytic Uremic Syndrome (HUS)	Rabies	

1 - HIV, AIDS, Suicide and Occupational Illness / Injury are reported through other mechanisms
2 - Frostbite, Immersion Foot, Hypothermia, or other cold injury resulting in a limited duty status.
3 - Heat Exhaustion/ Heat Stroke or other thermal injury resulting in a limited duty status.
4 - HPAI = Highly Pathogenic Avian Influenza / PI = Pandemic Influenza.

Medical Event Reporting Chart Within 7 Days

COMPLETE A MEDICAL EVENT REPORT IN NDRSI WITHIN 7 DAYS

Amebiasis	Influenza (AD ONLY)	Rubella
Campylobacteriosis	Lead Poisoning	Salmonellosis
Chancroid	Legionellosis	Schistosomiasis
Chlamydia trachomatis	Leishmaniasis	Shigellosis
Coccidioidomycosis	Leprosy	Streptococcal disease, Group A
Cryptosporiodiosis	Leptospirosis	Tetanus
Cyclosporiasis	Lyme Disease	Toxic Shock Syndrome
Dengue Fever	cMRSA Infection	Trichinosis
Ehrlichiosis	Mumps	Trypanosomiasis
Filariasis	Psittacosis	Typhoid Fever
Giardiasis	Relapsing Fever	Typhus Fever
Gonorrhea	Rheumatic Fever (AD ONLY)	Urethritis (non-gonococcal)
Hepatitis B	Rift Valley Fever	Vaccine Adverse Events
Hepatitis C	Rocky Mountain Spotted Fever	Varicella (AD ONLY)

(7) Commandant (CG-1121) will review all medical event reports in NDRSi on a weekly basis for medical trends and outbreaks.

(8) For all other MERS there is no need for health services personnel to contact Commandant (CG-1121), the only requirement is to enter MERS that are confirmed and final (no presumptive or preliminary diagnoses should be entered).

4. Sexually Transmitted Infection (STI) Program.

   a. Background. STIs, including the human immunodeficiency virus (HIV) are important and preventable causes of morbidity, mortality and associated lost-productivity and increased health care costs.

   b. Exposure information for non TRICARE beneficiaries.

   c. Exposure information for TRICARE beneficiaries.

   d. Duties of the Health Services Department. Health services department shall provide a coordinated, comprehensive STI control program including:

      (1) Education and prevention counseling of those at risk.

      (2) Detection of asymptomatically infected individuals.

      (3) Effective diagnosis and treatment of infected individuals.

      (4) Partner Services (PS) (formerly known as contact tracing).

      (5) Immunization of persons at risk for vaccine-preventable STIs.

      (6) Proper annotation and maintenance of health records.

      (7) Protection of confidentiality.

   e. Senior Medical Officer (SMO). The SMO oversees the medical management of the local STI control program; recommends STI control activities to the Commanding Officer; establishes and maintains liaison with local health authorities; and ensures confidentiality of the patient and his/her sexual partner(s).

   f. Medical Officer (MO). The MO who initially evaluates the patient shall perform appropriate diagnostic evaluation based on current CDC guidelines. The MO must fill out SF-602, Syphilis Record on all patients diagnosed with syphilis and file the SF-602, Syphilis Record in the patient's medical record. All patients (beneficiaries / active duty / reservists) presenting for evaluation of a possible STI will be tested for serological evidence of syphilis infection. All active duty / reservist presenting for evaluation of a possible STI shall be tested for serological evidence of HIV infection. Additionally all active duty members will be tested for HIV every two years. Reservists are required to have a current HIV test within 2 years of the date called to active duty if the CAD is for 30 days or more. Refer to, Coast Guard Human Immunodeficiency Virus (HIV) Program, COMDINST M6230.9 for more details on the CG's HIV program.

g. <u>Health Services Technician (HS) or Preventive Medicine Technician (PMT)</u>. An HS or PMT assigned to administer the local STI control program should be paygrade E-5 or higher. They shall perform the following actions:

   (1) Perform Partner Services (PS): PS is a set of activities intended to alert people exposed to STIs and facilitate appropriate, counseling, testing and treatment. Information about named partners shall be passed to the cognizant local or State public health function for partner notification. Valuable PS and STI resources are available on the internet from the Navy and Marine Corps Public Health Center's, Sexual Health and Responsibility Program (SHARP) at http://www-nehc.med.navy.mil/hp/sharp.

   (2) Annotate and sign the Chronological Record of Care, SF-600 in each patient's medical record to indicate he or she interviewed the patient, discussed symptoms, complications, treatment, and the importance of partner notification(s).

   (3) Determine whether a Test of Cure (TOC) is indicated for cases of gonorrhea or Chlamydia.

      (a) Gonorrhea - Patients who have symptoms that persist after treatment should be evaluated by culture for N. gonorrhea, and any gonococci isolated should be tested for antimicrobial susceptibility.

      (b) Chlamydia - Patients do not need to be retested for Chlamydia after completing treatment with doxycycline or azithromycin, unless symptoms persist or reinfection is suspected. A TOC may be considered 3 weeks after completion with erythromycin.

      (c) Active duty personnel will report to regular sick call for TOC. Place a suspense notice to check with the attending MO to ensure the patient receives TOC.

      (d) Dependents and retired personnel will be given regular appointments for local STI treatment.

   (4) Cross reference all positive STI cases from the clinic laboratory log book to ensure all STI patients have been contacted and interviewed. This should be performed on the first work day of each week.

   (5) Ensure security and confidentiality of all STI forms, reports and logs.

   (6) Complete timely reporting. HIV / AIDS (HIV /AIDS reporting must be consistent with the Coast Guard Human Immunodeficiency Virus (HIV) Program, COMDTINST M6230.9. Syphilis, gonorrhea, Chlamydia, and acute cases of hepatitis are reportable events in every state and the CG. The requirements for reporting other STIs differ by State. The National Coalition

of STI Directors website http://www.ncsddc.org/programsites.htm has links to state specific STI reporting requirements.

5. <u>STI Treatment</u>. MO should treat STIs according to the most current recommendation of the CDC.

6. <u>STI Drug Prophylaxis</u>. Drug prophylaxis for STI prevention is prohibited.

7. <u>STI Immunizations</u>. MO should review the immunization status of all patients presenting with a possible STI. All AD / reservists should receive Hepatitis A and Hepatitis B vaccines (unless vaccine series is complete). Other beneficiaries who seek evaluation for a possible STI should receive Hepatitis A and Hepatitis B if indicated (based on current CDC guidelines).

8. <u>STI Reporting</u>.

   a. <u>DoD/CG healthcare beneficiaries (TRICARE)</u>. Exposure information of DoD/CG healthcare beneficiary partners will be reported via the NDRSi as well as to any cognizant State or local health authority) using a State-specific form and process or using CDC Form 73.2936S – Field Record. Forms are available from the CDC at (404) 639-1819. (Local protocol will dictate which specific STI's need to be reported to the state, but all conditions in Figure B-1 and B-2 must be reported via the NDRSi system).

   b. <u>Non-DoD/CG healthcare beneficiaries (NON TRICARE)</u>. Exposure information of non-DoD/CG healthcare beneficiary partners will be reported to the cognizant public health authority. Health services personnel should follow local guidance for local reporting of partners. This may entail locally designated forms and procedures. For partners located outside the local area, partner identification information may be sent to the State public health authority (who will forward the report to the cognizant State or local health authority) using a State-specific form and process or using CDC Form 73.2936S – Field Record. Forms are available from the CDC at (404) 639-1819. Health services personnel should not expect confirmation of receipt or a disposition report. If a disposition report is desire, the health services personnel should state this on the Field Record, and provide a statement of justification and return address/phone number.

This page intentionally left blank.

Section C. Immunizations and Allergy Immunotherapy (AIT)

1. General 1
2. Unit Responsibilities 1
3. Equipment and Certification Requirement 1
4. Immunization Site Responsibilities 1
5. Immunization on Reporting for Active Duty for Training 4
6. Specific Vaccination Information 4

This page intentionally left blank.

C. Immunizations and Allergy Immunotherapy.

1. General. Immunizations and Chemoprophylaxis, COMDTINST M6230.4 (series), lists policy, procedure, and responsibility for immunizations and chemoprophylaxis. This section contains guidelines not specifically defined there. Immunizations for active duty and SELRES shall be documented in Medical Readiness Reporting System (MRRS) and P-GUI/AHLTA as outlined in Section 4-C. Vital signs are not required during immunization-only encounters.

2. Unit Responsibilities.

   a. Immunizing all individuals. Active duty and reserve unit Commanding Officers are responsible for immunizing all individuals under their purview and maintaining appropriate records of these immunizations. If local conditions warrant and pertinent justification supports, HSWL SC may grant authority to deviate from specified immunization procedures on request.

   b. Unit Commanding Officers. Unit Commanding Officers will arrange local immunizations for their unit's members. If this is not possible, he or she will request assistance from the CG clinic overseeing units in the geographic area.

3. Equipment and Certification Requirement.

   a. Immunization sites. All immunization sites must have the capability to administer emergency medical care if anaphylaxis or other allergic reactions occur. A designated CG Medical Officer must certify in writing that the registered nurse or HS selected to administer immunizations is qualified to do so because he or she has received instruction and displayed proficiency in these areas:

      (1) Vaccine dosages.

      (2) Injection techniques.

      (3) Recognizing vaccine contraindications.

      (4) Recognizing and treating allergic and vasovagal reactions resulting from the vaccination process.

      (5) Proper use of anaphylaxis medications and related equipment (e.g., oxygen, airways).

      (6) Verification the individual is currently certified in Basic Life Support (BLS).

   b. Supplies for immunization. The immunization site must have available: syringes with 1:1000 aqueous solution of epinephrine, emergency airways, oxygen, bag valve mask (BVM), and intravenous (IV) fluids with an IV injection set.

4. Immunization Site Responsibilities.

   a. Where available, a Medical Officer shall be present when routine immunizations are given.

b. <u>Medical Officer cannot be present</u>. In the event a Medical Officer cannot be present, a registered nurse or HS3 or above can be certified to administer the immunization process of active duty and reserve personnel when the following guidelines and procedures are met:

   (1) The designated CG Medical Officer who normally would oversee their independent activity must train and certify in writing registered nurses and HSs conducting immunizations in a Medical Officer's absence.

   (2) An emergency equipped vehicle must be readily available to transport patients to a nearby (within 10 minutes) health care facility staffed with an Advanced Cardiac Life Support (ACLS), certified physician or an EMS with ACLS capability must be within a 10-minute response time of the site.

   (3) Hypovolemic shock often is present in cases of anaphylaxis. Therefore medical personnel must be ready and able to restore fluid to the central circulation. In anaphylaxis treatment, epinephrine administration, airway management, summoning help are critical steps toward the treatment of this condition.

c. <u>Review and document immunizations</u>. The individual(s) administering the immunizations shall review MRRS and the MRRS generated an Adult Preventative and Chronic Care Flowsheet, DD Form 2766 (Immunization section). Only a Medical Officer has authority to immunize persons sensitive to an immunizing agent. Clinic personnel and IDHS must ensure immunizations have been accurately documented in MRRS.

   (1) Clinic personnel and IDHS must be cognizant of the use of the proper medical and administrative exemption codes within MRRS. Prior to selecting the exemption code in MRRS, select the information icon. The information icon provides a detailed explanation of the various codes. The cognizant medical administrator must ensure that all exemption codes are accurate within MRRS. Commandant (CG-1121) will review all medical permanent, medical reactive, medical declined and administrative refusal codes on a quarterly basis. Medical temporary codes and administrative temporary codes must be reviewed and verified by the medical administrator every 365 days and 90 days, respectively. The description of exemption codes can be found on the Commandant (CG-1121), Operational Medicine Web site.

   (2) Senior Health Services Officer (SHSO) must ensure all healthcare personnel receive appropriate training regarding the following – use of exemption codes, verifying accuracy of exemption codes of members in their clinics medical AOR, and <u>(NON TRICARE)</u> following up on temporary exemptions.

d. <u>Immunization Training</u>. Additional immunization training opportunities are offered by the Military Vaccine Agency (MILVAX).

e. Emergency immunizations. In some clinical situations, the medical indication may be to immunize even though the circumstances above cannot be met (e.g., tetanus toxoid for wound prophylaxis, gamma globulin for hepatitis A exposure, etc.). Such incidents commonly occur at sea and remote units or during time-sensitive situations (SAR, etc.). If the medical benefits outweigh the chance of a serious allergic reaction, take every available precaution possible, and administer the vaccine. Obtain radio, telephone, or message advice from the Flight Surgeon on call through the closest CG command center.

f. Adverse reaction. If an adverse reaction to a vaccine is suspected by anyone, including the vaccinee, the facility shall notify the Vaccine Adverse Event Reporting System (VAERS) using form VAERS-1. The likelihood of a causal relationship between the observed physical signs or symptoms and the vaccine does NOT need to be verified by a MO or anyone else. This reporting system is for anyone who suspects a vaccine adverse reaction. The VAERS form is obtained from the FDA on-line at http://vaers.hhs.gov/pdf/vaers_form.pdf or by calling 1-800-822-7967. Units providing vaccinations shall maintain a supply of these forms for vaccinees who request them. Alternatively, file the VAERS online at https://secure.vaers.org/scripts/VaersDataEntry.cfm. If filing online, be sure to print a copy of the form before clicking on the "submit" button. A copy of each submitted VAERS-1 will be forwarded to Commandant (CG-1121). Log the disclosure to VAERS in the Protected Health Information Management Tool (PHIMT); see Chapter 14, section B.2.e of this manual.

g. Vaccine Information Sheet (VIS). Every health care provider who administers vaccines shall provide a Vaccine Information Sheet (VIS) if available from the CDC. A current list of the vaccines for which VIS's are available and the VIS's themselves are found at http://www.cdc.gov/nip/publications/VIS. The list includes vaccines covered by the National Childhood Vaccine Injury Act, as well as several others. The VIS is available via MRRS. The VIS's are also available from the CDC, National Immunization Hotline, at telephone number (800) 232-2522 or at http://www.cdc.gov/nip/publications/VIS/default.htm.

h. Per the National Childhood Vaccine Injury Act (NCVIA) of 1986, health care providers are not required to obtain the signature of the vaccine recipient, parent or legal guardian acknowledging receipt of the VIS. However, to document that the VIS was given, health care providers must note in the patient's permanent medical record (1) the date printed on the VIS and (2) the date the VIS is given to the patient or legal guardian. In addition, the NCVIA requires, for all vaccines, that health care providers document in the patient's permanent medical record the following: (1) date the vaccine was given, (2) the vaccine manufacturer and lot number and (3) the name and address of the health care provider administering the vaccine. For all beneficiaries, the health care provider shall make a notation on the Chronological Record of Care, SF-600 stating that the vaccine recipient or legal guardian/representative has been given information on the vaccine(s) prior to the vaccine(s) being given, if applicable. For all vaccines, facilities administering vaccines must record the manufacturer and lot number of the vaccine, and the name, address and title of the person administering the vaccine in the recipient's health record and if requested in the service member's International Certificate of Vaccination, CDC-731.

5. <u>Immunization on Reporting for Active Duty for Training</u>.

    a. When a member reports for active duty training, the receiving unit shall review the individual's immunization information in MRRS, administer any delinquent immunizations whenever possible, and enter the information in MRRS and reprint out the Adult Preventative and Chronic Care Flowsheet, DD-2766.

    b. The individual's Reserve unit shall give the member a re-immunization schedule for the following year if one is needed for that period.

6. <u>Specific Vaccination Information</u>.

    a. <u>CG policy</u>. CG policy concerning immunizations follows the recommendations of the CDC and ACIP, unless there is a military relevant reason to do otherwise. Any immunizing agent licensed by the FDA or DHHS may be used. Privileged health care providers may make clinical decisions for individual beneficiaries to customize medical care to respond to an individual clinical situation.

    b. <u>Detailed information</u>. Detailed information on adult vaccines can be found in the Immunizations and Chemoprophylaxis, COMDTINST M6230.4 (series). Accessions include recruits, cadets, band members and Direct Commissioned Officer participants.

    c. <u>Anthrax</u>. Administer anthrax vaccine in accordance with the Coast Guard Anthrax Vaccine Immunization Program (AVIP), review COMDTINST M6230.3 (series).

    d. <u>Hepatitis A</u>. Administer hepatitis A to all AD and SELRES CG personnel (including accessions). Immunization may be accomplished with single-antigen hepatitis A vaccine or combined hepatitis A-hepatitis B vaccine (Twinrix). Ensure the accurate dosing schedule is followed for single antigen hepatitis A and/or Twinrix. The dosing schedule can be found on the Commandant (CG-1121) Operational Medicine website. The single-antigen hepatitis A dosing schedule is 0 and 6 months. Single-antigen hepatitis A is indicated for individuals 19 years and older. Ensure the pediatric dose of hepatitis A is given for individuals who are less than 19 years old. CG personnel who are less than 18 years of age cannot receive Twinrix. Performance of serology testing for accessions is recommended prior to administering the vaccine.

    e. <u>Hepatitis B</u>. Administer hepatitis B to all AD and SELRES CG personnel (including accessions). Immunization may be accomplished with single-antigen hepatitis B vaccine or combined hepatitis A-hepatitis B vaccine (Twinrix). Ensure the accurate dosing schedule is followed for single antigen hepatitis B and/or

Twinrix. The dosing schedule can be found on the Commandant (CG-1121) Operational Medicine website. The single-antigen hepatitis B dosing schedule is 0, 1 month and 6 months. Single-antigen hepatitis B is indicated for individuals 20 years and older. Ensure the pediatric dose of hepatitis B is given for individuals who are less than 20 years old. CG personnel who are less than 18 years of age cannot receive Twinrix. Performance of serology testing for accessions is recommended prior to administering the vaccine.

   (1) Healthcare personnel will have documentation of serological evidence of immunity against the hepatitis B virus (HBV) or a record of completion of the 2-dose hepatitis B (or Twinrix) vaccination series. All personnel who completed the series after 1 May 2008 will be tested for serological evidence of immunity. Those who completed the series prior to 1 May 2008 do not require serological evidence of immunity and should be tested only in the event of a potential HBV exposure.

   (2) New healthcare personnel who cannot provide documented serological evidence of immunity against HBV or a record of completion of the three dose hepatitis B (or Twinrix) vaccination series will begin the hepatitis B (or Twinrix) vaccination series, unless the vaccine is medically contraindicated.

   (3) For healthcare personnel, anti-HBs titers should be drawn 1 to 2 months after completion of the three dose hepatitis B (or Twinrix) vaccination series. If serological testing is delayed due to operational considerations, testing must be accomplished within one year after series completion.

   (4) Healthcare personnel who do not develop serological evidence of immunity after the initial vaccination series will complete a second 3-dose series.

   (5) Revaccinated healthcare personnel will be tested for anti-HBs titer 1 to 2 months after the last dose of vaccine. Personnel negative after a second vaccine series are considered non-responders to the hepatitis B (or Twinrix) vaccination (and likely still susceptible to HBV) and should be documented susceptible in MRRS.

f. Human Papilloma Virus (HPV). The HPV vaccine is not a mandatory immunization. It is highly recommended that healthcare providers recommend use of the HPV vaccine for all females within the appropriate age groups as part of a well-women examination.

g. Influenza A and B. Administer the influenza vaccine annually to all AD and SELRES CG personnel (including accessions).

h. Japanese encephalitis. Administer JEV to AD and SELRES CG personnel who will be stationed at least 30 days in rural areas of Asia where there is substantial risk of exposure to the virus, especially during prolonged field operations at night. Administer booster doses according to the manufacturer's recommendations if risk of exposure is still present. Under normal circumstances, personnel cannot embark on international travel within ten days of JEV immunization because of the possibility of delayed allergic reactions.

i. Measles, Mumps, and Rubella. Administer MMR vaccine to all AD and SELRES CG personnel born after 1957 (including accessions). Ensure they have received two lifetime doses of MMR vaccine or have positive serologic test results. Unless there is reason to suspect otherwise (e.g. childhood spent in a developing country, childhood immunizations not administered), a childhood dose of MMR vaccine may be assumed. Proof of immunity via serology testing or prior history of completed vaccination series (per medical documentation) will be accepted. Document immunization or results of proof of immunity in MRRS. For personnel whose records show receipt of bivalent measles-rubella vaccine, administration of MMR vaccine to achieve immunity against mumps is not necessary as a military requirement, but may be appropriate in exceptional clinical circumstances.

j. Meningococcal disease. Administer meningococcal vaccine (Menactra) to all accessions. Proof of vaccination with Menactra within one year of accession will be accepted. The need for, and timing of, a booster dose of Menactra will be determined in the coming years. Administer Menactra to personnel traveling for 15 or more days to regions subject to meningococcal outbreaks.

k. Pneumococcal disease. Administer pneumococcal vaccines per CDC and/or AFMIC guidelines.

l. Poliomyelitis. Administer a single booster dose of IPV to all CG accessions (IPV administration can be done within one year of arrival to the accession point). Personnel who have not received primary series must complete the series using IPV. Unless there is reason to suspect otherwise (for example, childhood in a developing country, childhood immunizations not administered), receipt of the basic immunizing series of IPV may be assumed.

m. Rabies. Administer rabies vaccines per CDC and/or AFMIC guidelines.

n. Smallpox. Administer the smallpox vaccine in accordance with the Coast Guard Smallpox Vaccine Program (SVP), COMDTINST M6230.10 (series).

o. Tetanus, Diphtheria, and Pertussis. Administer booster doses of Td or Tdap to all personnel every ten years. Adults 19 to 64 years old should substitute Tdap for one booster dose of Td. Td should be used for later booster doses. Tdap is not to be confused with Dtap which is administered in the pre-school age group (six years of age and younger).

p. Typhoid fever. Administer typhoid vaccine to military personnel before overseas deployment to typhoid-endemic areas.

q. Varicella. Administer varicella vaccine to all accessions who do not have medical documentation (proof of disease, prior immunization, serology). Serologic screening is the preferred means of determining those susceptible to varicella infection. Do not use a questionnaire.

r. <u>Yellow fever</u>. Administer yellow fever vaccine to all military personnel at accession. Boosters will be administered as per the Immunizations and Chemoprophylaxis, COMDTINST M6230.4 (series).

7. <u>Allergy Immunotherapy (AIT)</u>.

   a. AIT shall not be performed by IDHS in sickbays. AIT shall be restricted to clinics and shall only be given when Medical Officers (with current ACLS certification) are present in the clinic.

   b. AIT can only be performed by trained providers including HS, IDHS, nurses and Medical Officers who have completed one of three approved training courses:

      (1) United States Air Force's Introduction to Allergy/Allergy Extender Program.

      (2) United States Army's Walter Reed Immunization Technicians' Course.

      (3) United States Navy's Remote Site Allergen Immunotherapy Administration Course. For the Navy's remote course, the Medical Officer must provide face-to face training to the HS/IDHS. This course will be available on CG Central in the Commandant (CG-1121) Allergy Immunotherapy Administration Microsite.

   c. All personnel involved in the administration of allergen immunotherapy will participate in annual refresher training.

   d. All corpsman, nurses and Medical Officers must have completed the training and be designated in writing to administer AIT by the SMO/DSMO/SHSO. After receiving appropriate training, corpsman, nurses and Medical Officers are only authorized to give AIT to active duty members and only at maintenance doses. Clinical personnel should not initiate immunotherapy or give escalating doses.

This page intentionally left blank.

COMDTINST M6000.1E

CHAPTER 8

FISCAL AND SUPPLY MANAGEMENT

Section A. Resource Management.

1. Unit's Commanding Officers Responsibility 1
2. Health, Safety, and Work-Life Service Center (HSWL SC) 2
3. CG Headquarters 2

Section B. General Property Management and Accountability.

1. Basic Policies 1
2. Physical Property Classifications 1
3. Property Responsibility and Accountability 1
4. Expending Property Unnecessarily 1
5. Stock Levels, Reorder Points, and Stock Limits 1
6. Transferring and Loaning Property 3

Section C. Custody, Issues, and Disposition.

1. Transferring Custody 1
2. Storerooms 1
3. Issuing Material 1
4. Inspecting Storerooms 1
5. Disposing of Property 2

Section D. Health Services Supply System.

1. Health Services Control Point 1
2. Responsibility for General Stores Items 1
3. Supply Support Assistance 1
4. Authorized Allowances 2
5. Supply Sources 2
6. Health Care Equipment 3
7. Emergency Procurement 4
8. Factors for Replacing Equipment 4

Section E. Eyeglasses and Ophthalmic Services.

1. General 1
2. Personnel Authorized Refractions 1
3. Procuring and Issuing Standard Prescription Eyewear 1
4. Aviation Prescription Lenses 3
5. Contact Lenses 3

6. Sunglasses for Polar Operations 4
7. Safety Glasses 4

Section A. Resource Management

1. Unit Commanding Officer's Responsibility. 1
2. Health, Safety, and Work-Life Service Center (HSWL SC) 2
3. CG Headquarters...2

This page intentionally left blank.

CHAPTER EIGHT – FISCAL AND SUPPLY MANAGEMENT

Section A. Resource Management.

1. Unit Commanding Officer's Responsibility.

    a. CO's Responsibility. A unit Commanding Officer (CO) is charged with ensuring that all aspects of his/her unit operate effectively and efficiently. For units with health care facilities, this means using personnel, funds, equipment, expendable supplies and materials, health care spaces, and external health care providers economically and efficiently. The CO oversees all health care equipment maintenance. Commanding Officers will ensure that management of command resources provides the best amount of care to all eligible beneficiaries at the least possible cost to the Government.

        (1) Care provided in CG clinics is more cost-effective than any other source. The fixed cost of physical plant, staff, and equipment is divided by the number of beneficiaries served; thus, the more care provided, the lower the cost per visit. Therefore, units should set goals to provide the maximum amount of care possible. Achieve these goals by operating properly staffed clinics at times most convenient to beneficiaries, scheduling to decrease the time patients wait, efficiently managing health care providers' valuable time, and publicizing the availability of services to beneficiaries in the surrounding communities.

        (2) If the current level or mix of resources is inefficient, the Commanding Officer will report this fact through the chain of command and recommend corrections. Timeliness is extremely important in dealing with changes in resource requirements. Good resource planning should address these needs long before it becomes necessary for a unit Commanding Officer to deny care to any authorized beneficiary due to lack of resources.

    b. Reports. The unit Commanding Officer directly controls the unit's financial plan or budget, including unit health care resources. By the 5th working day of each month, the Commanding Officer reports medical, dental, pharmaceutical and equipment operating targets, adjustments to the targets, and actual expenditures to HSWL SC for inclusion in the monthly report forwarded to Commandant (CG-112). From an oversight or management review perspective, repeated or recurring amounts of unit Fund Code-57 (AFC-57) monies dedicated to health care are the "base" funds. Commanding Officers must justify additional unit operating funds above this base solely on the criterion of increased workloads.

    c. Review of funds. The unit Commanding Officer will review all uses of unit funds and reallocate funds during the current fiscal year. The unit Commanding Officer must first inform the chain of command before he/she can reduce the amount of care the unit's clinic provides to eligible beneficiaries. The CO will report the circumstances supporting the decision and identify what resources are required to ensure normal health care facility operations through the end of the fiscal year.

The District or Maintenance and Logistics Commander's Budget Review Board (for district or MLC units respectively) will address these current fiscal year AFC-57 unit requests.

2. Health, Safety, and Work-Life Service Center (HSWL SC).

    HSWL SC administers the health services program in their respective area of responsibility. Administrative functions include:

    a. Approving and funding care provided by non-Federal and Department of Veteran's Affairs sources.

    b. Health care equipment. Approving or disapproving requests to procure health care equipment costing more than $1500.00 for units with CG Clinics/AFC-57 funding and over $500.00 for sickbays with HS's assigned via AFC-57 funding; (See 8.D.7.d).

    c. Approving clinic budgets. Each clinic's parent command shall submit a zero-based AFC-57 direct care funding request to HSWL SC through the chain of command. This request should include predicted equipment procurement requests to Commandant (CG-83) using the automated ATU budget process according to current directives. The HSWL SC request should include a line item for each clinic, proposed equipment funding, and an estimate of non-Federal health care costs.

    d. Paying other agencies. Targeting AFC-57 and AFC-73 funds to pay the Department of Defense for all health care the Army, Navy, Air Force, TRICARE and USMTF programs provided to CG beneficiaries.

3. CG Headquarters.

    a. Commandant (CG-11) obtains health services program resources from the budget process for these purposes:

        (1) Targeting AFC-57 funds to HSWL SC to pay for all non-Federal and VA medical care provided in each region.

        (2) Targeting AFC-57 funds to HSWL SC to acquire health care equipment.

        (3) Targeting AFC-57 funds to allotted units in response to budget requests to HSWL SC.

    b. In charge of health care facilities. Commandant (CG-11) is also the Program Manager for replacing, expanding, or creating health care facilities with Acquisition, Construction, and Improvement Appropriation funds and works with Commandant (CG-924) and the Lant Area Facilities Design and Construction Center staffs on plans and layouts.

Section B. General Property Management and Accountability

1. Basic Policies. 1
2. Physical Property Classifications. 1
3. Property Responsibility and Accountability. 1
4. Expending Property Unnecessarily. 1
5. Stock Levels, Reorder Points, and Stock Limits. 1
6. Transferring and Loaning Property. 3

This page intentioanlly left blank.

B. General Property Management and Accountability.

1. Basic Policies. The Director of Health, Safety and Work-Life shall:

    a. Manage accounts. Establish procedures to manage and account for health care material pursuant to the personal property management policies contained in the Property Management Manual COMDTINST M4500.5 (series).

    b. Direct and coordinate the health care supply system;

    c. Determine requirements for health care material; and

    d. Establish allowance lists, advise, and assist field units.

2. Physical Property Classifications. Property is divided into two categories: real property and personal property. Health care material is personal property and is accounted for in accordance with Property Management Manual, COMDTINST M4500.5 (series).

3. Property Responsibility and Accountability.

    a. Clinic Administrators. Clinic Administrators are responsible for the accountability of the property for their facilities. Additionally, they serve as the health services finance and supply officer.

    b. In the absence of a Clinic Administrator, the senior commissioned health services department representative acts as the property custodian.

    c. If Health Services Technicians only are assigned to a facility, the senior Health Services Technician acts as the property custodian.

4. Expending Property Unnecessarily. All persons having custody of health care property shall avoid any unnecessary expenditures of such property within their authority's limits and shall prevent such expenditures by others.

5. Stock Levels, Reorder Points, and Stock Limits.

    a. General. Stock levels, reorder points, and stock limits discussed below apply to all health care facilities, especially those at major shore units (i.e. HQs units) such as the Academy, TRACEN Petaluma, TRACEN Yorktown, and Training Center Cape May. These large facilities with multiple components (e.g., pharmacy, laboratory, dental clinic, etc.) need to maintain a greater stock depth to serve their beneficiaries. Property Management Manual, COMDTINST M4500.5 (series) contains overall supply policy and procedures.

b. Terms.

   (1) Operating Stock. That quantity of material on hand needed to meet daily operating needs during the interval between delivery of replenishments.

   (2) Safety Stock. That amount of inventory in addition to operating stock needed to sustain operations if deliveries are delayed or demands unexpectedly heavy.

   (3) Reorder Point (Low Limit). Both terms mean the predetermined inventory level for a specific item at which it is reordered.

c. Stock Inventory and Transactions. All health care facilities shall maintain sufficient amounts of stock to prevent out-of-stock conditions. To do so, maintain stock inventory and transaction records, either electronically or by using stock cards, inventory records, etc.

   (1) Generally, health services supply activities at facilities with multiple components are authorized one month's safety stock. Experience may prove this level is not adequate for certain items or in certain circumstances. These units are authorized to maintain a larger supply if and wherever exceptional circumstances dictate. Establish procedures to ensure review of stock records periodically to identify items reaching a low limit (reorder point), the authorized allowance, and quantity to revise low limits if current usage so indicates.

   (2) Ships and small shore units may use the minimum quantities indicated in the Health Services Allowance List to establish reorder points. If the list does not indicate a minimum allowance, e.g. for "optional" items, establish reorder points for commonly used items based on current usage rates. Do not order excessive quantities of material.

   (3) When a ship receives orders to deploy or a station notice of a change in operating conditions that may require additional material, promptly review authorized allowance quantities to replenish critical items in time for the deployment or operational change.

   (4) Pharmacies procuring drugs through prime vendor systems (either directly or through pharmacy officer staffed clinics) should try to stock one-month quantities of regularly used items. Ongoing inventories of these limited quantities are not required except where applicable for controlled substances. Pharmacies shall "sight inventory" monthly before ordering.

6. <u>Transferring and Loaning Property</u>. Written approval is required from Commandant (CG-112) to loan health care property to any state, community, organization, or private individual. Property transferred to other military units is at the Commanding Officer's discretion. Obtain custody receipts in such instances. A Requisition and Invoice/Shipping Document, DD-1149 shall be used to transfer property locally, and from one activity to another according to the Property Management Manual, COMDTINST M4500.5 (series).

This page intentionally left blank.

Section C. Custody, Issues, and Disposition

1. Transferring Custody. 1
2. Storerooms. 1
3. Issuing Material. 1
4. Inspecting Storerooms. 1
5. Disposing of Property. 2

This page intentionally left blank.

COMDTINST M6000.1E

C. Custody, Issues, and Disposition.

1. Transferring Custody. When transferring custody of health services property and supplies a joint inventory is required conducted by both the departing and relieving custodians and an independent person who has no direct interest in the inventory outcome. If a joint inventory is impossible, the departing custodian shall conduct an inventory and submit a written report to the Commanding Officer before departing. As soon as possible after reporting, the relieving custodian also shall conduct an inventory, report the same to the Commanding Officer, and indicate any discrepancies noted between the two. In both cases, the inventories should include the participation of an independent person. Additionally, in all cases, an acknowledgment of inventory correctness must be entered in the unit Health Services Log. (See "Pharmacy Operations and Drug Control," Chapter 10, for detailed information on controlled substances).

2. Storerooms.

   a. Bulk stock. At large facilities, bulk stock of health care supplies and materials used by the various facility components (e.g., pharmacy, laboratory, dental clinic, etc.) shall be kept in a specifically designated storeroom. If facility layout permits, it may be advantageous to permit designated individuals responsible for a particular component (pharmacy, dental clinic, etc.) to manage their area's expendable supplies. The individual responsible for medical supply shall process their procurement requests. Otherwise, manage clinic supplies from a designated storeroom.

   b. Supply person. An individual familiar with supply procedures shall be in charge of the storeroom. He/she shall report directly to a Medical Administration Officer.

   c. Procurement request. In the interest of proper management, centralize clinic procurement request processing. Medical Administrators shall verify all procurement requests, including prime vendor "ZOA" documents, to ensure funds are available in their respective clinic's budget allocation.

3. Issuing Material.

   a. Supplies issued by or removed from the storeroom should be immediately recorded on the appropriate stock record. In large facilities where the health services storeroom is a distinct organizational entity, stores issued shall be made only upon receiving a properly prepared and authenticated local requisition document.

   b. Use the Requisition and Invoice/Shipping Document, DD-1149 to issue, return, or transfer equipment between activity components.

4. Inspecting Storerooms.

   a. Health services store items require periodic inspection (every three months for consumable supplies and equipment) to detect signs of deterioration or expiration.

COMDTINST M6000.1E

Accomplish such inspections by physically examining representative samples of various age groups of stock on hand.

b. It is extremely important to issue oldest stock first ("First in, First out"). This is true of all items but is mandatory for potency-dated items and those subject to spoilage.

5. Disposing of Property.

   a. In disposing of health services personal property, follow the Property Management Manual, COMDTINST M4500.5 (series) procedures regardless of the circumstances or conditions requiring disposal (e.g., over-ordering, decline in demand, fair wear and tear requiring survey, or damage requiring replacement).

   b. Certain conditions may require Board of Survey action. Property Management Manual, COMDTINST M4500.5 (series) contains procedures for this action.

      (1) Take precautions to assure compliance with local health and sanitation requirements when surveying and destroying poisonous chemicals (e.g., arsenic, strychnine, cyanide preparations).

         (a) Ordinarily, dispose of small amounts of liquid preparations and soluble substances through the local sewage system. Large quantities of soluble poisonous material may constitute pollution dangerous to public health or fish and wildlife.

         (b) If destroying large amounts of drugs (including controlled substances), coordinate this action with local air and water pollution control authorities. Then destroy by complete incineration with appropriate safeguards against toxic fumes or by such other methods as local health and sanitation officials recommend if disposal through sewage system or incineration are inappropriate.

         (c) Never deposit poisonous drugs and chemicals in dump piles or dumpsters.

      (2) Either burn or dissipate through the sewage system drugs requiring destruction other than poisonous chemicals.

   c. Dispose of used, contaminated, defective, or expired health care material in a manner that ensures it is both impossible to reuse and harmless to the environment. Completely destroy all drugs to preclude reusing them or any portion of them. Follow these specific procedures:

      (1) Sharps. Place all items likely to puncture or lacerate trash handlers in rigid plastic autoclavable disposable sharp containers. Do not attempt to sterilize or cover used blades or needles (this is hazardous to personnel), simply place them into the container. At appropriate intervals seal and dispose of containers as bio-hazardous material. These containers are NOT reusable.

(2) <u>Tablets, Capsules, Powders</u>. Remove from original container, crush or dissolve tablets and capsules, and flush into the local sewage system. Dispose of original container as ordinary trash. Follow bio-hazardous material disposal regulations when discarding chemotherapeutic and other hazardous agents (including biologicals).

(3) <u>Syrettes</u>. Cut along syrette's crimped end and discard contents into local sewage system. Place in a sharps disposable container.

(4) <u>Injectables/Parenterals</u>. Pour bottle contents into the local sewage system. Place empty vials in the trash. Follow bio-hazardous material disposal regulations when discarding chemotherapeutic and other hazardous agents (including biologicals).

(5) <u>Auto Injectors</u>. Activate the injector against a hard surface and discard contents into a suitable container. Dump container contents into the sewage system and then place the autoinjector in a sharps disposable container.

(6) Incinerate bio-hazardous materials, including used bandaging materials, or if sterilized, dispose of them as ordinary trash.

(7) Chapter 10 contains further detailed instructions on surveying and destroying controlled substances.

(8) Destroy the above materials in an appropriate area using appropriate personnel protective equipment (PPE): rubber gloves, protective goggles, and proper ventilation.

d. Do not dispose of medical materials at sea. Prepare materials for disposal and retain them onboard in a secure area until disposed of in accordance with Federal, State, and local laws.

e. Commandant Notices and other directives requiring disposal of defective material constitute authorization to immediately dispose of any suspect items on hand.

This page intentionally left blank.

Section D. Health Services Supply System

1. Health Services Control Point 1
2. Responsibility for General Stores Items 1
3. Supply Support Assistance 1
4. Authorized Allowances 2
5. Supply Sources 2
6. Health Care Equipment 3
7. Emergency Procurement 4
8. Factors for Replacing Equipment 4

This page intentionally left blank.

D. Health Services Supply System.

1. Health Services Control Point. Commandant (CG-1122) is the Health Services Control Point for CG health care material; in that capacity they:

   a. Prepare and distribute the Health Services Allowance List, COMDTINST M6700.5 (series), M6700.6 (series), and M6700.7 (series).

   b. Inform and assist field units.

   c. Review and respond to requests to change units' base operating funds allotment targets. Annually provides funds for routine health care supplies to the field as part of the recurring base of funds distributed through the Administrative Target Unit (ATU) budget process.

2. Responsibility for General Stores Items.

   a. Supply Officer.

      (1) Procures, receives, stores, issues, ships, transfers, and accounts for command stores and equipment;

      (2) Maintains specified records; and

      (3) Submits required reports for stores and equipment.

   b. Health Services Department Representative. Except where specific responsibility has been assigned, the Health Services Department Representative does not determine general supply requirements but acts in an advisory capacity for those items the department uses. The Health Services Department Representative will maintain close contact with the Supply Officer on special department needs and advise the latter when the requirement for any item will exceed the quantity normally carried in stock. The individual designated in writing as responsible for Health Services supply operations shall maintain a supply policy and procedures manual.

3. Supply Support Assistance.

   a. Direct problems with supply support of health care supplies (except controlled drugs) that cannot be resolved through the supply source, to HSWL SC. Direct problems with supply support of controlled drugs to Commandant (CG-112).

   b. Commandant (CG-112) will coordinate initial outfitting of new classes of units and vessels. HSWL SC will help in the initial outfitting process, limited to submitting requisitions and staging, when Commandant (CG-112) so requests through Commandant (CG-83).

4. Authorized Allowances. CG units are assigned specific minimum required allowances of health care supplies and equipment as described in COMDTINST M6700.5C (series), M6700.6F (series), and M6700.7A (series).

5. Supply Sources.

   a. Standard Items. Items listed in the DoD Medical Catalog (FEDLOG) are "standard". Obtain items with an Advice Acquisition Code (AAC) of "D" from the Defense Personnel Support Center (DPSC) through the Automated Requisition Management System (ARMS).

   (1) Non-Obtain "non-standard" items, i.e., those not described as above, from commercial sources.

   (2) All commercial procurements shall be made under the applicable acquisition regulations and CG Acquisition Procedures, COMDTINST M4200.19 (series). Commercial procurement of health care supplies, equipment, and repair and maintenance service is authorized in these conditions:

   (a) Time does not permit obtaining standard items from Government sources; or

   (b) A legitimate need exists for nonstandard items;

   (c) Equipment requires repair or maintenance.

   (3) These items are authorized:

   (a) Newly listed standard items not available from government sources;

   (b) Necessary non-standard health care supplies and equipment;

   (c) Medical Catalog (FEDLOG) items bearing the Acquisition Advice Code "L";

   (d) Equipment repair and maintenance (excluding installation); and

   (e) Health care technical books, publications, and professional journals.

   (4) Local or commercial procurement is not authorized for these items:

   (a) Non-standard items differing only slightly from standard items of identical capability; and

   (b) Preferred trade names and proprietary products in lieu of standard items.

b. Prime Vendor Items.

   (1) A prime vendor is one pre-arranged on behalf of the government procurement system. The Defense Personnel Support Center (DPSC) negotiates prime vendors, equivalent to Federal "depot" sources, for medical commodities.

   (2) Where available, DPSC prime vendors shall serve as the primary source of supply for pharmaceuticals. Use other sources if it is determined their price or service better meet the unit's needs.

6. Health Care Equipment.

   a. Factors for Initial Procurement. Due to changes in the beneficiary population or unit mission, a health care facility may require health care equipment not previously held by that facility. Units requesting an initial procurement shall provide justification on a U.S. Coast Guard Health Care Equipment Request, CG-5211.

   b. New Installations. The appropriate construction project (AC&I) funds normally will pay for equipment for newly constructed facilities. To ensure standardization, authorization and approval MUST be obtained from Commandant (CG-112) before requisitioning or procuring health care equipment for new installations.

   c. Health Care Equipment. All units with health care equipment (items with an original cost of more than $1500.00 or more for clinics and $500.00 or more for sickbays) shall verify their equipment annually (January) and submit the report to HSWL SC. Definitions for health care equipment, procurement procedures, and the criteria used for approval are outlined below.

      (1) Health care equipment. Any item of health care equipment which meets the following criteria:

         (a) Costs $1500.00 or more for clinics and $500.00 or more for sickbays.

         (b) Does not lose its identity when installed or placed into service.

         (c) Has a life expectancy of one year or more.

      (2) Units shall submit requests for health care equipment on form CG-5211, U.S. Coast Guard Health Care Equipment Request to HSWL SC. If the HSWL SC is unable to evaluate the CG-5211, U.S. Coast Guard Health Care Equipment Request within 15 working days of receipt, HSWL SC shall notify the requesting unit regarding the delay. HSWL SC shall

review the request and provide a forwarding endorsement that, as a minimum, addresses the following areas:

   (a) How the equipment is or is not appropriate for the requesting health care facility.

   (b) Why the purchase is or is not cost effective.

   (c) How the equipment will or will not impact on the quality of patient care.

(3) HSWL SC will evaluate health care equipment requests, and within 30 days of receipt of the CG-5211, U.S. Coast Guard Health Care Equipment Request will notify the unit that one of the following actions will be taken:

   (a) Purchase of the requested equipment.

   (b) Purchase of a substitute item of a different make or model in order to standardize health care equipment and/or ensure cost effectiveness.

   (c) Return the request via the chain of command with an explanation of why the equipment request was disapproved.

(4) Health care equipment costing less than $1500.00 for clinics and less than $500.00 for sickbays is a unit responsibility and shall be purchased using unit AFC-57 funds.

7. Emergency Procurement. A request for an emergency procurement may be relayed to the HSWL SC by telephone, followed by a faxed copy of a completed form U.S. Coast Guard Health Care Equipment Request, CG-5211.

8. Factors for Replacing Equipment. The fact that an item of health care equipment is approaching, or has passed, its normal life expectancy is not considered sufficient cause for replacement in and of itself. Units that request replacement equipment shall provide justification on the U.S. Coast Guard Health Care Equipment Request, CG-5211. Factors which are considered sufficient cause for equipment replacement include any of the following:

   a. Unreliability. Documented unreliability of equipment, demonstrated by unusual maintenance expenses or high frequency of repairs.

   b. Excessive repair costs, onetime or repetitive.

   c. Obsolete Equipment. Equipment is obsolete and new technology exists that reduces pain and discomfort, improves treatment, increases diagnostic accuracy, significantly reduces costs by conserving personnel, supplies, or utilities, or increases efficiency by reducing patient treatment time.

d. Receipts.

   (1) The unit shall retain one copy of signed receipts for health services material for record purposes.

   (2) Send one copy of signed receipts for all health care equipment to HSWL SC.

   (3) Maintain copies of receipts for controlled substances and security materials separately for record purposes.

e. Maintenance.

   (1) Each unit is responsible for maintaining health care equipment in optimum, safe operating condition. Maintenance shall include:

      (a) Measures necessary to ensure the equipment's operating safety and efficiency (preventive maintenance);

      (b) Manufacturer's representatives' required checks to meet warranty requirements;

      (c) Removing from service if deficiencies are detected; and

      (d) Replacing defective parts.

   (2) Preventive maintenance is systematic inspection of and service to equipment to maintain it in optimum operating condition. A properly executed program will detect and correct minor problems before they render the equipment inoperable. Manufacturers usually require preventive maintenance to maintain the warranty. Maintenance records are also valuable tools for evaluating equipment needs and justifying future equipment procurement requests.

   (3) Each clinic shall designate a Preventive Maintenance Coordinator who ensures the program is established and functions effectively. If a Biomedical Equipment Repair Technician (BMET) is assigned to the unit, he/she fills this role. If not, designate an individual with mechanical aptitude or a desire to work with equipment to fill this role. Clinics may contract for preventive maintenance services if funding permits and are encouraged to enter into cooperative agreements with DoD MTFs whenever possible. Each unit shall:

      (a) Establish a preventive maintenance schedule for all health care equipment. Each unit shall determine maintenance intervals based on manufacturers' recommendations and frequency of use.

(b) Maintain a written record of all preventive maintenance and repairs performed on health care equipment using a Medical/Dental Equipment Maintenance Record, NAVMED 6700/3CG. Use side A to record preventive maintenance and safety checks and side B to record repairs.

(c) Charge clinic health care equipment maintenance costs to unit AFC-57 funds and sickbay health care equipment maintenance costs to unit AFC-30 funds.

(d) HSWL SC and HQ units shall establish and maintain a program to replace their health care equipment.

Section E. Eyeglasses and Ophthalmic Services

1. General. 1
2. Personnel Authorized Refractions. 1
3. Procuring and Issuing Standard Prescription Eyewear. 1
4. Aviation Prescription Lenses. 3
5. Contact Lenses. 3
6. Sunglasses for Polar Operations. 4
7. Safety Glasses. 4

This page intentionally left blank.

E. Eyeglasses and Ophthalmic Services.

1. General. This section describes ophthalmic services (refractions and spectacle issue) provided.

2. Personnel Authorized Refractions.

    a. CG health care facilities and USMTFs. CG health care facilities and USMTFs to the extent of available facilities, including ophthalmologists' and optometrists' services, may furnish refractions to active duty and dependents not enrolled in TRICARE Prime on a "space available" basis and retired uniformed services members.

    b. No MTF. When USMTF's are not available, HSWL SC may authorize refractions at other facilities for active duty members only.

    c. USMTFs may furnish non-active duty eligible beneficiaries refractions if facilities are available. USMTFs may not furnish eyeglasses to dependents at government expense except as Section 8.E.3.b.(2)(b) authorizes.

    d. Reserve members on active duty for training for more than 30 days are authorized repair or replacement of standard eyeglasses during the active duty period.

3. Procuring and Issuing Standard Prescription Eyewear.

    a. CG units shall order standard eyewear from optical laboratories as outlined in this section.

        (1) Civilian sources are acceptable for procuring eyewear providing the prescription is for standard frames and lenses are available from fabrication labs. Transcribe this request onto a Eyewear Prescription, DD-771.

        (2) If fabrication would entail a prolonged delay (more than eight weeks) and the member's vision is so poor he/she cannot safely perform assigned duties, procure non-standard eyewear from local civilian sources using non-Federal health care funds.

        (3) Members requiring corrective lenses shall have two pair at all times, including eyeglasses issued from government sources or purchased at their own expense.

        (4) Requests for tinted eyewear for non-aviation members must be justified solely on the duties they perform, e.g. majority of duty time in bright sunlight, etc.

        (5) Replacement eyewear may be obtained without repeating a visual acuity check, provided the replacement prescription is less than two years old. If a corrected visual acuity check is required and indicates the current prescription is inadequate, patient must obtain a refraction.

    b. Available Eyewear and Standard Eyewear Sources of Supply.

        (1) These types of eyewear are available:

| | Cellulose acetate frame ||
Type of Correction	Glass Lens	Plastic Lens
Single Vision, white [1]	X	X
Single Vision, tinted [1,2]	X	X
Bifocal, 25mm segment, white [1]	X	X
Bifocal, 25mm segment, tinted [1,2]	X	X
Trifocal, white	X	
Cataract Aspheric		X
Trifocal, white and tinted [1,2]		X

(1) Eyewear provided in FG-58 (Flight Goggle) mounting for authorized personnel

(2) Only N-15 and N-32 tints authorized

Table 8-E-1

(2) Process all requests for standard prescription eyewear through the below military optical laboratory. This is the only optical laboratory from which CG units are authorized to order standard prescription eyewear.

> Naval Ophthalmic Support and Training Activity
> Yorktown, VA 23691-5071

Table 8-E-2

(a) It is extremely important to properly complete the Eyewear Prescription, DD-771 service identification block to indicate the patient's service affiliation.

(b) Dependent care in isolated areas. Spectacles may be furnished to command-sponsored dependents of uniformed services members assigned outside CONUS with the exception of Alaska, Hawaii and Puerto Rico.

(3) Procurement Procedures. Order all prescription eyewear using the Eyewear Prescription, DD-771. It is extremely important to accurately complete the prescription form. If the prescription is wrong the patient is inconvenienced. The CG is required to pay for eyewear even if it cannot be used. The supply activity will reject an improperly prepared prescription, resulting in delay. Use these guidelines to prepare a Eyewear Prescription, DD-771. See Section 4-B for more detailed instructions.

(a) Use a separate Eyewear Prescription, DD-771 for each type of eyewear.

(b) If no health services personnel are available at the unit, send the prescription obtained from the health record or local civilian source to the health record custodian to prepare and submit the Eyewear Prescription, DD-771.

(c) Submit all three Eyewear Prescription, DD-771 copies to the approving authority or supply activity; disregard the distribution instructions. Remove all carbon sheets before submission. File a photocopy of the Eyewear Prescription, DD-771 in the member's health record.

(d) TRACEN Cape May shall send recruits' eyewear prescriptions separately and mark the envelope, "RECRUIT—PLEASE EXPEDITE".

(4) Health Record Entries. Record on a separate Eyewear Prescription, DD-771 the current prescription, including frame measurements and all other data necessary to reorder eyewear, for each individual requiring eyeglasses.

4. Aviation Prescription Lenses. Aviation personnel are authorized two pair of clear aviation spectacles (FG-58) and one pair of tinted spectacles (N-15).

   a. Aviators Engaged in Actual Flight Operations. Aviation spectacles may be ordered for distant vision correction, or for distant vision and near vision correction (bifocal lenses). Those aviation personnel engaged in flight operation who desire near vision only correction in aviation frames must order bifocal lenses containing plano top portion and the near vision correction on the bottom. Spectacles containing only near vision correction are not authorized in aviation frames. This type correction will only be order in cellulose acetate frames.

   b. Landing Signal Officers (LSO).

   c. CG Ceremonial Honor Guard personnel.

   d. Small Boat Crew members are required to wear a helmet while performing their assigned duties.

5. Contact Lenses. Contact lenses are issued only to active duty personnel for postocular surgical difficulties or to enable a member to overcome a handicapping disease or impairment. HSWL SC will not approve contact lenses solely for cosmetic reasons with exception of the CG Honor Guard, where wearing of eye glasses may interfere with the performance of their duties.

   a. Submit letter requests for contact lenses to HSWL SC under Section 2-A-7.a.; include the type of lenses and cost.

   b. Approval. If HSWL SC approves they will provide an authorization number by return correspondence. Units will write this number on all correspondence and billings before submitting to HSWL SC.

6. <u>Sunglasses for Polar Operations</u>. Military fabrication laboratories no longer issue polar operation sunglasses. Activities requiring such glasses may use the process below to obtain them:

   a. <u>Non-prescription Lenses</u>. If issuing, the command must purchase and issue non-prescription lenses as part of the cold weather clothing allowance and pay the lenses' costs from operating expenses. The command should issue the lenses on a custodial basis, departing members should return them to the command for reissue.

   b. <u>Prescription Lenses</u>. Procure prescription lenses from NOSTRA.

      (1) Aviation-type frames.

      (2) Lenses must contain Type 1 or 1-A metallic coat.

7. <u>Safety Glasses</u>.

   a. <u>Standards</u>. Non-prescription or prescription safety glasses meeting American National Standards Institute Standard Z87.1 shall be for industrial wear to military and civilian personnel working in any environment hazardous to eyes, e.g., welders, machinists, mechanics, riggers, and grinders.

   b. Non-prescription safety glasses shall be furnished on a custody receipt when a prescription lenses are not required.

   c. Prescription safety glasses are no longer available from military optical laboratories. Prescription safety eyewear should be purchased with unit operating funds. Prescription safety glasses are only issued to personnel with a current eye exam within the last 12 months and costs incurred are chargeable to unit operating funds. Note: Government civilian employees requiring prescription safety eyewear must have their eye examination performed by an optometrist or ophthalmologist at no expense to the government.

COMDTINST M6000.1E

CHAPTER 9

HEALTH SERVICES TECHNICIANS ASSIGNED TO INDEPENDENT DUTY

Section A. Independent Duty Afloat.

1. Introduction 1
2. Mission and Responsibilities 1
3. Providing Health Care Afloat 5
4. Training 13
5. Supply and Logistics 17
6. Health Services Department Administration 23
7. Combat Operations 26
8. Environmental Health 27

Section B. Independent Duty Ashore at Sectors, Sector Field Offices, Air Stations, and Small Boat Stations.

1. Introduction 1
2. Mission and Responsibilities 1
3. Chain Of Command 2
4. Operation of the Health Services Division 2
5. Providing Health Care 5
6. Training 9
7. Supply and Logistics 11
8. Health Services Department Administration 17
9. Search and Rescue (SAR) Operations 20
10. Environmental Health 20

Section C. Independent Duty in Support of Deployable Specialized Forces (DSF)

1. Introduction 1
2. Mission and Responsibilities 1
3. Chain Of Command 2
4. Operation of the Health Services Division 2
5. Providing Health Care 5
6. Training 10
7. Supply and Logistics 12
8. Health Services Department Administration 18
9. Tactical Operations 21
10. Environmental Health 21

Section D. Quality Improvement Compliance Program (QICP)

1. Background 1
2. Purpose 1

Chapter 9 Contents

3. Overview 1
4. Program Elements 1
5. Collaborative Program 2
6. Monitoring the QICP 2
7. Assistance Program 2
8. Responsibility 2
9. QI Compliance Checklist 3
10. Compliance Certification Standards 3
11. Post Survey 4

Section E. Independent Duty Management of TRICARE

1. Introduction 1
2. Discussion 1
3. Access to Care 1
4. Access to Care Standards 1
5. Enrollment 2
6. Resources 2

Section A. Independent Duty Afloat

1. Introduction. 1
2. Mission and Responsibilities. 1
3. Providing Health Care Afloat. 5
4. Training. 13
5. Supply and Logistics. 17
6. Health Services Department Administration. 23
7. Combat Operations. 26
8. Environmental Health. 27

This page intentionally left blank.

CHAPTER NINE – HEALTH SERVICES TECHNICIANS ASSIGNED TO INDEPENDENT DUTY

Section A. Independent Duty Afloat.

1. Introduction. An independent duty health services technician (IDHS) is a Health Services Technician (HS) assigned to an afloat unit that has no attached Medical Officer. Assignment to independent duty is challenging. The role is one of tremendous responsibility and at times can tax even the most experienced HS's skill, knowledge and ability. Along with the increased responsibility and sometimes arduous duty comes the potential for personal satisfaction unsurpassed by any other job assignment.

2. Mission and Responsibilities.

    a. Mission. The Health Services Technician serving independently is charged with the responsibility for the prevention and control of disease and injury, and the treatment of the sick and injured.

    b. Responsibilities. The Commanding Officer (CO) is responsible for the health and physical readiness of the crew of the unit. In the absence of a permanently attached Medical Officer (MO) the vessel's Executive Officer (XO) will have direct responsibility for medical matters when no MO is attached to the vessel. The role of the IDHS is to assist the command in maintaining the good health and physical readiness of the crew. To accomplish this responsibility, the IDHS must be informed of planned operations and anticipate any operational demands resulting from such operations. To this end, the IDHS will consult and advise the command in all matters with potential to effect crew readiness or the health of personnel. Some of the duties of the IDHS include:

        (1) Assessment and treatment of illness and injury.

        (2) Prevention of illness and injury through an aggressive environmental health program. Such a program includes inspection of living and working spaces, food service and storage areas, and food storage and handling practices, integrated pest management practices, potable water quality surveillance, and recognition and management of communicable diseases.

        (3) Provision of Health Services training aligned with the needs and mission of the unit.

        (4) Security and proper use of health services supplies, material and property.

        (5) Maintenance and documentation of medical and dental readiness of unit personnel.

        (6) Supply and logistics to ensure supplies, materials and equipment necessary to carry out the mission of the Health Services Department are obtained and maintained in sufficient quantity and condition to

support the unit mission and operation.

(7) Health Services Department administration, maintenance, and security of health records.

(8) Strict adherence to Chapter 2 of this Manual which contains information about general and specific duties of the HS serving independently, including all required training in compliance with HIPAA privacy and security.

c. <u>Chain Of Command</u>. The IDHS will report directly to the Executive Officer (XO).

d. <u>Operation of the Health Services Department</u>. The IDHS is tasked with a wide variety and high volume of duties and responsibilities. This section sets forth policy and guidelines designed to assist the IDHS in carrying out assigned duties and responsibilities.

e. <u>Health Services Department Standard Operating Procedure</u>. In order to successfully manage the Health Services Department the IDHS must use time management and organizational skills and tools. One such tool is a written Standard Operating Procedure (SOP) for the Health Services Department. The SOP will govern the activity of the IDHS and has as its guiding precept the goals and missions of the unit. The SOP will be developed and submitted in written form to the CO for approval via the chain of command. In addition, the SOP will be reviewed at least annually by the IDHS, XO and CO. The approved SOP will be kept in the Health Services Department for easy referral. Copies of pertinent sections will be posted as appropriate. The SOP will include:

(1) A copy of the IDHS's letter of assumption of duties as Health Services Department Representative.

(2) A written daily schedule of events for both underway and inport periods.

(3) Copies of all letters of designation, assignment, and authority that directly impact upon the IDHS or Health Services Department. Examples include those granting "By direction" authority, designation as working Narcotics and Controlled Substances custodian, and assignment of a Designated Medical Officer Advisor (DMOA).

(4) A copy of the unit's organizational structure. This document will show graphically the IDHS's chain of command.

(5) A listing of duties and responsibilities assigned to the IDHS and the frequency that they are to be carried out. The listing will include both primary and collateral assigned duties.

(6) A listing of all required reports, the format required for submission, the frequency or date required, required routing and required "copy

addressees". Incorporation of this information in tabular format provides a quick and easy guide for reference purposes.

(7) A water bill, for the safe handling of potable water.

(8) A unit instruction or SOP for the management of rape or sexual assault cases. The document must provide policy for Health Services Department action in such cases, names of organizations, points of contact and telephone numbers for local resources as well as contact information for agencies and facilities which must be notified. CGIS must be notified on all cases of alleged rape or sexual assault. It must contain a prearranged mechanism for timely completion of a physical examination for the purpose of evidence gathering that meets requirements of all applicable law enforcement agencies. Additionally, it must define limitations that will exist if the unit is underway at the time the incident occurs.

(9) A unit instruction or SOP for the management of suicide threat or attempt. The document must provide policy for Health Services Department action in such cases, names of organizations, points of contact and telephone numbers for local resources, contact information for agencies and facilities which must be notified as well as a listing of required information, reports or actions.

(10) A unit instruction or SOP action required in the event of family violence. The document must provide policy for Health Services Department action in such cases, names of organizations, points of contact and telephone numbers for local resources, contact information for agencies and facilities which must be notified as well as a listing of required information, reports or actions.

f. <u>Other Necessary Documents</u>. The IDHS is an integral part of many unit activities and various unit bills and doctrines require specific action by the IDHS. Since these are changed frequently, incorporation of Health Services Department responsibilities contained in these various documents into the Health Services Department SOP is not recommended. Applicable portions should be kept in the Health Services Department for quick reference, however. These include:

(1) A battle doctrine for the unit.

(2) Portions of the unit mass casualty bill pertaining to Health Services Department responsibility.

(3) Portions of the unit general emergency bill pertaining to Health Services Department responsibility.

(4) Portions of the unit man overboard bill pertaining to Health Services Department responsibility.

(5) Portions of the unit replenishment at sea, special sea detail, flight

quarters and bomb threat bills pertaining to Health Services Department responsibility.

g. <u>Departure from the Daily Schedule of Events</u>. The day-to-day operation of the Health Services Department is complex and impacted by the operational needs of the unit. It will of necessity change when events of higher priority or concern occur. If deviation from the daily schedule of events is required, notification of the XO (IDHS's Division Officer) will be made at the earliest opportunity. When deviation from daily schedule of events occurs frequently, the daily schedule of events will be reviewed and if necessary, changed. Any changes will be incorporated into the Health Services Department SOP and approved by the Commanding Officer.

h. <u>Relief and Assumption of Duties as the IDHS</u>. Proper documentation of the status of the Health Services Department, the condition of its equipment, stores, and records is required at the time of relief and assumption of the duties and responsibilities as the IDHS. The process is complex and requires both the incoming and outgoing IDHS to jointly perform the following:

   (1) A complete inventory of all medical stores, spaces, and equipment, including durable medical equipment. The Health Services Allowance List Afloat, COMDTINST M6700.6 (series) provides a listing of supplies and the equipment required by each class of vessel.

      (a) A controlled substances inventory must be done. Use direction provided in Chapter 10 of this Manual.

      (b) A complete inventory of all unit property in custody of the Health Services Department.

   (2) A review of ongoing actions affecting the status of Health Services, e.g., outstanding requisitions, survey or repairs, and proper documentation of all such transactions.

   (3) A review of the Health Services Department SOP.

   (4) A review of the most recent HSWL SC Quality Assurance Assistance Survey for the unit. A copy of the survey annotated with any finding of incomplete or uncorrected discrepancies will be included as an enclosure to the letter of relief.

   (5) Review of all health records for completeness, accuracy, privacy and security.

   (6) A review of the most recent Tailored Annual Cutter Training evaluation. Paragraph 4 of this section provides the outline for the training program.

(7) A complete health, safety and sanitation inspection of the vessel, to include status of potable water systems (records of bacteriological, halogen content and pH testing), food stores inspections, and berthing and habitability of living and berthing spaces.

i. Letter of Relief and Assumption of Duties. Upon completion of the Health Services Department review a Coast Guard memorandum will be prepared and submitted by the oncoming IDHS via the chain of command and will advise the Commanding Officer of the status of the Health Services Department. A copy of the letter will be forwarded to the HSWL SC. The letter of Relief and Assumption of Duties will provide the following:

(1) Date of assumption of duties. A statement shall be signed by the oncoming IDHS, that the duties and responsibilities of the IDHS have been assumed; and a statement that a thorough review of the Health Services Department has been conducted. Any discrepancies of material or record keeping will be annotated on a copy of the unit's most recent HSWL SC Quality Assurance site survey and submitted as an enclosure to the letter of Relief and Assumption of Duties as IDHS for the vessel.

(2) Any discrepancies noted upon relief will be handled as a matter of individual command prerogative. Responsibility for correction, adjustment of account or inventory records, action required to replace missing items, as well as any necessary disciplinary action will be determined by the command.

(3) In cases in which no "on site" relief occurs, all of the preceding action will be completed. The supply officer of the unit will participate in the review process in place of the outgoing IDHS.

j. Actions upon Proper Relief. Upon assumption of duties as the unit's IDHS, one of the first tasks to complete is a thorough review of all SOPs and department instructions. Check the references; make contact with any listed points of contact. If possible, make visits and introductions in person. Find out how each system works and how it is accessed.

3. Providing Health Care Afloat. Provision of health care is undoubtedly the most challenging and rewarding part of the job of an IDHS. An IDHS bears a tremendous responsibility. This responsibility can never be taken lightly. This section is intended to provide a brief summary of the various facets of providing medical care afloat.

a. Designated Medical Officer Advisor (DMOA). All IDHS, and other HSs serving in training apprenticeship, shall be assigned a DMOA in accordance with Chapter 1 of this Manual. Good communication between all HSs and their DMOA can prevent problems affecting health care delivery to the crew. All HS will schedule a visit with the DMOA as soon as is practical after reporting aboard. The purpose of the visit is to allow first-hand communication of expectations, support facility requirements, and any unique needs or concerns. Open communication can be maintained through regular visits when practical, or at minimum, regular telephone calls. With regard to provision of direct care, the IDHS will seek DMOA or another MO's advice whenever there are questions about a patient's condition or when the following conditions exist:

(1) Return to sick call before assigned follow-up because of failure to improve or condition has deteriorated.

(2) Member cannot return to full duty status after 72 hours duration because of unresolved illness.

The IDHS shall contact the Flight Surgeon on call through the closest Coast Guard Command Center when any of the following emergency conditions exist:

(1) Undetermined fever of 102 degrees Fahrenheit or higher (when taken orally) persisting for 48 hours.

(2) Fever of 103 degrees Fahrenheit or higher (when taken orally).

(3) Unexplained pulse rate above 120 beats per minute.

(4) Unexplained respiratory rate above 28 breaths per minute or less than 12 breaths per minute.

(5) Depression with suicidal thoughts.

(6) Change in mental status.

(7) Chest pain or arrhythmia.

(8) Unexplained shortness or breath.

(9) Rape or sexual assault.

b. <u>Gender Considerations</u>. Chapter 1 Section B of this Manual provides specific direction for health services technicians about patient privacy, same gender attendant requirements, and examination restrictions.

c. <u>Avoiding Common Problems</u>. Scheduling and obtaining the routine medical care needed by crewmembers during short inport periods can tax the organizational skills of even the most experienced IDHS. There are, however, actions that the IDHS can take which will enhance the chances of getting the routine appointments needed for all members. Some of these are:

(1) Identify the routine medical and dental needs of the crew well in advance of return to port. The vessel's supporting clinic has an established appointment scheduling procedure within which the IDHS must work whenever operational schedules allow. Provide requests via message (or other written form as appropriate) for appointment scheduling ahead of "appointment schedule opening" for the inport

period whenever possible. Request reply by message prior to the vessel's scheduled return to port. When routine medical or dental care is to be made directly to a DOD MTF, the IDHS must determine the facility requirements for referral of patients and follow any local procedures.

(2) Communicate with the vessel's supporting clinic. Visit the supporting clinic, if practical, as soon as possible after return to port. Discuss the crew's medical and dental needs with the clinic supervisor and DMOA (if located at the facility).

(3) Perform as many preliminary tests and as much paperwork as possible before scheduling physicals at the supporting clinic.

(4) Post a listing of appointment dates and times as soon as it becomes available. Provide each division officer and shop chief a listing of the appointments applicable to the division or shop.

(5) Hold members accountable to be at their appointed place and time. Provide feedback to division officers and shop chiefs on any appointment failure. Notify XO of more than one failure.

d. <u>Consultations</u>. During the management of complex or protracted cases, consultations or specialty referral may be necessary. When such services are needed, the IDHS will normally contact a CG clinic or in some cases, a Department of Defense medical treatment facility (DOD MTF). When arranging for a patient to see a Medical Officer at a CG clinic, the IDHS shall ensure that a Chronological Record of Care, SF-600 entry is completed using the SOAP format and that an appointment is scheduled. The clinic will normally provide treatment or arrange care if treatment is beyond its scope. When consultations or referral for specialty care are required, the HS shall coordinate with the PCM. The IDHS must determine the facility requirements for referral of patients and follow any local procedures. Referrals to a DOD MTF will normally be documented using an SF-513, Consultation Sheet or a Referral for Civilian Medical Care, DD-2161. The consultation request shall provide a concise history of the condition to be evaluated as well as any pertinent findings and a provisional diagnosis. Chapter 4 Section B of this Manual provides direction on completion of a Consultation Sheet, SF 513. The patient should inform their supervisor of all referral appointment dates and times. Whenever possible, provide at least 24 hours notice for changes or cancellations.

e. <u>Medical Evacuation (MEDEVAC) of Injured or Ill Crewmembers</u>. Medical evacuation must be considered when care is needed by a patient to preserve life or limb, provide pain relief beyond capability onboard, or to provide other medical or dental treatment for which delay until the unit's next scheduled port call would provide undue hardship or pain for the patient. The unit's ability to MEDEVAC a patient will be affected by the vessel's current mission, availability of air transport assets, and location. When considering or executing a MEDEVAC:

(1) Keep the XO informed. At first indication that a MEDEVAC may become necessary, notify the XO.

(2) Request, via the XO, communication with the closest Coast Guard command center and request to consult with the Flight Surgeon on call. In addition to a thorough patient presentation, information about the unit's location in relation to medical resources ashore and realistic estimations of time requirements to reach a point that MEDEVAC is possible, must be available. Keep the Flight Surgeon advised of any change in the patient's condition.

(3) Thoroughly document the MEDEVAC process. Ensure that a complete patient record is maintained in the patient's health record. Maintain a complete record of events in the Health Services log. Make entries as events occur.

(4) Keep the patient informed. Explain in as much detail as possible the actions being taken and expected outcome of the actions. As time of departure approaches, describe for the patient what to expect during transport and upon arrival at destination. If a Coast Guard Beneficiary Representative is attached to the medical facility to which the patient is being MEDEVACed, provide this information to the patient.

(5) Ensure that all documentation about the patient's condition is contained in the health record and that it and any medication needed by the patient during transport are securely packaged and ready for transport with the patient. Ensure that information necessary for unit contact and contact of the unit's supporting clinic are provided and easily located by the receiving medical facility. Anticipate the patient's need for personal items, including a valid Armed Forces Identification Card, and ensure these are packaged for transport with the patient. Limit such items to those that are necessary. Encourage the patient to limit cash.

(6) Notify the unit's supporting clinic and DMOA of the MEDEVAC and any needed assistance for the patient.

(7) Provide an inpatient hospitalization notification e-mail in accordance with current directives. See Chapter 2 Section A of this Manual.

f. Surgical Procedures. Most routine minor surgical procedures will be delayed until the vessel is in port. Surgical procedures while underway will be limited to only those procedures that are needed in order to return a patient to a fit for full duty status. These procedures include:

(1) Placing and removing sutures in a wound.

(2) Incision and drainage.

(3) Unguinectomy.

(4) Paring down painful plantar warts.

g. Refusal of Treatment. Medical, dental, and surgical treatment will not be performed on a mentally competent member who does not consent to the recommended procedure except.

   (1) Emergency care is required to preserve the life or health of the member.

   (2) Isolation and quarantine of suspected or proven communicable diseases as medically indicated or required by law to ensure proper treatment and protection of the member or others.

h. Motion Sickness. Members that manifest chronic motion sickness, that do not respond to conventional therapy, and are unable to perform their duties as a result, will be considered for administrative separation from active duty as per the Personnel Manual, COMDTINST M1000.6 (series).

i. Antibiotic Therapy. The IDHS may prescribe and administer antibiotics included on the Health Services Allowance List Afloat. Whenever possible, the IDHS shall consult with his/her DMOA or a Medical Officer for a recommendation or concurrence prior to administering antibiotic therapy. If consultation is not possible prior to administration an e-mail must be sent to the DMOA providing case history, ICD9CM code and treatment provided.

j. Health Services Treatment Space. The Health Services treatment space will be manned at all times when patients are inside. All items are to be stowed in their proper place and secured. All medical records shall be locked in a cabinet. At no time should the Health Services space be left unlocked when the IDHS is not onboard.

k. Patient Berthing. Some units have facilities for close patient observation or treatment. Absolutely no person other than the sick or injured will be berthed in the Health Services Department. The IDHS may sleep in the Health Services Department when attending an injured or sick patient, but will have a regularly assigned berthing space. Personal gear and clothing are not to be stored in the Health Services Department. The Health Services Department will not be used as berthing spaces for augmented personnel.

l. Not Fit For Sea Duty. Members who are medically, surgically, or orthopedically unfit for sea duty (including wearing a cast or needing to use crutches) and unable to perform their duties will not be placed onboard the vessel. Personnel will either be placed on Limited Duty ashore or on Convalescent Leave.

m. Convalescent Leave/Sick Leave. Convalescent leave/Sick leave is a period of leave not charged against a member's leave account. It can be a recommendation to the command when a patient is Not Fit For Duty (usually for a duration expected to be greater than 72 hours) and whose recovery time can reasonably be expected to improve by freedom from the confines of quarters. It should be considered only when required as an adjunct to patient treatment. The command must evaluate each recommendation. Commands are authorized to grant convalescent leave as outlined in Chapter 7 of the Personnel Manual, COMDTINST M1000.6 (series).

n. <u>Controlled Substances</u>. Regulations for the handling, storage, and issue of narcotics and controlled substances are found in Chapter 10 of this Manual. The contents of this section are not intended to contradict the guidance provided there. This section serves to amplify policy provided with respect to medicinal narcotics and controlled substances onboard afloat units.

(1) Narcotics and controlled substances require special handling. All controlled substances shall be obtained through the unit's collateral duty Regional Pharmacy Executive (RPE).

(2) The CO will designate the Executive Officer as the controlled substances custodian (CSC). The CSC will follow the accounting procedure provided in Chapter 10 of this Manual. The IDHS will normally be assigned as custodian for narcotics and controlled substances working stock. Such assignment must be made in writing.

(3) All issues from working stock will be documented with a properly completed, written prescription. All non-emergent care requires contact with a Medical Officer before dispensing any controlled medication. The Medical Officer's orders will be documented on a prescription and in the patient's health record. The words "By verbal order of" will precede the ordering Medical Officer's initials, last name, and time of order and date of order both on the prescription and in the patient's health record. In the event of an emergency, a Medical Officer's order is not needed to dispense a controlled substance. Once the emergency situation is over or alleviated, the IDHS will contact a Medical Officer and detail the circumstances and the controlled substances that were administered. Upon concurrence by the Medical Officer, the prescription prepared for the patient will be annotated with the words "By concurrence of" the ordering physician's initials, last name, time of concurrence and date of concurrence.

(4) The XO will countersign all prescriptions prepared by the IDHS prior to issue of any controlled substance or narcotic.

(5) Controlled substances stored aboard cutters shall be limited to amounts in the Health Services Allowance List, Afloat, COMDTINST M6700.6 (series). If the need exists for the unit to carry additional quantities of controlled substances based on use or potential for operational need, a written request signed by the Commanding Officer will be forwarded to the IDHS's DMOA. The request must include nomenclature, quantity, and brief justification.

o. Dental. It is the duty of the IDHS to arrange for the necessary dental examinations of the crew. All personnel should be Class I or Class II prior to deployment and results shall be documented in DENCAS.

   (1) All personnel must receive an annual dental exam.

   (2) The IDHS will arrange, via e-mail or message, for the large group of dental appointments needed for crewmembers returning from deployment. A signup sheet and announcement to the crewmembers is advised, and early communication with the staff of the dental clinic is recommended in order to allow sufficient time for the scheduling of a large amount of dental visits. Urgent cases obviously are to be scheduled first, regardless of rank or position of the member. Once back in port, active communication with a designated POC in the dental clinic is advised in order to handle cancellations, substitutions and last minute appointment changes. Although it may be time consuming, it is easier to deliver patient reminders the morning of the scheduled appointment than to try and explain a group of no-show crewmembers to a dental officer or XO.

p. Rape or Sexual Assault. All victims of rape or sexual assault must be treated in a professional, compassionate and non-judgmental manner. Examination of rape and sexual assault victims will be limited to only visual examination of any wound or injury and treated according to present standards of care. In all cases, a Medical Officer and CGIS will be contacted for advice. In the event that no Medical Officer is available (underway), an IDHS may conduct the visual examination. A chaperone of the same gender as the patient will be present if such examination is conducted. All aspects of the patient encounter must be carefully documented. Physical examination to gather evidence of rape or sexual assault is strictly prohibited. The unit shall have a SOP for alleged rape and sexual assault. Refer to Reporting and Responding to Rape and Sexual Assault Allegations, COMDTINST 1754.10 (series).

q. Suicide Prevention. An encounter with a suicidal person is always a deeply emotional event. It is important for the IDHS to act in a caring and professional manner. Early intervention and good communication skills are essential. If suicidal ideation is suspected it is important to remember:

   (1) Take all threats and symptoms seriously. For any member considering suicide, immediately seek professional help from the nearest MTF or civilian emergency room with facilities appropriate to the situation. At no time should the person be left unattended. Once the patient is safe, contact the servicing Work-Life office for additional help or refer to Suicide Prevention COMDTINST 1734.1 (series).

   (2) Actively listen to the patient. Do not argue, judge, attempt to diagnose, or analyze the person's true intentions. It is important to provide a calm, caring, professional demeanor throughout the entire situation.

Thoroughly document the patient encounter using the SOAP format.

(3) Arrange for an escort and a driver to transport the patient to the nearest Coast Guard clinic, MTF or civilian emergency room with facilities appropriate to the situation. The unit's SOP for suicide threat or attempt should contain this information for ready use if needed. If underway, then a MEDEVAC must be considered. Contact a Flight Surgeon, the IDHS's DMOA or a Medical Officer familiar with the area of operation for advise on how to handle this patient.

r. <u>Decedent Affairs</u>. Chapter 5 of this Manual contains guidance about action that the Health Services Department must take when there is a death aboard a Coast Guard unit. Chapter 11 of the Personnel Manual, COMDTINST M1000.6 (series) contains further guidance concerning casualties and decedent affairs, as does the Decedent Affairs Guide, COMDTINST M1770.1 (series) . It is unlikely that the IDHS will be assigned as the Casualty Assistance Calls Officer (CACO) for the command, but the IDHS will undoubtedly be heavily involved with the process of proper disposition of remains, so familiarity with the information required is helpful. The IDHS should also perform the following:

(1) An entry in the Health Services Log will be made detailing all available information concerning the death.

(2) The health record of the deceased member will be terminated in accordance with Chapter 4 of this Manual.

s. <u>Disposition of Remains</u>. As soon as possible, remains will be transferred to the nearest Military Treatment Facility (MTF) for further disposition. When transfer cannot be accomplished immediately, the remains will be placed into a body pouch and refrigerated at a temperature of 36 to 40 degrees Fahrenheit to prevent decomposition. The space must contain no other items and must be cleaned and disinfected before reuse. Remains will be identified with a waterproof tag, marked with waterproof ink, and affixed with wire ties to the right great toe of the decedent and also to each end of the body pouch. The minimum information needed on each tag includes the full name, SSN and rate or rank of the decedent. Whenever possible, do not remove items attached to the deceased at time of death. Such items may include (for example) IV lines, needles, lengths of cord or line, etc. These may be important during an autopsy. Additionally, do not discard or launder clothing of the deceased. These items are sometimes important to surviving family members and in some cultures is part of the mourning process for the deceased. This is a cultural consideration but should be a part of the decision process.

t. <u>Physical Disability Evaluation System</u>. The medical board process is detailed in Chapter 17.A. of the Personnel Manual, COMDTINST M1000.6

(series) and the Physical Disability Evaluation Manual, COMDTINST

M1850.2 (series).

4. Training. The purpose of training provided to the crew of an afloat unit include: assurance that crewmembers are able to provide aid for themselves and their shipmates in an emergency or a combat situation and to promote the general health and well being of the crew. To this end, a written Health Services Department Training Plan will be prepared and submitted to the unit training officer for incorporation into the unit training plan.

   a. Health Services Department Training Plan. A plan for training of the crew will be established. The plan will be established in written form and kept on file. It will be based on a minimum 12 month cycle and be included in the cutter training schedule. At a minimum, the following training will be given annually:

      (1) Basic first aid.

      (2) Shock, hemorrhage control, bandaging.

      (3) Airway management and assisted ventilation.

      (4) Route to battle dressing stations (BDS), use of items in first aid kits, gunbags and boxes.

      (5) Personal and dental hygiene.

      (6) STI/HIV prevention.

      (7) Heat and cold stress programs, including hypothermia.

      (8) Respiratory protection program.

      (9) Hearing conservation.

      (10) Poisoning.

      (11) Sight conservation.

      (12) Blood borne pathogens.

   b. Documentation of Training. Documentation of the training is a Tailored Annual Cutter Training requirement as well as a requirement of several Coast Guard programs. The rule of thumb to remember is "If it isn't written down, it didn't happen." An outline must be prepared and kept on file for all training topics presented and a training log maintained for all training provided. The training log will contain a record of all HS training given to the crew, stretcher-bearers, and HSs. It will contain the following information:

      (1) Date.

      (2) Topic.

      (3) Duration.

      (4) Group or department receiving the training.

(5) Instructor's name.

(6) Names (signatures of those present) of members trained.

c. <u>Training Format</u>. Training will normally be presented in either lecture format or demonstration and practical application. Lecture format presentations should be limited to 15 to 20 minutes and demonstrations and practical application should not exceed 1 hour. Practical application must be of high priority in training the crew and stretcher-bearers in first aid, casualty evaluation, treatment, reports to damage control central, and transporting casualties to battle dressing stations. There is no substitute for "hands on" practice in developing effective first aid and patient transport skills.

d. <u>Departmental Training</u>. Specific training not applicable to the entire crew, but appropriate to individual departments, should be incorporated into the Health Services Training Plan. Such departmental training is normally needed because of workplace exposure to potential health hazards. Training subjects appropriate to various departments are listed in the following subparagraphs. The list is not all inclusive. It is provided as a guideline.

(1) Weapons department:

(a) Hearing conservation.

(b) Heat stress (ship's laundry personnel).

(c) Respiratory protection.

(d) Basic life support (fire control personnel).

(e) Review of prevention and treatment of electric shock casualties.

(f) Eyesight protection.

(2) Engineering department:

(a) Hearing conservation.

(b) Potable water.

(c) Heat stress.

(d) Respiratory protection.

(e) Eyesight protection.

(f) Hazards associated with human waste.

(3) Supply department:

(a) Food service sanitation (food service personnel).

(b) Heat stress (scullery personnel).

(4) Operations department:

(a) Basic life support (electronics shop personnel).

(b) Review of prevention and treatment of burns, electric shock and hemorrhage.

(5) Deck department:

(a) Eyesight protection.

(b) Hearing conservation.

(c) Heat stress.

(d) Respiratory protection.

e. <u>Drills</u>. Drills are a necessary part of unit training. Drills help to reinforce performance of skills and actions that must be completed during stressful or potentially dangerous situations. Drills that have close relation to health and safety of the crew will be incorporated into the Health Services Department Training Plan. The cutter training board should integrate Health Services Department Training Plan drills into the unit's training schedule.

(1) The following drills will be conducted semi-annually:

(a) Battle Dressing Station.

(b) Personnel casualty transportation.

(c) Mass casualty.

(2) The following drills, at minimum, will be conducted quarterly:

(a) Compound fracture.

(b) Sucking chest wound.

(c) Abdominal wounds.

(d) Amputation.

(e) Facial wounds.

(f) Electrical shock.

(g) Smoke inhalation.

(h) Casualty transport.

f. <u>Training and Assignment of Stretcher-Bearers</u>. No less than four stretcher-bearers will be assigned to the Primary Battle Dressing station (BDS). The training for stretcher-bearers will include all subjects given to the crew with emphasis on basic first aid, casualty evacuation, triage, use of all stretcher types maintained onboard the unit, casualty carrying methods, setup and organization and basic life support. Stretcher-bearers must also complete the advanced first aid portion of the Damage Control Personnel Qualification Standards (DC PQS).

g. Training for the IDHS. Careful study, practice, and concentration on all facets of the Health Services Technician are necessary to prepare an HS to be successful as an IDHS. In addition to the requirements of the rating, successful completion of certain training and "C" schools are required as per Cutter Training and Qualification Manual, COMDTINST M3502.4 (series) These are:

   (1) Coast Guard Independent Duty Health Services Technician, Air Force Medical Services Craftsman or Navy Surface Forces Independent Duty Technician.

   (2) Coast Guard Introduction to Environmental Health or Navy Basic Shipboard Series. (Note: This is not required for graduates of Navy Surface Forces Independent Duty Technician or Independent Duty Health Services Technician School).

   (3) Emergency Medical Technician – A Basic Level. IDHS assigned to a floating unit are required to maintain currency with the National Registry of Emergency Medical Technicians (NREMT) at the Basic level. Short Term Training Requests are to be completed in accordance with the Training and Education Manual, COMDTINST M1500.10 (series) and forwarded to Commandant (CG-1121). Funding will be provided by Commandant (CG-11). See the Emergency Medical Services Manual, COMDTINST M16135.4 (series) for additional information.

   (4) Instructor courses (Must maintain current certification in) CPR, BLS, AED and First Responder.

   (5) Field Management of Chemical and Biological Casualties. The Field Management of Chemical and Biological Casualties Course (FCBC) is conducted by the US Army Medical Research Institute of Chemical Defense (USAMRICD) at Aberdeen Proving Ground, Maryland. Classroom instruction, laboratory and field exercises prepare graduates to become trainers in the first echelon management of chemical and biological agent casualties. This course is required per Cutter Training and Qualification Manual, COMDTINST M3502.4 (series).

h. Training for the HS3 Aboard High Endurance Cutters. The HS3 assigned to a 378' is considered an apprentice for training purposes. The cutter HSC is responsible for the training and mentorship of the HS3. While assigned, the HS3 shall accomplish the following training requirements:

   (1) Completion of Enlisted Performance Quals for next paygrade.

   (2) While inport, attend weekly training sessions at supporting CG Clinic. This shall include spending clinical time working with their assigned DMOA. If cutter is not co-located with their DMOA Clinic, the HS3 should attend formal clinical training at a local MTF if available.

(3) Submit 100% of their record entries to the HSC for quality assurance review and training opportunities.

5. <u>Supply and Logistics</u>.

   a. <u>Custody of Health Services Equipment and Material</u>. As directed by the Commanding Officer, the IDHS is responsible and accountable for the health services material onboard the cutter. As such, the IDHS is the custodian of all health service equipment and material. The custodian will not permit waste or abuse of supplies or equipment and will use techniques such as stock rotation, planned replacement and preventive maintenance to minimize waste of resources.

   b. <u>Inventory</u>. An accurate record of medical stores and equipment must be maintained. The inventory of medical stores, spaces and equipment will be prepared using the NAVSUP-1114, Stock Record Card Afloat or in line item form (computerized database is an approved and preferred alternative if all necessary information is captured) and include

      (1) Quantity and shelf-life of each item currently on board.

      (2) Balance on hand, high-level, low-level (reorder point for each item).

      (3) Manufacturer, lot number and expiration date (pharmaceuticals).

      (4) Quantity placed on order, date received.

   c. <u>Unit Property</u>. Unit property in Health Services Department custody must also be safeguarded and accounted for. The unit property custodian should be contacted before transfer or destruction of such property.

   d. <u>Funding and Account Record Keeping</u>. Funds used to purchase supplies and equipment and to pay for the various expenses of operating the unit are broken down into Allotment Fund Control (AFC) expenditure categories. This method allows for efficient budgeting and accounting. Fund categories generally used by an IDHS fall within the AFC subhead 30 or 57 expenditure categories.

      (1) AFC-30 is a general ship fund used by the supply department to purchase generally needed operating supplies and services. Examples include pens, paper, books, training aids, etc. AFC-30 funding can be used to pay for Health Services Department supplies and equipment not obtainable through Defense Supply Center Philadelphia Prime Vendor Program (via the unit's supporting clinic) or the major medical equipment request process (see Chapters 6 and 8 of this Manual). Restrictions exist on what may be purchased with AFC-30 funds. Specific questions can be answered by unit supply personnel.

      (2) AFC-57 is a funding category used to purchase health care related supplies and equipment, and to pay for health care. AFC-57 funds are

distributed to the HSWL SC and further allocated by them to the units within their areas of responsibility with HS's assigned.

(3) With the full implementation of the Prime Vendor programs for Pharmaceuticals and for Medical and Surgical Supplies, AFC-57 fund allocations will be made to the Prime Vendor ordering point assigned for the unit.

e. Budgets and Budgeting. In general, IDHSs do not need to plan and submit an AFC-57 budget request because medical supplies and equipment funding are controlled by the HSWL SC and Prime Vendor ordering points. If additional AFC-57 resource needs are anticipated, the IDHS's supporting clinic should be contacted for direction on how the resources are to be requested. The budget build process does have value for the IDHS however. AFC-30 funds will need to be planned for and requested and medical equipment in need of planned replacement must be identified and a Coast Guard Health Care Equipment Request, CG-5211 submitted. The budget build process is a good way to handle these needs. AFC-30 fund budget planning is relatively straight forward, although it can be time consuming. AFC-30 expenditures for Health Services should be broken into general use categories. Examples of categories are books and publications, non-consumable goods and services such as hydro testing and replacement of oxygen cylinders, and travel for continuing education. Budgeting categories can be as simple or complicated as the IDHS desires to make it. Once categories have been established, a ledger for the Health Services Department should be "opened" and the expenditure categories entered into it. The use of a "spreadsheet" program is an efficient way to keep an accounting record, but a ledger book works just as well. Attention to detail is the key. In general, a system using four to five categories works well.

(1) In preparing a budget for the upcoming year, it is important to look back over what was purchased in the previous year. To do this, collect all records of AFC 30 orders and expenditures. Review each line item and record the amount spent into the appropriate budget category. The following is a timeline on how to prepare a budget.

| March | Look back process. Review amount of funds spent over the first two quarters of the fiscal year as well as spending patterns for the previous fiscal year. Note general categories on which funds were spent and in which quarter items were ordered. This will allow projection of quarterly funding needs into the upcoming year. |

April/May	Review status of the Health Services Department medical library and determine which texts and references must be updated.
	Review status of HS certifications and continuing medical education. Funding for training, conferences or seminars not normally funded by AFC 56 funds must be budgeted for as AFC 30 budget line items.
	Review preventive maintenance records and include cost projections in AFC 30 budget. Prepare and submit any Coast Guard Health Care Equipment Request, CG-5211 for medical equipment to be replaced.
	Seek guidance from XO on known or planned activities outside normal operations. An example is a yard period (which will require higher than normal supplies of various personal protective equipment (PPE)) or extended deployments in which normal supply is difficult.
June	Submit finalized budget proposal through chain of command. AFC 30 budget information will be added to the unit budget. Be prepared to "defend" the budget request submitted. Documentation of the data gathering process and retrieval of the raw data used to justify the funding requested will likely be required. AFC 56 funds requests will be consolidated by the command and forwarded to the unit's district, HSWL SC or Area commander, as appropriate.

    (2) Careful stewardship, good record keeping and accounting make existing funding and justification for increased funding levels easier.

f. <u>Obtaining Pharmaceuticals, Medical and Surgical Supplies</u>. Chapter 8 of this Manual provides policy applicable to the management of Health Services supplies. Prime Vendor programs for both Pharmaceuticals and Medical/Surgical Supplies have been established and it is through these programs that essentially all pharmaceuticals and supplies will be obtained. Medical Prime Vendor Program Implementation within the Coast Guard, COMDTINST M6740.2 (series) provides detailed instruction about this program. From an "afloat" perspective important aspects of the program include:

    (1) Each afloat unit has been assigned a Prime Vendor ordering point for Pharmaceuticals and for Medical/Surgical Supplies. The HSWL SC assigns the POCs and periodically updates the information. The Prime Vendor ordering point may be different for each of the programs.

(2) Funding for both Prime Vendor for Pharmaceuticals and Prime Vendor for Medical/Surgical Supplies is provided to the assigned Prime Vendor ordering point by the HSWL SC. Internal accounting procedures vary among Prime Vendor ordering points. Some have established individual "accounts" for the units they are responsible for while others manage funds from a central account. Regardless of the accounting method used by the Prime Vendor ordering point, the IDHS must establish and maintain a system to track expenditures.

(3) Prime Vendor ordering points establish pharmaceutical and medical/surgical supply ordering procedures for their assigned units. Pharmaceutical and medical supply items ordered will be those required by the Health Services Allowance List (HSAL) in quantities required for the unit type. Deviation from the HSAL requirements will normally occur only after justification of the need is made by the IDHS to the DMOA for the unit. It will be made in writing and kept on file for review during a HSWL SC site surveys.

g. Health Services Supporting Clinic. The supporting clinic for a vessel is the IDHS's partner in providing health care for the vessel's crew. Local agreements and resources may be available to allow the supporting clinic to provide a broader range of services to the IDHS and the vessel's crew but at a minimum, the following will be provided.

(1) All supplies and equipment (under $500.00) listed in the HSAL for the class of vessel and on the HS Core Formulary. The unit no longer receives AFC-57 funding for the operation of the Health Services Department. These funds are provided instead to the vessel's supporting clinic with the intent that the supporting clinic will provide all required items for the IDHS to operate the Health Services Department.

(2) Assign the IDHS a DMOA in writing. The DMOA shall be available for questions about patient care, as well as completing record reviews quarterly.

(3) Perform medical boards for the IDHS unit as necessary.

(4) Provide a resource for advice and support in all administrative areas of health care provision to include medical administration, physical examination review (within the approving authority of the Clinic Administrator), health benefits, medical billing and bill payment processing assistance, dental care pharmacy administration, supply and logistics, bio-medical waste management, IDHS continuing education, and quality assurance support. Any services provided at the clinic shall be extended to the IDHS to the maximum extent possible.

h. Preventive Maintenance of Health Services Equipment. Chapter 8 of this

Manual details the preventive maintenance program for Health Services equipment. Chapters 1 and 2 of the Health Services Allowance List Afloat, COMDTINST M6700.6 (series) provide guidance on the maintenance of specific items carried onboard ship (i.e. gunbags, portable medical lockers, stokes litter, etc.). An important part of medical readiness is a program of preventive maintenance and planned equipment replacement. Repair and routine replacement part costs should be recorded on side B of NAVMED 6700/3CG, Medical/Dental Equipment Maintenance Record. Capture of this data will allow more accurate forecasting of AFC-30 funding needs for preventive maintenance.

i. Replacement of Health Care Equipment. Chapter 8 of this Manual provides direction on how to obtain replacement of health care equipment. An effectively managed planned equipment replacement program minimizes repair costs and avoids loss of critical equipment at unscheduled times. Additionally, used but still serviceable equipment can be used by other facilities by "turn-in and reissue" through the Defense Reutilization Management Office (DRMO). At least annually, normally during the budgeting process, review the preventive maintenance costs for each piece of health care equipment. When repair and maintenance costs for the year exceed 50 percent of the current replacement cost of the equipment, then a CG-5211, U. S. Coast Guard Health Care Equipment Request should be submitted to the HSWL SC requesting replacement.

j. Disposal of Unserviceable or Outdated Medical Material.

   (1) Equipment and Supplies. The Property Management Manual, COMDTINST M4500.5 (series) provides guidance on when a formal survey is required. In general, a formal survey is not required except when equipment has been lost or stolen. If uncertain about whether or not a formal survey should be done, the unit's supply officer should be consulted.

   (2) Pharmaceuticals and Medicinals. Destruction of pharmaceuticals and medicinals will rarely be required. Chapter 8.C. of this Manual directs that materials will not be disposed of at sea, but prepared for destruction and held in a secure area until the vessel's return to port where they can be disposed of in accordance with federal, state and local laws.

      (a) Prime Vendors provide a partial credit for some materials returned to them. IDHSs and supporting clinics will establish local policy for transfer of expired or short shelf-life pharmaceuticals. A transfer and replacement of pharmaceuticals within 6 months of expiration should be made with the supporting clinic to minimize waste.

      (b) If destruction is required, it will be accomplished in a well-ventilated area. Liquid substances present potential exposure through splash back. At a minimum, splash proof goggles and neoprene rubber gloves will be worn when working with liquid substances that may be absorbed through the skin. The wearing of protective equipment such as a splash apron is also encouraged. Thorough hand washing after the destruction process must be accomplished. Medical material must be disposed of in a manner so as to ensure that the material is rendered non-recoverable for use and harmless to the environment. Destruction must be complete, to preclude the use of any portion of a pharmaceutical. Chapter 8. C. of this Manual provides detailed information about destruction and disposal of unsuitable medications.

k. <u>Disposal of Medical Waste</u>. Federal regulation defines how medical waste must be stored and disposed of, and the records that must be kept to document the storage and disposal. The information in the following paragraphs is provided as a general explanation of program requirements rather than an in-depth instruction on handling of medical waste. Medical waste must be classed in one of two categories: potentially infectious or non-infectious waste. In depth guidance about storage, disposal and required record keeping for medical waste can be found in Chapter 13 of this Manual, in Quality Improvemnt Implementation Guide (QIIG) 16, and in Chapter 5 of the Safety and Environmental Health Manual, COMDTINST M5100.47 (series). An additional source of information is the unit's hazardous material control officer. In general, the disposal and record keeping requirements for the waste depend on the waste category and are:

(1) Potentially infectious waste is defined as an agent that may contain pathogens that may cause disease in a susceptible host. Used needles, scalpel blades, ("sharps"), syringes, soiled dressings, sponges, drapes and surgical gloves will generate the majority of potentially infectious waste. Potentially infectious waste (other than sharps) will be double bagged in biohazard bags, autoclaved if possible and stored in a secure area until disposed of ashore.

(2) Used sharps will be collected in an approved "sharps" container and retained on board for disposal ashore. "Sharps" will not be clipped. Needles will not be recapped.

(3) An adequate supply of storage and disposal material (containers, bags, etc.), must be maintained on board to ensure availability even on a long or unexpected deployment.

(4) A medical bio-hazardous waste log must be establish and maintained, and must be kept on file for a period of 5 years. A medical bio-hazardous waste log must include the following information:

(a) Date of entry.

(b) Type of waste.

(c) Amount (in weight or volume).

(d) Storage location.

(e) Method of disposal.

(f) Identification number (if required by the state regulating authority). If such a number is required, the authority will provide it.

(5) Non-infectious waste includes disposable medical supplies that do not fall into hazardous waste. Non-infectious waste will be treated as general waste and does not require autoclaving or special handling. It should be placed into an appropriate receptacle and discarded with other general waste.

6. Health Services Department Administration.

   a. Required Reports, Logs, and Records. Clear, accurate record keeping is of paramount importance for the IDHS. The quality of care provided to the unit's crew is reflected in the thoroughness of record and log entries completed by the IDHS. During compliance inspections, Tailored Annual Cutter Training and customer assistance visits, the IDHS and the unit will be evaluated at least in part on the accuracy and completeness of the reports and records created and maintained by the IDHS. The following records will be maintained in the Health Services Department. They will be in book/log form and in sufficient detail to serve as a complete and historical record for actions, incidents and data.

   (1) Health Services Log. A Health Services Department log will be maintained by the IDHS. This log is a legal document. Entries will be clearly written in a concise, professional manner. The log may be either hand written or prepared using a standard workstation but must be kept on file in "hard copy" form. It is used to document the daily operation of the Health Services Department. Chapter 1. Section B. of this Manual provides the requirement for this log. At a minimum, it will contain the names of all individuals reporting to sickcall for treatment, inspections, inventories conducted, and the results of potable water testing. The log will be signed daily by the IDHS. It is worth noting that the Health Services Log will provide the information used in the Binnacle List (see required reports in this Chapter and Chapter 4 of this Manual), so a complete record containing information required in the binnacle list as well as other information of interest will streamline preparation of the report. All protected health information in the log must be kept private and secure in compliance with HIPAA.

   (a) Training Log. See "Training" in this chapter.

(b) Potable Water Quality Log. This log will document the date, location and results of free available Chlorine residual or Bromine testing and bacteriological testing. Such logs will be maintained in chronological order, record the date and time of test, type of test, collection site, and results of testing. Potable water quality logs must be kept onboard for 2 years. A sample Potable Water Quality Log is available for local reproduction in Chapter 1, Appendix 1.A of the Water Supply and Wastewater Disposal Manual, COMDTINST M6240.5 (series).

(c) Biohazard Waste Log. This log will contain information as provided in Chapter 13 of this Manual.

(d) Health Records. Health records will be maintained and checked for accuracy as outlined as outlined in Chapter 4 of this Manual. A Health Record Receipt Form, NAVMED 6150/7 will be used whenever a Health Record leaves the custody of the IDHS. A quarterly check using the unit's alpha roster will ensure that any oversight is identified in a reasonably timely manner. All records checked out and not returned shall be reported to the command. In the event of Abandon Ship, make necessary arrangements to retrieve health records, if possible. Retrieving health records will be secondary to treating and evacuating casualties.

(2) Required Reports. Numerous reports are required at various intervals. A brief explanation along with a reference is provided for those not mentioned elsewhere in this chapter. Additionally, the information is provided in tabular format at the end of this section.

(a) Binnacle List. The binnacle list is normally a part of the Health Services Department Log. It is a listing of the names of the members provided treatment and the duty status determination resulting from the treatment. The list must be kept daily and submitted to the command for review as directed by the CO. It is normally reviewed each week by the XO and signed by the CO.

(b) Injury Reports. See paragraph 8. of this section.

(c) Disease Alert Reports. See Chapter 7 Section B. of this Manual for requirements.

(d) Inpatient Hospitalization Report. See Chapter 2 Section A. of this Manual.

(e) Food Service Sanitation Inspection Report. See the Food Service Sanitation Manual, COMDTINST M6240.4 (series) and paragraph 10.a. (2) of this chapter.

(f) Potable Water Quality Discrepancy Report. Required by chapter 1-K.6 of the Water Supply and Wastewater Disposal Manual, COMDTINST M6240.5 (series) when potable water quality fails to meet requirements or is suspect.

Reports Required Weekly

Report Name	Format or Form Required	Reference	Frequency or Date
Binnacle List	locally designed form	COMDTINST M6000.1 (series) Chap 1. Section B.	Compiled daily, submitted weekly (or as directed by command).
Food Service Establishment Inspection Report	CG-5145	COMDTINST M6240.4 (series) Chap 11.	

Reports Required Quarterly

Report Name	Format or Form Required	Reference	Frequency or Date
Controlled Substances Audit Board	Perpetual Inventory of Narcotics, Alcohol and Controlled Drugs, NAVMED 6710/5 and CG5353.	Chapter 10. Section B of this Manual	No later than 5th working day of the month following end of quarter.

Reports Required "As Needed"

Report Name	Format or Form Required	Reference	Frequency or Date
Injury Report for Not Misconduct and In-Line-of-Duty Determination	CG-3822	See paragraph 8 l of this section	As needed. See aragraph 8 l of this section.
Disease Alert Reports	RCN 6000-4	See chapter 7 Section B. of this Manual	As needed
Inpatient Hospitalization Report	Message format	See chapter 2. Section A. of this Manual	As needed
Report of Potential Third Party Liability	CG 4889	COMDTINST 6010.16 (series) and Chapter 11 Section B of this Manual	As needed
Potable Water Quality Discrepancy Report		COMDTINST M6240.5 (series)	when potable water quality fails to meet require-ments or is suspect
Emergency Medical Treatment Report	CG 5214	COMDTINST M16135.4 (series)	As needed

Table 9-A-1

7. Combat Operations.

    a. Battle Dressing Station (BDS). The Health Services Allowance List contains a list of all items required in the BDS and provides information about required frequency of inventory and documentation.

    b. Route and Access Marking to the BDS. On cutters that have a BDS, the routes to the BDS shall be marked in accordance with the Coatings and Color Manual, COMDTINST M10360.3 (series). In general:

        (1) Self adhering Red Cross decals in both photo-luminescene (internal) and nonphoto-luminescene (exterior marking) are authorized.

        (2) When establishing and marking the routes to the various stations throughout the cutter, the markers shall be located frequently enough to enable the person following the route to have a clear view of the next marker of the route to be followed.

            (a) On the interior surfaces of the cutter, the signs shall be placed not less than 12 inches above the deck and no higher than 36 inches above the deck.

            (b) On exterior surfaces, signs shall be placed approximately 60 inches above the deck.

        (3) Label plates with red letters will be installed at each direct access to BDS.

        (4) An adhesive reflective marking system will be used and maintained. The purpose of this system is to provide emergency information during a situation involving the loss of lighting.

    c. Use of BDS. On cutters with separate BDSs, the BDS is not to be used for any purpose other than the treatment of injured personnel in an emergency situation. No items are to be placed in a manner which will block access or restrict use of the BDS.

    d. First Aid Kits, Gun Bags and Portable Medical Lockers.

        (1) Supplies stored in emergency medical kits (first aid kits, gun bags, and portable medical lockers) must be protected from weather and pilferage, and will be maintained as directed in the Health Services Allowance List. An inventory list for each kit will be maintained and a monthly inspection of all first aid kits, gun bags and portable medical lockers will be performed by the IDHS. Each kit will be secured with a wire seal or other anti-pilferage device that will indicate when it has been accessed. Each kit will be inspected for tampering (seal intact). The inspection will be noted in the Health Services Log. Once per quarter, the contents of all first aid kits, gun bags and portable medical lockers will be inventoried. The inspection will be noted in the Health Services Log.

e. <u>Oxygen Cylinders</u>. Ensure that oxygen handling and storage precautions are posted next to all oxygen cylinders onboard the vessel. Oxygen is considered a drug and under no circumstances will oxygen be used for any purpose other than patient care. Oxygen cylinders (for ready use) must have the content level read every morning by the HS in order to ensure readiness in case of an emergency. Empty cylinders will be clearly tagged as empty and stored separately from full cylinders. Oxygen cylinders must be hydrostatically tested every 5 years. Damage Control Department personnel will be a good source of information on where to have Oxygen cylinders refilled or hydrostatically tested. Oxygen for medical use must be grade D.

8. <u>Environmental Health</u>. Environmental health program related activities make up a large percentage of the daily responsibility of the IDHS. The link between environmental health and mission accomplishment cannot be over-emphasized. From a military perspective, environmental health and environmental health related problems accounted for almost eighty percent of personnel losses during past conflicts in which the United States was involved. For the purposes of this chapter, environmental health encompasses the disciplines of preventive medicine, sanitation and occupational health. An effective environmental health program requires the IDHS to have a working knowledge of a large number of unit systems and work processes. An aggressive program of inspection and observation is required. These include:

   a. <u>Environmental Health Inspection</u>. The IDHS will make routine daily messing and berthing space "walk through inspections" and make note of any conditions that require immediate action. These "walk through inspections" should be done in an informal manner but items requiring correction will be brought to the attention of the department head responsible for the berthing area.

   b. <u>Food Service Sanitation</u>. The Food Service Sanitation Manual, COMDTINST M6240.4 (series) provides in-depth information regarding food service sanitation. This section is intended to provide information specific to the duties of an IDHS on an afloat unit. In general, the IDHS will monitor the food service operation to ensure the protection of the crew from food borne illnesses. The duties of the IDHS will include:

      (1) Maintain sanitary oversight of the galley and all food service, preparation, storage and scullery spaces. Such oversight includes stores on-load, storage, preparation, and serving of food; disposal of garbage; proper cleaning and sanitizing of equipment and utensils; personal hygiene of food handlers; proper storage temperature of food products, and the condition and cleanliness of the spaces.

      (2) Food service areas will be inspected weekly and the findings will be reported on a Food Services Establishment Inspection Report, CG-5145.

(3) Conduct an inspection of the subsistence items and food for fitness for human consumption. Ensure that subsistence items were received from sources approved by the U.S. Department of Agriculture (USDA) or an approved source from a foreign port that complies with all laws relating to food and food labeling.

(4) Conduct an initial physical screening of food service personnel for detection of any condition or communicable disease that could result in transmission of disease or food borne illness.

c. Storage of Food Items. Proper storage procedures play a major part in preventing food borne illnesses. The IDHS will make routine inspections of food storage areas to ensure that spaces are properly maintained to prevent supplies from being:

(1) Infested by insects and rodents.

(2) Contaminated by sewage, chemicals, or dirt.

(3) Subsistence items will be inspected by the HS upon receipt to determine food quality and ensure the stores are free from insect or rodent infestation. The results of this inspection will be recorded in the Health Services Log.

d. Coffee Mess. Food consumption, with the exception of coffee and condiments, will be limited to messing areas and lounges. Coffee messes provide a potential food source for insects and rodents if they are not properly located and kept scrupulously clean. For these reasons, permission to establish a coffee mess must be obtained from the Commanding Officer by the department desiring to establish a mess prior to its establishment. Messes will be physically located in a place that can be easily cleaned. Food contact areas (surrounding counter or table tops) must be non porous and kept free of spillage and food debris. Strict sanitary measures are to be used. Coffee mess regulations specifying sanitary operation of the mess will be posted. Use of community cups and spoons are prohibited. Inspection of coffee messes may be documented using a Food Service Sanitation Inspection Report, CG-5145 or through a locally generated inspection report form.

e. Water Supply. Water is used by all members of ship's company and so a tremendous potential exists for ship wide illness should potable water not be properly loaded from sources free from contamination, protected from contamination onboard, and a halogen residual maintained in the potable water tanks and throughout the distribution system. The IDHS will be notified whenever the potable water distribution system is opened for maintenance or repair. Establishment of a working relationship with the ship's engineering company and the "water king" will aid the IDHS in maintaining a proactive stance in regard to prevention of contamination of the vessel's potable water. The IDHS will make a monthly inspection of the potable water system and report conditions with potential to affect the health of the crew to the Commanding Officer.

(1) Halogen Residual Testing. Chlorine/Bromine residual testing will be performed before receiving any water onboard, and also about 30 minutes after an initial halogenation has been accomplished. A water log shall be kept and the results of the daily halogen testing recorded in it. The Color Comparator Test set is used for determining Halogen and pH levels. Nomenclature and ordering information is available in the HSAL. Four test sites should be selected: forward, aft, amidships and as far above the 0-1 deck as possible. This will give the widest range of sample points. Lack of a residual or a residual reading that is significantly lower than results at the other locations indicate possible contamination. Systematic testing from areas with low residuals "backward" to areas with "average" residuals will help locate the source or general area of contamination.

(2) Bacteriological Test of Water. Weekly, a potable water sample for bacteriological analysis will be collected from one of the four test sites selected for halogen residual testing. This includes a sample(s) collected directly from the potable water tanks and potable water retained in storage tanks when under direct service from shorelines. Samples of ice must also be collected from any machines making ice used for human consumption and tested for bacteriological growth. The results of bacteriological testing will be entered into the Potable Water Quality Log.

f. Habitability. The need for sanitary and hygienic living and working spaces is essential for good health and morale of the crew. General guidance on habitability standards can be found in the Safety and Environmental Health Manual COMDTINST M5100.47 (series), 5.D.1. Habitability inspection can most easily be accomplished if it is made a part of the material inspection of all ship's spaces normally scheduled by each command.

g. Barber Shops. Any space used for cutting hair may be designated a barber shop by the command. It will not be located in food service areas or berthing areas. Sanitation inspection of the ship's barber shop will be performed on a schedule determined by the command. General guidance on standards can be found in the, Safety and Environmental Health Manual, COMDTINST M5100.47 (series), 5.D.1.d.(6).

h. Ship's Laundry. Laundry spaces will be maintained in a clean and sanitary condition. Because of the potential for elevated temperature and high humidity within the space when laundry equipment is in operation, the ship's laundry will be identified as a heat stress monitoring space and monitored accordingly. Sanitation inspection of the ship's laundry will be performed on a schedule determined by the command. General guidance on standards can be found in the Safety and Environmental Health Manual

COMDTINST M5100.47 (series), 5.D.1.d.(5).

i. <u>Fitness and Exercise Facilities</u>. The fitness and exercise facility will be inspected for cleanliness and compliance with general sanitation standards on a schedule determined by the command. General guidance on standards can be found in Chapter 2 of Manual of Naval Preventive Medicine, NAVMED P-5010 (series).

j. <u>Insect Control</u>. Roaches, stored product pests, and to a lesser degree flies, can have significant impact on the health and general morale of a ship's company. Insect control starts in the warehouse from which stores are received. When practical, a visit by the IDHS to assess storage conditions can help decrease numbers of pests brought on board. Dockside inspection of all food stores brought on board is a must if insects are to be excluded. Produce with "loose" husks or skin such as onions provide common harborage for roaches as does the corrugation of cardboard boxes. Careful inspection with a good light and adjuncts such as an aerosolized flushing agent can identify harborages from which cans and stores can be removed prior to their being brought aboard. General guidance on standards can be found in the Safety and Environmental Health Manual COMDTINST M5100.47 (series), 5.D.3.

   (1) <u>Roach Control</u>. A ship provides myriad harborages for roaches. Frequent and regular surveillance by the IDHS using a good light and a flushing agent can pinpoint areas of infestation. Roach traps containing pheromones work well in areas with small or isolated infestations. Larger or more widespread areas must be controlled initially with insecticide. Insecticide application will be made only by HSs that hold current certification to apply pesticides. Such personnel have been properly trained in pesticide selection, application, safety and handling precautions. This training is available through Navy Environmental Preventive Medicine Units (NEPMU)s. Pesticide application may be available through Coast Guard Integrated Support Commands with attached Preventive Medicine Technicians. Any insect surveillance activity, general report of findings, or pesticide application, will be reported in the Health Services Log. Pest control services may also be contracted for from civilian pest control firms. Such services are paid for from ships AFC-30 funds and are contracted in the same manner as any other contract for services. While proper selection and application of the materials used is the legal responsibility of the licensed pest control operator, the IDHS must be informed of all applications made. The contractor must provide a report of pest control operations which includes, trade and chemical name of product used, strength and formulation applied, type of application (crack and crevice, etc), location of application. Requirement for such a report will be included in the contract for services. Report of pest control operations will be held on file for 3 years.

(2) Stored Products Pests. A relatively small infestation of flour, grains, beans and cereals with stored products pests can spread quickly and lead to the loss of most or all of such products in a storage area if an infestation is not identified quickly and action taken to control it. In general, such action consists of identifying infested or suspect lots, removing them from storage with other food stuffs with the potential to become infested, and application of pesticide to control flying insects. Underway, control is limited to identification of infested or suspect lots and their removal.

(3) Rodent Control.

  (a) Exclusion is by far the most effective means of rodent control available to the IDHS. Proper installation of rat guards is required on all mooring and service lines when the vessel is in port. Information about proper installation of rat guards can be found in Chapter 8 of the Manual of Naval Preventive Medicine, NAVMED P-5010 (series) and in the Safety and Environmental Health Manual, COMDTINST M5100.47 (series). The IDHS will inspect all mooring and service lines upon arrival in any port, including home port, to verify the proper placement of rat guards on all of the lines.

  (b) In the event that rodents do gain access to the vessel, an aggressive campaign using traps and/or poisoned bait (if the IDHS has been properly trained to apply and use such substances) must be undertaken. Trapping is the preferred method. Assistance may be available from Coast Guard Integrated Support Commands with attached Preventive Medicine Technicians or through the HSWL SC.

  (c) A current deraterization exemption certificate (CDC 75.5(F.4.452)) must be kept onboard at all times. The certificate may be obtained from Coast Guard Integrated Support Commands with attached Preventive Medicine Technician; Navy units or bases with attached Preventive Medicine Technicians or NEPMUs. The deraterization certificate must be renewed every 6 months and must be included as a pre-deployment checklist item.

k. Immunizations and Prophylaxis. The IDHS will ensure that all personnel receive required immunizations in accordance with Immunizations and Chemoprophylaxis, COMDTINST 6230.4 (series). IDHS are only authorized to immunize active duty and reserve personnel. HSWL SC and NEPMUs can provide up to date information on immunization requirements, disease intelligence and preventive medicine precautions required for vessels deploying to OUTCONUS ports.

l. Safety. A ship is a very dangerous place and dangers inherent to the shipboard environment are heightened by worker's lack of attention, short-cuts, "horseplay," inadequate training or understanding of a job or process, fatigue or over-familiarity. The IDHS must remain vigilant in regard to the safety and safe work practices of the crew. A safe work environment can't be maintained from the Health Services Department space. The IDHS must become familiar with the work processes that are on-going and be able to recognize when they are not being done in the proper manner or with the proper materials.

   (1) Mishap Reporting. When accidents or mishaps do occur, certain reports or action may be required. The Safety and Environmental Health Manual, COMDTINST M5100.47 (series) contains requirements and guidance about mishap reporting. Such reports are not normally completed by the IDHS, but input may be required regarding severity of injury and required treatment.

   (2) Accident Reports. The Administrative Investigations Manual, COMDTINST 5830.1 (series) contains a requirement that a Injury Report for Not Misconduct and In-Line-of-Duty Determination, CG-3822 be completed whenever an injury results in temporary or permanent disability. This report is referred to in the Physical Disability Evaluation System, COMDTINST M1850.2 (series) as a "Line of Duty (LOD) Report" and must be completed for all initial medical boards involving or resulting from trauma. Since it is difficult to determine the outcome of a serious injury in the early stages of treatment, a Injury Report For Not Misconduct and In Line of Duty Determination, CG-3822 (also commonly known as an "Accident Report") is usually completed in such cases. It is not necessary to complete an "Accident Report" for any and all injuries unless command policy dictates otherwise.

m. Vessel's Safety Board. The IDHS is a required member of the vessel's Safety Board. The IDHS should strive to be an active participant in the board, to identify potential problems or accident trends and suggest solutions to current or potential safety problems. Be proactive. Educate supervisors whenever possible.

n. Hazard Communication. The Hazard Communication Program is a unit wide program. Each unit will have appointed a Hazardous Materials Control Officer with overall responsibility for carrying out the program. Safety and Environmental Health Manual, COMDTINST M5100.47 (series) and Hazard Communication for Workplace Materials, COMDTINST 6260.21 (series) contain in-depth information about this program. The IDHS must be aware of the program requirements and its impact upon the operation of the Health Services Department. Additionally, the IDHS must know the location of the unit's central MSDS file and have immediate access to product information which may be needed to render proper treatment to exposed crewmembers. Computerized databases available on

CD-ROM are acceptable for this purpose if the Health Services Department contains appropriate access to the information.

o. Heat Stress Program. Cutter Heat Stress Program, COMDTINST M6260.17 (series) provides details about this program. All areas of the vessel that expose crewmembers to extreme heat will have a dry bulb thermometer installed. Such areas normally include (but are not limited to) ship's laundry, scullery and engine room spaces. Wet Bulb Globe Thermometer (WBGT). A WBGT apparatus must be used to determine stay times of personnel working within heat hazardous spaces or areas and so familiarity with this equipment is required. The apparatus is normally operated by the IDHS or member of the engineering department. Recommendations for safe work rest cycles will be provided by the IDHS to the Engineering Watch Officer (EWO). Cutter Heat Stress Program, COMDTINST M6260.17 (series) provides information about the program. The WGBT is listed on the Health Services Allowance List (HSAL) and is procured as health care equipment. A Coast Guard Health Care Equipment Request, CG-5211 should be submitted to the HSWL SC. Current calibration of the ship's WGBT apparatus is a Tailored Annual Cutter Training "critical" item. Delinquent calibration can result in cancellation of some or all TACT drills by the training evaluation team. Contact the HSWL SC for locations to send WGBTs for calibration.

p. Sight Conservation Program. Eye protection and safety should be stressed in the workplace. Safety glasses or goggles will be provided for all crewmembers involved in eye-hazardous tasks. Tools with strong potential for eye hazard will be identified with an adhesive warning label. Fixed machinery with eye hazard potential will have posted nearby an easily visible warning placard, and eye protection will be easily accessible and clearly visible.

q. Eyewash Stations. Eyewash stations will be located in any space or work area with strong potential for splashes to, or foreign body injury of the eye. Eyewash stations will be maintained in accordance with the station's manufacturer requirements. Eyewash stations shall be flushed weekly for 15 seconds and flushed and drained according to the recommendations of the biostat ingredient manufacturer used in the station. This interval is usually every six months. Eyewash stations will be "tagged" with a maintenance record tag and inspection or maintenance activities will be recorded when performed. Inspections of eyewash stations will be recorded in the Health Services Log.

This page intentionally left blank.

COMDTINST M6000.1E

Section B. Independent Duty Ashore at Sectors, Sector Field Offices, Air Stations, and Small Boat Stations

1. Introduction 1
2. Mission and Responsibilities 1
3. Chain of Command 2
4. Operation of the Health Services Division 2
5. Providing Health Care 5
6. Training 9
7. Supply and Logistics 11
8. Health Services Department Administration 17
9. Search and Rescue (SAR) Operations 20
10. Environmental Health 20

This page intentionally left blank.

B. Independent Duty Ashore at Sectors, Sector Field Offices, Air Stations, and Small Boat Stations.

1. Introduction. An Independent Duty Health Services (IDHS) Ashore is a Health Services Technician assigned to an ashore unit such as a Sector, Sector Field Office, Air Station, or Small Boat Station which has no permanently attached Medical Officer. The IDHS's role at an ashore unit is one of tremendous responsibility. It requires superior organizational and networking skills and sound technical knowledge of the Health Services rating. Assignment to independent duty at one of the aforementioned units can be challenging but very rewarding. Along with the increased responsibility comes the potential for great personal satisfaction.

2. Mission and Responsibilities.

    a. Mission. The Health Services Technician serving at an ashore unit is charged with the responsibility for the prevention and control of disease and injury, and the treatment of the sick and injured. It is recognized that IDHSs assigned to an ashore unit are responsible for ensuring personnel assigned to units within their parent command's area of responsibility (AOR) maintain their fitness for duty and medical readiness. This oversight requires the IDHS to work closely with unit Executive Officers (XO)/Executive Petty Officers (XPO) to ensure unit personnel are up to date on medical readiness items such as, immunizations, required lab tests, physical and dental exams and are receiving the necessary medical training in order to perform their jobs.

    b. Responsibilities. The Commanding Officer (CO) is responsible for the health and medical/dental readiness of the unit. In the absence of a permanently assigned Medical Officer (MO), or when no MO is assigned to the unit, the CO will designate a CG officer to have direct responsibility for medical matters. The role of the Independent Health Services Technician (IDHS) is to assist the command in maintaining the good health and medical/dental readiness of the unit and units in their AOR. To accomplish this responsibility, the IDHS must be informed of planned operations and anticipate any operational demands resulting from such operations. To this end, the IDHS will consult and advise the command in all matters with potential to effect unit readiness or the health of personnel. The duties of the IDHS include but are not limited to:

    (1) Assessment and treatment of illness and injury.

    (2) Prevention of illness and injury through an aggressive environmental health program. Such a program includes inspection of living and working spaces as well as food service and storage areas; food storage and handling practices; integrated pest management practices; potable water quality surveillance; and recognition and management of communicable diseases.

(3) Security and proper use of Health Services supplies, material and property.

(4) Supply and logistics to ensure supplies, materials and equipment necessary to carry out the mission of the Health Services Division are obtained and maintained in sufficient quantity and condition to support the unit mission and operation.

(5) Health Services Division administration, maintenance and security of health records.

(6) Maintenance and documentation of medical and dental readiness of personnel at their unit and units within their command's AOR.

(7) Strict adherence to Chapters 1 and 2 of this Manual, which contain information about general and specific duties of the HS serving independently, including all required training on compliance with HIPAA privacy and security.

3. <u>Chain Of Command</u>. The IDHS will report directly to the Executive Officer (XO).

4. <u>Operation of the Health Services Division</u>. The IDHS Ashore Health Services Division is classified as a 1-D (ashore) sickbay. The unit may request a waiver from maintaining the full allowance list. This request will be routed to the assigned Designated Medical Officer advisor (DMOA) for approval. The IDHS is tasked with a wide variety and high volume of duties and responsibilities. This section sets forth policy and guidelines designed to assist the IDHS in carrying out assigned duties and responsibilities.

   a. <u>Health Services Division Standard Operating Procedure</u>. In order to successfully manage the Health Services Division, the IDHS must use time management and organizational skills and tools. One such tool is a written Standard Operating Procedure (SOP) for the Health Services Division. The SOP will govern the activities of the IDHS, and has as its guiding precept, the goals and missions of the unit. The SOP will be developed and submitted in written form to the CO for approval via the chain of command. In addition, the SOP will be reviewed, updated to reflect current policies and procedures and signed at least annually by the IDHS, DMOA, XO and CO. The approved SOP will be kept in the Health Services Division for easy referral. Copies of pertinent sections will be posted as appropriate. The SOP will include:

      (1) A copy of the IDHS's letter of assumption of duties as Health Services Division Representative.

      (2) A copy of the IDHS's prescribing formulary approved by the DMOA.

      (3) A written daily schedule of events for both on base and deployed periods.

(4) Copies of all letters of designation, assignment, and authority that directly impact upon the IDHS or Health Services Division. Examples include those granting " By direction" authority, designation as working Narcotics and Controlled Substances custodian, written certification to provide immunizations (see Chapter 7 Section C) and assignment of a DMOA.

(5) A copy of the unit's organizational structure. This document will show graphically the IDHS's chain of command.

(6) A listing of duties and responsibilities assigned to the IDHS and the frequency that they are to be carried out. The listing will include both primary and collateral assigned duties.

(7) A listing of all required reports, the format required for submission, the frequency or date required, required routing and required "copy addressees". Incorporation of this information in tabular format provides a quick and easy guide for reference purposes.

(8) Guidance on how any change in a member's duty status is relayed from the member through the IDHS to the XO.

(9) A unit instruction or SOP section for the management of sexual assault cases. The document must provide policy for Health Services Division action in such cases; names of organizations, points of contact and telephone numbers for local resources as well as contact information for agencies and facilities which must be notified. It must contain directions on how to complete a Victim Reporting Preference Statement, CG-6095. Additionally, it must define the unrestricted and restricted reporting procedures as outlined in the Sexual Assault Prevention and Response Program (SAPRP), COMDTINST 1754.10 (series).

(10) A unit instruction or SOP section for the management of suicide threat or attempt. The document must provide policy for Health Services Division action in such cases, names of organizations, points of contact and telephone numbers for local resources, contact information for agencies and facilities which must be notified as well as a listing of required information, reports or actions.

(11) A unit instruction or SOP section for the management of family violence. The document must provide policy for Health Services Division action in such cases, names of organizations, points of contact and telephone numbers for local resources, contact information for agencies and facilities which must be notified as well as a listing of required information, reports or actions.

b. <u>Departure from the Daily Schedule of Events</u>. The day-to-day operation of the Health Services Department is complex and has the potential to be impacted by the operational needs of the unit. It will, of necessity, change when events of higher priority or concern occur. When deviation from the daily schedule of events is required, notifying the chain of command will be made at the earliest opportunity. When deviation from the daily schedule of events occurs frequently, the daily schedule of events will be reviewed and if necessary, changed. Any changes will be incorporated into the Health Services Division SOP and approved by the Commanding Officer.

c. Relief and Assumption of Duties as the IDHS. Proper documentation of the status of the Health Services Division and the condition of its equipment, stores, and records is required at the time of relief and assumption of the duties and responsibilities as the IDHS. The process is complex and requires both the incoming and outgoing IDHS to jointly perform the following:

(1) A complete inventory of all medical stores, spaces, and equipment, including durable medical equipment. Health Services Allowance List, Ashore COMDTINST M6700.5 (series) provides a listing of supplies and the equipment required.

(a) A controlled substances inventory must be done. Use direction provided in Chapter 10 of this Manual.

(b) A complete inventory of all unit property in custody of the Health Services Division if the IDHS is the custodian of the property.

(2) A review of ongoing actions affecting the status of the Health Services Division such as, outstanding requisitions, survey or repairs, and proper documentation of all such transactions.

(3) A review of the Health Services Division SOP.

(4) A review of the most recent HSWL SC Quality Improvement Survey for the unit. A copy of the survey annotated with any finding of incomplete or uncorrected discrepancies will be included as an enclosure to the letter of relief.

(5) An account and review of all health records for completeness, accuracy, privacy and security.

d. Letter of Relief and Assumption of Duties. Upon completion of the Health Services Division review, a memorandum will be prepared and submitted by the incoming IDHS via the chain of command and will advise the Commanding Officer of the status of the Health Services Division. A copy of the letter will be forwarded to the HSWL SC. The letter of Relief and Assumption of Duties will provide the following:

(1) Date of assumption of duties; a statement that the duties and responsibilities of the IDHS have been assumed; and a statement that a thorough review of the Health Services Division has been conducted. Any discrepancies of material or record keeping will be annotated on a copy of the unit's most recent HSWL SC Quality Improvement Survey

and submitted as an enclosure to the letter of Relief and Assumption of Duties as IDHS.

    (2) Any discrepancies noted upon relief will be handled as a matter of individual command prerogative. Responsibility for correction, adjustment of account or inventory records, action required to replace missing items, as well as any necessary disciplinary action will be determined by the command.

    (3) In cases in which no "on site" relief occurs, all of the preceding action will be completed. The supply officer of the unit will participate in the review process in place of the outgoing IDHS.

  e. Actions upon Proper Relief. Upon assumption of duties as the unit's IDHS, one of the first tasks to complete is a thorough review of all SOPs and department instructions. A check of the references should be accomplished in order to ensure established point of contacts for the local area are verified and updated as needed. If possible, make visits and introductions in person. The IDHS must find out how each system works and how it is accessed.

5. Providing Health Care. Delivery of health care is undoubtedly the most challenging and rewarding part of the job of any IDHS. The IDHS assigned to an ashore unit will face the challenges of determining when to deliver care to patients and when it is necessary for he/she to refer patients to a higher level of care at a local health care facility (military or civilian). At times, the IDHS will be called upon to assist his/her command or a unit in his/her command's AOR in determining a member's fitness for duty. This section is intended to provide a brief summary of the various facets of providing this medical care.

  a. Designated Medical Officer Advisor (DMOA). Each IDHS ashore shall be assigned a physician DMOA in accordance with Chapter 1 of this Manual. Good communication between the IDHS and DMOA can prevent many problems affecting health care delivery to personnel. The IDHS shall schedule a visit to the DMOA as soon as is practical after reporting to their unit or upon completion of IDHS school. The purpose of the visit is to allow first-hand communication between the DMOA and IDHS on expectations, support facility requirements, and any unique needs or concerns. This visit will normally be scheduled for a period of at least two weeks. This time frame will allow for the DMOA to evaluate the IDHS's performance factors and qualifications, and to develop a formulary for the IDHS. Open communication should be maintained through regular site visits when practical, or at minimum, regular telephone calls. With regard to provision of direct care, the IDHS will seek his DMOA's or another Medical Officer's (MO) advice whenever there are questions about a patient's condition or when the following conditions exist:

    (1) Return to sick call before assigned follow-up because of failure to improve or condition has deteriorated.

(2) Member cannot return to full duty status after 72 hours duration because of unresolved illness or injury.

The IDHS should contact the Flight Surgeon on call through the closest Coast Guard Command Center when any of the following emergency conditions exist:

(1) Undetermined fever of 102 degrees Fahrenheit or higher (when taken orally) persisting for 48 hours.

(2) Fever of 103 degrees Fahrenheit or higher (when taken orally).

(3) Unexplained pulse rate above 120 beats per minute.

(4) Unexplained respiratory rate above 28 breaths per minute or less than 12 breaths per minute.

(5) Depression with or without suicidal thoughts.

(6) Change in mental status.

(7) Chest pain or arrhythmia.

(8) Unexplained shortness of breath.

(9) Rape or sexual assault.

b. Gender Considerations. Chapter 1.Section B of this Manual provides specific direction for health services technicians about patient privacy, same gender attendant requirements, and examination restrictions.

c. Avoiding Common Problems. Scheduling and obtaining the routine medical care required by personnel can tax the organizational skills of even the most experienced IDHS. There are, however, actions that the IDHS can take which will enhance the chances of getting the routine appointments needed for all members. Some of these are:

(1) Identify the routine medical and dental needs of unit personnel. The IDHS's supporting Coast Guard (CG) clinic, Department of Defense Medical Treatment Facility (DoD MTF) or civilian primary care manager have established appointment scheduling procedures which the IDHS must work within whenever time allows. Follow the requirements for scheduling all appointments. When routine medical or dental care is to be made directly to a DoD MTF, the IDHS must determine the facility's requirements for referral of patients and follow any local procedures.

(2) Communicate with the supporting clinic often. Discuss the unit's medical and dental needs with the clinic supervisor and DMOA (if located at the facility).

(3) Perform all preliminary tests and complete all necessary paperwork before scheduling physical exams at the supporting clinic.

(4) Post a listing of appointment dates and times as soon as they become available. Provide each Department/Division Chief with a listing of the appointments applicable to their division or shop.

(5) Hold members accountable for being at their appointed place and time. Provide feedback to division officers and shop chiefs on appointment failures. Notify the XO or XPO if members fail to show for more than one appointment.

d. Consultations. During the management of complex or protracted cases, consultations or specialty referral may be necessary. When such services are needed, the IDHS will normally make referral to a CG clinic, or in some cases, a DoD MTF. When referring a patient to see a Medical Officer at a CG clinic, the IDHS shall ensure that a Chronological Record of Care, SF-600 entry is completed using the SOAP format and that an appointment is scheduled. The clinic will normally provide treatment or arrange care if treatment is beyond its scope. When consultations or referral for specialty care are made directly to a DoD MTF, the IDHS must determine the facility requirements for referral of patients and follow any local procedures. Referrals to a DoD MTF will normally be documented using a Consultation Sheet, SF-513 or a Referral for Civilian Medical Care, DD-2161. The consultation will provide a concise history of the condition to be evaluated as well as any pertinent findings. A provisional diagnosis is normally expected by the consultant. Chapter 4 Section B. of this Manual provides direction on completion of a Consultation Sheet, SF-513. The patient and the patient's supervisor must be informed of all consultation or referral appointment dates and times. Professional courtesy is an important part of maintaining good working relationships with the facilities that the IDHS accesses for consultation and referral. Timely notification to the referral facility when appointment changes or cancellations occur (along with a brief explanation of why the change is required) helps maintain those relationships. Whenever possible, provide at least 24 hours notice for changes or cancellations.

e. Antibiotic Therapy. The IDHS may prescribe and administer antibiotics included on the Health Services Allowance List. Whenever possible, the IDHS shall consult with their DMOA or other Medical Officer for a recommendation or concurrence prior to administering antibiotic therapy. If consultation is not possible prior to administration, electronic notification, via email or message, must be sent to the DMOA providing case history, ICD9CM code and treatment provided.

f. Health Services Division Treatment Space. The Health Services Division treatment space will be manned at all times when patients are inside. All items are to be stowed in their proper place and secured. All medical records shall be locked in a cabinet. At no time should the Health Services space be left unlocked when the IDHS is not in the space.

g. Convalescent Leave/Sick Leave. Convalescent leave/Sick leave is a period of leave not charged against a member's leave account. It can be a recommendation to the command when a patient is Not Fit For Duty (usually for a duration expected to be greater than 72 hours) and whose recovery time can reasonably be expected to improve by freedom from the confines of quarters. It should be considered only when required as an adjunct to patient treatment. The command must evaluate each recommendation. Commands are authorized to grant convalescent leave as outlined in Chapter 7 of the Personnel Manual, COMDTINST M1000.6 (series).

h. Dental. The IDHS is responsible for arranging for the necessary dental examinations of unit personnel. All personnel must receive an annual dental exam and the results must be documented in DENCAS. See Chapter 2 of this Manual for guidance on obtaining dental services from contract dental providers.

i. Sexual Assault. All victims of sexual assault must be treated in a professional, compassionate and non-judgmental manner. The unit shall have an SOP for dealing with reported cases of sexual assault. Refer to the Sexual Assault Prevention and Response Program (SAPRP), COMDTINST 1754.10 (series) for further guidance.

j. Suicide Prevention. An encounter with a suicidal person is always a deeply emotional event. It is important for the IDHS to act in a caring and professional manner. Early intervention and good communication skills are essential. If suicidal ideation is suspected it is important to remember:

   (1) Take all threats and symptoms seriously. Immediately seek professional help from the nearest MTF or local health care facility for any member considering suicide. At no time should the person be left unattended. Once the patient is safe, contact the servicing Work-Life office for additional help or refer to Suicide Prevention COMDTINST 1734.1 (series).

   (2) Actively listen to the patient. Do not argue, judge, attempt to diagnose, or analyze the person's true intentions. It is important to provide a calm, caring, professional demeanor throughout the entire situation. Thoroughly document the patient encounter using the SOAP format.

   (3) Arrange for an escort and a driver to transport the patient to the nearest CG clinic, DoD MTF or civilian emergency room with facilities appropriate to the situation. The unit's SOP for suicide threat or attempt should contain this information for ready use if needed.

k. Decedent Affairs. Chapter 5 of this Manual contains guidance about action that the Health Services Division must take when there is a death of a CG member. Chapter 11 of the Personnel Manual, COMDTINST M1000.6 (series) contains further guidance concerning casualties and decedent affairs, as does the Decedent Affairs Guide, COMDTINST M1770.1 (series). It is unlikely that the IDHS will be assigned as the Casualty Assistance Calls Officer (CACO) for the command, but the IDHS will undoubtedly be heavily involved with the process of proper disposition of remains, so familiarity with the information required is helpful. The IDHS should also perform the following:

(1) Make an entry in the Health Services Log will be made detailing all available information concerning the death.

(2) Terminate the deceased member's health record in accordance with Chapter 4 of this Manual.

l. Disposition of Remains. As soon as possible, remains will be transferred to the nearest Military Treatment Facility (MTF) for further disposition. When transfer cannot be accomplished immediately, the remains will be placed into a body pouch and refrigerated at a temperature of 36 to 40 degrees Fahrenheit to prevent decomposition. The space must contain no other items and must be cleaned and disinfected before reuse. Remains will be identified with a waterproof tag, marked with waterproof ink, and affixed with wire ties to the right great toe of the decedent and also to each end of the body pouch. The minimum information needed on each tag includes the full name, SSN and rate or rank of the decedent. Whenever possible, do not remove items attached to the deceased at time of death. Such items may include (for example) IV lines, needles, lengths of cord or line, etc. These may be important during an autopsy. Additionally, do not discard or launder clothing of the deceased. These items are sometimes important to surviving family members and in some cultures is part of the mourning process for the deceased. This is a cultural consideration but should be a part of the decision process.

m. Physical Disability Evaluation System. The medical board process is detailed in Chapter 17.A. of the Personnel Manual, COMDTINST M1000.6 (series) and the Physical Disability Evaluation System, COMDTINST M1850.2 (series).

6. Training. The purpose of training for both the assigned IDHS and that provided to the unit includes: assurance that the IDHS and crewmembers are able to provide aid for themselves and their shipmates in an emergency situation and to promote the general health and well being of the unit.

a. Training for the IDHS. In addition to the requirements of the rate, the ashore IDHS must complete certain "C" schools. These are:

(1) CG Independent Duty Health Services Technician, Air Force Medical Services Craftsman or Navy Surface Forces Independent Duty Technician.

(2) CG Introduction to Environmental Health or Navy Basic Shipboard Series. (Note: This is not required for graduates of Navy Surface

Forces Independent Duty Technician or Independent Duty Health Services Technician School).

- (3) Emergency Medical Technician – Basic Level. IDHS are required to maintain currency with the National Registry of Emergency Medical Technicians (NREMT) at the Basic level. Short Term Training Requests are to be completed in accordance with the Training and Education Manual, COMDTINST M1500.10 (series) and forwarded to Commandant (CG-1121). Funding will be provided by Commandant (CG-11). See the Emergency Medical Services Manual, COMDTINST M16135.4 (series) for additional information.

- (4) Instructor courses (Must maintain current certification in) CPR, BLS, AED and First Responder.

- (5) Field Management of Chemical and Biological Casualties. The Field Management of Chemical and Biological Casualties Course (FCBC) is conducted by the US Army Medical Research Institute of Chemical Defense (USAMRICD) at Aberdeen Proving Ground, Maryland. Classroom instruction, laboratory and field exercises prepare graduates to become trainers in the first echelon management of chemical and biological agent casualties.

b. Health Services Department Training Plan. A plan for training of unit personnel will be established in written form and kept on file. It will be based on a minimum 12 month cycle and be included in the unit training schedule. At a minimum, the following training will be given:

- (1) Basic first aid (to include shock, hemorrhage control, dressing, airway management and assisted ventilation and the use of items in first aid kits).
- (2) Personal and dental hygiene.
- (3) STI/HIV prevention.
- (4) Heat and cold stress programs, including hypothermia.
- (5) Respiratory protection program.
- (6) Hearing conservation.
- (7) Sight conservation.
- (8) Blood borne pathogens.

c. Documentation of Training. Documentation of the training is a requirement. An outline must be prepared and kept on file for all training topics presented and a training log maintained for all training provided. The training log will contain a record of all HS training given to unit personnel. It will contain the following information:

- (1) Date.

(2) Topic.

(3) Duration.

(4) Instructor's name.

(5) Names and signatures of members attending training.

d. Training Format. Training will normally be presented in either lecture format or demonstration and practical application. Lecture format presentations should be limited to 15 to 20 minutes and demonstrations and practical application should not exceed 1 hour. Practical application must be of high priority in training unit personnel in first aid, casualty evaluation, and treatment. There is no substitute for "hands on" practice in developing effective first aid skills.

7. Supply And Logistics.

   a. Custody of Health Services Equipment and Material. As directed by the Commanding Officer, the IDHS is responsible and accountable for the health services material onboard the unit. As such, the IDHS is the custodian of all health service equipment and material. The custodian will not permit waste or abuse of supplies or equipment and will use techniques such as stock rotation, planned replacement and preventive maintenance to minimize waste of resources.

   b. Inventory. An accurate record of medical stores and equipment must be maintained. The inventory of medical stores, spaces and equipment will be prepared using the Stock Record Card Afloat, NAVSUP-1114 or in line item form (computerized database is an approved and preferred alternative if all necessary information is captured) and include:

      (1) Quantity and shelf-life of each item currently on board.

      (2) Balance on hand, high-level, low-level (reorder point for each item).

      (3) Manufacturer, lot number and expiration date (pharmaceuticals).

      (4) Quantity placed on order, date received.

   c. Unit Property. Unit property in Health Services Department custody must also be safeguarded and accounted for. The unit property custodian should be contacted before transfer or destruction of such property.

   d. Funding and Account Record Keeping. Funds used to purchase supplies and equipment, and to pay for the various expenses of operating the unit are broken down into Allotment Fund Control code (AFC) expenditure categories. This method allows for efficient budgeting and accounting. Fund categories generally used by IDHSs fall within the AFC subhead 30 or 57 expenditure categories.

(1) AFC-30 is a general unit fund used by the supply department to purchase generally needed operating supplies and services. Examples include pens, paper, books, training aids, etc. AFC-30 funding can be used to pay for Health Services Department supplies and equipment not obtainable through Defense Supply Center Philadelphia Prime Vendor Program (via the unit's supporting clinic) or the major medical equipment request process (see Chapters 6 and 8 of this Manual). Restrictions exist on what may be purchased with AFC-30 funds. Unit supply personnel can answer specific questions.

(2) AFC-57 is a funding category used to purchase health care related supplies and equipment, and to pay for health care. AFC-57 funds are distributed to the HSWL SC and further allocated by them to the units within their areas of responsibility with IDHSs assigned.

(3) With the full implementation of the Prime Vendor programs for Pharmaceuticals and for Medical and Surgical Supplies, AFC-57 fund allocations will be made to the Prime Vendor ordering point assigned for the unit.

e. <u>Budgets and Budgeting</u>. In general, IDHSs do not need to plan and submit an AFC-57 budget request because medical supplies and equipment funding are controlled by the HSWL SC and Prime Vendor ordering points. If additional AFC-57 resource needs are anticipated, the IDHS's supporting clinic should be contacted for direction on how the resources are to be requested. The budget build process does have value for the IDHS however. AFC-30 funds will need to be planned for and requested from your unit. Medical equipment in need of replacement costing less than $500.00 must be requested from the supporting clinic. Medical equipment in need of replacement costing $500.00 or more must be requested from the HSWL SC via a Health Care Equipment Request, CG-5211. The budget build process is a good way to handle these needs. AFC-30 fund budget planning is relatively straight forward, although it can be time consuming. AFC-30 expenditures for Health Services should be broken into general use categories. Examples of categories are books and publications, non-consumable goods and services such as hydro testing and replacement of oxygen cylinders, and travel for continuing education. Budgeting categories can be as simple or complicated as the IDHS desires to make it. Once categories have been established, a ledger for the Health Services Division should be "opened" and the expenditure categories entered into it. The use of a "spreadsheet" program is an efficient way to keep an accounting record, but a ledger book works just as well. Attention to detail is the key. In general, a system using four to five categories works well.

(1) In preparing a budget for the upcoming year, it is important to look back over what was purchased in the previous year. To do this, collect all records of AFC-30 orders and expenditures. Review each line item and record the amount spent into the appropriate budget category. The

steps for preparing a budget and carrying it out along with general timelines are contained in this paragraph. They are:

March	Look back process. Review amount of funds spent over the first two quarters of the fiscal year as well as spending patterns for the previous fiscal year. Note general categories on which funds were spent and in which quarter items were ordered. This will allow projection of quarterly funding needs into the upcoming year.
April/May	Review status of the Health Services Division medical library and determine which texts and references must be updated. Review status of HS certifications and continuing medical education. Funding for training, conferences or seminars not normally funded by AFC-56 funds must be budgeted for as AFC 30 budget line items. Review preventive maintenance records and include cost projections in AFC-30 budget. Prepare and submit CG 5211s for medical equipment to be replaced. Seek guidance from XO on known or planned activities outside normal operations.
June	Submit finalized budget proposal through chain of command. AFC 30 budget information will be added to the unit budget. Be prepared to "defend" the budget request submitted. Documentation of the data gathering process and retrieval of the raw data used to justify the funding requested will likely be required. AFC-56 funds requests will be consolidated by the command and forwarded to the unit's district, HSWL SC or Area commander, as appropriate.

Table 9-B-1

    (2) Careful stewardship, good record keeping and accounting make existing funding and justification for increased funding levels easier.

f. <u>Obtaining Pharmaceuticals, Medical and Surgical Supplies</u>. Chapter 8 of this Manual provides policy applicable to the management of Health Services supplies. Prime Vendor programs for both Pharmaceuticals and

Medical/Surgical Supplies have been established and it is through these programs that essentially all pharmaceuticals and supplies will be obtained. Medical Prime Vendor Program Implementation within the Coast Guard, COMDTINST M6740.2 (series) provides detailed instruction about this program. From an IDHS's perspective important aspects of the program include:

(1) Each unit has been assigned a Prime Vendor ordering point for Pharmaceuticals and for Medical/Surgical Supplies. The HSWL SC assigns the POCs and periodically updates the information. The Prime Vendor ordering point may be different for each of the programs.

(2) Funding for both Prime Vendor for Pharmaceuticals and Prime Vendor for Medical/Surgical Supplies is provided to the assigned Prime Vendor ordering point by the HSWL SC. Internal accounting procedures vary among Prime Vendor ordering points. Some have established individual "accounts" for the units they are responsible for while others manage funds from a central account. Regardless of the accounting method used by the Prime Vendor ordering point, the IDHS must establish and maintain a system to track expenditures.

(3) Prime Vendor ordering points establish pharmaceutical and medical/surgical supply ordering procedures for their assigned units. Pharmaceutical and medical supply items ordered will be those required by the Health Services Allowance List (HSAL) in quantities required for the unit type. Deviation from the HSAL requirements will normally occur only after justification of the need is made by the IDHS to the DMOA for the unit. It will be made in writing and kept on file for review during HSWL SC site surveys.

g. Health Services Supporting Clinic. The supporting clinic is the IDHS's partner in providing health care for the crew. Local agreements and resources may be available to allow the supporting clinic to provide a broader range of services to the IDHS and the crew but at a minimum, the following will be provided.

(1) All supplies and equipment (under $500.00) listed in the HSAL for the type of unit and on the HS Core Formulary. The unit no longer receives AFC-57 funding for the operation of the Health Services Division. These funds are provided instead to the supporting clinic with the intent that the supporting clinic will provide all required items for the IDHS to operate the Health Services Division.

(2) Assign the IDHS a DMOA in writing. The DMOA shall be available for questions about patient care, as well as completing record reviews quarterly.

(3) Perform medical boards for the IDHS unit as necessary.

(4) Provide a resource for advice and support in all administrative areas of health care delivery to include medical administration, physical

examination review (within the approving authority of the Clinic Administrator), health benefits, medical billing and bill payment processing assistance, dental care, pharmacy administration, supply and logistics, bio-medical waste management, IDHS continuing education, and quality assurance support. Any services provided at the clinic shall be extended to the IDHS to the maximum extent possible.

h. Preventive Maintenance of Health Services Equipment. Chapter 8 Section D of this Manual details the preventive maintenance program for Health Services equipment. An important part of medical equipment readiness is a program of preventive maintenance and planned equipment replacement. Repair and routine replacement part costs should be recorded on side B of NAVMED 6700/3CG, Medical/Dental Equipment Maintenance Record. Capture of this data will allow more accurate forecasting of AFC-30 funding needs for preventive maintenance.

i. Replacement of Health Care Equipment. Chapter 8 Section D of this Manual provides direction on how to obtain replacement of health care equipment. An effectively managed planned equipment replacement program minimizes repair costs and avoids loss of critical equipment at unscheduled times. Additionally, used but still serviceable equipment can be used by other facilities by "turn-in and reissue" through the Defense Reutilization Management Office (DRMO). At least annually, normally during the budgeting process, review the preventive maintenance costs for each piece of health care equipment. When repair and maintenance costs for the year exceed 50 percent of the current replacement cost of the equipment, then a CG-5211, U. S. Coast Guard Health Care Equipment Request should be submitted to the HSWL SC, through the supporting clinic, requesting replacement.

j. Disposal of Unserviceable or Outdated Medical Material.

   (1) Equipment and Supplies. Property Management Manual, COMDTINST M4500.5 (series) provides guidance on when a formal survey is required. In general, a formal survey is not required except when equipment has been lost or stolen. If uncertain about whether or not a formal survey should be done, the unit's supply officer should be consulted.

   (2) Pharmaceuticals and Medicinals. Destruction of pharmaceuticals and medicinals will rarely be required. When disposal is necessary it must be done in accordance with federal, state, and local laws as well as applicable CG policy, if any (e.g. AVIP, SVP).

      (a) Prime Vendors provide a partial credit for some materials returned to them. IDHSs and supporting clinics will establish local policy for transfer of expired or short shelf-life pharmaceuticals. A transfer and replacement of pharmaceuticals within 6 months of expiration should be made with the supporting clinic to minimize waste.

 (b) If destruction is required, it will be accomplished in a well-ventilated area. Liquid substances present potential exposure through splash back. At a minimum, splash proof goggles and neoprene rubber gloves will be worn when working with liquid substances that may be absorbed through the skin. The wearing of protective equipment such as a splash apron is also encouraged. Thorough hand washing after the destruction process must be accomplished. Medical material must be disposed of in a manner so as to ensure that the material is rendered non-recoverable for use and harmless to the environment. Destruction must be complete, to preclude the use of any portion of a pharmaceutical. Chapter 8 Section C of this Manual provides detailed information about destruction and disposal of unsuitable medications.

k. <u>Disposal of Medical Waste</u>. Federal regulation defines how medical waste must be stored and disposed of, and the records that must be kept to document the storage and disposal. The information in the following paragraphs is provided as a general explanation of program requirements rather than an in-depth instruction on handling of medical waste. Medical waste must be classed in one of two categories: potentially infectious or non-infectious waste. In-depth guidance about storage, disposal and required record keeping for medical waste can be found in Chapter 13 of this Manual, in Quality Improvement Implementation Guide (QIIG) 16, and in Chapter 5 of the Safety and Environmental Health Manual, COMDTINST M5100.47 (series). An additional source of information is the unit's hazardous material control officer. In general, the disposal and record keeping requirements for the waste depend on the category of the waste:

 (1) Potentially infectious waste is defined as an agent that may contain pathogens that may cause disease in a susceptible host. Used needles, scalpel blades, ("sharps"), syringes, soiled dressings, sponges, drapes and surgical gloves will generate the majority of potentially infectious waste. Potentially infectious waste (other than sharps) will be double bagged in biohazard bags, autoclaved if possible and stored in a secure area until disposed of.

 (2) Used sharps will be collected in an autoclavable "sharps" container. "Sharps" will not be clipped. Needles will not be recapped.

 (3) An adequate supply of storage and disposal material (containers, bags, etc.) must be maintained to ensure availability even on a long or unexpected deployment.

 (4) A medical bio-hazardous waste log must be established and maintained, and must be kept on file for a period of 5 years. The

medical bio-hazardous waste log must include the following information:

    (a) Date of entry.

    (b) Type of waste.

    (c) Amount (in weight or volume).

    (d) Storage location.

    (e) Method of disposal.

    (f) Identification number (if required by the state regulating authority). If such a number is required, the authority will provide it.

(5) Non-infectious waste includes disposable medical supplies that do not fall into hazardous waste. Non-infectious waste will be treated as general waste and does not require autoclaving or special handling. It should be placed into an appropriate receptacle and discarded with other general waste.

8. <u>Health Services Department Administration</u>.

   a. <u>Required Reports, Logs, and Records</u>. Clear, accurate record keeping is of paramount importance for the IDHS. The quality of care provided to the unit's crew is reflected in the thoroughness of record and log entries completed by the IDHS. During compliance inspections and customer assistance visits, the IDHS and the unit will be evaluated at least in part on the accuracy and completeness of the reports and records created and maintained by the IDHS. The following records will be maintained in the Health Services Division. They will be in book/log form and in sufficient detail, to serve as a complete and permanent historical record for actions, incidents and data.

     (1) <u>Health Services Log</u>. A Health Services Division log will be maintained by the IDHS. This log is a legal document. Entries will be clearly written in a concise, professional manner. The log may be either hand written or prepared using a typewriter or word processor but must be kept on file in "hard copy" form. It is used to document the daily operation of the Health Services Division. Chapter 1.Section B. of this Manual provides the requirement for this log. At a minimum, it will contain the names of all individuals reporting to sickcall for treatment, inspections, inventories conducted, and the results of potable water testing (if required). The log will be signed daily by the IDHS. It is worth noting that the Health Services Log will provide the information used in the Binnacle List (see required reports in this Chapter and Chapter 6 of this Manual), so a complete record containing

information required in the binnacle list as well as other information of interest will streamline preparation of the report. All protected health information in the log must be kept private and secure in compliance with the Health Insurance Portability and Accountability Act of 1996 (HIPAA).

(a) Training Log. See "Training" in this chapter.

(b) Biohazard waste log. This log will contain information as provided in Chapter 13 of this Manual.

(c) Health Records. Health records will be maintained and checked for accuracy and completeness as outlined in Chapter 4 of this Manual. The NAVMED 6150/7, Health Record Receipt Form will be used whenever a Health Record leaves the custody of the IDHS. A quarterly check using the unit's alpha roster will ensure that any oversight is identified in a reasonably timely manner. All records checked out and not returned shall be reported to the command. No health record is to be taken to the field. If necessary for deployment, a battle record will be made up consisting of the following at a minimum:

1. One Chronological Record of Care, SF-600.

2. A copy of the Medical Readiness Reporting system printout of Immunization and Medical Readiness records

3. A copy of the Adult Preventive and Chronic Care Flow Sheet, DD-2766.

(2) Required reports. Numerous reports are required at various intervals. A brief explanation along with a reference is provided for those not mentioned elsewhere in this chapter. Additionally, the information is provided in tabular format at the end of this section.

(a) Binnacle List. The binnacle list is normally a part of the Health Services Department Log. It is a listing of the names of the members provided treatment and the duty status determination resulting from the treatment. The list must be kept daily and submitted to the command for review as directed by the CO. It is normally reviewed each week by the XO and signed by the CO.

(b) Disease Alert Reports. See Chapter 7 of this Manual for requirements.

(c) Inpatient Hospitalization Report. See Chapter 2 Section A. of this Manual.

(d) <u>Food Service Sanitation Inspection Report</u>. (Required for units with food service facilities) See the Food Service Sanitation Manual and paragraph A.10.a.(2) of this chapter.

(e) Potable Water Quality Discrepancy Report (when not using a community based water source) required by Water Supply and Wastewater Disposal Manual, COMDTINST M6240.5 (series) Chapter 2.N.2 when potable water quality fails to meet requirements or is suspect.

Reports Required Weekly

Report Name	Format or Form Required	Reference	Frequency or Date
Binnacle List	Locally designed form	COMDTINST M6000.1 (series) Chap 1. Section B.	Compiled daily, submitted weekly (or as directed by command).
Food Service Establishment Inspection Report	CG 5145	COMDTINST M6240.4 (series) Chap 11.	

Table 9-B-2

Reports Required Quarterly

Report Name	Format or Form Required	Reference	Frequency or Date
Controlled Substances Audit Board	Perpetual Inventory of Narcotics, Alcohol and Controlled Drugs, NAVMED 6710/5	Chapter 10.B. of this Manual	5th working day of the month

Table 9-B-3

Reports Required "As Needed"

Report Name	Format or Form Required	Reference	Frequency or Date
Injury Report for Not Misconduct and In-Line-of-Duty Determination	CG-3822	See paragraph 10.c of this section.	As needed. See paragaph 9.c of this chapter
Disease Alert Reports	RCN 6000-4	See Chapter 7. Section B. of this Manual	As needed
Inpatient Hospitalization E-Mail	E-mail	See Chapter 2. Section A. of this Manual	As needed
Report of Potential Third Party Liability	CG-4889	COMDTINST 6010.16 (series) and chapter 6 of this Manual	As needed
Potable Water Quality Discrepancy Report	COMDTINST M6240.5 (series)		when potable water quality fails to meet requirements or is suspect
Emergency Medical Treatment Report	CG-5214	COMDTINST M16135.4 (series)	As needed

Table 9-B-4

9. <u>Search and Rescue (SAR) Operations</u>. In order for SAR units to provide the necessary level of medical support during SAR operations, COs must ensure personnel are trained to provide lifesaving measures in adverse and austere environments. The IDHS ashore may be called upon to play an integral role in the training and certification of unit personnel in first aid and cardiopulmonary-nary resuscitation (CPR). IDHSs who are certified as a First Aid and CPR Instructor by one of the following organizations: American Red Cross, National Safety Council, or American Safety and Health Institute have the ability to positively impact local units by providing the required medical training to boat crewmembers {Note: Personnel who serve as boat crewmembers aboard CG small boats are required to be certified in First Aid and CPR by one of the aforementioned organizations in accordance with the Boat Crew Seamanship Manual, COMDTINST M16114.5 (series) and the U.S. Coast Guard Boat Operations and Training (BOAT) Manual, Volume II, COMDTINST M16114.33 (series).

10. <u>Environmental Health</u>. Environmental health program related activities make up a large percentage of the daily responsibility of the IDHS. The link between environmental health and mission accomplishment cannot be over-emphasized.

From a military perspective, environmental health and environmental health related problems accounted for almost eighty percent of personnel losses during past conflicts in which the United States was involved. For the purposes of this chapter, environmental health encompasses the disciplines of preventive medicine, sanitation and occupational health.

a. <u>Environmental Health Program Components</u>. An effective environmental health program requires the IDHS to have a working knowledge of a large number of unit systems and work processes. An aggressive program of inspection and observation is required. These include:

   (1) Environmental Health Inspection.

   (2) Immunizations and Prophylaxis. The IDHS will ensure that all personnel receive required immunizations in accordance with Immunizations and Chemoprophylaxis, COMDTINST 6230.4 (series) and other relevant Commandant policy. Commandant (CG-1121), HSWL SC, and NEPMUs can provide up to date information on immunization requirements, disease intelligence, and preventive medicine precautions required for vessels deploying to OCONUS ports.

b. <u>Safety</u>. The IDHS must become familiar with the work processes that are on-going at the unit and be able to recognize when they are not being performed in the proper manner or with the proper materials. The IDHS should report any safety related findings to the unit Safety Officer.

c. <u>Accident Reports</u>. The Administrative Investigations Manual, COMDTINST M5830.1 (series) contains a requirement that a CG-3822, Injury Report for Not Misconduct and In-Line-of-Duty Determination be completed whenever an injury results in temporary or permanent disability. This report is referred to in the Physical Disability Evaluation System, COMDTINST M1850.2 (series) as an "Line of Duty (LOD) Report" and a requirement is made that it be completed for all initial medical boards involving or resulting from trauma. Since it is difficult to determine the outcome of a serious injury in the early stages of treatment, a CG-3822, Injury Report for Not Misconduct and In-Line-of-Duty Determination (also commonly known as an "Accident Report") is usually completed in such cases. It is not necessary to complete an "Accident Report" for any and all injuries unless command policy dictates otherwise.

d. <u>Hazard Communication</u>. The Hazard Communication Program is a unit wide program. Each unit will have appointed a Hazardous Materials Control Officer with overall responsibility for carrying out the program. Safety and Environmental Health Manual, COMDTINST M5100.47 (series) and Hazard Communication for Workplace Materials, COMDTINST 6260.21 (series) contain in-depth information about this program. The IDHS must be aware of the program requirements and its impact on the operation of the Health Services Division. Additionally, the IDHS must know the location of the unit's central MSDS file and have immediate access to product information which may be needed to render proper treatment to exposed crewmembers. Computerized databases available on CD-ROM are acceptable for this purpose if the Health Services Division contains appropriate access to the information.

Section C. Independent Duty in Support of Deployable Specialized Forces (DSF)

1. Introduction. 1
2. Mission and Responsibilities. 1
3. Chain of Command. 2
4. Operation of the Health Services Department. 2
5. Providing Health Care 5
6. Training. 10
7. Supply and Logistics. 12
8. Health Services Department Administration. 18
9. Tactical Operations. 21
10. Environmental Health. 21

This page intentionally left blank.

C. **Independent Duty in Support of Deployable Specialized Forces.**

1. **Introduction.** The Deployable Specialized Forces (DSF) provides waterborne and a modest level of shoreside antiterrorism force protection for strategic shipping, high interest vessels, and critical infrastructure. DSFs are a quick response force capable of rapid, nationwide and international deployment via air, ground or sea transportation in response to changing threat conditions and evolving Maritime Homeland Security (MHLS) mission requirements. An assignment to one of these units requires additional knowledge, skills, and physical abilities beyond that of a general duty Health Services Technician (HS) as the DSF may be deployed to areas that pose a great hazard from armed conflict and Weapons of Mass Destruction (WMD) agents (nuclear, chemical, and biological) as well as specific health care needs due to lack of local medical support. Along with the increased responsibility comes the potential for great personal satisfaction.

2. **Mission and Responsibilities.**

    a. **Mission.** The Health Services Technician serving with a DSF is charged with the responsibility for ensuring the personnel of the DSF are qualified for deployment. They will provide routine independent duty level medical care plus WMD knowledge and treatment of traumatic (e.g. gunshot) wounds if deployed with the team. It is recognized that HSs assigned to DSFs may participate in the same basic tactical training as non-HS DSF unit members, thus necessitating close coordination between the Executive Officer (XO) and Designated Medical Officer Advisor (DMOA) to ensure that both medical and tactical training needs are met.

    b. **Responsibilities.** The Commanding Officer (CO) is responsible for the health and medical/dental readiness of the crew of the unit. In the absence of a permanently assigned Medical Officer (MO), the DSF's CO will designate the Executive Officer (XO) to have direct responsibility for medical matters when no medical officer is assigned to the unit. The role of the Independent Health Services Technician (IDHS) is to assist the command in maintaining the good health and medical/dental readiness of the crew. To accomplish this responsibility, the IDHS must be informed of planned operations and anticipate any operational demands resulting from such operations. To this end, the IDHS will consult and advise the command in all matters with potential to effect crew readiness or the health of personnel. Some of the duties of the IDHS include:

    c. Assessment and treatment of illness and injury.

    d. Prevention of illness and injury through an aggressive environmental health program. Such a program includes inspection of living and working spaces as well as food service and storage areas; food storage and handling practices; integrated pest management practices; potable water quality surveillance; and recognition and management of communicable diseases.

e. Train DSF personnel in the Coast Guard's Tactical Combat Casualty Care Self-Aid / Buddy-Aid program or any other medical training to meet the mission of the unit.

f. Security and proper use of Health Services supplies, material and property.

g. Supply and logistics to ensure supplies, materials and equipment necessary to carry out the mission of the Health Services Department are obtained and maintained in sufficient quantity and condition to support the unit mission and operation.

h. Health Services Department administration, maintenance and security of health records.

i. Maintenance and documentation of medical and dental readiness of unit personnel.

j. Strict adherence to Chapters 1 and 2 of this Manual, which contain information about general and specific duties of the HS serving independently, including all required training on compliance with HIPAA privacy and security.

3. Chain Of Command. The IDHS will normally be assigned to the Administrative Department and will report directly to the XO.

4. Operation of the Health Services Department. The DSF Health Services Department is classified as a 1-D (ashore) sickbay. The unit may request a waiver from maintaining the full allowance list. This request will be routed through the assigned DMOA to the HSWL SC for approval. The IDHS is tasked with a wide variety and high volume of duties and responsibilities. This section sets forth policy and guidelines designed to assist the IDHS in carrying out assigned duties and responsibilities.

   a. Health Services Department Standard Operating Procedure. In order to successfully manage the Health Services Department, the IDHS must use time management and organizational skills and tools. One such tool is a written Standard Operating Procedure (SOP) for the Health Services Department. The SOP will govern the activity of the IDHS and has as its guiding precept the goals and missions of the unit. The SOP will be developed and submitted in written form to the CO for approval via the chain of command. In addition, the SOP will be reviewed at least annually by the IDHS, DMOA, XO and CO. The approved SOP will be kept in the Health Services Department for easy referral. Copies of pertinent sections will be posted as appropriate. The SOP will include:

      (1) A copy of the IDHS's letter of assumption of duties as Health Services Department Representative.

      (2) A copy of the HSs prescribing formulary approved by the DMOA.

(3) A written daily schedule of events for both on base and deployed periods.

(4) Copies of all letters of designation, assignment, and authority that directly impact upon the IDHS or Health Services Department. Examples include those granting "By direction" authority, designation as working Narcotics and Controlled Substances custodian, written certification to provide immunization (see Chapter 7 Section C) and assignment of a DMOA.

(5) A copy of the unit's organizational structure. This document will show graphically the IDHS's chain of command.

(6) A listing of duties and responsibilities assigned to the IDHS and the frequency that they are to be carried out. The listing will include both primary and collateral assigned duties.

(7) A listing of all required reports, the format required for submission, the frequency or date required, required routing and required "copy addressees". Incorporation of this information in tabular format provides a quick and easy guide for reference purposes.

(8) Guidance on how any change in a member's duty status is relayed from the member through the HS to the XO.

(9) A unit instruction or SOP for the management of rape or sexual assault cases. The document must provide policy for Health Services Department action in such cases, names of organizations, points of contact and telephone numbers for local resources as well as contact information for agencies and facilities which must be notified. CGIS must be notified on all cases of alleged rape or sexual assault. It must contain a prearranged mechanism for timely completion of a physical examination for the purpose of evidence gathering that meets requirements of all applicable law enforcement agencies. Additionally, it must define limitations that will exist if the unit is deployed at the time the incident occurs.

(10) A unit instruction or SOP for the management of suicide threat or attempt. The document must provide policy for Health Services Department action in such cases, names of organizations, points of contact and telephone numbers for local resources, contact information for agencies and facilities which must be notified as well as a listing of required information, reports or actions.

(11) A unit instruction or SOP action required in the event of family violence. The document must provide policy for Health Services Department action in such cases, names of organizations, points of contact and telephone numbers for local resources, contact information for agencies and facilities which must be notified as well as a listing of required information, reports or actions.

b. <u>Departure from the Daily Schedule of Events</u>. The day-to-day operation of the Health Services Department is complex and impacted upon by the operational needs of the unit. It will of necessity change when events of higher priority or concern occur. If deviation from the daily schedule of events is required, notification to the chain of command will be made at the earliest opportunity. When deviation from daily schedule of events occurs frequently, the daily schedule of events will be reviewed and if necessary, changed. Any changes will be incorporated into the Health Services Department SOP and approved by the Commanding Officer.

c. <u>Relief and Assumption of Duties as the IDHS</u>. Proper documentation of the status of the Health Services Department and the condition of its equipment, stores, and records is required at the time of relief and assumption of the duties and responsibilities as the IDHS. The process is complex and requires both the incoming and outgoing IDHS to jointly perform the following:

   (1) A complete inventory of all medical stores, spaces, and equipment, including durable medical equipment. The Health Services Allowance List, Ashore COMDTINST M6700.5 (series) provides a listing of supplies and the equipment required.

      (a) A controlled substances inventory must be done. Use direction provided in Chapter 10 of this Manual.

      (b) A complete inventory of all unit property in custody of the Health Services Department if the HS is the custodian of the property.

   (2) A review of ongoing actions affecting the status of Health Services, e.g., outstanding requisitions, survey or repairs, and proper documentation of all such transactions.

   (3) A review of the Health Services Department SOP.

   (4) A review of the most recent HSWL SC Quality Improvement Assistance and Deployable Operations Group Ready for Operations Surveys for the unit. A copy of the surveys annotated with any finding of incomplete or uncorrected discrepancies will be included as an enclosure to the letter of relief.

   (5) A review of all health records for completeness, accuracy, privacy and security.

d. <u>Letter of Relief and Assumption of Duties</u>. Upon completion of the Health Services Department review, a memorandum will be prepared and submitted by the oncoming IDHS via the chain of command and will advise the Commanding Officer of the status of the Health Services Department. A copy of the letter will be forwarded to the HSWL SC. The letter of Relief and Assumption of Duties will provide the following:

(1) Date of assumption of duties; a statement that the duties and responsibilities of the IDHS have been assumed; and a statement that a thorough review of the Health Services Department has been conducted. Any discrepancies of material or record keeping will be annotated on a copy of the unit's most recent HSWL SC Quality Improvement site survey and submitted as an enclosure to the letter of Relief and Assumption of Duties as IDHS.

(2) Any discrepancies noted upon relief will be handled as a matter of individual command prerogative. Responsibility for correction, adjustment of account or inventory records, action required to replace missing items, as well as any necessary disciplinary action will be determined by the command.

(3) In cases in which no "on site" relief occurs, all of the preceding action will be completed. The supply officer of the unit will participate in the review process in place of the outgoing IDHS.

e. Actions upon Proper Relief. Upon assumption of duties as the unit's IDHS, one of the first tasks to complete is a thorough review of all SOPs and department instructions. Check the references; make contact with any listed points of contact. If possible, make visits and introductions in person. Find out how each system works and how it is accessed.

5. Providing Health Care. Delivery of health care is undoubtedly the most challenging and rewarding part of the job of any IDHS. The IDHS assigned to a DSF will have the challenges of having to deliver this care, at times, in remote locations during deployments as well as ensuring that any medical condition is evaluated to determine a member's status for deployment. This section is intended to provide a brief summary of the various facets of providing this medical care.

a. Designated Medical Officer Advisor (DMOA). Each DSF HS shall be assigned a physician DMOA. in accordance with Chapter 1 of this Manual. Good communication between the IDHS and the unit DMOA can prevent many problems affecting health care delivery to the crew. The IDHS will schedule a visit to the DMOA as soon as is practical after reporting aboard or upon completion of IDHS training. The purpose of the visit is to allow first-hand communication of expectations, support facility requirements, and any unique needs or concerns. This visit will normally be scheduled for a period of at least two weeks. This will allow the time required for the DMOA to evaluate the HS's performance factors and qualifications, and to develop a formulary for the HS. Open communication can be maintained through regular visits when practical, or at minimum, regular telephone calls. With regard to provision of direct care, the IDHS will seek DMOA or another MO's advice whenever there are questions about a patient's condition or when the following conditions exist:

(1) Return to sick call before assigned follow-up because of failure to

improve or condition has deteriorated.

    (2) Member cannot return to full duty status after 72 hours duration because of unresolved illness or injury.

    (3) The IDHS shall contact the Flight Surgeon on call through the closest Coast Guard Command Center when any of the following emergency conditions exist:

    (1) Undetermined fever of 102 degrees Fahrenheit or higher (when taken orally) persisting for 48 hours.

    (2) Fever of 103 degrees Fahrenheit or higher (when taken orally).

    (3) Unexplained pulse rate above 120 beats per minute.

    (4) Unexplained respiratory rate above 28 breaths per minute or less than 12 breaths per minute.

    (5) Depression with or without suicidal thoughts.

    (6) Change in mental status.

    (7) Chest pain or arrhythmia.

    (8) Unexplained shortness of breath.

    (9) Rape or sexual assault.

b. <u>Gender Considerations</u>. Chapter 1 Section B of this Manual provides specific direction for health services technicians about patient privacy, same gender attendant requirements, and examination restrictions.

c. <u>Avoiding Common Problems</u>. Scheduling and obtaining the routine medical care needed by crewmembers during non-deployed times can tax the organizational skills of even the most experienced IDHS. There are, however, actions that the IDHS can take which will enhance the chances of getting the routine appointments needed for all members. Some of these are:

    (1) Identify the routine medical and dental needs of the crew. The DSF's supporting clinic has an established appointment scheduling procedure within which the IDHS must work whenever operational schedules allow. Follow the supporting clinics requirements for scheduling all appointments. When routine medical or dental care is to be made directly at a DoD MTF, the IDHS must determine the facility requirements for referral of patients and follow any local procedures.

    (2) Communicate with the supporting clinic. Discuss the crew's medical and dental needs with the clinic supervisor and DMOA (if located at the facility).

    (3) Perform all preliminary tests and complete all necessary paperwork before scheduling physicals at the supporting clinic.

    (4) Post a listing of appointment dates and times as soon as it becomes

available. Provide each Department/Division Chief a listing of the appointments applicable to the division or shop.

    (5) Hold members accountable to be at their appointed place and time. Provide feedback to division officers and shop chiefs on any appointment failure. Notify XO of more than one failure.

d. <u>Consultations</u>. During the management of complex or protracted cases, consultations or specialty referral may be necessary. When such services are needed, the IDHS will normally make referral to a Coast Guard clinic, or in some cases, a Department of Defense medical treatment facility (DoD MTF). When referring a patient to see a Medical Officer at a CG health services clinic, the IDHS shall ensure that a SF-600, Chronological Record of Care entry is completed using the SOAP format and that an appointment is scheduled. The clinic will normally provide treatment or arrange care if treatment is beyond its scope. When consultations or referral for specialty care are made directly to a DoD MTF, the IDHS must determine the facility requirements for referral of patients and follow any local procedures. Referrals to a DoD MTF will normally be documented using an SF-513, Consultation Sheet or a DD-2161, Referral for Civilian Medical Care. The consultation will provide a concise history of the condition to be evaluated as well as any pertinent findings. A provisional diagnosis is normally expected by the consultant. Chapter 4 Section B of this Manual provides direction on completion of a SF 513, Consultation Sheet. The patient and the patient's supervisor must be informed of all consultation or referral appointment dates and times. Courtesy is an important part of maintaining good working relationships with the facilities that the independent duty HS accesses for consultation and referral. Timely notification to the referral facility when appointment changes or cancellations occur (along with a brief explanation of why the change is required) helps maintain those relationships. Whenever possible, provide at least 24 hours notice for changes or cancellations.

e. <u>Antibiotic Therapy</u>. The IDHS may prescribe and administer antibiotics included on the Health Services Allowance List. The IDHS should consult with their DMOA or other Medical Officer for a recommendation or concurrence prior to administering antibiotic therapy. If consultation is not possible prior to administration, electronic notification, via email or message, must be sent to the DMOA providing case history, ICD9CM code and treatment provided.

f. <u>Health Services Treatment Space</u>. The Health Services treatment space will be manned at all times when patients are inside. All items are to be stowed in their proper place and secured. All medical records shall be locked in a cabinet. At no time should the Health Services space be left unlocked when the IDHS is not in the space.

g. <u>Convalescent Leave/Sick Leave</u>. Convalescent leave/Sick leave is a period of leave not charged against a member's leave account. It can be a recommendation to the command when a patient is Not Fit For Duty (usually for a duration expected to be greater than 72 hours) and whose recovery time can reasonably be expected to improve by freedom from the confines of quarters. It should be considered only when required as an adjunct to patient treatment. The command must evaluate each recommendation. Commands are authorized to grant convalescent leave as outlined in Chapter 7 of the Personnel Manual, COMDTINST M1000.6 (series).

h. <u>Controlled Substances</u>. Regulations for the handling, storage, and issue of narcotics and controlled substances are found in Chapter 10 of this Manual. The contents of this section are not intended to contradict the guidance provided there. This section serves to amplify policy provided with respect to medicinal narcotics and controlled substances as they pertain to the DSF. Narcotics and controlled substances require special handling. All controlled substances shall be obtained through the unit's collateral duty pharmacy officer.

(1) The CO will designate a commissioned officer as the controlled substances custodian (CSC). The CSC will follow the accounting procedure provided in Chapter 10 of this Manual. The IDHS will normally be assigned as custodian for narcotics and controlled substances working stock. Such assignment must be made in writing.

(2) All issues from working stock will be documented with a properly completed, written prescription. All non-emergent care requires contact with a Medical Officer before dispensing any controlled medication. The Medical Officer's orders will be documented on a prescription and in the patient's health record. The words "By verbal order of" will precede the ordering Medical Officer's initials, last name, time of order, and date of order both on the prescription and in the patient's health record. In the event of a true emergency, a Medical Officer's order is not needed to dispense a controlled substance. Once the emergency situation is over or alleviated, the IDHS will contact a Medical Officer, detail the circumstances and the controlled substances that were administered. Upon concurrence by the Medical Officer, the prescription prepared for the patient will be annotated with the words "By concurrence of" the ordering physician's initials, last name, time of concurrence and date of concurrence.

(3) The XO will countersign all prescriptions prepared by the IDHS prior to issue of any controlled substance or narcotic.

(4) Controlled substances shall be limited to amounts in the Health Services Allowance List for a 1-D unit. If the need exists for the unit to carry additional quantities of controlled substances based on use or potential for operational need, a written request signed by the Commanding Officer will be forwarded to the HSWL SC through the unit's DMOA. The request must include nomenclature, quantity, and

brief justification.

i. Dental. It is the duty of the IDHS to arrange for the necessary dental examinations of the crew. All personnel should be Class I or Class II prior to deployment and all personnel must receive an annual dental exam and results must be documented in DENCAS.

j. Rape or Sexual Assault. All victims of rape or sexual assault must be treated in a professional, compassionate and non-judgmental manner. Examination of rape and sexual assault victims will be limited to only visual examination of any wound or injury and treated according to present standards of care. In all cases, a Medical Officer and CGIS will be contacted for advice. In the event that no Medical Officer is available (deployed), an IDHS may conduct the visual examination. A chaperone of the same gender as the patient will be present if such examination is conducted. All aspects of the patient encounter must be carefully documented. Physical examination to gather evidence of rape or sexual assault is strictly prohibited. The unit shall have a SOP for alleged rape and sexual assault. Refer to Reporting and Responding to Rape and Sexual Assault Allegations, COMDTINST 1754.10 (series).

k. Suicide Prevention. An encounter with a suicidal person is always a deeply emotional event. It is important for the IDHS to act in a caring and professional manner. Early intervention and good communication skills are essential. If suicidal ideation is suspected it is important to remember:

   (1) Take all threats and symptoms seriously. Immediately seek professional help from the nearest MTF for any member considering suicide. At no time should the person be left unattended. Once the patient is safe, contact the servicing Work-Life office for additional help or refer to Suicide Prevention, COMDTINST 1734.1 (series).

   (2) Actively listen to the patient. Do not argue, judge, attempt to diagnose, or analyze the person's true intentions. It is important to provide a calm, caring, professional demeanor throughout the entire situation. Thoroughly document the patient encounter using the SOAP format.

   (3) Arrange for an escort and a driver to transport the patient to the nearest Coast Guard clinic, DoD MTF or civilian emergency room with facilities appropriate to the situation. The unit's SOP for suicide threat or attempt should contain this information for ready use if needed.

l. Decedent Affairs. Chapter 5 of this Manual contains guidance about action that the Health Services Department must take when there is a death of a Coast Guard member. Chapter 11 of the Personnel Manual, COMDTINST M1000.6 (series) contains further guidance concerning casualties and decedent affairs, as does the Decedent Affairs Guide, COMDTINST 1770.1 (series). It is unlikely that the IDHS will be assigned as the Casualty Assistance Calls Officer (CACO) for the command, but the IDHS will undoubtedly be heavily involved with the process of proper disposition of remains, so familiarity with the information required is helpful. The IDHS should also perform the following:

(1) An entry in the Health Services Log will be made detailing all available information concerning the death.

(2) The health record of the deceased member will be terminated in accordance with Chapter 4 of this Manual.

m. Disposition of Remains. As soon as possible, remains will be transferred to the nearest Military Treatment Facility (MTF) for further disposition. When transfer cannot be accomplished immediately, the remains will be placed into a body pouch and refrigerated at a temperature of 36 to 40 degrees Fahrenheit to prevent decomposition. The space must contain no other items and must be cleaned and disinfected before reuse. Remains will be identified with a waterproof tag, marked with waterproof ink, and affixed with wire ties to the right great toe of the decedent and also to each end of the body pouch. The minimum information needed on each tag includes the full name, SSN and rate or rank of the decedent. Whenever possible, do not remove items attached to the deceased at time of death. Such items may include (for example) IV lines, needles, lengths of cord or line, etc. These may be important during an autopsy. Additionally, do not discard or launder clothing of the deceased. These items are sometimes important to surviving family members and in some cultures contribute to the mourning process of the deceased. This is a cultural consideration but should be a part of the decision process.

n. Physical Disability Evaluation System. The medical board process is detailed in Chapter 17.A. of the Personnel Manual, COMDTINST M1000.6 (series) and the Physical Disability Evaluation System, COMDTINST M1850.2 (series).

6. Training. The purpose of training for both the assigned HS and that provided to the crew includes: assurance that the HS and crewmembers are able to provide aid for themselves and their shipmates in an emergency or a tactical/combat situation; and to promote the general health and well being of the crew.

a. Training for the DSF HS. In addition to the requirements of the rate, the support HS will attend all general DSF training required of members of the DSF. In addition to this general DSF training the DSF HSs must successfully complete certain "C" schools is required. These are:

(1) Coast Guard Independent Duty Health Services Technician School, Navy Surface Forces Independent Duty Technician School or the Air Force Medical Services Craftsman School.

(2) Coast Guard Introduction to Environmental Health or Navy Basic Shipboard Series. (Note: This is not required for graduates of the CG IDHS School or Navy Surface Forces Independent Duty Technician).

(3) Emergency Medical Technician - Basic Level. IDHSs assigned to deployable units are required to maintain currency with the National Registry of Emergency Medical Technicians (NREMT) at the Basic level. Short Term Training Requests are to be completed in accordance with the Training and Education Manual, COMDTINST M1500.10 (series) and forwarded to Commandant (CG-1121). Funding will be provided by Commandant (CG-11). See the Emergency Medical Services Manual, COMDTINST M16135.4 (series) for additional information. (This is part of the CG IDHS School).

(4) Tactical Combat Casualty Care Live Tissue Training. The specific course and funding is to be determined. For guidance contact Commandant (CG-1121).

(5) Instructor courses (must maintain current certification in) CPR, BLS, AED and First Responder

(6) Field Management of Chemical and Biological Casualties course. HSs assigned in support of DSFs must complete this training. Funding will be provided by Commandant (CG-1121).

(7) Recognition and Treatment of Dive Injuries. HSs assigned to DSFs that support dive operations must complete this training. Funding will be provided by Commandant (CG-11).

b. <u>Health Services Department Training Plan</u>. A plan for training of the crew will be established in written form and kept on file. It will be based on a minimum 12 month cycle and be included in the unit training schedule. At a minimum, the following training will be given:

(1) Basic first aid.

(2) Shock, hemorrhage control, dressing.

(3) Airway management and assisted ventilation.

(4) Use of items in Individual First Aid Kits.

(5) Personal and dental hygiene.

(6) STI/HIV prevention.

(7) Heat and cold stress programs, including hypothermia.

(8) Respiratory protection program.

(9) Hearing conservation.

(10) Sight conservation.

(11) Blood borne pathogens.

(12) Additionally, at least one member of each boat crew will be trained as a Combat Lifesaver.

c. <u>Documentation of Training</u>. Documentation of the training is a requirement. An outline must be prepared and kept on file for all training topics presented and a training log maintained for all training provided. The training log will contain a record of all HS training given to the crew. It will contain the following information:

(1) Date.

(2) Topic.

(3) Duration.

(4) Instructor's name.

(5) Names (signatures of those present) of members trained.

d. <u>Training Format</u>. Training will normally be presented in either lecture format or demonstration and practical application. Lecture format presentations should be limited to 15 to 20 minutes and demonstrations and practical application should not exceed 1 hour. Practical application must be of high priority in training the crew in first aid, casualty evaluation, and treatment. There is no substitute for "hands on" practice in developing effective first aid skills.

7. <u>Supply And Logistics</u>.

a. <u>Custody of Health Services Equipment and Material</u>. As directed by the Commanding Officer, the IDHS is responsible and accountable for the health services material onboard the unit. As such, the IDHS is the custodian of all health service equipment and material. The custodian will not permit waste or abuse of supplies or equipment and will use techniques such as stock rotation, planned replacement and preventive maintenance to minimize waste of resources.

b. <u>Inventory</u>. An accurate record of medical stores and equipment must be maintained. The inventory of medical stores, spaces and equipment will be prepared using the NAVSUP-1114, Stock Record Card Afloat or in line item form (computerized database such as the IDHS inventory tool is an approved and preferred alternative if all necessary information is captured) and include:

(1) Quantity and shelf-life of each item currently on board.

(2) Balance on hand, high-level, low-level (reorder point for each item).

(3) Manufacturer, lot number and expiration date (pharmaceuticals).

(4) Quantity placed on order, date received.

c. <u>Unit Property</u>. Unit property in Health Services Department custody must also be safeguarded and accounted for. The unit property custodian should be contacted before transfer or destruction of such property.

d. Funding and Account Record Keeping. Funds used to purchase supplies and equipment, and to pay for the various expenses of operating the unit are broken down into Allotment Fund Control code (AFC) expenditure categories. This method allows for efficient budgeting and accounting. Fund categories generally used by IDHSs fall within the AFC subhead 30 or 57 expenditure categories.

   (1) AFC-30 is a general unit fund used by the supply department to purchase generally needed operating supplies and services. Examples include pens, paper, books, training aids, etc. AFC-30 funding can be used to pay for Health Services Department supplies and equipment not obtainable through Defense Supply Center Philadelphia Prime Vendor Program (via the unit's supporting clinic) or the major medical equipment request process (see Chapters 6 and 8 of this Manual). Restrictions exist on what may be purchased with AFC-30 funds. Unit supply personnel can answer specific questions.

   (2) AFC-57 is a funding category used to purchase health care related supplies and equipment, and to pay for health care. AFC-57 funds are distributed to the HSWL SC and further allocated by them to the units within their areas of responsibility with HS's assigned.

   (3) With the full implementation of the Prime Vendor programs for Pharmaceuticals and for Medical and Surgical Supplies, AFC-57 fund allocations will be made to the Prime Vendor ordering point assigned for the unit.

e. Budgets and Budgeting. In general, IDHSs do not need to plan and submit an AFC-57 budget request because medical supplies and equipment funding are controlled by the HSWL SC and Prime Vendor ordering points. If additional AFC-57 resource needs are anticipated, the IDHS's supporting clinic should be contacted for direction on how the resources are to be requested. The budget build process does have value for the IDHS however. AFC-30 funds will need to be planned for and requested and medical equipment in need of planned replacement must be identified and a CG-5211, Health Care Equipment Request submitted. The budget build process is a good way to handle these needs. AFC-30 fund budget planning is relatively straight forward, although it can be time consuming. AFC-30 expenditures for Health Services should be broken into general use categories. Examples of categories are books and publications, non-consumable goods and services such as hydro testing and replacement of oxygen cylinders, and travel for continuing education. Budgeting categories can be as simple or complicated as the IDHS desires to make it. Once categories have been established, a ledger for the Health Services Department should be "opened" and the expenditure categories entered into it. The use of a "spreadsheet" program is an efficient way to keep an accounting record, but a ledger book works just as well. Attention to detail is the key. In general, a system using four to five categories works well.

(1) In preparing a budget for the upcoming year, it is important to look back over what was purchased in the previous year. To do this, collect all records of AFC-30 orders and expenditures. Review each line item and record the amount spent into the appropriate budget category. The steps for preparing a budget and carrying it out along with general timelines are contained in this paragraph. They are:

March	Look back process. Review amount of funds spent over the first two quarters of the fiscal year as well as spending patterns for the previous fiscal year. Note general categories on which funds were spent and in which quarter items were ordered. This will allow projection of quarterly funding needs into the upcoming year.
April/May	Review status of the Health Services Department medical library and determine which texts and references must be updated. Review status of HS certifications and continuing medical education. Funding for training, conferences or seminars not normally funded by AFC-56 funds must be budgeted for as AFC-30 budget line items. Review preventive maintenance records and include cost projections in AFC 30 budget. Prepare and submit CG-5211, Health Care Equipment Request for medical equipment to be replaced. Seek guidance from XO on known or planned activities outside normal operations.
June	Submit finalized budget proposal through chain of command. AFC-30 budget information will be added to the unit budget. Be prepared to "defend" the budget request submitted. Documentation of the data gathering process and retrieval of the raw data used to justify the funding requested will likely be required. AFC-56 funds requests will be consolidated by the command and forwarded to the unit's district, HSWL SC or Area commander, as appropriate.

Table 9-C-1

(2) Careful stewardship, good record keeping and accounting make existing funding and justification for increased funding levels easier.

f. Obtaining Pharmaceuticals, Medical and Surgical Supplies. Chapter 8 of this Manual provides policy applicable to the management of Health Services supplies. Prime Vendor programs for both Pharmaceuticals and Medical/Surgical Supplies have been established and it is through these programs that essentially all pharmaceuticals and supplies will be obtained. Medical Prime Vendor Program Implementation within the Coast Guard, COMDTINST M6740.2 (series) provides detailed instruction about this program. From an IDHS's perspective important aspects of the program include:

(1) Each unit has been assigned a Prime Vendor ordering point for Pharmaceuticals and for Medical/Surgical Supplies. The HSWL SC assigns the POCs and periodically updates the information. The Prime Vendor ordering point may be different for each of the programs.

(2) Funding for both Prime Vendor for Pharmaceuticals and Prime Vendor for Medical/Surgical Supplies is provided to the assigned Prime Vendor ordering point by the HSWL SC. Internal accounting procedures vary among Prime Vendor ordering points. Some have established individual "accounts" for the units they are responsible for while others manage funds from a central account. Regardless of the accounting method used by the Prime Vendor ordering point, the IDHS must establish and maintain a system to track expenditures.

(3) Prime Vendor ordering points establish pharmaceutical and medical/surgical supply ordering procedures for their assigned units. Pharmaceutical and medical supply items ordered will be those required by the Health Services Allowance List (HSAL) in quantities required for the unit type. Deviation from the HSAL requirements will normally occur only after justification of the need is made by the IDHS to the DMOA for the unit. It will be made in writing and kept on file for review during HSWL SC site surveys.

g. Health Services Supporting Clinic. The supporting clinic for a DSF is the IDHS's partner in providing health care for the crew. Local agreements and resources may be available to allow the supporting clinic to provide a broader range of services to the IDHS and the crew but at a minimum, the following will be provided.

(1) All supplies and equipment (under $500.00) listed in the HSAL for the type of unit and on the HS Core Formulary. The unit no longer receives AFC-57 funding for the operation of the Health Services Department. These funds are provided instead to the supporting clinic with the intent that the supporting clinic will provide all required items for the IDHS to operate the Health Services Department.

(2) Assign the IDHS a DMOA in writing. The DMOA shall be available for questions about patient care, as well as completing record reviews

quarterly.

(3) Perform medical boards for the IDHS unit as necessary.

(4) Provide a resource for advice and support in all administrative areas of health care delivery to include medical administration, physical examination review (within the approving authority of the Clinic Administrator), health benefits, medical billing and bill payment processing assistance, dental care, pharmacy administration, supply and logistics, bio-medical waste management, IDHS continuing education, and quality assurance support. Any services provided at the clinic shall be extended to the IDHS to the maximum extent possible.

h. Preventive Maintenance of Health Services Equipment. Chapter 8 Section D of this Manual details the preventive maintenance program for Health Services equipment. An important part of medical equipment readiness is a program of preventive maintenance and planned equipment replacement. Repair and routine replacement part costs should be recorded on side B of NAVMED 6700/3CG, Medical/Dental Equipment Maintenance Record. Capture of this data will allow more accurate forecasting of AFC-30 funding needs for preventive maintenance.

i. Replacement of Health Care Equipment. Chapter 8 Section D of this Manual provides direction on how to obtain replacement of health care equipment. An effectively managed planned equipment replacement program minimizes repair costs and avoids loss of critical equipment at unscheduled times. Additionally, used but still serviceable equipment can be used by other facilities by "turn-in and reissue" through the Defense Reutilization Management Office (DRMO). At least annually, normally during the budgeting process, review the preventive maintenance costs for each piece of health care equipment. When repair and maintenance costs for the year exceed 50 percent of the current replacement cost of the equipment, then a CG-5211, U. S. Coast Guard Health Care Equipment Request should be submitted to the HSWL SC, through the supporting clinic, requesting replacement.

j. Disposal of Unserviceable or Outdated Medical Material.

(1) Equipment and Supplies. Property Management Manual, COMDTINST M4500.5 (series) provides guidance on when a formal survey is required. In general, a formal survey is not required except when equipment has been lost or stolen. If uncertain about whether or not a formal survey should be done, the unit's supply officer should be consulted.

(2) Pharmaceuticals and Medicinals. Destruction of pharmaceuticals and medicinals will rarely be required. When disposal is necessary it must be done in accordance with federal, state, and local laws as well as applicable CG policy, if any (e.g. AVIP, SVP).

(a) Prime Vendors provide a partial credit for some materials returned to them. IDHSs and supporting clinics will establish local policy for transfer of expired or short shelf-life pharmaceuticals. A transfer and replacement of pharmaceuticals within 6 months of expiration should be made with the supporting clinic to minimize waste.

(b) If destruction is required, it will be accomplished in a well-ventilated area. Liquid substances present potential exposure through splash back. At a minimum, splash proof goggles and neoprene rubber gloves will be worn when working with liquid substances that may be absorbed through the skin. The wearing of protective equipment such as a splash apron is also encouraged. Thorough hand washing after the destruction process must be accomplished. Medical material must be disposed of in a manner so as to ensure that the material is rendered non-recoverable for use and harmless to the environment. Destruction must be complete, to preclude the use of any portion of a pharmaceutical. Chapter 8 Section C of this Manual provides detailed information about destruction and disposal of unsuitable medications.

k. Disposal of Medical Waste. Federal regulation defines how medical waste must be stored and disposed of, and the records that must be kept to document the storage and disposal. The information in the following paragraphs is provided as a general explanation of program requirements rather than an in-depth instruction on handling of medical waste. Medical waste must be classed in one of two categories: potentially infectious or non-infectious waste. In-depth guidance about storage, disposal and required record keeping for medical waste can be found in Chapter 13 of this Manual, in Quality Improvement Implementation Guide (QIIG) 16, and in Chapter 5 of the Safety and Environmental Health Manual, COMDTINST M5100.47 (series). An additional source of information is the unit's hazardous material control officer. In general, the disposal and record keeping requirements for the waste depend on the category of the waste:

(1) Potentially infectious waste is defined as an agent that may contain pathogens that may cause disease in a susceptible host. Used needles, scalpel blades, ("sharps"), syringes, soiled dressings, sponges, drapes and surgical gloves will generate the majority of potentially infectious waste. Potentially infectious waste (other than sharps) will be double bagged in biohazard bags, autoclaved if possible and stored in a secure area until disposed of:

(2) Used sharps will be collected in an autoclavable "sharps" container. "Sharps" will not be clipped. Needles will not be recapped.

(3) An adequate supply of storage and disposal material (containers, bags,

etc.) must be maintained to ensure availability even on a long or unexpected deployment.

(4) A medical bio-hazardous waste log must be established and maintained, and must be kept on file for a period of 5 years. A medical bio-hazardous waste log must include the following information:

(a) Date of entry.

(b) Type of waste.

(c) Amount (in weight or volume).

(d) Storage location.

(e) Method of disposal.

(f) Identification number (if required by the state regulating authority). If such a number is required, the authority will provide it.

(5) Non-infectious waste includes disposable medical supplies that do not fall into hazardous waste. Non-infectious waste will be treated as general waste and does not require autoclaving or special handling. It should be placed into an appropriate receptacle and discarded with other general waste.

8. Health Services Department Administration.

a. Required Reports, Logs, and Records. Clear, accurate record keeping is of paramount importance for the IDHS. The quality of care provided to the unit's crew is reflected in the thoroughness of record and log entries completed by the IDHS. During compliance inspections and customer assistance visits, the IDHS and the unit will be evaluated at least in part on the accuracy and completeness of the reports and records created and maintained by the IDHS. The following records will be maintained in the Health Services Department. They will be in book/log form and in sufficient detail, to serve as a complete and permanent historical record for actions, incidents and data.

(1) Health Services Log. A Health Services Department log will be maintained by the IDHS. This log is a legal document. Entries will be clearly written in a concise, professional manner. The log may be either hand written or prepared using a typewriter or word processor but must be kept on file in "hard copy" form. It is used to document the daily operation of the Health Services Department. Chapter 1.Section B of this Manual provides the requirement for this log. At a minimum, it will contain the names of all individuals reporting to sickcall for treatment, inspections, inventories conducted, and the results of potable water testing (if required). The log will be signed daily by the IDHS. It

is worth noting that the Health Services Log will provide the information used in the Binnacle List (see required reports in this Chapter and Chapter 6 of this Manual), so a complete record containing information required in the binnacle list as well as other information of interest will streamline preparation of the report. All protected health information in the log must be kept private and secure in compliance with HIPAA.

(2) Training Log. See "Training" in this chapter.

(3) Biohazard Waste log. This log will contain information as provided in Chapter 13 of this Manual.

(4) Health Records. Health records will be maintained and checked for accuracy and completeness as outlined in Chapter 4 of this Manual. The NAVMED 6150/7, Health Record Receipt Form will be used whenever a Health Record leaves the custody of the IDHS. A quarterly check using the unit's alpha roster will ensure that any oversight is identified in a reasonably timely manner. All records checked out and not returned shall be reported to the command. No H/R is to be taken to the field. If necessary for deployment, a battle record will be made up consisting of the following at a minimum:

(a) One Chronological Record of Care, SF-600

(b) MRRS printout of Immunization and Medical Readiness records,

(c) Copy of completed Adult Preventative and Chronic Care Flowsheet, DD-2766.

b. Required reports. Numerous reports are required at various intervals. A brief explanation along with a reference is provided for those not mentioned elsewhere in this chapter. Additionally, the information is provided in tabular format at the end of this section.

(1) Binnacle List. The binnacle list is normally a part of the Health Services Department Log. It is a listing of the names of the members provided treatment and the duty status determination resulting from the treatment. The list must be kept daily and submitted to the command for review as directed by the CO. It is normally reviewed each week by the XO and signed by the CO.

(2) Disease Alert Reports. See Chapter 7 of this Manual for requirements.

(3) Inpatient Hospitalization Report. See Chapter 2 Section A. of this Manual.

(4) Food Service Sanitation Inspection Report. (Required for units with food service facilities) See the Food Service Sanitation Manual and paragraph A.10.a.(2) of this Chapter.

(5) Potable Water Quality Discrepancy Report (when deployed and not

using a community based water source) required by Water Supply and Wastewater Disposal Manual, COMDTINST M6240.5 (series) Chapter 2.N.2 when potable water quality fails to meet requirements or is suspect.

a. Reports Required Weekly

Report Name	Format or Form Required	Reference	Frequency or Date
Binnacle List	locally designed form	COMDTINST M6000.1 (series) Chap 1. Section B.	Compiled daily, submitted weekly (or as directed by command).
Food Service Establishment Inspection Report	CG-5145	COMDTINST M6240.4 (series) Chap 11.	

Reports Required Quarterly

Report Name	Format or Form Required	Reference	Frequency or Date
Controlled Substances Audit Board	Perpetual Inventory of Narcotics, Alcohol and Controlled Drugs, NAVMED 6710/5	Chapter 10.B. of this Manual	5th working day of the month

Reports Required "As Needed"

Report Name	Format or Form Required	Reference	Frequency or Date
Injury Report for Not Misconduct and In-Line-of-Duty Determination	CG-3822	See paragraph 10.c of this section.	As needed. See paragraph 9.c of this chapter
Disease Alert Reports	RCN 6000-4	See Chapter 7. Section B of this Manual	As needed

Inpatient Hospitalization Report	Message format	See Chapter 2. Section A of this Manual	As needed
Report of Potential Third Party Liability	CG-4889	COMDTINST 6010.16 (series) and chapter 6 of this Manual	As needed
Potable Water Quality Discrepancy Report		COMDTINST M6240.5 (series)	When potable water quality fails to meet requirements or is suspect.
Emergency Medical Treatment Report	CG-5214	COMDTINST M16135.4 (series)	As needed

9. <u>Tactical Operations</u>. In order to provide the necessary level of medical support during tactical operations the HS and assigned DMOA will ensure that each team has personnel trained to provide lifesaving measures in adverse and austere environments. This can be accomplished by training a minimum of one member of each operational team as a Combat Lifesaver. In addition the HS will train each member of the operational team in tactical self/buddy aid including the use of both hemostatic agents in the IFAK. The IDHS must also ensure the Combat Lifesavers maintain profiency in their skills i.e. at least 2 saline locks per month in locations other than antecubital. The HS must also attend all aspects of operational training to ensure that they are prepared to respond with the team in a high threat deployment where the COr feels the threat to the team requires a level of medical training above that of the regular team members.

10. <u>Environmental Health</u>. Environmental health program related activities make up a large percentage of the daily responsibility of the IDHS. The link between environmental health and mission accomplishment cannot be over-emphasized. From a military perspective, environmental health and environmental health related problems accounted for almost eighty percent of personnel losses during past conflicts in which the United States was involved. For the purposes of this chapter, environmental health encompasses the disciplines of preventive medicine, sanitation and occupational health.

    a. <u>Environmental Health Program Components</u>. An effective environmental health program requires the IDHS to have a working knowledge of a large number of unit systems and work processes. An aggressive program of inspection and observation is required. These include:

    (1) Environmental Health Inspection.

    (2) Immunizations and Prophylaxis. The IDHS will ensure that all

personnel receive required immunizations in accordance with Immunizations and Chemoprophylaxis, COMDTINST 6230.4 (series) and other relevant Commandant policy. Commandant (CG-1121), HSWL SC and NEPMUs can provide up to date information on immunization requirements, disease intelligence and preventive medicine precautions required for vessels deploying to OCONUS ports.

b. Safety. The support HS must become familiar with the work processes that are on-going at the DSF and be able to recognize when they are not being done in the proper manner or with the proper materials. The support HS should report any safety related findings to the DSF Safety Officer.

c. Accident Reports. The Administrative Investigations Manual, COMDTINST M5830.1 (series) contains a requirement that a CG-3822, Injury Report for Not Misconduct and In-Line-of-Duty Determination be completed whenever an injury results in temporary or permanent disability. This report is referred to in the Physical Disability Evaluation System, COMDTINST M1850.2 (series) as an "Line of Duty (LOD) Report" and requirement is made that it be completed for all initial medical boards involving or resulting from trauma. Since it is difficult to determine the outcome of a serious injury in the early stages of treatment, a CG-3822, Injury Report for Not Misconduct and In-Line-of-Duty Determination (also commonly known as an "Accident Report") is usually completed in such cases. It is not necessary to complete an "Accident Report" for any and all injuries unless command policy dictates otherwise.

d. Hazard Communication. The Hazard Communication Program is a unit wide program. Each unit will have appointed a Hazardous Materials Control Officer with overall responsibility for carrying out the program. The Safety and Environmental Health Manual, COMDTINST M5100.47 (series) and Hazard Communication for Workplace Materials, COMDTINST 6260.21 (series) contain in-depth information about this program. The IDHS must be aware of the program requirements and its impact upon the operation of the Health Services Department. Additionally, the IDHS must know the location of the unit's central MSDS file and have immediate access to product information which may be needed to render proper treatment to exposed crewmembers. Computerized databases available on CD-ROM are acceptable for this purpose if the Health Services Department contains appropriate access to the information.

Section D. Quality Improvement Compliance Program.

1. Background 1
2. Purpose 1
3. Overview 1
4. Program Elements 1
5. Collaborative Program 2
6. Monitoring the QICP 2
7. Assistance Program 2
8. Responsibility 2
9. QI Compliance Checklist 3
10. Compliance Certification Standards 3
11. Post Survey 4

This page intentionally left blank.

D. Quality Improvement Compliance Program (QICP).

1. Background. The CG established an internal healthcare quality improvement (QI) program in the early 1990s to monitor the quality of healthcare delivered at its clinics and sickbays. The HSWL SC have historically administered the program by conducting QI surveys at each facility on a pre-determined schedule. However, in recent years the CG has moved to an external accreditation for it's clinics, but sickbays are not subject to the accreditation program. The need for a QI program that ensures sickbay compliance with CG specific healthcare issues and health readiness still exists. CG specific QI and operational health readiness issues are monitored by the HSWL SC under the Quality Improvement Compliance Program (QICP).

2. Purpose. The intent of the QICP is to assist with and ensure all Independent Duty Health Services Technicians (IDHS) comply with and maintain CG specific healthcare-related requirements and unit operational health readiness.

3. Overview.

    a. Definitions.

        (1) Operational Readiness. Standards established by the CG that determine whether individual members and units are prepared to meet their assigned missions.

        (2) Quality Improvement. See Chapter 13 Section A.5.a-d.

4. Program Elements. The QICP is designed to monitor healthcare-related QI requirements for sickbays and to ensure units within their area-of-responsibility (AOR) are operationally ready in accordance with CG standards. Elements that are applicable in the QICP for sickbays are:

    a. Unit Demographics

    b. Administration

    c. Record Maintenance

    d. Fiscal and Supply Management

    e. Preventive Maintenance

    f. Health Care Delivery

    g. TRICARE

    h. Professional Education

    i. Pharmacy Services

    j. Environmental Health and Safety

    k. Operational Readiness

5. <u>Collaborative Program</u>. The primary mission of CG sickbays is to maintain the operational health readiness of active duty and reserve personnel by assuring their availability to physically and mentally meet worldwide deployment standards in accordance with the Medical Manual COMDTINST M6000.1 (series). Maintaining a high level of health readiness involves collaboration between providers, commands, clinics, sickbays and the HSWL SC.

6. <u>Monitoring the QICP</u>. The IDHS must review the operational health readiness of active duty/reserve members within their AOR on a regular basis. It is the Command's responsibility to ensure medical and dental readiness of the active duty/reserve members in their AOR. It is the responsibility of the unit Independent Duty Health Services Technician to develop and maintain a plan that ensures optimal health readiness for all active duty/reserve members within the designated AOR in accordance with guidance provided in this instruction. The HSWL SC will review CG-specific QI and operational health readiness issues on a continual basis and provide needed assistance to sickbays to ensure a high level of health readiness. Quality Improvement compliance will be accomplished through HSWL SC assist visits. A post-visit evaluation report will be provided to the unit CO through the Designated Medical Advisor Officer and supporting Clinic Administrator.

7. <u>Assistance Program</u>. The QICP is designed to provide an environment in which QI and operational health readiness of sickbays are monitored on a continuous, versus retroactive, basis. The QICP is an assistance program designed to ensure a high level of care is provided at CG sickbays and that a high level of operational health readiness is maintained. The program assists sickbays in meeting both CG readiness and QI standards.

8. <u>Responsibility</u>.

    a. HSWL SC.

        (1) Ensure the Commandant's Health Care QI Program is executed at the field level.

        (2) Ensure that Independent Duty Health Services Technicians (IDHS's) are performing their duties in strict adherence to this manual.

        (3) Conduct site visits on an appropriate schedule (usually on a two-year cycle) to verify standards compliance and to provide assistance in meeting the expectations of the Quality Improvement Compliance Program.

        (4) Develop and maintain health services support program guides necessary to provide operational guidance for IDHS activities.

        (5) Develop and maintain Quality Improvement Self Assessment Checklists for assist visits.

        (6) Provide technical and professional advice regarding health services to units, as required.

(7) Ensure the IDHS's Operational Integration Form has been filled out and signed by the IDHS and DMOA.

b. Units.

(1) Ensure the unit actively pursues health services standards for independent duty as set forth in this manual and the HSWL SC Quality Improvement Compliance Program.

(2) Develop and maintain a plan that ensures optimal health readiness for all active duty/reserve members within the designated unit AOR in accordance with guidelines provided in this instruction.

(3) Continually monitor all sickbay QA activities by reviewing the HSWL SC QI Checklist.

9. <u>QI Compliance Checklist</u>. The compliance checklist shows QI and/or operational readiness tasks that sickbays must address on a regular basis. The checklist is used to assess compliance with Quality Improvement standards. There are *Basic Elements* and *Key Elements* that hold pre-determined weighted values and will allow the HSWL SC surveyor to assign the appropriate certification based on the compliance level. To view the most current QI Compliance Checklist, go to the following web site in CG Central: <Our CG><Organizational Information><MLCA or MLCP Division><Health and Safety ><KOM Operational Medicine>IDHS QI Checklist (Independent Duty)>.

10. <u>Compliance Certification Standards</u>. Because sickbays are not subject to an external accreditation, continued oversight by the HSWL SC is critical to ensure that IDHS's are performing all duties required of them. This oversight is achieved through site visits every 2 years. HSWL SC will use the Compliance Checklist and evaluate the performance level of each IDHS site. A detailed report will be provided with a summary of any discrepancies or recommendations for improvement. Based on the result, the HSWL SC surveyor will determine the appropriate re-visit rotation as follows:

a. Full Certification: Full certification is obtained by achieving at least ninety percent (90%) for compliance. Sickbays in compliance with at least ninety percent (90%) of the key elements and at least ninety percent (90%) of the basic elements will be fully certified. Full Certification requires no re-visit and the certification is good for 2 years.

b. Provisional Certification: Provisional certification is given when a sickbay's compliance falls below 90%. Sickbays in compliance with at least eight (80%) of the key elements and at least eighty percent (80%) of the basic elements will be provisionally certified. A Provisional Certification requires a re-visit in 6 months or 1 year as determined by the surveyor.

c. Non-Certification: A Non-Certified status is given when a sickbay's compliance falls below 75%. Sickbays falling below 75% compliance will not be certified and require a 3-month follow-up assessment.

11. <u>Post Survey</u>. A detailed report describing all discrepancies and an Executive Summary outlining the findings and recommendations will be provided to the command no later than 30 days following the date of survey. A written plan of corrective action shall be sent to HSWL SC within 30 days of receipt of the survey results. The plan shall be vetted through the assigned DMOA and address all items listed under the Summary of Pertinent Findings.

Section E. Independent Duty Management of TRICARE.

1. Introduction 1
2. Discussion 1
3. Access to Care 1
4. Access to Care Standards 1
5. Enrollment 2
6. Resources 2

This page intentionally left blank.

E. Independent Duty Management of TRICARE.

1. Introduction. Working within the Military Health System (MHS): What is the role of the MHS? To enhance DoD and our Nation's security by providing health support for the full range of military operations and sustaining the health of all those entrusted to our care, which includes all active duty service members (ADSM). The MHS supports the military mission by fostering, protecting, sustaining and restoring health.

2. Discussion. The IDHS needs to be aware of the policies and concepts that surround the Military Health System (MHS). The MHS includes all Department of Defense Military Treatment Facilities (MTF), USCG Clinics, and the civilian network providers contracted by the Managed Care Support Contractors known as TRICARE providers. Additionally Veteran's Administration facilities while not a part of the MHS do allow access to health care for active duty members. Depending on the location of your command you may work with all of these entities in the coordination of primary and specialty health care for your crew. How you choose where you get primary care is outlined in Chapter 2.A.1 of this Manual. (Note section 2.A.1.c. states that "Health care in civilian healthcare facilities for non-emergent conditions is not authorized without HSWL SC approval".) This should state that "Health care in civilian health care facilities other than from the assigned PCM for non-emergent conditions and is not authorized without prior authorization from the PCM through the MTF or TRICARE Managed Care Support Contractor."

3. Access to Care. There are four basic steps that will ensure almost seamless access to health care for your crew.

    a. The first step is simply having a check-in process in place for new arrivals to your unit. Every member should be required to visit your office or sick bay.

    b. Secondly, each member must be properly enrolled to a PCM, either military or civilian, depending on your local policy. It is required by law (32CFR) and DOD/CG policy that all active duty personnel with a permanent duty assignment of 180 days or more to enroll in a TRICARE Prime Program. The enrollment process requires the member to fill out a form and choose a Primary Care Manager (PCM). Enrollment forms can be obtained from your local TRICARE Service Center which typically are co-located with the MTF or can be found online at www.tricare.mil

    c. ADSM are required to get all non-emergent health care from their PCM

    d. ADSM are required to get pre-authorization for specialty care from their PCM.

4. Access to Care Standards. The MHS has specific access standards to care that are important for the IDHS to understand to ensure your ADSM crew is getting the

appropriate care in a timely manner. It is important to note that the access standards for family members and retirees are slightly different. They are as follows:

   a. Urgent care appointment—24 hours or less

   b. Routine appointment—One week or less

   c. Specialty appointment or wellness visits— Within four weeks or 28 days

   d. Travel time may not exceed 60 minutes from work to your PCM office.

   e. You should not have to travel more than one hour from your home for referred specialty care.

   f. If the service is not available at the MTF within the appropriate access standards, you should be referred to a TRICARE network provider if available.

5. Enrollment. Managing your crew's enrollment outside the catchment of a CG or DoD MTF. In this situation your crew will be enrolled into what is known as TRICARE Prime Remote or TPR. It is wise in this case to limit crew's choice to only a few civilian network providers in your area. This helps ease the burden of training civilian providers and their staff on the nuances of the service specific requirements. For example: duty status chits, reporting potential fitness for duty issues, access to health record and readiness information as HIPPA rules are followed and helps keep track of specialty care referrals from the PCM to other civilian providers.

6. Resources. It is important for the IDHS to understand that there are plenty of CG, DOD and TRICARE resources available to assist them with challenges and issues both for the individual as well as systemic concerns with regards to health care.

   a. Beneficiary Counseling and Assistance Coordinator (BCAC). Located at all MTF locations as well at the HSWL SC. For the CG BCAC call 1-800-9-HBAHBA (1-800-942-2422). Their job is to improve customer service and satisfaction, enhance beneficiary education troubleshoot complicated, delayed, and mishandled issues, and respond to phone, e-mail, and written correspondence

   b. Debt Collection Assistance Officer. Located at all MTF locations as well at the HSWL SC. For the CG BCAC call 1-800-9-HBAHBA (1-800-942-2422). Their job is to assist with TRICARE-related collection (debt) problems, assist with negotiations with collection agencies, credit bureaus, and agencies, research the problem and recommend appropriate actions to resolve the problem. Contact DCAO when a collection notice is received.

   c. The Military Medical Support Office (MMSO). MMSO was established to serve as the centralized Service point of contact (SPOC) for customer service and medical case management for all eligible Active Duty military and Reserve component service members within the 50 United States and District of Columbia. MMSO also coordinates all civilian health care services outside of the cognizance of a Military Treatment Facility for TRICARE Prime Remote (TPR). HSWL SC has a detached billet at the CG SPOC and can be reached at 1-888-647-6676, option 7 ext. 6716.

This page intentionally left blank.

COMDTINST M6000.1E

CHAPTER 10

PHARMACY OPERATIONS AND DRUG CONTROL

Section A. Pharmacy Administration.

1. Responsibilities 1
2. Prescribers 4
3. Prescriptions 6
4. Prescribing in the Medical Record 8
5. Signatures 11
6. Dispensing 11
7. Labeling 16
8. Drug Stock 17
9. Credit Return Program (Reverse Distribution Program) 19
10. Pharmacy and Therapeutics Committee 20
11. Figure 10-A-1 Clinic Non-Prescription Medication Program 22

Section B. Controlled Substances.

1. General 1
2. Custody and Controlled Substance Audits 1
3. Drug Enforcement Administration (DEA) Registration 4
4. Reporting Theft or Loss 4
5. Procuring, Storing, Transferring, and Disposing of Controlled Substances 5
6. Prescribing Practices 7

Section C. Forms and Records.

1. General 1
2. Prescription Forms 1
3. Quality Control Forms 2
4. Controlled Drug Forms 2
5. Forms Availability 5

Section D. Drug Dispensing Without a Medical Officer.

1. General 1
2. Child-Resistant Containers 1
3. Controlled Substances 1
4. Formulary 1
5. Non-prescription Medication Program 2

COMDTINST M6000.1E

This page intentionally left blank

Chapter 10 Contents

Section A. Pharmacy Administration.

1. Responsibilities 1
2. Prescribers 4
3. Prescriptions 6
4. Prescribing in the Medical Record 8
5. Signatures 11
6. Dispensing 11
7. Labeling 16
8. Drug Stock 17
9. Credit Return Program (Reverse Distribution Program) 19
10. Pharmacy and Therapeutics Committee 20
11. Figure 10-A-1 Clinic Non-Prescription Medication Program 22

This page intentionally left blank.

COMDTINST M6000.1E

CHAPTER TEN – PHARMACY OPERATIONS AND DRUG CONTROL

Section A. Pharmacy Administration.

1. Responsibilities.

    a. Duties of designated person. The person designated in writing as responsible for the pharmacy is accountable to the Senior Health Services Office (SHSO), or the Executive Officer, for properly storing and dispensing drugs, record keeping, and maintaining a pharmacy policy and procedures manual, including HIPAA complaint privacy and security provisions, and ensuring limited access into the pharmacy during and after hours.

    b. Responsibility. The person in charge of the pharmacy shall acquire, store, compound, and dispense medications according to applicable Federal laws (principally Title 42, United States Code [42 USC] and Title 21, Code of Federal Regulations [21 CFR]) and observe the highest standards of professional practice and established pharmaceutical procedures to ensure the best possible in patient safety and/or patient medication safety practices. This responsibility includes maintaining appropriate inventory and monitoring of expiration dates of all pharmaceuticals. Specific units have been/will be tasked by Commandant (CG-11) to maintain special stocks of pharmaceuticals. Quarterly, all units maintaining pharmaceuticals used for the purpose of anthrax prophylaxis or pandemic influenza prophylaxis are to provide summary data to the HSWL SC Pharmacy Officer to include name(s) of pharmaceutical agent, amount on hand, lot number, and expiration date. The HSWL SC Pharmacy Officer shall maintain this information and provide to Commandant (CG-11) when directed.

    c. Pharmacy references. The person in charge of the pharmacy shall ensure adequate and appropriate current pharmacy references, hardbound and/or online access (e.g., Drug Facts and Comparison, a drug information handbook, a drug interaction reference, a drug identification reference, Sanford Guide to Anitmicrobial Therapy, Mosby's Nursing Drug Reference, a pediatric dosage handbook, a drugs during pregnancy and lactation reference, etc.).

    d. Request funding. Through medical administration, persons responsible for daily pharmacy operations shall request adequate funding to provide the level of pharmaceutical care required in Section 10.A.2.

    e. Senior Health Services Officer (SHSO)/Regional Practice Director (RP DIR). The SHSO/RP DIR shall ensure that all short term, interim, or temporarily assigned pharmacy personnel have successfully completed the Quality Improvement Implementation Guide #41, Pharmacy Watch Stander Qualification Guide (PWQG). In addition, all regular assigned pharmacy personnel shall have completed pharmacy technician "C" school training. These minimum standards of qualifications must be documented in the training file of all pharmacy watch standers. The PWQG does not replace the requirement for "C" school trained pharmacy technicians, but will assist clinic personnel in becoming more productive members of the CG health services team and therefore enhance CG mission support. For clinics without a Pharmacy Officer or "C" School Trained Pharmacy Technician on site, as training tabs permit, units must send a qualified health services technician to pharmacy "C" School or all prescriptions must be double checked by a pharmacy "C" School trained technician or by a privileged medical provider for product and labeling accuracy prior to dispensing. In addition, appropriate patient counseling will be provided prior to the dispensing of medication. Information regarding alternate pharmacy sources, such as Tricare Mail Order Pharmacy, Civilian Retail Pharmacy Network or a Department of Defense Military Treatment Facility will be provided to direct eligible beneficiaries to alternative points of service. Information for enrollment and how the Tricare Mail Order Pharmacy Program operates can be found at www.tricare.mil/mybenefit and clicking on the "prescription" tab found at the top of the page. When providers issue a prescription to be filled at an alternative location, they shall note the medications prescribed in the comments section of the PGUI/POE notation and provide the patient with a written prescription on a DD-1289 or equivalent prescription blank. Prescriptions should not be entered in the "MED" tab of the PGUI as this will prevent the prescription from being filled at an alternative point of service. Clinics will be advised they shall ensure pharmacy technicians receive pharmacy "C" school training in order to provide the highest quality pharmaceutical service and ensure patient and medication safety to our beneficiaries. Facilities are advised the availability of a Pharmacy Officer or a "C" school trained technician is a risk management tool. Many medications have a narrow therapeutic index, especially those for pediatric and elderly patients, placing considerable responsibility upon a non-pharmacy "C" school trained pharmacy technician, the SHSO, the CG Health Care System, and ultimately the safety of the patient.

f. Pharmacy Officer Oversight. Pharmacy Officer collateral duty oversight shall be provided for all clinics and sickbays that do not have Pharmacy Officers assigned. The details of the Pharmacy Officer Collateral Duty Program are delineated in QIIG 45, which shall be administered by the HSWL SC, who shall:

(1) Determine cost requirements for the Pharmacy Officer collateral duty program and submit funding requests to Commandant (CG-112) in the annual operating summary of budget estimates process.

(2) Provide direction and funding to Pharmacy Officers for matters relating to assignments in pharmacy officer collateral duty program.

(3) Develop work plans specifying units for which the Pharmacy Officer is responsible.

(4) Ensure visit schedule will be:

   (a) The most cost effective.

   (b) Feasible to maintain responsibilities at the unit where the pharmacy billet is assigned.

   (c) Coordinated with the unit CO possessing the billet.

(5) Ensure that rating officers of Pharmacy Officers on assignment in the pharmacy collateral duty program obtain input for completing the USPHS Commissioned Officers' Effectiveness Report from the other units where the Pharmacy Officer provides oversight.

(6) Oversees the following responsibilities of collateral duty Pharmacy Officers who:

   (a) Report to the SHSO of the unit to which they are assigned.

   (b) Follow the established chain of command.

   (c) Serve as a member of the Pharmacy and Therapeutics Committee, and assist those units to which they are assigned with developing and maintaining a drug formulary based on the Department of Defense Basic Core Formulary. This formulary shall be standardized to provide a list of medications stocked in the "therapeutic category" format.

   (d) Provide direct assistance for all aspects of the Pharmaceutical Prime Vendor Program.

   (e) Assist each unit in eliminating or minimizing the purchase of medication through nonfederal sources by using formulary process and redistributing medication as needed.

   (f) Develop an inventory of limited use pharmaceuticals and/or pharmaceutical supplies for distributing to each unit.

   (g) Serve as the point of contact for redistribution of medication due to expire or are in excessive supply.

   (h) Identify special order medication, label them for each patient and assure that they are not considered formulary items. These should be marked for a specific patient only and removed when the patient no longer requires them.

(i) Analyze and develop the most cost effective methods for providing non-formulary medication for chronic conditions.

(j) Provide oversight to the Health Services Technician(s) who normally operate the unit pharmacy and assist in dispensing operation as required.

(k) Provide and document in-service training to the clinic staff.

(l) Review all pharmacy operations and policies including controlled substance activities.

(m) Assist the unit in preparation of the pharmacy, and other areas of the clinic under the responsibility of the pharmacy, for AAAHC and HSWL SC Quality Improvement Surveys.

(n) Provide current information as obtained from the DoD Shelf Life Extension Program (SLEP) and Medical Material Quality Control (MMQC) messages. Pharmacy personnel can refer to the website for subscribing information at: http://www.usamma.army.mil/apps/nala_qaweb/nala_index.cfm. Pharmacies shall document review of MMQC messages that contain information on medication recall or warnings and the appropriate actions taken as described in the message. Documents shall be retained for a period of three years after which they may be destroyed. Ensure messages include initial, date of review, and action taken.

(o) Submit a report of the content and frequency established by HSWL SC

(p) QIIG 45, Collateral Duty Pharmacy Program provides additional guidelines.

2. Prescribers.

   a. Authorized prescribers include:

   (1) Medical Officers and Dental Officers as defined in Sections 1.B.1. and 1.B.4. of this Manual.

   (2) Civilian medical and dental providers employed by the CG.

   (3) HSs may prescribe drugs listed in the Standardized Health Services Technician Drug Formulary, COMDTINST 6570.1 (series). While performing isolated duty at LORAN stations or underway, HSs may prescribe additional drugs listed in Health Services Allowance List Afloat, COMDTINST 6700.6 (series). HSs in these situations shall

seek medical advice from their assigned Designated Medical Officer Advisor (DMOA).

(4) Civilian physicians, dentists, and allied health care providers (nurse practitioners, physician assistants, optometrists, etc.) as authorized by State law in their licensing jurisdiction to write prescriptions in practicing their profession.

(5) Uniformed service medical and dental officers/providers, other than CG, authorized by their service to write prescriptions in practicing their profession

b. <u>Non-clinic issued prescriptions</u>. Prescriptions by uniformed service or civilian medical and dental officers/providers, other than CG, shall be honored whenever possible and only at CG clinics where a registered pharmacist or pharmacy officer is physically present. For example, DoD prescription policies (TRICARE) shall be observed to the fullest extent possible within the scope of the primary care nature of CG Health Care facilities and based on the DoD Basic Core Formulary. Prescriptions by these providers shall be written on the prescription forms authorized by their service. Prescriptions written by outside providers (providers not billeted or assigned to the clinic) will only be honored at CG facilities with a Registered Pharmacist physically present at the clinic. If a Registered Pharmacist is not available, new outside prescriptions will not be filled. Pharmacy personnel working in the pharmacy for that day shall inform the patient that a pharmacist is not available for the day and may give the patient the opportunity to decide to return, if a Pharmacist is expected within a reasonable time frame, or seek pharmacy services at another location. This policy was implemented in 2002 in order to meet the reasonable standard of care existing in the civilian and other federal sectors. AUTOPENED (electronically signed) outside prescriptions will not be honored at CG pharmacies.

c. <u>Formulary medications</u>. Prescriptions for eligible beneficiaries from licensed uniformed, civilian or outside physicians, dentists, or podiatrists shall be honored for products on the clinic's formulary provided a Pharmacist is available. Clinic formularies are to be based on DoD Basic Core Formulary (BCF) guidelines and the prescribing habits of the providers assigned to that clinic.

(1) For those CG clinics with a Pharmacy Officer permanently assigned, the BCF contains the minimum drugs that each pharmacy must have on its formulary and provide to all eligible beneficiaries.

(2) For those CG clinics without a Pharmacy Officer permanently assigned, there are no requirements to stock the entire contents of the BCF. Military practitioners or contract providers shall not countersign

civilian/outside prescriptions nor shall civilian/outside prescriptions be rewritten during cursory outpatient visits with the intent of authorizing the prescription for dispensing at the facility.

(3) In the case of multiple strength BCF drugs, all strengths need not be stocked but all prescriptions for that agent will be filled, regardless of strength. Pharmacists shall use discretion to determine if the prescribed dose can be filled using the available strengths the pharmacy carries (e.g. hydrochlorothiazide 25 mg can be filled with 50 mg strength with pharmacy instruction on the label to read "take ½ tablet").

(4) If additional funding is required for specific, high cost drugs, it shall be requested via the AFC-57 budget process via the HSWL SC.

(5) For CG patients referred out of the clinic for specialty care: Patients shall be advised by their referring CG provider/clinic that prescriptions written by the consulting provider may be filled at the CG clinic pharmacy location where the consultation was generated, at a DoD Military Treatment Facility (MTF) pharmacy, or at a Tricare Retail Network Pharmacy. After completing the consult appointment, patients shall return to their referring CG provider with a consultation brief to maintain continuity of care and assess a treatment plan. If medications prescribed by the consulting provider are not on the referring CG clinic pharmacy's formulary and the patient prefers to obtain the medication at this location, the CG provider will review the consulting provider's brief and determine if a medication on the formulary may be an appropriate therapeutic substitute. If not, the CG provider shall generate a CG special order medication request to be presented at the CG clinic pharmacy for procurement. The request shall also be submitted for review at the next Group Practice Pharmacy and Therapeutics Committee (PTC) meeting.

d. Self Prescribing. Authorized prescribers shall not prescribe controlled medications for themselves and/or their family members. If such medication is required and no other prescriber is assigned to the facility, the CO, or XO, shall review, approve, and countersign each controlled prescription before it is filled by pharmacy personnel.

3. Prescriptions.

a. Prescriptions written by CG providers. Prescriptions written by CG providers shall be filled at the facility where written. In cases of emergencies where it is advisable for a patient to start a prescription immediately and it is not available at the pharmacy, prescriptions may be written on form DD-1289 so that the patient may have the prescription filled outside of the clinic. Prescriptions written by Health Services Technicians shall be filled only at the facility where written. CG clinics may agree amongst themselves to honor another CG clinic's Physician Assistants' or Nurse Practitioners' prescriptions if stock shortages so necessitate. Other CG facilities may honor CG physician assistants' and nurse practitioners' refills (for other than controlled substances) if the patient presents his or her health care record containing the original entry.

b. Telephoned and verbal prescriptions. At the Pharmacy Officer's discretion, telephoned and verbal prescriptions may be accepted only in emergencies. CG clinics without a Pharmacy Officer shall not accept telephone prescriptions.

c. Facsimile prescriptions. At the Pharmacy Officer's discretion, faxed prescriptions may be accepted in the best interest of the patient's care. Faxed prescriptions for controlled/narcotics will not be accepted. CG clinics without a Pharmacy Officer will not accept faxed prescriptions.

d. Transferring prescriptions. Prescriptions may be transferred at the discretion of the Pharmacist. The transferring of prescriptions shall only be conducted between licensed Pharmacists. If a licensed Pharmacist is not available, patients shall be requested to obtain a new prescription. ONLY a one time transfer of the same prescription number is authorized. Multiple transfers of the same prescription number are not authorized.

e. Contacting providers. Health Services Technicians shall not contact civilian/outside prescribers to resolve prescription problems but return the problem prescription to the patient and explain why he or she cannot dispense it. The HS may provide the names of suggested available products to the patient.

f. Prescriptions shall be personalized. If more than one member of a family is prescribed the same drug, a separate prescription shall be generated for each member.

g. Scope of practice. Items prescribed must treat conditions within the normal scope of professional practice and the ethics of the prescriber.

h. Cosmetic conditions. Prescriptions for medications to treat cosmetic conditions (baldness, wrinkles, etc.) and for weight loss will not be honored nor shall medications for these conditions be stocked at CG facilities.

i. Prescriptions for animals. Prescriptions for animals other than Government owned shall not be filled.

j. Physician Assistant. If a Physician Assistant has clinical privileges at a local DoD facility, he or she may use its prescription form to write prescriptions to be filled at that facility, provided the form contains the statement "To be filled only at [insert designated DoD facility]."

k. Responsibility of prescribing facility. The prescriber's facility has the responsibility to procure and dispense all medications its staff members (including in-house contract prescribers) prescribe. In the rare event a patient must carry a prescription elsewhere for dispensing, the prescriber shall write the facility's name in addition to the other required information on the form (i.e., facility address, phone number, provider's DEA or National Provider Identifier (NPI) number, date of prescription).

l. Special order medications. Providers are tasked with the cost effective use of medications. The DoD Basic Core Formulary (BCF) serves as the basis of all CG clinics' formulary. Pharmaceuticals ordered that are not on the clinic formulary are considered Special Order Medications. A Special Order Medication is defined as: a medication for a specific patient for which the provider has completed a Special Order Medication Request form submitted to the pharmacy and reviewed during the next convening Group Practice Pharmacy and Therapeutics Committee meeting; a medication chosen due to a patient's treatment failure to a BCF drug in the same therapeutic category as the special order medication; and/or, a medication not therapeutically available from the BCF and clearly indicated as a medical necessity for a specific patient. In the rare event a patient must carry a prescription elsewhere for dispensing, the prescriber shall include the facility's name, facility's address, phone number, provider's DEA or NPI number, and date of prescription on the prescription blank along with all other pertinent information in order for the patient to have the prescription filled outside of the clinic.

4. Prescribing in the Medical Record.

a. Process. The CG method of prescribing for Medical Providers is the Provider Graphic User Interface (PGUI) and Point of Entry (POE) as per Chapter 14 of this Manual. At all clinics and sickbays, patient medications will be ordered by utilizing the Chronological Record of Care, SF-600 or when appropriate an Emergency Care and Treatment, SF-558. The medical record thus becomes a more comprehensive repository for all patient health information and ensures the pharmacy staff has access to the necessary clinical information (age, weight, allergies, laboratory values, vital signs, etc.). In the case of dental care, Dental Providers shall write prescriptions in the dental record on Dental Record Continuation, SF-603A. For controlled prescriptions written by Dental Providers, a single hard copy of the prescription (e.g., DD-1289) is required as well. For medical providers utilizing PGUI or POE an additional DD-1289 is not required. However for proper documentation and accountability of the controlled substance, the Pharmacy Staff will generate a duplicate pharmacy label of the ordered controlled substance medication, placing it on a prescription blank. The patient shall sign the back of this "generated prescription" with the appropriate documentation as designated in MEDMAN Chapter 10-B.6.b.4.

b. Procedures.

   (1) Document in subjective, objective, assessment, and plan (SOAP) format the patient visit on a Chronological Record of Care, SF-600 or Emergency Care and Treatment, SF-558 in the chart. Under the "Plan" section, list the drug name, strength, directions, quantity, and refills. Prescriptions shall be legibly written. Abbreviated names of medications and unapproved acronyms should be avoided to prevent medication errors and enhance patient safety.

   (2) In the "Plan" section, state a disposition to assist pharmacy staff in coordinating quantities of all chronic medications until the next appointment. Complete the entry with the authorized prescriber's signature.

   (3) The terms chronic and maintenance medications are synonymous. A maintenance medication is defined as any medication used to treat a chronic condition. The term "maintenance" implies that a prescriber and patient have gone through a dosage titration process and have determined that the patient should be "maintained" on an effective dose of a medication that is well tolerated. Ultimately, the individuals in a position to make such a determination are the patient and the prescriber. The standard quantity issued for chronic conditions is a 90-day supply. If it is necessary to deviate from this amount, prescribe quantities in 30-day increments (30, 60, 90, etc.) if possible. If pharmacy staff, in consultation with the prescriber, deems it advantageous to the patient due to travel, deployment, operational commitments, packaging, etc., they may dispense larger quantities (up to 180 days). Active Duty members deploying outside the continental United States (OCONUS) for greater than 180 days will be advised and instructed to use the Tricare Mail Order Program (TMOP).

   (4) For in-house prescriptions and prior to dispensing, in the event of a medication error, incomplete entry, or question/concern regarding a medication, pharmacy staff shall contact/notify the prescriber for further guidance. Upon confirmation/clarification from the prescriber, completely draw a single horizontal line through errors or changes and conspicuously write "Error" next to the item. The person changing the entry shall initial the change or error. If the provider requires further review before making a change, return incorrect or incomplete entries to the prescriber for revision/review. The medication error shall be documented in a Medication Error Report.

   (5) Pharmacy staff will adhere one-part of the multi-part strip of the prescription label that designates the patient name, drug, and quantity on the PGUI or POE generated Chronological Record of Care, SF-600 and all members will initial in ink to signify who prepared the

(6) Pharmacy staff shall write the manufacturer's name, lot number, and expiration date to the right of the drug prescription (not required with CHCS). Sickbays not on CHCS also shall maintain a drug dispensing log containing prescription number, patient's name, patient's SSN, drug name, drug manufacturer, and lot number. Retain this log for record purposes for 3 years.

(7) In addition to the SF-600, Chronological Record of Care or SF-558, Emergency Care and Treatment entry, written prescriptions are required for all prescriptions (including controlled substances) when a prescription must be taken to another pharmacy for dispensing. When controlled substance prescriptions are processed in-house, separate documentation shall be maintained and filed appropriately (i.e., CII file and CIII-V file) in the pharmacy by the pharmacy staff.

(8) All prescriptions generated from sources outside the clinic shall be filled or refilled using CHCS or the procedures specified in this chapter and maintained on file in the pharmacy. The pharmacy need not maintain a health care record if the patient receives only basic pharmaceutical care from the facility. Offer such patients the HIPAA MHS Notice of Privacy Practices. Pharmacy personnel shall ensure DEERS eligibility with every visit.

(9) At clinics where a Pharmacy Officer/Pharmacist is available, the Pharmacy Officer/Pharmacist should make a significant effort to ensure all prescriptions are double-checked by a pharmacist. At clinics where the Pharmacy Officer/Pharmacist is unavailable, the RPE may allow a "C" school trained Pharmacy Technician to prepare and dispense prescriptions, double checked by either another "C" school trained technician or a pharmacy technician who is Watchstander qualified. At clinics where neither a pharmacist or "C" school trained Pharmacy Technician is available, a Pharmacy Technician Watchstander may prepare and dispense prescriptions, after the prescriptions have been double-checked by a medical provider. In cases where neither a pharmacist, "C" school trained Pharmacy Technician, or Pharmacy Technician Watchstander is available, ashore CG units shall instruct patients to have their prescriptions dispensed by either a civilian pharmacy, a Military Treatment Facility Pharmacy or through the

TRICARE Mail Order Pharmacy; afloat CG units staffed by CG IDHS Corpsmen shall be exempt from the double-check prescription requirement (but are required to complete requirements to become a Pharmacy Technician Watchstander through their RPE; however if a Medical Officer (MO) is aboard, the IDHS corpsman shall have prescriptions double-checked by the MO.

5. <u>Signatures</u>. No prescription or order shall be filled unless it bears the signature of an individual authorized to write prescriptions. All prescriptions shall include the printed or stamped name, rank, and professional discipline (MD, DDS, HS2, etc.) of the prescriber. Prescriptions for controlled substances shall also provide the NPI or DEA number of the prescriber. Pharmacy personnel shall maintain signature examples for in-house and contract prescribers. Professional judgment shall be used to verify authenticity of When prescriptions from other sources. CG provider order entry is utilized, electronic signature satisfies this requirement.

6. <u>Dispensing</u>.

    a. The pharmacy shall serve as the source of supply from which clinics or satellite activities normally obtain required pharmaceuticals and related supplies. In addition, the pharmacy dispenses required, authorized preparations directly to patients.

    b. <u>Prescription verification</u>. Except for approved OTC program items, the pharmacy/sickbay will dispense all stocked items only on receiving a properly written, verified prescription. If pharmacy staff receives an illegible prescription or questions its authenticity, dosage, compatibility, or directions to the patient, staff shall obtain clarification from the prescriber before dispensing the medication(s). In the case of outside prescriptions, the Pharmacist is the only authorized pharmacy staff to contact an outside provider for clarification of a prescription.

    c. <u>Medication recall</u>. Clinics/Sickbays shall have a system (computerized, written, etc.) in place to ensure they can retrieve prescriptions in case of a product recall, segregate recalled product until receipt of further guidance on disposition, and make appropriate notification based on the recall level.

    d. <u>Adverse medication reaction reporting</u>. Clinics shall submit all pertinent patient adverse reactions or product quality problems on the FDA MEDWATCH system on FDA Form 3500. Obtain MEDWATCH forms and information from the FDA at 1-800-FDA-1088 or at www.fda.gov. VAERS (Vaccine Adverse Event Reporting System) forms can also be obtained at the same website. When it becomes necessary to complete a VAERS form, clinics are responsible for submitting, via fax, a completed copy to Commandant (CG-1121) at (202) 475-5172, ATTN: Epidemiologist and to HSWL SC (OM).

e. Patient identification. When dispensing medication, the dispenser shall identify the patient through a military identification card and ensure his or her DEERS eligibility, via CHCS and particularly on new outside prescriptions presented to the pharmacy for filling.

f. Medication information. Pharmacy personnel shall ensure patients receive a printed copy of the medication's patient education monograph with all new prescriptions that accompanies the CHCS generated prescription label. Additionally, FDA required Medication Guides that are currently not included in the patient education monograph shall be made available to the patient. These can be obtained from the FDA website at http://www.fda.gov/cder/Offices/ODS/medication_guides.htm.

g. Medication Error. In the event of a medication error (i.e. an error discovered after a prescription has been dispensed to the patient), a Pharmacy Error Report including pertinent information relevant to the error (name of discoverer, date of discovery, a brief statement describing error, and steps taken to prevent recurrence) shall be completed. A copy of the report shall be submitted for review during the next convening Group Practice Pharmacy and Therapeutics Committee (PTC) meeting and a copy of the completed PTC meeting minutes will be forwarded for review and inclusion in the minutes of the next convening Group Practice Quality Improvement Focus Group meeting.

h. Medication containers. Child-resistant containers shall be used to dispense all prescription legend medications except for sublingual nitroglycerin tablets, which are dispensed in the original packaging. The practitioner or patient may specifically request a conventional closure. A practitioner must so indicate on the prescription order. If the patient requests such a closure, enter a statement so saying on the back of the prescription and have the patient sign it. When refilling prescriptions, the pharmacy must ensure the safety closure still functions and the label is legible before dispensing in the original container. In the case where a particular patient is requesting all of his/her prescriptions be conventional (non-child resistant) closures, pharmacy shall ensure a signature card containing the statement: "I request non-child proof closures for all medications prescribed for me" is completed and signed by the patient. Signature cards shall include date, printed name of patient, and initials of pharmacy personnel and shall be maintained at the pharmacy until patient permanently leaves the area or has not used the facility within one year of original date of signature card. Patient's CHCS profile shall be annotated in Pharmacy Patient Comment (PPC) to reflect the request

i. Refills. Prescriptions (except for controlled substances-see 10-B-4.c.) may be refilled when authorized by the prescriber. The maximum quantity shall be a year's supply of medication. No prescription shall be refilled after more than one year from the date it was written. PRESCRIPTIONS SHALL NOT BE REFILLED FROM THE LABEL ON THE CONTAINER ONLY

j. Non-prescription Medication Program. CG clinics are encouraged to establish non-prescription medication programs under the following guidelines:

(1) CO of CG units assigned with health care personnel may elect to operate a nonprescription drug program. Units not staffed with an HS may operate a nonprescription medication program with oversight provided by a CG Pharmacist or supporting Independent Duty HS. Units electing to offer a nonprescription drug program shall request authorization through HSWL SC, and verify that they will operate within the guideline.

(2) All CG health care facilities shall make condoms available to beneficiaries even if they elect not to offer a nonprescription drug program. Condoms shall be made available to beneficiaries under 18 years of age unless specifically forbidden by law.

(3) Items available shall be limited to those specifically identified (authorized) in the Nonprescription Medication Program (see Enclosure 1). Units may elect not to offer every product from this list but shall not add unauthorized products.

(4) A beneficiary family shall be limited to a maximum of two items per week from the program. Occasionally, it may be necessary to extend this limit due to family size. Pharmacy and Therapeutics Committees (if available) and collateral duty Pharmacy Officers shall provide guidance and monitor any such extensions.

(5) Items shall only be available during normal operating hours of the pharmacy, sick bay or facility.

(6) Pharmacy or sick bay personnel shall monitor the program for perceived overuse. Individuals suspected of this shall be referred to a Medical Officer and may have their access to this privilege denied.

(7) All products must be dispensed in the Manufacturer's FDA approved packages with required instructions and warnings. Other locally packaged items are not authorized. Local Pharmacy and Therapeutics Committees may develop supplemental information on sheets to provide additional dosage or drug information to the patient.

(8) Nonprescription drug program items shall not be dispensed to pregnant patients or non active duty beneficiaries under 18 years of age. Local Flight Surgeons, via the Pharmacy and Therapeutics Committee, shall

determine which products may be acquired and which products are restricted to personnel on flight status.

(9) Facilities offering this service shall keep monthly statistics as to the quantity of items dispensed. This figure shall be separated from regular pharmacy workload statistics and not be counted as a prescription number, but will be added to monthly pharmacy statistics report as requested by the Clinic Administrator. Once collected, request forms may be shredded and disposed. Over the counter medication forms that contain pseudoephedrine will be retained for 3 years. Only those items which have been dispensed by a written prescription shall be counted in the facility prescription number totals.

(10) Beneficiaries are responsible for providing an authorized picture identification card to verify their eligibility (e.g., military identification card).

(11) To receive a nonprescription item, patients must sign a log or complete a request form which certifies the following:

 (a) "I do not wish to see a physician or other health care provider for advice before receiving these medications. I understand that the medication is for minor illness or conditions and that if symptoms worsen or persist longer than 48 hours, the person for whom this medication is intended should be seen by a health care provider.

 (b) "I am not pregnant or under 18 years of age (unless active duty). If on flight status, I understand that I am only authorized to receive over-the-counter items approved by the Flight Surgeon.

 (c) The person for whom this medication is intended does not have high blood pressure/cardiac problems, diabetes, thyroid problems, is not taking blood thinners, or is not pregnant.

(12) Individuals suspected of returning for medication for a non-resolving problem shall be referred to a Medical Officer for evaluation.

(13) The log sheet or request form shall also contain the date, patient's name, and the name and quantity of the item(s) received.

(14) Pharmacy personnel shall ensure positive control and tracking mechanism for any items on the OTC list containing pseudoephedrine. Pharmacy personnel shall ensure that all beneficiaries, requesting any items on the OTC containing pseudoephedrine, have signed the request form prior to dispensing. These request forms shall be segregated from the other OTC request forms and maintained in the pharmacy for a period of three years, after which they may be destroyed by shredding.

(15) Beneficiaries requesting medical advice that, in the opinion of the pharmacy or sick bay personnel, is beyond their expertise shall be referred to the Medical Officer.

(16) Funding for independent duty HS assigned units (vessel, Sector, etc.) deciding to offer this service shall be from their supporting pharmacy's AFC-57 account.

(17) Enclosure one (1) provides a sample form for the Non Prescription Medication Program with a current list of authorized items.

k. When the pharmacy is closed, a Medical or Dental Officer, or a person so authorized, shall dispense medication only from a locked cabinet or locker containing pre-packaged or limited supplies of after-hours medications. The after hours locker shall be maintained in a secured location outside of the pharmacy and shall contain limited pharmaceuticals required to treat acute medical conditions to stabilize the patient until he/she can return during normal clinic hours. This procedure shall prevent the need for access into the pharmacy after hours. These drugs are dispensed under the same procedures required when the pharmacy is open, including appropriate labeling and complete entry in the health record. Prescriptions from civilian or outside providers shall not be filled after hours. Patients presenting with the above will be advised they can return during normal pharmacy hours or shall be referred to another pharmacy source including a Military Treatment Facility or Tricare Retail Network Pharmacy.

l. Bulk items for use in the clinic may be issued on authorized prescription forms or locally approved requisition forms.

m. A sign shall be posted outside of the pharmacy in a highly visible location stating "Please inform our pharmacy staff if you are breast feeding or may be pregnant." Clinic pharmacies shall maintain a written drug information system (USP, FDA, CHCS) to provide information to patients when appropriate. Post the MHS Notice of Privacy Practices in an accessible location.

n. Pharmacies shall adhere to applicable state laws governing generic dispensing of civilian prescriptions. Civilian prescribers may provide the facility with a written statement giving "blanket approval" to dispense generics for their prescriptions.

o. Drug samples are not authorized at CG facilities.

p. For guidance on pharmaceutical gifts, the CG Ethics Program can be found in Standards of Ethical Conduct, COMDTINST M5370.8 (series), specifically 2.C.

7. Labeling.

   a. Requirements. A label will be prepared for each prescription dispensed to individuals and will be securely affixed to the container prior to dispensing. The label or appropriate auxiliary labeling will show as a minimum:

      (1) Facility identity, including the pharmacy address and telephone number.

      (2) Consecutive identifying number.

      (3) Prescribers name.

      (4) Definite, concise directions to the patient.

      (5) Drug name and strength, unless prescriber directs otherwise.

      (6) Quantity dispensed.

      (7) Patient's first and last name.

      (8) Inked initials of person preparing the prescription label and the person double checking the prepared prescription.

      (9) The legend "KEEP OUT OF THE REACH OF CHILDREN" on all prescription labels.

      (10) Date prescription filled.

      (11) Indication of refills.

      (12) Expiration date for prepared and compounded prescriptions (e.g. liquid antibiotics, dermatologic products, etc.).

      (13) The legend "CAUTION: FEDERAL LAW PROHIBITS THE TRANSFER OF THIS DRUG TO ANY PERSON OTHER THAN THE PATIENT FOR WHOM IT WAS PRESCRIBED" (for controlled substances only).

      (14) Necessary supplemental or auxiliary labels.

   b. Directions on labels. If prescription contents are for external use only or require further preparation(s) for use (shaking, dilution, temperature adjustment, or other manipulation or process) include the appropriate directions on the label or affix an additional label to the container. If liquid preparations for external use are poisonous, affix a "poison" label to the container. If medicines prescribed for internal use are poisonous, use sound judgment whether to label them "poison" based on the finished preparation's potency in each case.

c. <u>Generic names</u>. Medicinal preparations compounded or packaged in the pharmacy for subsequent issue will be identified and labeled with the full generic name, except that trade or brand names may be used provided trade or brand name product actually is in the container. The manufacturer's name, lot number, and expiration date, if any, will be shown on the label.

d. <u>Labeling Medications for Transfer</u>. Drugs issued to clinics for subsequent reissue to outpatients shall bear appropriate pharmacy label with space available to write in the patient's name, prescriber, date issued and prescribing instructions. The pharmacy shall ensure these medications are in FDA approved packaging such as commercially available pre-packed or unit of use bottles.

e. <u>Multiple Dose Injectables</u>. All multiple dose injectable vials shall be dated upon opening. The expiration date will be thirty days from the date of opening unless the manufacturer's product information indicates a shorter or longer expiration date.

8. <u>Drug Stock</u>.

    a. <u>Source of medications</u>. The Defense Supply Center, Philadelphia (DSCP) is the primary source of medications for either the "Depot" system or prime vendor contracts. Other Federal sources (Perry Point IHS Depot, Federal Supply Schedules, HSWL SC negotiated purchase agreements, etc.) may be used when, due to price or service advantages, it is determined to be the most cost-effective procurement method to meet the needs of the unit. Drug procurement from retail sources shall be done only when absolutely required for urgent patient needs and when other, less costly, sources cannot meet this need.

    b. <u>Nutritional/Herbal/Dietary Supplements/Medications and Performance Enhancing Substances</u>. Scientific information (quality and production control, adverse effects, drug interaction, side effects) regarding these products are often times scanty or nonexistent. Often, these products interact with each other and with prescribed medications in unpredictable ways. The possible/potential side effects from these agents are hard to predict, occur with irregularity, and may be different in any given population. Side effects may be manifested in any body system and may affect the central nervous system, cardiovascular system, vision, balance, mood, behavior, learning and cognitive ability. Active duty personnel are required to be operationally ready, stand watch/post, and/or perform special duties. Because active duty personnel are required to remain alert with full use of all senses and reasoning powers, active duty members may neither possess, use, nor purchase (via any venue) herbal supplements, dietary products, or alternative health care substances banned or not approved by the FDA for sale or use in the United States. Only those items that have been licensed and approved by the Food and Drug Administration (with the exception of vitamins with an established RDA) are authorized for use in CG health care facilities. CG health care facilities shall not purchase or dispense "herbal supplements" or "dietary supplements". Patients should inform their healthcare providers if taking any type of herbal supplements to avoid potential drug interactions. Aviators and flight crew members shall follow guidance provided in the Aviation Manual, Chapter 12, Section B.3.h. Commands can contact the Collateral Duty Pharmacy Officer or HSWL SC Pharmacy Officer for further guidance.

c. <u>Separation of dosage forms</u>. In storage, separate external use medications from internal use medications and ophthalmic and otic preparations. Caustic acids such as glacial acetic, sulfuric, nitric, concentrated hydrochloric, or oxalic acid shall not be issued to clinics, but shall be stored in separate lockers, clearly marked as to contents. Methyl alcohol shall not be stored, used, or dispensed by the pharmacy.

d. <u>Refrigerated items</u>. Pharmaceuticals requiring refrigeration shall be stored in proper refrigeration equipment that meets the criteria for storing pharmaceuticals requiring specific temperature control/storage process. Refrigerators will be installed with temperature monitoring devices that provides constant temperature recording and shall be connected to an emergency power supply to protect refrigerated medications in the event of an electrical malfunction or power surge. Manual temperature readings will be checked and recorded twice daily. Temperatures that register outside the acceptable storage range will be immediately reported to the RPE, the Clinic Administrator (if ashore) or the Executive Officer (if afloat). The HSWL SC Pharmacy Officer can be contacted for further guidance and information on sources for obtaining refrigerators and temperature monitoring devices. Vaccines shall not be stored in the same refrigerator used to store food as the potential increased access to the (food) refrigerator will not provide a stable temperature environment for the vaccines. Additionally, the potential hazard of vaccines contaminated by food spill or spoilage could compromise the vaccine. Additional guidance can be found at http://www2.cdc.gov/nip/isd/shtoolkit/006Chap5.pdf or at http://www.methodistmd.org/pdf/pi/PI2 Leb.pdf.

e. <u>Hazardous substances</u>. Store flammable drugs according to accepted fire safety regulations. Additional information regarding hazardous materials can be found at: http://www.uscg.mil/ccs/cit/cim/directives/CI/CI_6260_21B.pdf.

f. <u>Doors</u>. Solid core doors with one-inch (minimum), throw key-operated, dead-bolt locks shall be used for all pharmacy and medical supply areas and shall be secured at the end of the day. On Dutch doors, both sections shall have this type lock. Pharmacy doors shall have a second keylock or cipher lock to remain secured at all times.

g. <u>Shelf Life Extension program</u>. Remove from stock drugs under testing in the FDA/DoD Shelf Life Extension Program; label them with the project number until results are received. While pending, use these items only in emergencies to offset medical allowance list requirements. Upon return of results, items should be destroyed or marked with FDA approved labels with new expiration dates and returned to stock. Oral contraceptives, ophthalmics, otics, and inhaler medications should not be extended.

    h. <u>Poison antidotes</u>. The pharmacy shall maintain, in the pertinent clinic areas, an adequate supply of emergency medications (or kits), poison antidotes, and the National Poison Control Center telephone number (1-800-222-1222). Containers for these items shall be closed with break-away seals to prevent the unreported removal of items. The outside of the container shall post an inventory list with their expiration dates.

9. <u>Credit return program (Reverse Distribution Program)</u>. Clinics shall establish a credit return program through a pharmaceutical returns vendor that accepts expired pharmaceuticals and disposes of them in accordance with federal law. The company shall coordinate and issue refunds from the respective manufacturers of the returned products directly to the clinic's prime vendor who will issue it as available credit for the specific clinic. Expired medications not accepted by the returned goods vendor shall be disposed of as biohazard waste. DSCP currently has an established contract with several reverse distribution or returned goods vendor. Participating facilities shall select from one of the contracted vendors following guidance as provided by DSCP. Prior to transfer of drugs to the returns vendor, pharmacy personnel shall ensure an inventory of all returned pharmaceuticals is prepared and retained at the pharmacy before the shipment leaves the facility. Quarterly, preferably prior to next scheduled P&T Committee meeting, Pharmacy Officer will review returned pharmaceuticals data for trends that indicate a need to modify inventory levels or ordering practices and make recommendations to the committee. If controlled substances are included in the pharmaceutical returns, pharmacy personnel shall ensure appropriate documentation has been completed (e.g., DD-1149, Requisition And Invoice/Shipping Document and NAVMED 6710, Perpetual Inventory).

10. <u>Pharmacy and Therapeutics Committee (PTC)</u>.

    a. This is a mandatory advisory committee in all CG health service treatment facilities which have assigned Medical Officers and shall meet quarterly face-to-face, video or teleconference. The PTC will be conducted centrally as a function of the Regional Practice for that district and each clinic in the district will participate in the meeting. The committee is composed of, but not limited to, the following members and will constitute a quorum: the Senior Medical Executive (SME) or representative, the Senior Dental Executive (SDE) or representative, the Regional Pharmacy Executive (RPE), the Regional Manager (RM) or representative, and one representative from each clinic within the district. Clinic Administrators are strongly encouraged to attend. The chairman will be the SME and the RPE will be the secretary.

b. The committee is an advisory group on all matters relating to the acquisition and use of medications. Its recommendations are subject to the approval of the SHSO. The basic responsibilities of this committee are to:

(1) Use the Department of Defense Basic Core Formulary (DOD BCF) as guidance to develop and maintain a clinic drug formulary as specified in 10-A-2.c., review newly requested items, and delete unnecessary items.

(2) Maintain a unit formulary ensuring items authorized for Health Service Technicians (based on the authorized CG Standardized Health Services Technician Formulary) are properly notated.

(3) Ensure the unit formulary does not include items based primarily on civilian prescriber demand.

(4) Prevent unnecessary therapeutic duplications of formulary products.

(5) Conduct an ongoing review of all non-formulary items the pharmacy procures and dispenses. To accomplish this, the Group Practice and/or P&T committee reviews:

(a) A list of all clinic formulary items not currently in the DoD BCF.

(b) A list of all special order items (Special Order Medication Request forms) and the patients for whom procured.

(6) Conduct an ongoing drug usage evaluation (DUE) program for selected medications.

(7) Monitor the facility's controlled drug prescribing and usage.

(8) Review pharmacy policies and procedures as necessary.

(9) Monitor the quality and accuracy of prescriptions and patient information the pharmacy provides and enacts any quality assurance measures it deems necessary (double checks, etc.).

(10) Reviews any adverse reaction or product quality reports (VAERS or MEDWATCH).

(11) Monitors compliance with HIPAA privacy and security mandates.

c. Documentation for the upcoming PTC will be forwarded to the RPE in the first month of each quarter for inclusion to the PTC agenda, which will be prepared and forwarded to the SHSO for approval prior to the meeting. The PTC meeting will be conducted in the second month of the quarter. Minutes of the meeting will be prepared and forwarded to the SHSO for approval by the end of the third month of the quarter and then returned to the RPE for retention and uploaded to the CG's online CG Portal Microsite. A copy of the minutes will be forwarded to the Regional Manager.

d. Quality Improvement Implementation Guide (QIIG) #5, Pharmacy and Therapeutics Committee provides additional guidelines.

COMDTINST M6000.1E

Figure 10-A-1
CLINIC NON-PRESCRIPTION MEDICATION PROGRAM
USCG (may insert name of clinic or location here)
Limited to TWO (2) Items Per Family Per Week

This program is for military beneficiaries only. MILITARY ID CARD IS REQUIRED. Please read and sign the following statement:

_____ I do not wish to see a physician or other health care provider for advice before receiving these medications. I understand that these medications are for minor illnesses or conditions and that if symptoms worsen or persist longer than 48 hours, the person for whom this medication is intended should be seen by a health care provider.

_____ I am not under 18 years old (unless active duty). If on flight status, I understand that I am only authorized to receive non-prescription items approved by the Flight Surgeon.

_____ I will inform the pharmacy staff if the person for whom this medication is intended has high blood pressure, cardiac problems, diabetes, thyroid problems, is taking blood thinners, or is pregnant.

Signature: _____

Printed name: _____

Date: _____

Address:(Required only for products containing Pseudoephedrine)
_____
_____

NOTE: Items listed are not guaranteed to always be available.

- ___ Acetaminophen 325mg tabs, 50 count
- ___ Acetaminophen 80 mg chewable tabs, 30 count
- ___ Acetaminophen 160mg/5ml liquid, 120ml
- ___ Acetaminophen 0.8mg/0.8ml drops
- ___ Ibuprofen 200mg tabs, 24 count
- ___ Ibuprofen 100mg/5ml, solution
- ___ Pseudoephedrine 30mg tabs, 24 count
- ___ Pseudoephedrine 30mg/5ml, 120ml
- ___ Triprolidine/Pseudoephedrine tabs, 24 count
- ___ Brompheniramine/Phenylephrine solution, 120ml
- ___ Guaifenesin 100mg/5ml, 120ml
- ___ Guaifenesin 100mg/Dextromethorphan 5mg, 120ml
- ___ Diphenhydramine 25mg capsules, 24 count
- ___ Diphenhydramine liquid, 120ml
- ___ Cetylpyridinium AnestheticLozenge
- ___ Liquid Antacid, 150ml
- ___ Loperamide caplets, 12 count
- ___ Antichap Lipstick
- ___ Bacitracin Ointment, 30gm
- ___ Analgesic Balm, 30gm
- ___ Saline Nasal Spray, 45ml
- ___ Clotrimazole Topical cream, 30gm
- ___ Hydrocortisone 1% topical cream, 30gm
- ___ Tolnaftate powder, 45gm
- ___ Calamine Lotion
- ___ Male Condoms

Section B. Controlled Substances.

1. General 1
2. Custody and Controlled Substance Audits 1
3. Drug Enforcement Administration (DEA) Registration 4
4. Reporting Theft or Loss 4
5. Procuring, Storing, Transferring, and Disposing of Controlled Substances 5
6. Prescribing Practices 7

This page intentionally left blank.

B. Controlled Substances.

1. General.

   a. Controlled substances, as used here, are defined as.

      (1) Drugs or chemicals in DEA Schedules I-V: (for example, the manufacturers label for Acetaminophen with Codeine #3(30 mg.) carries the DEA symbol for Schedule III (C-III) and will be treated as a Schedule III by Coast Guard units.). NOTE: The use of Schedule I, II, III, IV, and V is synonymous to CI, CII, CIII, CIV, and CV, respectively.

      (2) Precious metals.

      (3) Ethyl alcohol (excluding denatured).

      (4) Other drugs or materials the local CO or Pharmacy and Therapeutics Committee determine to have significant abuse potential.

   b. CG authorized uses for controlled substances are one of the following.

      (1) Medicinal purposes.

      (2) Retention as evidence in legal or disciplinary actions.

      (3) Other uses CG Regulations specifically authorize.

   c. Controlled substances not authorized.

      (1) Amphetamines for fatigue management or performance enhancement (go-pills).

      (2) Ephedra derivatives including ephedrine.

      (3) Controlled substances for weight loss including human chorionic gonadotropin (HCG).

   d. Quantity Definitions. Due to the potential for abuse and associated audits required, and the DoD Pharmaceutical Prime Vendor ordering advantage, CG units should strive to maintain minimal quantities of controlled substances based solely on the prescribing habits of its providers.

2. Custody and Controlled Substance Audits.

   a. Controlled Substance Custodian (CSC).

(1) Pharmacy Officers, when assigned, shall be appointed in writing as the CSC by the CO (Air Stations), Base Commanders, or the HSWL Regional Manager.

(2) In the absence of a Pharmacy Officer, COs (Air Stations) or Regional Manager (RM) shall designate the Clinic Administrator as CSC.

(3) Medical and Dental Officers may not serve as alternate CSC's to avoid possible conflict of interest.

(4) Temporarily assigned personnel shall not serve as CSCs or alternates.

(5) Under United States Coast Guard Regulations 1992, COMDTINST M5000.3 (series), Chapter 6-2-3-A.(6), the XO is directly responsible for medical matters if a Medical Officer is not assigned. For sickbays, the CO shall designate a commissioned officer as the CSC.

(6) An audit of all controlled substances is required when the CSC is changed. The results of this inventory shall be filed in the command's permanent file and in the Health Services Log. All keys should be transferred and/or combination locks changed at the time of this inventory.

b. Unit Controlled Substance Audits.

(1) Controlled Substance Audit Boards (CSAB). Each unit procuring, storing, or dispensing controlled substances shall have a CSAB.

(a) Membership: The CSAB shall consist of two or more disinterested members, E-6 or above, designated in writing by the CO (Air Stations) or the Regional Manager. CSAB letters of designation will remain in effect until the members are relieved in writing or detached from the command. In no case may the controlled substance custodian be a member of the CSAB. A DISINTERESTED MEMBER is defined as one not assigned or directly involved in daily clinic operations.

(b) The CSAB shall conduct monthly audits of controlled substances at clinics (quarterly at ashore or afloat sickbays) and submit its report to the CO (Air Stations) or the Regional Manager within 5 working days after the completed audit for signature. The command/Regional Manager will sign the report, make a copy for their files, upload to the online CG Portal Microsite, and forward the signed original back to the pharmacy for retention. The pharmacy will retain for three (3) years.

(c) Monthly, CSABs shall audit all working and bulk stock of C-II through C-V controlled substances, precious metals, ethyl alcohol, and drugs or other items locally designated as controlled substances due to abuse potential and report all quantities on Monthly Report for Narcotics and Other Controlled Drugs, CG-5353.

(d) During monthly audits, CSABs shall inspect controlled substances for expiration, deterioration, and inadequate or improper labeling. Expired products or those with other discrepancies shall be removed for disposal.

(e) The CSAB shall count required controlled substances, review a representative random sample of prescriptions, receipts and issue documents, and report the results on Monthly Report for Narcotics and Other Controlled Drugs, CG-5353. For sealed containers, a bottle count is sufficient; for open containers an exact count is required. For open liquid containers, an estimate other than an exact volume measurement is adequate. CSABs may use tamper-proof seals on open containers to avoid future counting of partial quantities.

(f) CSAB members shall be advised that the CG health care program is committed to the privacy of patient health information. Federal laws (the Privacy Act and the Health Insurance Portability and Accountability Act [HIPAA]) govern uses and disclosures of medical information.

(g) During the CSAB process, respect patient privacy: do not access information you do not need for CSAB tasks, do not discuss patient information with anyone outside the CSAB. HIPAA is Federal law and violations may mean civil penalties up to $50,000 and/or criminal penalties. It is to be reminded that these laws also govern how ones information is protected while even a patient in any CG/DoD health care facility.

(2) DEA Biennial Inventories. To comply with DEA requirements, all controlled substances shall be inventoried by the custodian during May of even-numbered years. This copy of the Monthly Report for Narcotics and Other Controlled Drugs, CG-5353 shall be maintained on file locally and labeled "FOR DEA BIENNIAL INVENTORY" at the top of the form.

3. <u>Drug Enforcement Administration (DEA) Registration</u>.

   a. DEA registration is required for those CG clinics with Prime Vender Ordering capability. Purchase of controlled substances from commercial sources is prohibited unless approved and procured by pharmacy officers. Sickbays shall not register with the DEA unless in-house physician services are provided. The unit's Drug Enforcement Agency Registration Form, DEA-244A shall be signed by the Commanding Officer. By direction signature is not authorized. Forward the signed form to the HSWL SC Pharmacy Officer. The HSWL SC Pharmacy Officer is the approving authority for Fee Exempt Status of clinic DEA certificate.

- b. The HSWL SC shall forward the Drug Enforcement Agency Registration Form, DEA-244A to the DEA and provide a copy to the originating unit. The DEA will issue the registration to the unit.

- c. In the case of DEA renewals, (CLINIC RENEWALS ONLY [NOT INDIVIDUAL PROVIDERS]), do not complete. Send the entire renewal application to the HSWL SC Pharmacy Officer via traceable means (e.g. DHS authorized Commercial Carriers FedEx or UPS); US Postal Service (USPS): 1) Express Mail or 2) Proof of Delivery using Extra Services which are either Certified, Delivery Confirmation, or Signature Confirmation, who will electronically complete and submit the renewal application. For questions regarding renewal of clinic DEA certificates, contact the HSWL SC Pharmacy Officer for further guidance.

4. Reporting Theft or Loss. Theft or loss of controlled substance is defined as any discrepancy for which all accountability process has been exhausted with negative results. NOTE: Overage or underage of a newly opened bottle of controlled substance does not constitute theft or loss but shall be notated in the Perpetual Inventory as manufacturer's bottling overage or underage. Immediately, upon discovery of theft of loss, notify the HSWL SC Pharmacy Officer.

- a. If discovered during the course of a monthly CSAB, a designated command member shall contact the HSWL SC Pharmacy Officer, discuss the circumstances of the discrepancy, and request guidance for further action. The HSWL SC Pharmacy Officer will advise the command in writing or by e-mail of the guidance provided. Should the HSWL SC Pharmacy Officer determine an investigation is warranted, the command shall appoint one or more members of the command to investigate the discrepancy. The command shall not appoint CSAB members or interested members to investigate an incident they have reported.

- b. If discovered other than during the course of a monthly CSAB, the CSC, via the clinic's proper chain of command, shall notify the HSWL SC Pharmacy Officer and request guidance for further action. Guidelines as indicated in 4.a. above may be followed, if warranted.

    (1) Review and send to the HSWL SC Pharmacy Officer the findings of the investigation.

(2) The HSWL SC Pharmacy Officer shall determine if the theft or loss warrants further action or DEA notification via Report of Theft or Loss of Controlled Substances, DEA Form 106. A copy of all Report of Theft or Loss of Controlled Substances, DEA Form 106 reports submitted to DEA shall be sent to Commandant (CG-112).

5. Procuring, Storing, Transferring, and Disposing of Controlled Substances.

    a. Procurement.

        (1) Clinics shall procure controlled substances from the DSCP prime vendor source. CG vessels shall obtain authorized controlled substances through their collateral duty Pharmacy Officer.

        (2) Schedule I controlled substances and alcoholic beverages are prohibited and shall not be procured or stocked in CG health care facilities.

        (3) Upon receipt, controlled substances shall immediately be placed in the custody of the designated custodian. The invoice shall be checked against the requisition to verify receipt of all quantities listed on the invoice. The custodian shall acknowledge receipt by signing the invoice. Controlled substance procurement documents shall be maintained in the pharmacy for three years.

    b. Storage.

        (1) Controlled substances shall be stored in an all-purpose GSA Class V safe. Chapter 11 of the Physical Security and Force Protection Manual, COMDTINST M5530.1 (series), offers in depth guidance regarding storage of Controlled Substances.

        (2) In the case of CANA (Diazepam 10mg Auto Injectors), required quantities are often too bulky to feasibly store in Class V safes. Therefore, storage in a secured locked cabinet in a controlled access area is authorized. For field deployments, CANA may be stored in a secured portable container under the control and custody of the unit CO or the Designated Controlled Substance Custodian and, if possible, in a controlled access area. CANA should be stored between 59-86 degrees Fahrenheit. If this temperature cannot be controlled, a log must be maintained indicating storage temperature and conditions. Disposition of CANA shall be documented on the Perpetual Inventory of Narcotics, Alcohol, and Controlled Drugs, NAVMED 6710/5, from time of receipt to issuance to the primary user. For field deployments, an issue log signed by the recipient is an acceptable form of documentation. Transfer of CANA between units shall be documented via Requisition

and Invoice/Shipping Document, DD-1149. Units are required to include CANA in its Controlled Substance Audits.

(3) Afloat units may use existing "built in" containers to store controlled substances. Such "built in" units shall be secured at all times with positive control.

c. Transfer.

(1) Controlled substances may be transferred between CG and other government facilities using the Requisition and Invoice/Shipping Document, DD-1149. When completed, the document shall include:

(a) Names of issuing and receiving facility or unit.

(b) Name, strength, and quantity of each drug.

(c) Date.

(d) Signatures of the issuing and receiving custodians.

(2) Both units shall adjust inventories as required and file copies of the Requisition and Invoice/Shipping Document, DD-1149 for three years.

(4) When the transaction cannot be done in person, it shall be done via traceable means (e.g. DHS authorized Commercial Carriers FedEx or UPS); US Postal Service (USPS): 1) Express Mail or 2) Proof of Delivery using Extra Services which are either Certified, Delivery Confirmation, or Signature Confirmation. The Registered Mail Return Receipt (PS Form 3806), or tracking document, shall be maintained by the issuing unit until a signed copy of the Requisition and Invoice/Shipping Document, DD-1149 is returned.

(5) A copy of the Requisition and Invoice/Shipping Document, DD-1149 shall be sent to the Pharmacy Officer with collateral duty responsibility for the facility.

d. Disposal.

(1) Expired, contaminated, excessive, inadequately labeled, or otherwise unusable controlled substances shall be destroyed by the CSAB in accordance with 10.A.8. CSAB reports shall include the drug name, quantity, reason for destruction, and mechanism of destruction. These shall be maintained on file for three years. In the case of full or partially full bottle of expired controlled substances, they shall be properly labeled as expired, isolated in the Controlled Safe from usable or in-date items, and included in the next shipment of pharmaceutical returns via the contracted pharmaceutical returns good vendor.

Pharmacy personnel shall document return of controlled items via Requisition and Invoice/Shipping Document, DD-1149 as well as documents as required by the returned goods vendor.

(2) If any controlled pharmaceutical is dropped or damaged, it shall be recovered, isolated, and stored, with adequate labeling to identify the contents, and labeled as "To be Destroyed by CSAB", in the controlled pharmaceuticals safe until the next CSAB at which time it shall be destroyed by the audit board in accordance with 10.A.8. and 10.B.5.d.(1) above.

6. Prescribing Practices.

   a. Authorized (Active Duty) prescribers (see 10-A-2.a). are exempt from registration under provision of 21 CFR 1301.25. The officer's social security number may be used in lieu of a DEA or NPI registration number. The exemption does not apply when the officer prescribes controlled substances outside of his or her official duties. In that case, the prescriber is required to register with the DEA, at his or her own expense, and comply with applicable state and federal laws.

   b. Signatures.

      (1) All prescriptions for controlled substances shall be signed by a medical or dental provider. For medical provider prescriptions generated in PGUI or by POE and signed electronically in the CHCS system, the pharmacy staff will generate a duplicate pharmacy label of the ordered controlled substance, placing it on a prescription blank and have the patient annotate the back of the prescription as designated in Chapter 10.B.6.b.(4). If none is assigned, the prescription shall be signed by the senior health services department representative and countersigned by the XO.

      (2) All schedule II controlled substance prescriptions by Physician Assistant or Nurse Practitioners shall be countersigned quarterly by their supervising Medical Officer.

      (3) All controlled substance quantities used in the preparation of other products (compounding, etc.) shall be accounted for on a prescription form and signed by the Pharmacy Officer or custodian.

      (4) The back of all controlled substance prescriptions shall include the wording "RECEIVED BY:" followed by the patient's signature, address, the date dispensed, and quantity received by the patient. It is recommended the patient observes the amount dispensed during the course of the second (dual integrity) count or at time of dispensing, if time permits.

c. Quantities and Refills.

   (1) Controlled substances shall be prescribed in minimal quantities consistent with proper treatment of the patient's condition. Outside prescriptions for controlled substances may only be honored at facilities where a Pharmacy Officer is available and at the discretion of the Pharmacy Officer.

   (2) Out-of-state controlled substance prescriptions may be dispensed if, in the professional judgment of the Pharmacy Officer, the prescription appears legitimate. These prescriptions should invoke special scrutiny by the Pharmacist

   (3) Schedule II prescriptions shall not be accepted more than seven days after the date the prescription was written. For Schedule III through V, 30 days shall be the limit.

   (4) Schedule II prescriptions shall be limited to a maximum of 30 day quantity and shall not be refilled. The only exception shall be medication for Attention Deficit Disorder (ADD) where quantities may be dispensed in up to a 90 day supply with no refills.

   (5) Schedule III, IV, and V prescriptions shall be limited to 30-day quantities with up to five refills only as authorized by the prescriber. The only exception shall be for chronic seizure medications, which may be dispensed in up to 90-day quantities with one refill (six months' total supply). Outside prescriptions for these medications shall only be honored for these quantities, at the discretion of the Pharmacist. Patients shall be informed of this quantity/refill limit and be offered the opportunity to have the prescriptions filled elsewhere.

   (6) Controlled prescriptions shall not be commonly filled until the patient, for whom it is intended, is available to pick up the medication. This should also include refills. However, if a pharmacy's workload is such that in the opinion of the Pharmacist it is in the best interest to maintain pharmacy flow, refill of controlled substances may be done in advance as long as the pharmacy personnel ensures positive and secured control until the patient picks up the medication. These refills shall be bagged and/or sealed in such a way to ensure tamper resistance. Additionally, they shall be housed in a central location such that at the end of the day, those controlled prescriptions not picked up shall be returned to the narcotics safe for storage.

d. <u>Filing Prescriptions</u>.

   (1) Controlled substance prescriptions shall be serially numbered and maintained in two files:

   (2) File #1: All C-II, precious metals, and alcohol prescriptions.

   (3) File #2: All C-III, C-IV, and C-V prescriptions.

   (4) All prescriptions shall be maintained on file for three years after which they may be destroyed by shredding.

   (5) All controlled prescriptions shall be posted on Perpetual Inventory of Narcotics, Alcohol, and Controlled Drugs, NAVMED 6710/5 at the time of each transaction. A physical back count of the opened container from which the prescription was dispensed will be conducted to verify the remaining balance. The prescription shall then be diagonally lined across and initialed by the pharmacy staff member completing the transaction.

This page intentionally left blank.

Section C. Forms and Records

1. General. 1
2. Prescription Forms. 1
3. Quality Control Forms. 2
4. Controlled Drug Forms. 2
5. Forms Availability. 5

This page intentionally left blank.

C. Forms and Records.

1. General. Records shall be maintained for certain procedures conducted within all CG Clinics. Among mandatory requirements for record keeping are the prescribing of drugs, handling of controlled substances, and quality control procedures. Standardized forms are available for all procedures except quality control.

2. Prescription Forms.

    a. Clinic providers shall write prescriptions on the DoD Prescription blank, DD-1289 or equivalent, when chart prescribing, PGUI or POE is not available.

    b. All prescriptions shall be filed in one of three files:

        (1) All non-controlled drug prescriptions;

        (2) Schedule II prescriptions; and

        (3) Schedule III, IV, and V prescriptions.

    c. Prescriptions in black or blue ink, indelible pencil, or typewritten must show the information:

        (1) Patient's full name.

        (2) Date the prescription was written.

        (3) Full generic name (or trade name with substitution instructions), dosage form desired, and dosage size or strength written in the metric system. The quantity dispensed shall be clearly specified numerically ("one bottle" or "one package" are not acceptable). When writing for controlled prescriptions, the numeric quantity shall also be written out and in parentheses next to the numeric amount (e.g. Disp. 12 (twelve) tablets). Standard pharmacy abbreviations may be used in writing dispensing and dosage instructions but not in specifying the drug to be dispensed.

        (4) Complete, explicit directions to the patient are required. Expressions such as "take as directed," "label," etc. are not adequate directions and not allowed.

        (5) Prescriber's legible, legal signature (initials not permitted) with printed or stamped name and professional discipline (MD, DO, DMD, DDS, PA, HS2, etc.). When CG provider order entry is utilized, electronic signature satisfies this requirement.

        (6) All additional requirements when prescribing controlled substances:

            (a) Patients complete address.

            (b) Prescriber's SSN, DEA or NPI number.

            (c) NOTE: Alterations on prescriptions for CII controlled substances are prohibited.

d. Multiple prescription forms, such as Poly Prescription, NAVMED 6710/6 or Prescription Limited, Poly, NAVMED 6710/10 which are intended for use when prescribing a number of non-controlled drugs for one patient, are authorized.

e. Maintain all prescriptions on file, including all "prescription logs" related to chart prescribing, for three (3) years, after which they may be destroyed by shredding.

f. The pharmacy shall have ready access to the patient's medical information including provider's current patient visit entry, patient's current medications, age, allergies, weight, etc., when preparing and dispensing prescriptions.

3. Quality Control Forms. Quality control is important for proper conformity and safety of drug products to be dispensed. The two main areas that benefit from quality control are compounding and prepackaging. A locally prepared form shall be used which will provide clearly definable material sources (manufacturer's name, lot numbers, and expiration dates), procedures used, intermediary and final checks by supervisory personnel, and sample labeling.

4. Controlled Drug Forms.

   a. Narcotic and Controlled Drug Inventory-24 Hours, NAVMED 6710/4. This record shall be maintained at CG facilities providing inpatient care.

      (1) The Narcotic and Controlled Drug Inventory-24 Hours, NAVMED 6710/4 shall be signed by the senior health services technician on each watch after the drugs have been checked prior to relief. The drugs shall be checked concurrently by the HS reporting for duty as well as by the HS being relieved. Any discrepancies noted shall be reported immediately. The record is used for two (2) weeks, with a one (1) week period on each side. The night HS shall initiate the record.

      (2) The serial numbers of new Narcotic and Controlled Drug Account Record, NAVMED 6710/1 received from the pharmacy during each watch shall be entered. The serial numbers of completed Narcotic and Controlled Drug Account Record, NAVMED 6710/1 returned to the pharmacy shall be entered and the Pharmacist or authorized representative shall acknowledge receipt by initialing in the appropriate column.

      (3) At the time specified in local instructions, the senior health services technician shall audit the clinic controlled substances supplies. After the audit, the senior health services technician shall date and sign the Narcotic and Controlled Drug Inventory-24 Hours, NAVMED 6710/4.

   b. Narcotic and Controlled Drug Account Record, NAVMED 6710/1.

      (1) Upon receipt of a properly completed prescription requisition, a separate Narcotic and Controlled Drug Account Record, NAVMED 6710/1 shall be prepared by the pharmacy for each Schedule II through

Schedule V drug, and any other drug which, in the opinion of the CO, requires control procedures.

(2) All Narcotic and Controlled Drug Account Records, NAVMED 6710/1 shall be kept in a controlled drug book.

(3) All entries shall be made in blue or black ink. Errors shall be corrected by drawing a single line through the erroneous entry and having the person making the correction sign the entry. The correct entry shall be recorded on the following line, if necessary.

(4) If a new issue is received before the old issue is completely expended, the new Narcotic and Controlled Drug Account Record, NAVMED 6710/1 shall be inserted in back of the current record. The serial number of the new Narcotic and Controlled Drug Account Record, NAVMED 6710/1 shall be entered on the Narcotic and Controlled Drug Inventory-24 Hours, NAVMED 6710/4.

(5) The heading for each Narcotic and Controlled Drug Account Record, NAVMED 6710/1 shall be completed at the time of issue. The body shall be used for recording expenditures and balances only.

(6) Each time a drug is used, complete information shall be recorded: date, time, patient, prescriber's name, dispenser, amount used, and balance remaining on hand on the Narcotic and Controlled Drug Account Record, NAVMED 6710/1.

   (a) Record all amounts in Arabic numerals. Where the unit of measure is a milliliter (ml) and the amount used is less than one ml, it shall be recorded as a decimal (e.g., 0.5 ml) rather than a fraction.

   (b) When a fraction of the amount is expended to the patient, it shall be placed in parentheses before the amount recorded in the expended column; [e.g., an entry of (0.0005)1 on the morphine sulfate 16 mg/ml record indicates that one-half ml was expended and that 0.008 gm was administered].

   (c) If a single dose of a controlled substance is accidentally damaged or contaminated during preparation for administration or the patient refuses after preparation, the dose shall be destroyed and a brief statement of the circumstances shall be entered on the Narcotic and Controlled Drug Account Record, NAVMED 6710/1. Such statements shall be signed and witnessed by a second health care provider.

   (d) If multiple doses of a controlled substance are damaged, another senior HS shall record the disposition of the drug, including date, amount of drug, brief statement of disposition, and new balance. Both the senior and witnessing HS shall sign the Narcotic and Controlled Drug Account Record, NAVMED 6710/1.

(e) Deteriorated drugs shall be returned to the pharmacy for disposal.

(f) The completed Narcotic and Controlled Drug Account Record, NAVMED 6710/1, along with the counter-type dispenser, shall be returned to the pharmacy.

(g) Monthly, the pharmacy shall report all Narcotic and Controlled Drug Account Records, NAVMED 6710/1 still outstanding 30 days from date of issue. The report shall be verified and returned to the pharmacy for reconciliation. Discrepancies shall be reported to the CO via the Controlled Substances Audit Board Inventory Report.

c. <u>Narcotic and Controlled Drug Book</u>.

(1) Each activity drawing controlled substances from the pharmacy shall maintain a loose leaf notebook containing Narcotic and Controlled Drug Inventory-24 Hours, NAVMED 6710/4 in the first section and individual Narcotic and Controlled Drug Account Record, NAVMED 6710/1 in the latter sections.

(2) The senior HS shall remove all filled Narcotic and Controlled Drug Inventory-24 Hours, NAVMED 6710/4 over three (3) months old from the Narcotic and Controlled Drug Book and return them to the pharmacy.

d. <u>Perpetual Inventory of Narcotics, Alcohol, and Controlled Drugs, NAVMED 6710/5</u>. Separate Perpetual Inventory of Narcotics, Alcohol, and Controlled Drugs, NAVMED 6710/5 forms are not required for each controlled substance (C-II through C-V) when electronic records or documentation are available via the Composite Health Care System (CHCS) or equivalent software programs. The requirement for hard copy monthly substance audit board report, Monthly Report For Narcotics and Other Controlled Drugs, CG-5353 is still required, however the CHCS software prepares and automates controlled substance inventory reports which are acceptable and can be used as an equivalent to the Monthly Report For Narcotics And Other Controlled Drugs, CG-5353. If software is not consistently available, prepare a separate Perpetual Inventory of Narcotics, Alcohol, and Controlled Drugs, NAVMED 6710/5 for each controlled substance (C-II through C-V). All boxes and columns below are self-explanatory except as noted:

(1) Drug Name. Enter generic or proprietary drug name as appropriate, e.g., "Codeine Sulfate.

(2) Strength. Express as gm, mg, etc.

(3) Unit. Enter dosage form as appropriate.

(4) Prescription or Requisition Number. Enter appropriate prescription or requisition (voucher) number. For issues returned to the pharmacy, enter the source.

(5) Recipient. Enter "pharmacy" for receipts. Enter clinic or patient name, as appropriate, for expenditures.

(6) Narcotic and Controlled Drug Account Records, NAVMED 6710/1 Returned. The date the Narcotic and Controlled Drug Account Records, NAVMED 6710/1 is returned to the pharmacy shall be entered on the appropriate line bearing the same serial number or prescription number.

5. Forms Availability.

   a. Obtain DEA forms from the nearest DEA office. Consult with a pharmacy officer for more information.

   b. Prescription Blanks. Prescription blanks DoD Prescription, DD1289 can be found at the following web site: http://www.dtic.mil/whs/directives/infomgt/forms/formsprogram.htm.

This page intentionally left blank.

COMDTINST M6000.1E

Section D. Drug Dispensing Without a Medical Officer

1. General. 1
2. Child-Resistant Containers. 1
3. Controlled Substances. 1
4. Formulary. 1
5. Non-Prescription Medication Program 2

This page intentionally left blank.

Section D. **Drug Dispensing Without a Medical Officer**.

1. **General**. Health Services Technicians (HSs) dispensing prescriptions without a Medical Officer's direct supervision, (e.g., at independent duty shore stations or vessels), shall be conducted in accordance with provisions of this manual and the Health Services Allowance List. These services shall be provided for active duty personnel only. HSs in these situations are encouraged to seek consultation with their assigned collateral duty Pharmacy Officer when necessary.

2. **Child-Resistant Containers**. Prepackaged OTC products should be issued in their original container. For vessels, limited quantities of prescription drugs may be issued in labeled plastic zip-lock bags while underway with proper labeling including name of patient, name of medication, exact instructions, precautions, and warnings regarding the medication, date dispensed, and initials of dispenser. These bags must be inserted in a child resistant container with proper labeling if they are removed from the vessel.

3. **Controlled Substances**.

    a. All drugs shall be dispensed under the supervision of a Health Services Technician at activities where there are no officers of the health services department.

    b. An officer (usually the XO), designated by the CO, shall serve as the Controlled Substance Custodian (CSC) and keep in a separate locked compartment, all bulk un-issued controlled substances, alcohol, or items otherwise controlled. The CSC shall always maintain positive control of the keys or combination. The CSC shall arrange for the care and safe custody of all keys and require strict compliance with instructions concerning the receipt, custody, and issue of controlled substances and alcohol as contained in the law, CG Regulations, and this manual.

    c. The CSC or the designated Sickbay/Medical personnel shall retain the keys or combination to the working stock storage area while on duty. When relieved, they shall deliver the keys to their relief or to a responsible person designated by local instructions. A copy of the combination of a safe, if used, shall be sealed in an envelope and deposited with the CO.

    d. COs may authorize temporary deviations from the controls established in this Chapter due to operational and/or emergency situations.

    e. Controlled Substance Audit Board (CSAB) at these units (e.g., Cutters) shall be conducted at least quarterly by two disinterested members. CSAB shall also be conducted when there is a change in designation of the CSC and when there is a permanent change in Sickbay/Medical personnel. Chapter 10.B. provides detailed instructions regarding CSAB.

4. **Formulary**. Health Services Technicians on independent duty shall maintain drug formularies consisting of:

    a. Standardized Health Services Drug Formulary items.

    b. Health Services Allowance List requirements.

c. Chronic medications prescribed by a physician for active duty members currently assigned to the duty station.

d. Other drugs the HS has been authorized in writing by the DMOA to stock for their active duty members. A copy of the DMOA's written approval of these medications will be forwarded to the collateral duty pharmacist (RPE) for review and approval. The review will ensure compliance with the DoD Basic Core Formulary.

5. <u>Non-Prescription Medication Programs</u>. Sickbays are encouraged to operate non-prescription medication programs as described in paragraph 10-A-6.j. of this Manual. HSs shall contact their collateral duty Pharmacists for guidance and additional support.

COMDTINST M60001.E

CHAPTER 11

HEALTH CARE PROCUREMENT

Section A. Contracting For Health Care Services.

1. General 1
2. Type of Services 1
3. Eligibility For Contract Health Care Services 2
4. Approval to Contract for Services 2
5. Funding 3
6. Pre-contract Award Actions 4
7. Award Evaluation Factors 6
8. Post-Contract Award Actions 6

Section B. Health Care Services Invoice Review and Auditing.

1. General 1
2. Invoices Subject to Review and Audit 1
3. Review and Audit Procedures 1
4. Report of Potential Third Party Liability (RCN 6000-2) 2

Section C. Claims Processing.

1. General 1
2. Certification 1
3. Administrative Screen 1
4. Technical Screen 2
5. Appropriateness Review 3
6. Peer Review 4
7. Guidelines for Initial Appropriateness and Peer Reviews 5

COMDTINST M6000.1E

This page intentionally left blank

Chapter 11 Contents

Section A. Contracting For Health Care Services.

1. General 1
2. Type of Services 1
3. Eligibility for Contract Health Care Services 2
4. Approval to Contract for Services 2
5. Funding 3
6. Pre-Contract Award Actions 3
7. Award Evaluation Factors 5
8. Post-Contract Award Actions 6

This page intentionally left blank.

A. Contracting For Health Care Services.

1. General. Commandant (CG-11) has fiscal responsibility for health care for all CG beneficiaries. The necessary care can be obtained through contracts with private concerns and individuals and interagency and other agreements with military facilities. COs are responsible for obtaining the necessary services for each fiscal year, subject to HSWL SC review and approval. HSWL SC first authorizes all non-emergency, non-Federal health care. The HSWL SC is responsible for all health services contracting in its area and shall comply with Federal Acquisition Regulations Part 37. The HSWL SC oversees all non-Federal care acquired and minimizes expenses by ensuring competitive contracting procedures take place.

2. Type of Services. The following services may be procured by contract as determined by the HSWL SC.

    a. Allergist.

    b. Dental Prosthetic Laboratory.

    c. Dentist, Dental Hygienist, or chairside Dental Assistant.

    d. General medicine (Physician or Midlevel Providers).

    e. Group Practice Hospital.

    f. Gynecologist.

    g. Medical Laboratory.

    h. Neurologist.

    i. Nurse (Registered or Licensed Practical).

    j. Obstetrician.

    k. Occupational Health Services (for OCCMED Physicals).

    l. Optometrist.

    m. Orthopedist.

    n. Pharmacist.

    o. Physical Therapist or Certified Athletic Trainer.

    p. Psychiatrist or Psychologist.

    q. Radiologist.

3. <u>Eligibility For Contract Health Care Services</u>. Eligibility for contract health care services is the same as described in Chapter 2.

   a. The following persons are NOT eligible for health care services rendered by contract providers:

      (1) Family members of CG personnel and retired and retired members of the CG (however, they may receive health care services when the contractor performs the service at a CG Clinic or sickbay and/or if the CG has contracted with a health care provider as a demonstration project).

      (2) Active duty beneficiaries separated from the Service while undergoing treatment (eligibility for treatment terminates and becomes the member's responsibility).

      (3) CG civilian employees except for required Occupational Medical Surveillance and Evaluation Program (OMSEP) physical examinations and required pre-appointment examinations, all funded using HSWL SC funds.

   b. Dental laboratory fees for non-active duty beneficiaries:

      (1) <u>Retirees</u>. Retirees are authorized to use private sector dental laboratories. Pay retirees' dental laboratory fees in the same manner as for active duty members.

      (2) <u>Dependents</u>. The dependent receiving the treatment shall pay all private sector laboratory fees resulting from space-available treatment . A suggested way to handle such payments is to require dependents to submit a check or money order payable to the private sector laboratory before delivery of appliances. The attending Dental Officer then photocopies the check or money order, pays the laboratory, and retains the photocopy in the dental record.

4. <u>Approval to Contract for Services</u>.

   a. Units shall submit letter requests for contract health care services through the appropriate chain of command to the HSWL SC. All requests must contain this information:

      (1) Description of services required (e.g., general health care, pharmacy, lab, or specialty care such as OB/GYN, optometry, or psychiatry), including desired days and hours of availability.

      (2) A justification of the need for the service.

      (3) Estimated annual cost of the required services.

(4) A list of USMTFs within 40 miles of the unit and whether they could perform the desired service.

(5) A list of CG units benefiting from the services.

(6) The number of active duty members assigned to each unit.

(7) Either the names and mailing addresses of all interested, recommended providers or a justification of other than full, open competition (see paragraph 11-A-7, Pre-contract Award Actions, below).

(8) Preferred solicitation area and the rationale for it (e.g. "provider must be located within 20 miles of the unit", etc.).

(9) Estimated number of annual CG visits to the provider.

(10) A list (by type) of any other approved or requested health care contracts.

b. Each request must be able to stand on its own merits and fulfill cost-to-benefit criteria. HSWL SC will analyze each request and provide written approval or disapproval (with alternative proposals) to the requesting unit through the chain of command. If approved, the HSWL SC Contracting Officer will undertake procurement.

c. HSWL SC will not renew existing contracts simply as a matter of convenience. Each contract must continue to prove its value annually on a cost-to-benefit basis before its renewal. HSWL SC will review each contract's current fiscal year activity. If the contract passes review, it may be renewed; if it does not, HSWL SC will so advise the unit receiving the contract services.

5. Funding.

a. The HSWL SC shall budget, review, and pay for all HSWL SC authorized non-Federal health care obtained in its area. These documents contain detailed instructions:

(1) HSWL SC Standing Operating Procedures (HSWL SC SOP), Annex D.

(2) Maintenance and Logistics Command, Pacific Instruction M6000.1 (series).

b. Charge all HSWL SC authorized non-Federal health care expenditures to the HSWL SC AFC-57 account. HSWL SC can find detailed object class and cost center information in the Accounting Manual, COMDTINST M7300.4 (series).

6. Pre-contract Award Actions.

a. The Contracting Officer issues solicitations to obtain supplies and services from industry on a competitive (more than 1 source) or non-competitive (1 source) basis. The Competition in Contracting Act of 1984 (PL-98-369) requires the Government to contract for supplies and services by means of full, open competition to the maximum extent possible. This means all responsible firms or individuals who can provide the supplies or services must be allowed to compete for a government contract. Contracting Officers locate potential contractors by publishing the proposed procurement in the *Commerce Business Daily* as required by Federal Acquisition Regulation (FAR), Part 5.

   (1) <u>Non-competitive Procurements</u>. Pre-awarding a firm a Government contract violates the Competition in Contracting Act of 1984. If it is claimed only one firm can provide the supplies or service, the purchasing office must justify in writing other than full, open competition, setting forth the facts and rationale (see FAR, Part 6) to support this claim. The justification must be certified that it is accurate and complete and send it with the purchase request when sending it to the contracting officer for procurement action.

   (2) <u>Competitive Procurements</u>. The Contracting Officer also may require certain information before contracting on a competitive basis. The Contracting Officer may request the types of information below to determinate responsibility within the meaning of Federal Acquisition Regulation, Part 9.

       (a) Organizational structure and plan to accomplish the service.

       (b) Summary of experience in performing the same or similar work.

       (c) Evidence of pertinent state and local licenses.

       (d) Evidence of professional liability insurance, or that the offeror can obtain such insurance.

       (e) Membership in professional organizations.

       (f) Resume of key personnel with particular emphasis on academic achievements pertinent to the proposed services.

       (g) Information about the firm or its key individuals that reflects their status or professional recognition in their field, e.g., awards, published articles, and the like.

b. <u>Pre-award survey</u>. Subject to the Contracting Officer's approval, a visit may be made to the offeror's facility before the award (pre-award survey) to review some of the above data to reduce submitted data. The following paragraphs are examples of the information that may be required from an offer or

   (1) Brief description of the facility, how long established, where located relative to the required mile radius, daily operating hours, weekly operating hours (include holidays, Saturdays, and Sundays).

   (2) Brief description of similar work performed under Government contracts including the government agency's name, contract number, contract price, and name and telephone number of the agency's contracting officer.

   (3) A resume, X pages maximum, including education, past and present experience over the last X years, certificates, association membership, etc., of the key persons who will perform the work under the contract and their letter of intent indicating they intend to work for the offeror if it is awarded the medical services contract.

   c. Qualifications. Minimum qualifications required to perform the contract may be stated; however, these qualification requirements must be justified. For example:

   (1) Personnel.

      (a) Physician. At a minimum, a X year degree in medicine from an accredited college, license to practice medicine in the location where the services will be performed, member of the AMA; X years' experience in practicing general medicine.

      (b) Nurse. RN or LPN. B.S. degree (or equivalent) in nursing from an accredited college; ANA-certified or equivalent; X years' experience in handling patients, administering patient records, etc.

      (c) Laboratory Technician. HHS certified, ASCP or eligible, X years' experience in all phases of laboratory work; e.g., x-rays, blood samples, etc.

   (2) Facility.

      (a) Within a X mile radius of the CG facility requiring the services.

      (b) Capable of accommodating or rendering services for at least X patients simultaneously.

7. Award Evaluation Factors.

   a. State the steps or procedures to be used to evaluate the proposals.

b. List the evaluation criteria in the descending order of relative importance and state whether one factor will have predominant consideration over another. For example:

   (1) Personnel.

   (2) Experience.

   (3) Facility.

   (4) Price.

c. Establish the criteria to be used in evaluating the proposal. They must be the same as the evaluation factors for award the solicitation cited. The weights assigned to the factors may be in any form, e.g., adjective (acceptable, outstanding), numerical (50). Give this information to the Contracting Officer, preferably before he or she issues the solicitation, but in any event before receiving the proposals for evaluation.

8. <u>Post-Contract Award Actions</u>.

   a. <u>Referring for Contract Services</u>. Before referring any person to a medical services contractor, the cognizant authority shall determine whether:

      (1) The person is eligible.

      (2) Services are available in-house.

      (3) Services are available from a USMTF.

      (4) Services are available from another Federal facility, e.g., Department of Veterans Affairs, under an interagency support agreement.

   b. <u>Contracting Officer's Technical Representative</u>. The contracting office that awarded the contract administers it. If the requiring office requests, a Contracting Officer's Technical Representative (COTR) may be assigned to the contract. The COTR is preferably a health services program manager or medical administration officer having jurisdiction in the contract services area. The Contracting Officer designates the Contracting Officer's Technical Representative in a written, signed letter of appointment describing the COTR's responsibilities and limitations. These responsibilities and limitations must strictly be adhered to avoid any conflicts with the contractor about changes to contract terms and conditions.

   c. <u>Health Care Invoices</u>.

      (1) Contractor Invoices.

         (a) All invoices for health care services contractors by contractors shall be processed for payment under the applicable contract's terms and conditions. This Manual's Chapter 2 describes certifying and processing non-Federal health care invoices. The Contracting Officer is responsible for including the applicable invoice and payment clauses (e.g., Federal Acquisition Regulations 52.204-3, Taxpayer Identification, 52.232-25, Prompt Payment, etc.) in the contract. Ensure the contracting officer also includes these invoice requirements in the contract so the invoice is proper for payment:

(1) An itemized, priced list of the services by contract or order line item number.

(2) Any additional information deemed necessary to process the invoice for payment.

(b) In addition to the invoice requirements above any invoice without the following supporting documentation will not be paid.

(1) Services Rendered Under Non-Emergent Conditions. A referral slip or written confirmation of patient's eligibility from cognizant health services department representative.

(2) Services Rendered Under Emergent Conditions. A written statement from the patient describing the emergent condition(s). The cognizant health services department representative must certify the patient's eligibility and emergent condition.

(c) If the eligible patient pays the contractor for services rendered under a contract and requests reimbursement, the reimbursement claim must be submitted to the appropriate accounting office on Public Voucher for Purchases and Services Other Than Personal SF-1034,. A patient's invoice cannot be reimbursed from funds obligated under a contract even though the contractor rendered the services. These documents must accompany the claim:

(1) The contractor's itemized invoice.

(2) A copy of the invoice and receipt showing payment to the contractor.

(3) The patient's written statement of the circumstances justifying the claim.

(4) The cognizant health services department representative's approval of the claim.

(2) Invoices outside the CONUS.

(a) The nearest CG facility having an authorized certifying officer shall process invoices for emergency health care from civilian facilities furnish to CG members. The invoices and justification explaining the reasons for the emergency health care must be attached to the Claim for Reimbursement for Expenditures on Official Business, SF-1164.

(b) Every attempt to pay for emergency health care should be made before departing from a foreign port to reduce paperwork and pay at the exchange rate. For emergency care under $2500.00 the Imprest Fund may be used. If payment prior to departure is not feasible, advise the facility rendering the service to send all invoices to the United States Embassy or appropriate consular office for the area.

Figure 11.A.1

STATEMENT OF WORK

1. Scope. Provide all labor, materials, and facilities necessary to perform the tasks herein.

2. Definitions.

    a. Patient. An eligible CG military member.

    b. Emergency. Treatment required to curtail the patient's undue suffering or loss of life or limb.

    c. Non-Elective Condition. A condition that, if untreated, would render the patient unfit for duty.

    d. Elective Procedure. Treatment the patient *desires*, e.g., vasectomy, tubal ligation, sterility test, contact lenses, orthodontics, etc.

    e. Duty Status. A determination of the patient's ability to perform the assigned tasks at the assigned work station. These statuses apply:

        (1) Fit for Full Duty (FFD). Patient is not physically restricted or limited.

        (2) Fit for Limited Duty (FLD). Patient is physically restricted or limited, e.g., office work only; no lifting, stooping, prolonged standing, walking, running, jumping, sea duty, etc.

        (3) Not Fit for Duty (NFD). Patient cannot perform any assigned tasks at assigned work station.

3. The contractor shall perform these tasks:

    a. Task I - Eligibility Determination. Provide service to the CG military personnel listed below. Each patient must show the required authorizations before the Contractor renders service.

    b. Task II - Physical Examinations. Examine the patient according to Attachment (1) requirements. [Attach copy of appropriate section of Medical Manual, COMDTINST M6000.l (series).]

    c. Task III - Immunization. Immunize the patient and document appropriately on Standard Form 601 (Immunization Record) or Public Health Form 731 (International Certificate of Vaccination) in the CG Health Record the patient presents the contractor. Record also any sensitivity reactions to the immunization. The contractor shall use only those immunizing agents approved by the Department of Health and Human Services. Immunize the patient at the time intervals Attachment 2 specifies. [Attach a copy of Immunization and Chemoprophylaxis, COMDTINST M6230.4 (series).]

d. Task IV - Emergency Hospitalization. Provide all necessary services to patient while he or she is hospitalized, to a maximum of seven days. If the patient requires hospitalization for eight or more days, the contractor shall notify the CG point of contact by telephone. If the CG elects to transfer the patient to a military hospital, the contractor shall complete all necessary documents the civilian hospital may require to effect the transfer.

e. Task V - Prosthetic and Orthopedic Appliances. The contractor shall provide prosthetic or orthopedic appliances to the patient only under emergency conditions (required immediately due to his or her condition). The contractor shall document the emergency condition on the CG Health Record. Under non-emergency conditions, the contractor shall refer the patient to a military hospital to obtain these appliances.

f. Task VI - Communicable Disease. The contractor shall report all communicable diseases and recommended control measures to the CG health care provider or CO immediately after detecting the disease. The contractor also shall report to local authorities as required by local regulations.

g. Task VII - Notification. The contractor shall notify the CG health care provider or patient's CO if a patient is seriously ill, injured, or dies.

h. Task VIII - Records and Reports. For all patients the contractor shall maintain a record with this information:

   (1) Outpatient Record. Record the name, rank or rating, Social Security Number, address, date of treatment, history of present illness, physical findings, diagnostic procedures including x-rays and laboratory, therapy provided, fitness for duty determination, duration and limitations if unfit or fit for limited duty, and the contractor's printed name and signature.

   (2) Inpatient Report. On discharge from the hospital, furnish the patient's medical report written using diagnostic nomenclature (standard disease and operation nomenclature) to summarize the course of the case, laboratory and x-ray findings, surgeries and treatments, complications, current condition, final diagnosis, and a fitness for duty determination with duration and limitations if unfit or fit for limited duty.

i. Task IX - Certificate of Services. After rendering services to the patient, complete Attachment (3) and obtain the patient's signature before he or she departs from the contractor's facility or location where the services were rendered. [Attach copy of certification form.]

4. The contractor shall not execute any oral or written agreements with the patient to render a more expensive type of service than that described in the contract in which the patient pays the difference in price between the contract unit price and the price the contractor charges (for eyeglasses, see Chapter 8 Section E).

5. The contractor must obtain written authority from the patient's CG unit before filling any prescriptions.

6. The contractor must obtain written authority from the patient's CG unit before performing any elective procedure.

Personnel	Required Authorization
Active Duty	1. Valid Common Access I.D. Card 2. A referral slip signed by an authorized CG official
Reservists (Active Duty)	1. Valid Common Access I.D. Card 2. Copy of active duty orders 3. A referral slip signed by an authorized CG official
Reservists	1. Valid Common Access I.D. Card 2. A Notice of Eligibility. See Reserve Policy Manual, COMDTINST M1001.28 (series) for further details.
PHS Commissioned Officers on CG Active Duty	1. Valid Common Access I.D. Card
Prospective CG Recruit	A letter signed by an authorized official at the CG recruiting unit
The contractor shall not provide services under this contract to personnel who do not have the required authorizations listed above.	

Table 11-A-1

This page intentionally left blank.

COMDTINST M6000.1E

Section B. Health Care Services Invoice Review and Auditing.

1. General 1
2. Invoices Subject to Review and Audit 1
3. Review and Audit Procedures 1
4. Report of Potential Third Party Liability (RCN 6000-2) 2

This page intentionally left blank.

B. Health Care Services Invoice Review and Auditing.

1. General.

   a. Review and audit. All health care invoices are subject to review and audit to ensure the CG pays only for necessary, appropriate health care for its beneficiaries.

      (1) The auditing process ensures the contractor's invoice charges for services provided at either reasonable fees or those in agreement with the contract.

      (2) The review process determines the appropriateness of care for the diagnosis.

   b. Discrepancies. Personnel performing the review and audit functions must remember if they find discrepancies, they must give the care provider the opportunity to comment on the findings.

   c. Conduct. The process of health care invoice auditing and review is complex and lends itself to errors; thus, most reviews and audit inquiries are not dismissed. Finding must be presented in a non-threatening manner, demonstrating the CG's willingness to cooperate with our health care providers in determining fair, equitable charges.

2. Invoices Subject to Review and Audit. These contract and non-contract health services invoices are subject to review and audit. The unit processing the invoice should review bills in these categories before paying them:

   a. All outpatient invoices contractors submit;

   b. All inpatient and outpatient supplemental care.

3. Review and Audit Procedures. The personnel processing health care invoices should perform these procedures:

   a. Review.

      (1) Is the diagnosis compatible with the prescribed care?

      (2) Are ancillary services (e.g., lab, x-ray, pharmacy, electrodiagnostic tests, etc.) prescribed appropriately in amount and frequency?

      (3) Is the length of care appropriate for the diagnosis?

   b. Audit. Does the contractor's invoice meet the contract definition of a proper invoice? If not, notify the Contracting Officer immediately.

      (1) Is the bill mathematically correct?

(2) Does it bill only for authorized care and services?

(3) Were services and billed care actually furnished?

(4) Do the charges agree with the provider's regular fee schedule or the prices listed in the contract?

(5) Does the bill give credit for incomplete, canceled, or partial treatments?

(6) Do dates of care match the time period the patient received the care or services?

(7) Have previous audits of this provider demonstrated billing errors?

4. <u>Report of Potential Third Party Liability, RCN 6000-2</u>. Under the Federal Medical Care Recovery Act the CG will collect the cost of health care provided to any eligible beneficiary from the appropriate insurance carrier or eligible third party. Refer to Health Care Third Party Claims Recovery, COMDTINST 6010.16 (series) for current policy. Submit this report on Report of Potential Third Party Liability, CG-4899.

Section C. Claims Processing

1. General 1
2. Certification 1
3. Administrative Screen..1
4. Technical Screen..2
5. Appropriateness Review 3
6. Peer Review 4
7. Guidelines for Initial Appropriateness and Peer Reviews 5

This page intentionally left blank.

C. Claims Processing.

1. General. The HSWL SC is responsible for processing Federal and nonfederal health care claims in compliance with the Federal Law and CG Regulations.

2. Certification. Certification ensures that only authorized payment services to eligible beneficiaries receiving health care within their entitlements and the care and related charges are appropriate. The HSWL SC shall:

    a. Administratively screen each claim and supporting documents according to paragraph 3 below. Claims submission procedures from field units are provided by the HSWL SC Standard Operating Procedures.

    b. Technically screen claims and supporting document according to paragraph 4 below. In screening, perform these actions:

        (1) Refer claims that do not satisfy the Technical Screen criteria to a medical audit staff for Appropriateness Review and/or audit.

        (2) Enter information from these claims into the Non-Federal Invoice Processing System (NIPS) data base and approve them for payment in this manner:

            (a) Claims that satisfy Administrative and Technical Screen criteria (including Active Duty Claims Program (ADCP) claims coded through a TRICARE Fiscal Intermediary).

            (b) Claims referred for Appropriateness Review and/or audit recommended for payment.

    c. Transmit payment data electronically to the CG Finance Center.

    d. Certify batch transmissions.

    e. Correct batch errors.

    f. Update vendor files.

3. Administrative Screen.

    a. Administrative screening. Administrative screening of a claim package determines the patient's authorization and eligibility to receive billed services and also ensures the package contains all appropriate, necessary documents. At a minimum, administrative screening includes:

        (1) Patient information is present and complete.

        (2) Public Voucher for Purchases and Services other than Personal, SF-1034 is completed for reimbursement requests.

(3) The claim is a complete, itemized original.

(4) A copy of the Report of Potential Third Party Liability, CG-4899 is attached if a third party is potentially liable.

(5) Verification of pre-authorization number.

(6) Support documentation is complete for Reservists' bills.

(7) Claims for formal contracts have the Contracting Officer's signature and amount to be paid.

(8) Claims for clinic support contracts have a CG beneficiary breakdown.

b. Ensure that all claims that fail to satisfy the administrative screening are corrected by the unit through the most expeditious means possible.

4. Technical Screen.

a. Health care claims must be reviewed to ensure they comply with Federal regulations. Part of that process compares claim packages to standard criteria to withstand the scrutiny of Departmental Accounting and Financial Information System (DAFIS) for payment. Technical screening of claim packages includes:

(1) Comparing charges against contract fee schedules, pre-authorizations, blanket purchase agreements, or the geographic area's usual and customary fees; claims falling within ADCP guidelines are exempt from fee review.

(2) Entering relevant claim information into NIPS.

(3) Determining whether services were appropriate for the diagnosis.

(4) Identifying claims requiring further review under these circumstances.

(a) Unrelated charges to the initial diagnosis or injury.

(b) Duplicate charges for services received on a given day.

(c) Care was unauthorized or unnecessary.

(d) Claims submitted by different providers for the same service (e.g., anesthesiology charges from more than one provider).

(e) NIPS "flagged" the claim.

(f) The reviewer "feels" a need for further review.

b. Claims a Technical Screen identifies for further review and/or audit require:

(1) Documentation of the problem.

(2) A recommended course of action.

5. Appropriateness Review.
    a. An Appropriateness Review is performed under these circumstances:

    (1) The HSWL SC selects or NIPS flags a claim for further review and/or audit for a Technical Screen; and/or

    (2) Periodically for quality assurance.

    b. An Appropriateness Review requires:

    (1) An itemized claim.

    (2) A patient's signed Request for Medical Records, DD-877 or its' equivalent, to request medical records and other information about an individual's care. Various records, which may include.

        (a) Hospital records.

        (b) Physician's orders.

        (c) Physician and nursing progress notes.

        (d) Lab and x-ray reports.

        (e) Operative or endoscopic reports.

        (f) Admission records (history and physical examinations).

        (g) Discharge summaries.

    c. Appropriateness Review. An Appropriateness Review process often involves these activities:

    (1) Reviewing records to verify treatment of therapy was:

        (a) Appropriate for the diagnosis.

        (b) Consistent with currently accepted medical practice.

        (c) Not duplicated unnecessarily.

        (d) The length of inpatient hospitalization was appropriate for the diagnosis and course of care.

(e) The charges were reasonable; claims falling within ADCP guidelines are exempt from fee review.

(2) Obtaining additional documentation and/or correspondence from health care providers.

(3) Initially notifying health care providers of this information:

(a) Their claims are being reviewed and audited.

(b) The audit is a normal part of the CG's health care review process and does not indicate or allege the health care provider committed an offense.

(c) If reviewing cases for longer than 30 days, periodically communicate with health care providers to inform them of claim status.

d. <u>An Appropriateness Review may recommend</u>.

(1) Full payment for services. Enter data into and process through NIPS.

(2) Partial payment for services. Attach decision documents; recommend the amount of payment; and enter data into NIPS. Initiate a reimbursement request if the claim initially was overpaid.

(3) Consulting a specialist for peer review.

(4) Referral to a contractor for further review or an on-site hospital audit.

(5) Closing the case with no further action.

e. <u>An Appropriateness Review includes</u>.

(1) Fully documenting the decision process.

(2) Initiating payment or the provider's reimbursement.

(3) Drafting appropriate correspondence.

6. <u>Peer Review</u>.

a. A Peer Review will be performed under one of these circumstances:

(1) A health care provider objects to under these other reviews' findings.

(2) An Appropriateness Review reveals the need for a more sophisticated evaluation of the diagnosis, prognosis, or specific medical procedures employed.

b. Send the case and health care provider's additional documentation (if any) to a qualified medical, pharmaceutical, or dental specialist for review. These services should be contracted if in-house specialists are not available. Obtain a business associate agreement that the privacy, confidentiality and security of protected health information will be safeguarded in compliance with Federal and State laws.

c. Peer Review may include these detailed examinations:

   (1) Diagnosis.

   (2) Prognosis.

   (3) Appropriateness of the care provided.

   (4) Claims submitted to a Fiscal Intermediary for pricing are exempt from fee review.

   (5) Selection of the most cost-effective therapy.

d. Among other things a Pharmacist's review of pharmaceutical bills and supporting documents may include one of the following:

   (1) Determine the efficacy of prescribed medication.

   (2) Identify cost-effective choices.

   (3) Recommend stocking pharmaceuticals for future issuance.

7. Guidelines for Initial Appropriateness and Peer Reviews. These common health care services guidelines are not all-inclusive. Appropriateness and Peer Reviews should be used to assist reviewers in deciding whether in-hospital audits or contracted review services are required.

   a. Trauma. Answer these questions:

      (1) Does the level of care correspond to the diagnosis?

      (2) Were appropriate facilities used?

      (3) Were laboratory and x-ray procedures appropriate? Include justification for:

         (a) Repeating procedures on a given day.

         (b) Repeating normal procedures.

         (c) Failing to follow up abnormal tests.

(4) Were iatrogenic complications were identified appropriately? Include:

    (a) Sepsis.

    (b) Wound dehiscence.

    (c) Hemorrhage.

    (d) Pulmonary complications.

    (e) Cardiovascular complications (thrombophlebitis, etc.).

    (f) Urinary tract infection.

    (g) Anesthetic or other drug reactions (appropriate drug and dosage, known allergies).

    (h) Other associated injuries.

(5) The length of stay was appropriate for the diagnosis and indicated complications.

(6) The discharge diagnosis was compatible with admission diagnosis and the patient's history.

(7) The patient's physical status on discharge:

    (a) Alive.

    (b) Complications were controlled.

    (c) Wound(s) condition was satisfactory.

    (d) Required follow-up arrangements are listed.

    (e) Medications were prescribed.

(8) Follow-up care was appropriate, including:

    (a) Therapy.

    (b) Office visits.

    (c) Additional hospitalization was for a good reason, e.g., iatrogenic complications, continued therapy, or additional surgeries.

(9) Fees are usual and customary for the geographic area (claims falling within ADCP guidelines are exempt from fee review).

(10) The use of multiply providers is explained.

(11) Providers' and reviewers' differences in medical opinion (particularly involving altered treatment and length of hospital stay) are significant enough to warrant negotiation.

b. <u>Laboratory Services</u>. Answer these questions:

(1) Are tests related to or necessary for the diagnosis?

(2) Were ICU standing orders in effect?

(3) Were tests repeated excessively?

(4) Were charges duplicated for the same procedure on the same day?

(5) Were tests repeated due to equipment or operator error?

(6) Were tests repeated despite normal previous test(s) (justification is required)?

(7) Were there multiple charges for the same or similar tests?

(8) Were multiple tests performed in a logical sequence (i.e., the most invasive or sophisticated performed last)?

(9) Were fees usual and customary (claims falling within ADCP guidelines are exempt from fee review)?

(10) For a laboratory under CG contract, were:

(a) Tests covered by the contract?

(b) Charges within fee schedule?

c. <u>Radiology Services</u>. Considerations:

(1) Was the examination required given the diagnosis?

(2) Were charges for portable radiology of an ambulatory patient?

(3) Were examinations repeated?

(4) Were bilateral x-rays appropriate (patients over 12 years of age)?

(5) Were charges or exams of the same anatomical part duplicated?

(6) Do examinations and in-patient dates coincide?

(7) Were examinations repeated despite normal findings in previous examinations?

d. Physical Therapy. Considerations:

(1) Was the injury or diagnosis properly documented? Did it include:

(a) Objective findings?

(b) Functional findings?

(c) Multiple provider discrepancies?

(d) Documentation of improvement?

(2) Did a physician prescribe treatment?

(3) Were injury management and treatments reasonable and necessary? Did they cover these:

(a) Was the treatment plan documented?

(b) Did objective findings permit the therapist and/or physician to monitor treatment results?

(c) Were changes in the treatment program due to unsuccessful results?

(d) Was treatment only for subjective complaints?

(e) Was the treatment related to diagnosis?

(f) Did the treatment follow standard procedures and protocols?

(g) Did the treatment plan include goals and objectives?

(4) Was the length or number of treatments excessive?

(5) Was treatment consistent or continuous or did patient attend sporadically?

(6) Did therapy continue after "Fit-For-Duty" status?

(7) Did therapy charges continue during stays in cardiac or intensive care units.

(8) Were charges duplicated for same-day, apparently inappropriate treatments?

(9) Was therapy frequency within accepted standards?

(10) Were same-day charges for three or more modalities during a single therapy session?

(11) Were charges usual and customary (claims falling within ADCP guidelines are exempt from fee review).

e. Dentistry.

(1) For provider contract care, were:

(a) Services within the contract scope?

(b) Charges within fee schedules?

(2) For emergency care, were:

(a) Services within the scope of entitlements?

(b) Charges reasonable and customary?

(3) For care pre-authorized in Chapter 2-A-6, did any of these occur?

(a) Did the HSWL SC assign a pre-authorization number?

(b) Were services within the authorized, standard treatment plan?

(c) Were treatments split to circumvent pre-authorization requirements?

(4) For all dental services, do any of these apply?

(a) Were services duplicated?

(b) Were billings for the same service duplicated?

(c) Were diagnosis charges consistent with services received?

(d) Were crowns constructed of precious metals?

(e) Are laboratory charges consistent with the service provided (bridges, crowns, partial or full dentures)?

f. Pharmacy.

(1) For contract providers, were services within the scope of the contract?

(2) For inpatient care, do any of these apply?

(a) Were billings duplicated?

(b) Was credit received for returned or unused medications?

(c) Did medication and in-patient dates coincide?

(d) Did medications' costs exceed 250 percent of Annual Pharmacists' Reference ("Red Book") average wholesale price (Note: This equals a 150 percent markup.)? Claims falling within ADCP guidelines are exempt from fee review.

CHAPTER 12

OCCUPATIONAL MEDICAL SURVEILLANCE AND EVALUATION PROGRAM (OMSEP)

Section A. General Requirements.

1. Description 1
2. Enrollment 1
3. Reporting Requirements 3
4. Medical Removal Protection 4
5. Roles and Responsibilities 4

Section B. Administrative Procedures.

1. General 1
2. Examination Types 1
3. Use of OMSEP Forms 5
4. Medical Removal Standards 6
5. Reporting of Examination Results 6

Section C. Medical Examination Protocols.

1. General 1
2. Asbestos, CG-6203 1
3. Benzene, CG-6204 4
4. Chromium Compounds, CG-6202 6
5. Hazardous Waste, CG-6206 8
6. Lead, CG-6207 10
7. Noise, CG-6205 and CG-6215 12
8. Pesticides, CG-6209 17
9. Respirator Wear, CG-6208 19
10. Respiratory Sensitizers, CG-6210 21
11. Solvents, CG-6213 23
12. Tuberculosis, CG-6212 26
13. Bloodborne Pathogens, CG-6211 27
14. Radiation (Ionizing/Non-ionizing), CG-6214 32

COMDTINST M6000.1E

This page intentionally left blank

Chapter 12 Contents

Section A. General Requirements.

1. Description 1
2. Enrollment 1
3. Reporting Requirements 3
4. Medical Removal Protection 4
5. Roles and Responsibilities. 4

This page intentionally left blank.

A. General Requirements.

1. Description.

    a. Introduction. The work environment and occupational activities inherent to CG missions can expose personnel to health hazards with the potential for disease or injury. The Occupational Medical Surveillance and Evaluation Program (OMSEP) is designed to identify work related diseases or conditions, through baseline and periodic examinations, at a stage when modifying the exposure or providing medical intervention could potentially arrest disease progression or prevent recurrences. The fundamental purpose of this program is to identify pre-existing health conditions, provide risk specific periodic screenings, and monitor clinical laboratory tests and biologic functions suggestive of work related environmental exposures. All OMSEP enrollees receive periodic physical examinations, in accordance with Occupational Safety and Health Administration (OSHA) requirements, for the duration of their health hazard exposure or end of their employment. Individuals are released from active surveillance at the end of their exposure. In accordance with OSHA regulations, the OMSEP personnel tracking database containing the name, social security number, billet or occupation code, applicable examination protocols, and next physical examination due date remains active for an additional 30 years.

    b. The OMSEP is the physical examination process for the CG's Occupational Health Program. The guidance for this program is outlined in the Safety and Environmental Health Manual, COMDTINST M5100.47 (series). OMSEP replaces the present version of the physical exam process described in the SEH Manual as the Occupational Medical Monitoring Program (OMMP).

2. Enrollment.

    a. CG Medical Surveillance Action Level: The medical surveillance action level (MSAL) is the level of worker exposure, determined by workplace sampling, at or above which occupational medical surveillance examinations will be performed. The CG MSAL will be 50% of the most stringent of the current OSHA permissible exposure limit (PEL), or the most current American Conference of Governmental Industrial Hygienists (ACGIH) Threshold Limit Value (TLV).

    b. Determination of Occupational Exposure.

        (1) An employee is considered occupationally exposed for OMSEP purposes if an exposure or hazardous condition is likely to occur 30 or more days per year. Documentation of the exposure must meet the following criteria: quantitative work-site sampling measurements indicate hazard levels at or above the MSAL or that the exposure can

reasonably be determined, in the absence of quantitative sampling, to exceed the MSAL.

(2) Quantitative sampling is the primary and definitive means to characterize workplace health hazards, although personal sampling measurement is preferred to workplace sampling. CG Safety and Environmental Health Officers (SEHOs) using guidance contained in the Safety and Environmental Health Manual, COMDTINST M5100.47 (series) will generally perform this function. SEHOs will normally characterize workplaces by frequency of exposure, type of exposure, and risk groups.

(3) Certain occupations or exposures may require surveillance by federal statutes, DOT regulations, or Safety and Environmental Health Manual, COMDTINST M5100.47 (series) without regard to the 30-day exposure threshold.

(4) Competent environmental health authority is considered to be the cognizant SEHO but the authority may be delegated to other recognized and approved personnel with the necessary technical training and abilities. Qualitative assessments must be based on expected type, frequency, mode, and duration of hazard exposure, and are considered temporary until validated by quantitative means.

(5) Unit Directives and/or Standard Operating Procedures (SOP's) enrollment guidelines and monitoring criteria developed and approved, at the unit level, by ALL cognizant parties (Health Services Division; Safety and Environmental Health; Industrial Hygiene-Unit Command) are acceptable so long as they comply, with the enrollment criteria set forth in Section A-2, b (1-4) above.

c. <u>Enrollment Criteria</u>. Recommendations for enrollment are based on specific job assignments and the level of worker exposure. This process is initiated at the unit level and must be finalized by the IH or cognizant SEHO, with recommendations from the supervising Medical Officer (if necessary), before forwarding to the HSWL SC via the OMSEP database (see section 12-A-3-(a)-3). Personnel will be enrolled in the OMSEP if either of the following criteria are met:

(1) Personnel identified as occupationally at risk/exposed to hazardous chemicals or physical agents at levels documented or reasonably determined to be above the CG Medical Surveillance Action Level (MSAL) for that hazard.

(2) Personnel actively engaged for 30 or more days per calendar year in the following occupations will be enrolled in OMSEP, unless an IH investigation determines individuals are not exposed to toxic chemicals

or physical hazards: resident inspectors, pollution investigators, marine safety (general), port safety (general), vessel inspectors or marine investigators; and firefighters.

(3) Note: New OMSEP enrollees may be considered for enrollment under the guidelines of the Hazardous Waste Protocol, which provides the most thorough surveillance for those with unknown hazardous risks and no prior history of exposures. However, the unit IH or cognizant SEHO may recommend enrollment using the medical surveillance protocol considered most appropriate.

3. <u>Reporting Requirements</u>.

   a. <u>Examination Reports</u>.

      (1) Required forms. OMSEP Initial/Baseline and Exit/Separation physical examinations require completion of the most current version of History and Report of OMSEP Examination, CG-5447 in addition to Report of Medical Examination, DD-2808 and Report of Medical History, DD-2807-1. Periodic examinations require completion of the most current version of the Periodic History and Report of OMSEP Examination, CG-5447A and any Acute Exposure requires completion of the Acute Exposure Information Form. Other OMSEP specific forms and their uses are presented in Chapter 4 of this Manual.

      (2) Record keeping. OMSEP personnel records will be handled in the same manner as other medical records (see Chapter 4 of this Manual) with the following exceptions: all x-ray, laboratory test, and related reports of examinations or procedures done for OMSEP purposes, as well as the medical record cover, shall be clearly labeled "OMSEP." All OMSEP examination reports, including all laboratory data, must be entered into the individual's health record and maintained in accordance with OSHA regulations. The member's medical record custodian will maintain all OMSEP medical records on file for the duration of employment. Upon separation or retirement, all records concurrently labeled "OMSEP" will be maintained, for an additional 30 years, as required by OSHA regulations [29 CFR 1915.1020].

      (3) OMSEP database. The HSWL SC will maintain an electronic database of all OMSEP enrollees based on enrollment information provided by the local units and will be accessible to the commands in accordance with privacy act requirements. The OMSEP personnel tracking database should include, at a minimum, the member's name, social security number (SSN), billet or occupation code, applicable examination protocols, and next physical examination due date. The handling of all data in the OMSEP database will comply with Privacy Act requirements.

COMDTINST M6000.1E

(4) Substitutions. OMSEP examination forms may not be substituted for other examination forms. If another examination is anticipated/required, (i.e. FLIGHT, RELAD) at the same time as the OMSEP examination the appropriate forms for each particular examination should be provided to the examiner so they may be completed at the same time. Duplicate laboratory tests are not required, so long as all specific tests and procedures required for each exam are completed and reported.

(5) Exposure data records. Any available exposure data, from workplace surveys, industrial hygiene personal or area monitoring, material safety data sheets, or assigned IH/SEHO other appropriate sources, will be provided by OMSEP coordinator to the examining Medical Officer as part of the examination packet. These data should be supplied by the local unit, in coordination with the supporting industrial hygienist, prior to the examination. The protocols in Section 12-C, in addition to OSHA regulations, specify what exposure surveillance data must be maintained and made available to the examining Medical Officer.

b. Individual unit's responsibilities. Individual units, in coordination with the cognizant SEHO, are responsible for creating and managing a roster of all OMSEP enrollees, and providing this information to the Designated Medical Officer Advisor (DMOA)/clinic and the HSWL SC. This information may be accessed at any time through the database. No written reports are required.

c. Sentinel Occupational Health Event Reporting. The occurrence of a new illness or disease, which is likely associated with an occupational exposure or condition, may be considered a "sentinel event." Such an event may serve as a warning signal that the quality of preventive measures may need to be improved. In order to facilitate timely intervention, the initial diagnosis of any such diseases must be reported IAW Section 7-B of this Manual. A complete list of reportable occupational diseases is found in Figure 7-B-2.

4. Medical Removal Protection. It is the responsibility of the CO to assure a safe and healthy working environment. The finding of a work-related illness or injury, which could be further exacerbated by continued exposure to a workplace hazard or condition, requires immediate evaluation to determine whether the worker must be at least temporarily removed from further exposure. A recommendation to remove the member should be made to the unit's CO by the examining Medical Officer in coordination with the cognizant SEHO (see section 12-B-4-b.).

5. Roles and Responsibilities. The OMSEP is part of a larger and more comprehensive surveillance process requiring the coordinated effort of various district units and local commands working to secure the safety and health of CG workers. Key personnel have been identified as essential in maintaining a sound

occupational health prevention program. Following is a description of their expected roles and responsibilities in this process: NOTE: For the purposes of this Chapter all references to employees, workers, personnel will be assumed to be part of the ONE CG TEAM concept. Rules, regulations, and directives apply equally to ALL unless otherwise specified.

a. Units/Commands. Each unit must appoint an OMSEP coordinator, usually the Safety Coordinator (SC) or the Safety and Occupational Health Coordinator (SOHC), or Independent Duty Corpsman. Even if units are under one servicing clinic, the unit is still required to appoint an OMSEP coordinator. The OMSEP coordinator is responsible for updating the database of OMSEP enrollees, ensuring OMSEP examinations are completed in a timely fashion, and ensuring all available exposure data is available to the Medical Officer at the time of the OMSEP examination. The OMSEP coordinator is responsible for assuring the privacy, confidentiality and security of the OMSEP records and reports.

b. HSWL SC. The HSWL SC will ensure that SEHO work-site monitoring and reporting is completed and entered into the appropriate database. Additionally they will provide oversight to the local units ensuring the accuracy and completeness of the OMSEP personnel database. The HSWL SC Medical Officers will provide oversight over the physical examination consultation and referral process. The HSWL SC will also provide indicated guidance and or training to HS personnel on examination practices and procedures.

c. SEHO's. SEHO's are required to review all requested OMSEP enrollments from the unit OMSEP Coordinators. SEHOs will approve or disapprove requested enrollments through the on-line database. Disapprovals need to be explained to the requesting unit. To substantiate enrollments, SEHOs are required to conduct and update quantitative and/or qualitative IH assessments of their units' workplace environment. SEHOs are required to have these written assessments available to the Medical Officer for review, if requested, to determine the appropriate medical surveillance protocol to use. SEHOs are also required to provide training and day-to-day consultation with their unit OMSEP Coordinators on database management, enrollment criteria and reporting requirements.

d. Commandant (CG-113). Commandant (CG-113) will provide planning, development, and expertise on occupational health issues. Commandant (CG-113) is responsible for policy making, procedural decisions, and ensuring currency of Chapter 12 of the Medical Manual with OSHA standards. The Commandant (CG-113) occupational medicine Medical Officer will provide support on physical examination problems and review all diagnosed occupational health related abnormalities encountered by the on-site provider, will be provided to onsite providers. Commandant (CG-113) is the final authority on decisions of any OMSEP related problems.

e. Medical Officer's Responsibilities.

   (1) Medical Diagnosis coding. The examining Medical Officer is responsible for explaining and/or following any abnormalities through to a resolution. All diagnoses made must be appropriately coded using the International Classification of Diseases (ICD), clinical modification's most current revision. ICD codes should be noted in parentheses next to the diagnosis on the examination report and be reported to the fifth digit.

   (2) Written assessment or opinion. Whenever a physical exam is performed, the examining Medical Officer must include the following information in writing as part of the record of each examination. This information should be included in the appropriate blocks.

      (a) The occupationally pertinent results of the medical examination.

      (b) An opinion about adequacy of the information available to support any diagnosed occupational disease(s), if appropriate.

      (c) Any recommended limitations to the employee's assigned work.

      (d) A statement that the employee has been informed about the results of the examination. (see Section 12-B-3-j.).

      (e) Any additional written information required by the protocols listed in Section 12-C.

f. Medical Administrators.

   (1) Support. Medical Administrators are responsible for providing administrative assistance on all OMSEP related matters. This support should extend to :

      (a) All units within the designated AOR.

      (b) Contracted medical providers and their respective facilities.

      (c) IDT's.

   (2) OMSEP report/worksite data. Medical Administrators should interact with OMSEP coordinators within their AOR to ensure currency of the roster of enrollees and ensure that work-site information is received in a timely manner. Worksite exposure information, reported history of past exposures and Material Safety Data Sheets (if needed) should precede the physical examination to give the Medical Officer ample time to reach an educated decision.

(3) Physical Examinations/Medical Records. The Medical Administrator is responsible for the following clinic functions in support of OMSEP:

    (a) Timely scheduling of physicals and entry of completed examination date in the OMSEP database.

    (b) Providing qualified technicians to perform the indicated laboratory and radiological procedures.

    (c) Ensuring proper calibration of equipment, and

    (d) Compliance with quality assurance standards.

g. <u>Civilian and Auxiliary Personnel</u>. Civilian employees and Auxiliary personnel (participating in the Trident program 30 or more days per year) may be entitled to OMSEP services provided by CG medical facilities should a determination be made by the Safety and Environmental Health Officer and confirmed by a medical provider, that an adverse health condition resulted from a work place exposure. Employees are expected to report and explain any illnesses or injuries resulting from exposure sources outside their primary duty station or from other non-occupational settings. Should a determination of an injury or illness, resulting from an exposure at the workplace, be made by a medical provider, civilian appropriated fund employees should contact their servicing civilian Command Staff Advisor (CSA) for assistance in making a claim with the Department of Labor. Non-appropriated fund employees (NAF) should contact their immediate supervisor and/or personnel liaison office. The services provided by the CG facilities will be only to establish an occupationally-related illness/injury. Further medical care should be provided by the civilian employee's health care provider.

h. <u>Others</u>. In the event of an emergency situation with heavy exposure (e.g., fire, spill), 24-hour assistance is available from the Agency for Toxic Substances Disease Registry (ATSDR) at the Centers for Disease Control and Prevention. Call (770) 488-7100.

LIST OF ABBREVIATIONS

ACGIH	American Conference of Governmental Industrial Hygienists
ALT	Alanine aminotransferase
AST	Aspartate amino transferase
BUN	Blood urea nitrogen
CBC	Complete blood count
CNS	Central nervous system
CXR	Chest x-ray
DOT	Department of Transportation
EL	Excursion limit (OSHA mandated maximal "safe" airborne concentration of a substance)
FVC	Forced vital capacity
FEV-1	Forced expiratory volume at one second
ICD-9	International Classification of Diseases, (coding system for medical diagnoses.)
IH	Industrial hygiene or industrial hygienist
LDH	Lactic dehydrogenase
MCV	Mean corpuscular volume
MCH	Mean corpuscular hemoglobin
MCHC	Mean corpuscular hemoglobin concentration
MO	Medical Officer (physician, physician's assistant or nurse practitioner)
MSAL	Medical surveillance action level (Defined in 12-A-3)
OMSEP	Occupational Medical Surveillance and Evaluation Program
OSHA	Occupational Safety and Health Administration
PEL	Permissible exposure limit (The OSHA mandated TWA airborne exposure limit)
PFTs	Pulmonary function tests

Table 12-A-1

LIST OF ABBREVIATIONS (continued)

RBC	red blood cell
SC	Safety Coordinator
SEHO	Safety and Environmental Health Officer
SOHC	Safety and Occupational Health Coordinator
STEL	Short-term exposure limit (The maximal "safe" airborne concentration of a substance)
STEL/C	Short-term exposure limit/ceiling (maximal "safe" airborne concentration of a substance)
STS	Significant threshold shift
TB	Tuberculosis
TLV	Threshold limit value (ACGIH) (The TWA airborne concentration of a substance)
TST	tuberculin skin test (Mantoux)
TWA	time-weighted average
U/A	Urinalysis

Table 12-A-1 (cont.)

This page intentionally left blank.

COMDTINST M6000.1E

Section B. Administrative Procedures.

1. General 1
2. Examination Types 1
3. Use of OMSEP Forms 5
4. Medical Removal Standards 6
5. Reporting of Examination Results 6

This page intentionally left blank.

B. Administrative Procedures.

1. General. All medical examinations and procedures required under the OMSEP shall be performed by or under the supervision of a licensed Medical Officer and an accredited laboratory shall perform all laboratory tests. Timely completion and monitoring of scheduled examinations is essential in identifying work related health hazards and any specific health effects. All tests required as part of an OMSEP examination should be completed prior to and the results made available to the health care provider at the time of the physical examination. This requirement may be waived if travel or time costs make separate visits impractical. The provider is required to review, approve (sign), and explain any abnormalities. Any unexplained, examination finding, laboratory abnormality, or test result must be referred to a certified Occupational Health Clinic/provider for further evaluation.

2. Examination Types.

    a. Initial/baseline. Baseline examinations are required before placement in a specific job in order to assess whether the worker will be able to do the job safely, to meet any established physical standards, and to obtain baseline measurements for future comparison. Each baseline examination shall consist of all of the elements specified under the appropriate surveillance protocol(s) in Section 12-C. In the event that the employee is being monitored under more than one protocol, each unique form or test need only be completed once for a particular examination.

        (1) An initial examination is required for all employees prior to employment. The employee may not be exposed to a potential health hazard until the physical examination is completed. In the event of scheduling delays, this requirement may be waived, if the employee completes ALL the necessary laboratory tests specified under the appropriate surveillance protocol(s). The physical examination must still be completed at the earliest possible date, but not beyond 30 days after the initial date of employment. Longer delays will require temporary removal. Workers, who transfer from operational to administrative positions on a frequent basis during the same duty assignment may, with Medical Officer approval, receive a periodic physical vice a complete baseline examination upon re-entering the hazardous work site.

        (2) All employees must have an initial physical examination prior to reassignment to any position with an occupational health hazard exposure as defined in Section 12-A-2-b. This requirement is subject to the stipulation described above in Section 12-B-2-a-1.

b. Underline: Periodic.

   (1) Periodic examinations are generally provided at twelve-month intervals, though under some protocols, the period between examinations may vary. Once enrolled in the OMSEP periodic examinations will be performed at the required interval for the duration of the health hazard. Members being monitored under more than one exposure protocol need to complete the Periodic History and Report of OMSEP Examination, CG-5447A only once during a particular examination. The member should review the last History and Report of OMSEP Examination, CG5447 on record and annotate any changes, which may have occurred since the last examination. Each periodic examination shall consist of all of the elements specified under the appropriate surveillance protocol(s).

   (2) Any OMSEP enrollee actively monitored, identified as a risk of exposure to a new health hazard requiring additional protocols, must complete all the required laboratory tests and procedures specified under the appropriate surveillance protocol(s). The employee must also complete the Periodic History and Report of OMSEP Examination, CG-5447A. The employee may not be placed at risk of exposure until the examination is completed. This requirement is subject to the stipulation described above in Section 12-B-1.

   (3) Employees, who transfer from operational to administrative positions on a frequent basis may, with Medical Officer approval, receive a periodic physical examination vice a complete exit (end of exposure) examination. This does not preclude a complete exit/separation examination upon the end of employment.

   (4) Laboratory tests are required for most exposure protocols as part of the periodic surveillance examination. Laboratory tests are usually performed in accordance with the specific protocol. Members being monitored under more than one exposure protocol need to have similar laboratory test (i.e. CBC; U/A; Chem panel) performed only once during a particular examination. The medical provider may perform additional tests as often and as deemed necessary.

c. Acute Exposure.

   (1) An acute health hazard exposure examination is required, when the applicable short-term exposure limit (STEL) ceiling limit of the substance(s) in question is exceeded. The requirement applies whether or not the employee exhibits any overt symptoms of acute exposure. Specific requirements, if any, for an acute exposure examination are found under the protocols in Section 12-C.

(2) An acute health hazard exposure examination is required if the employee exhibits any adverse effects following an acute exposure to a suspected hazardous substance. If the substance(s) is identified, an examination should be performed following the specific protocol(s) for that substance(s). In the event no specific substance is identified, an examination should be directed according to the "Hazardous Waste" examination protocol and presenting symptoms. The Acute Exposure Information Form, CG-6000-1 should be used to collect and organize information when an acute exposure occurs. The information on this form must accompany the employee to his/her examination.

(3) All HAZMAT response personnel with a documented exposure event, including CG Strike Team members and firefighters, must complete an Acute Exposure Information Form, CG-6000-1 at the end of each HAZMAT response. Special attention must be provided to the type, duration and degree of toxicity of the agent(s) encountered as well as the type of contact (inhalation, skin absorption, ingestion). The type of PPE utilized, type of respirator (if any), and protective clothing worn should also be noted. This information is to be reviewed by the cognizant medical provider before entering into the medical record. Based on this information as well as any additional information from the exposure event, the medical provider may choose to direct an acute health hazard exposure examination. Specific requirements, if any, are found under the protocols in Section 12-C.

d. Exit/Separation (Employment/Exposure). Exit exams are designed to assess pertinent aspects of the worker's health when the worker leaves employment or when exposure to a specific hazard has ceased. Results may be beneficial in assessing the relationship of any future medical problem to an exposure in the workplace. Exit physical examinations must be completed within 30 days of the last day of exposure or employment. The worker may not be re-assigned to a hazardous area once the examination is completed. In the event the worker is exposed to a hazardous substance, after completing the examination, ALL laboratory tests required by the specific protocol for that particular substance must be repeated. The following conditions also apply:

(1) End of Exposure:

(a) OMSEP enrollees assigned to a non-hazardous work environment but likely to be assigned to a designated area later in their career should receive an end of exposure examination including completion of the Periodic History and Report of OMSEP Examination, CG-5447A.

(b) Individuals enrolled in the OMSEP, with exposures to known carcinogens or agents with prolonged latency periods for disease development (e.g., asbestos, benzene), will receive an end of exposure exam including completion of the Periodic History and Report of OMSEP Examination, CG-5447A upon reassignment to non-hazardous area and continue to receive periodic annual physicals according to the designated protocol(s). These individuals will be monitored for the duration of their CG career unless the responsible supervising Medical Officer or other cognizant medical authority determines such monitoring is not required.

(2) End of Employment:

(a) OMSEP enrollees permanently separating from CG employment should receive an end of employment examination; including completion of the History and Report of Examination Form, CG-5447 specified laboratory tests and procedures and any required consultations and referrals.

(b) At the time of the examination the member's permanent home of record and phone number must be secured for notification of any abnormalities. A copy of the member's occupational health history, including all potential exposure agents, severity and duration of exposure, and any recommendations on future protocol testing or examinations, must be placed in the member's medical record. A personal copy should also be provided to the member. (see Section 12-B-3-j). All copies that become part of the member's medical record fall under the privacy and security provisions of HIPAA.

(c) All members must be provided with a personal copy of the "Separation Letter" in addition to the one placed in the member's medical record. Upon request, the member should also be provided with a copy of the "Medical Officer's Report," part 2 of the History and Report of Examination Form, CG-5447.

e. <u>Timing of next examination</u>. The default interval between examinations is one year for all protocols except respirator wear and prior (not current) exposure to asbestos, in which case the default interval is five years. However, a Medical Officer may recommend for any individual patient a shorter interval between examinations than the default period, if such is medically indicated. Any recommendation on the timing of the next examination should be included as part of the physician's written assessment.

3. Use of OMSEP Forms.

   a. History and Report of OMSEP Examination, CG-5447. This form must be completed whenever an OMSEP (initial or separation) physical examination is required, except when only annual hearing conservation program is needed. Ensure that the examinee and Medical Officer identifying information are accurately recorded, including phone numbers. All history sections on the History and Report of Examination Form, CG-5447 must be completed.

   b. Periodic History and Report of OMSEP Examination, CG-5447A. This form must be completed whenever a periodic OMSEP physical examination is required. The examinee must review the last History and Report of Examination Form, CG-5447 form or record and note any changes, which may have occurred since the last examination. If there have been no changes during the interval from the last examination, the examinee should mark the appropriate box in each of the sections.

   c. OSHA Respirator Medical Evaluation Questionnaire-(mandatory). This questionnaire is to be completed by any worker who is to be issued a respirator or assigned to a task that may require a respirator.

   d. Audiometric Biological Calibration Check, CG-5140. This form is to be used to record calibration of the audiometric equipment.

   e. Reference Audiogram, DD-2215. This form is used to record initial audiometric test results.

   f. Hearing Conservation Data, DD-2216. This form is used to record the results of periodic and follow-up audiometry for individuals routinely exposed to hazardous noise. This form should be preceded by a Reference Audiogram, DD-2215 or other record already on file in the individual's health record.

   g. Notification of Summary Results. A sample of this form is provided in (Figure 12-B-2). A photocopy or a locally generated form may be used to provide the required notification to the enrollee of the results of his/her OMSEP examination.

   h. Acute Exposure Information Form, CG-6000-1. This form is used to record the results of any unexpected exposures and for verification of notification of the appropriate agencies.

   i. Separation Letter. This letter serves as notification of the member's documented exposure(s) while serving in the CG. It provides the nature and levels of exposure(s), if known, and the medical provider's comments and recommendations. Copies of this letter should be placed in the official health record and also provided directly to the member.

j. Patient Notification. The Medical Officer is responsible for notifying the patient of any and all abnormalities found or diagnoses made, whether or not they are occupationally related or simply an incidental finding. Notification must be made within 30 days of completion of the examination and should be documented as a medical record entry.

4. Medical Removal Standards.

   a. Laboratory finding. The following abnormal laboratory findings during an OMSEP examination mandate immediate removal of the employee from further workplace exposure to the hazard listed, pending resolution of the abnormality or a determination that the abnormality is not due to a workplace exposure. The Medical Officer should coordinate all medical removal recommendations with the cognizant SEHO before forwarding to the CO.

      (1) Benzene (any of the following):

         (a) The hemoglobin/hematocrit falls below the laboratory's normal limit and/or these indices show a persistent downward trend from the individual's pre-exposure norms; provided these findings cannot be explained by other means.

         (b) The thrombocyte (platelet) count varies more than 20% below the employee's most recent prior values or falls below the laboratory's normal limit.

         (c) The leukocyte count is below 4,000 per mm3 or there is an abnormal differential count.

      (2) Lead: A blood lead level at or above 40μg/100 ml of whole blood.

      (3) Noise: A loss of hearing of $\geq$ 25 dB in either ear at one or more of the speech frequencies (500, 1,000, 2000, or 3000 Hz), compared with the current reference audiogram.

      (4) Organophosphate pesticides: cholinesterase level at or below 50% of the pre-exposure baseline.

   b. Pregnancy is not a reason for automatic medical removal from the workplace. A decision to remove or restrict a pregnant woman must be based on sound clinical judgment after careful consideration of the workplace environment and the woman's physical capabilities. The woman's pre-natal health care provider (obstetrician) should be apprised early of any/all potential hazards and safety precautions available.

5. Reporting of Examination Results.

   a. CG Medical Officers will have 30 days from completion of the examination to meet all Medical Officer responsibilities in Section 12-B-4.

b. Contractual providers, Independent Duty Technicians (IDT), and other detached HSs/units must forward all OMSEP examination questions, problems, and any unresolved matters, with accompanying supporting information, to the assigned CG Medical Officer for review within 15 days of receipt (includes the examination and any additional testing or consultations).

c. All records must be forwarded to the record custodian upon compliance with Sections 12-B-6- (a) and 12-B-6 (b) above.

This page intentionally left blank.

Section C. Medical Examination Protocols.

1. General..1
2. Asbestos, CG-6203……..............…………………………………………… 1
3. Benzene, CG-6204……...……………………………………………………4
4. Chromium Compounds, CG-6202……...……………………………………6
5. Hazardous Waste, CG-6206……………………………………………….…8
6. Lead, CG-6207….....…………………………………………………………10
7. Noise, CG-6205 and CG-6215………….………………………...…………12
8. Pesticides, CG-6209……..……………………………………………...……17
9. Respirator Wear, CG-6208…….....…………………………………….…… 19
10. Respiratory Sensitizers, CG-6210……..………………………………….…21
11. Solvents, CG-6213……..……………………………………………………23
12. Tuberculosis, CG-6212.......…………………………………………………26
13. Bloodborne Pathogens, CG-6211…….....…………………………………. 27
14. Radiation (Ionizing/Non-ionizing), CG-6214……..……………………..…32

This page intentionally left blank.

COMDTINST M6000.1E

C. Medical Examination Protocols.

1. General.

   a. The following protocols follow the same format. Each contains a brief description of the hazard and its possible effects; the conditions required for an individual to be surveyed under that protocol; information which must be provided to the examining Medical Officer; specific requirements of the history and physical, including laboratory tests and special procedures; and any additional written requirements on the part of the examining Medical Officer. The protocols are summarized in forms CG-6202 through CG-6215. Copies of these forms may be locally reproduced. The unit OMSEP coordinator should complete the information in the first eight blocks at the very top, and the appropriate protocol summary forms should be provided to the examining Medical Officer with the examination packet.

   b. Multiple protocols for a single individual. In the event that an individual is being monitored on more than one protocol (e.g., asbestos and noise), the final examination packet must include each of the required items for each of the protocols. However, each required form or test need only be completed once.

   c. Past exposure. Personnel who have a documented history of workplace exposure to known carcinogens, but who are not currently exposed, shall be offered an annual medical examination, according to this protocol until end of employment. Undergoing this examination is strictly voluntary.

2. Asbestos, CG-6203.

   a. Exposure effects. Asbestos exposure can cause asbestosis, bronchogenic carcinomas, mesothelioma, and gastric carcinoma. It may also be associated with multiple myeloma and renal carcinoma. Disease risk is dose dependent. There is a synergistic effect between asbestos exposure and cigarette smoking, so that the risk of lung cancer is roughly ten times greater in asbestos-exposed workers who smoke as opposed to nonsmoking asbestos-exposed workers. The primary route of exposure is inhalation, though ingestion of fibers may also occur.

   b. Required surveillance.

      (1) All personnel with current employment exposure to airborne asbestos, who meet the MSAL criteria in Section 12-C-2-b (4) below, shall undergo medical surveillance. These personnel shall be included in the OMSEP and be examined according to the protocol in Section 12-C-2.d below. Medical examinations shall be provided upon enrollment and at least annually thereafter, throughout the duration of exposure or until end of employment, whichever comes first. Under current Coast Guard policies for management of asbestos, very few non-shipyard workers should be currently exposed at or above the PEL or STEL.

(2) Construction worker standard. The OSHA standard for asbestos applies to, but is not limited to, workers who demolish, remove, alter, repair, maintain, install, clean up, transport, dispose of, or store asbestos containing materials.

(3) The current MSALs are based on the OSHA exposure standard for shipyards [29 CFR 1915.1001].

(4) Medical surveillance is required for those workers who are exposed at or above 50% of the PEL or STEL for a combined total of 30 or more days per year.

c. Information to Medical Officer. The following information must be provided to the examining Medical Officer, by the OMSEP coordinator, prior to the examination taking place:

(1) A copy of the OSHA asbestos standards [29 CFR 1915.1001], with appendices D and E.

(2) A description of the affected employee's duties as they relate to the employee's exposure.

(3) The employee's representative exposure level or anticipated exposure level.

(4) A description of any personal protective or respiratory equipment used or to be used.

d. Examination protocol.

(1) Each initial, periodic, and exit examination shall include, as a minimum:

(a) A medical and work history. Emphasis should be placed on the member's history of tobacco use (smoking), and associated symptoms of dyspnea on exertion, recurrent epigastric discomfort, pleuritic chest pains or unexplained cough.

(b) Completion of the OSHA Respiratory Medical Evaluation Questionnaire Appendix C to RP Standard 29CFR 1910.134. Note: additional information on asbestos reporting guidelines may be found at www.osha.gov.

(c) A complete physical examination of all systems, with emphasis on the respiratory system, the cardiovascular system, and digestive tract.

(d) A stool guaiac test, if the patient is age 35 or over.

(e) Pulmonary Function Tests (PFT), including Forced Vital Capacity (FVC) and Forced Expiratory Volume in One Second (FEV1).

(f) Routine screening labs, including a complete blood count (CBC), multichemistry panel (including glucose, blood urea nitrogen (BUN), creatinine, total protein, total bilirubin, aspartate aminotransferase (AST), alanine aminotransferase (ALT), Lactate dehydrogenase (LDH), and alkaline phosphatase), and urinalysis (U/A) with microscopic.

(g) A postero-anterior (PA) chest x-ray (CXR), in accordance with the schedule and interpretation requirements in Section 12-C-2-d(2) below;

(h) Any other tests or procedures deemed appropriate by the examining physician, including specialty consultations.

(2) Chest x-ray requirements:

(a) A PA CXR shall be performed at the initial examination and then according to the following schedule:

Years since: First exposure	Age of examinee: 15 to 35	36 to 45	over 45
0 to 10	Every 5 yrs.	Every 5 yrs.	Every 5 yrs.
Over 10	Every 5 yrs.	Every 2 yrs.	Annually

(b) A PA chest-x-ray shall be performed at the exit examination.

(c) All CXRs shall be interpreted and classified in accordance with a professionally accepted classification system and recorded following the format of the CDC/NIOSH (M) 2.8 form. A B-reader or a board eligible/certified radiologist using the ILO-U/C International Classification of Radiographs for Pneumoconiosis references shall only do the interpretation.

(d) Assistance in obtaining the location of the nearest B-reader is available from the HSWL SC.

e. Specific written requirements. In addition to the general requirements specified in Section 12-B-4-b, the examining physician must address the following in writing:

(1) Any detected medical conditions placing the employee at increased risk of health impairment from further asbestos exposure.

(2) The employee's ability to use respiratory and other personal protective equipment (see Section 12-C-9), and any limitations thereof.

(3) Employee notification of the results of the examination and any medical conditions resulting from asbestos exposure that might require follow-up.

(4) Employee notification of the increased risk of lung cancer attributable to the synergistic effects of asbestos and smoking.

3. <u>Benzene, CG-6204</u>.

   a. <u>Exposure effects</u>. Benzene exposure can cause central nervous system depression, leukemia, aplastic anemia, and dermatitis. The primary route of exposure is inhalation of vapors, though skin absorption may also occur. Within the CG most benzene exposure occurs among marine inspectors and oil spill responders.

   b. <u>Required surveillance</u>.

   (1) The CG MSALs are based on the OSHA action level and PEL standards. Enrollment in the OMSEP is required for all personnel:

   (a) who are or may be exposed to benzene at or above the current average exposure action level 30 or more days per year,

   (b) who are or may be exposed to benzene at or above the current short-term exposure action level 10 or more days per year, or

   (c) who served as resident inspectors, pollution investigators, marine safety officers, port safety officers, vessel inspectors, or marine investigators prior to 1990. These personnel are considered to have been exposed at/or above the MSAL unless otherwise documented.

   (2) In addition to routine surveillance requirements above, if an employee is exposed to benzene in an emergency (fire, spill) situation, a urine specimen will be collected as soon as possible thereafter, but not later than 24 hrs. after the exposure, and an acute exposure examination will be performed within 72 hrs. of the exposure. Such an examination must contain a urinary phenol test on the collected urine specimen.

   c. <u>Information to Medical Officer</u>. The following information must be provided to the examining physician, by the OMSEP coordinator, prior to the examination taking place:

   (1) A description of the affected employee's duties as they relate to the employee's exposure.

   (2) The employee's representative exposure level or anticipated exposure level.

COMDTINST M6000.1E

(3) A description of any personal protective or respiratory equipment used or to be used.

d. Examination protocols.

(1) Each routine (non-acute exposure) initial, periodic, and exit examination shall include, as a minimum:

(a) A detailed history which includes:

(1) Past occupational exposure to benzene or any other hematological toxins, at work or at home.

(2) A family history of blood dyscrasias, including hematological neoplasms.

(3) A personal history of blood dyscrasias, including genetic hemoglobin abnormalities, bleeding abnormalities, abnormal function of formed blood elements; and of renal or liver dysfunction.

(4) History of exposure to ionizing radiation.

(5) Smoking history, alcohol usage history, and all medicinal drugs routinely taken.

(6) Any current history of headache, difficulty concentrating, decreased attention span, short-term memory loss, mood lability, fatigue, dry skin, abnormal bleeding, anemia, or weight loss.

(b) A complete physical examination, (Ensure the patient is examined for mental status changes, dermatitis, and pallor).

(c) A CBC and differential, with platelet count and RBC indices (MCV, MCH, MCHC).

(d) A multichemistry panel (includes glucose, BUN, creatinine, total protein, total bilirubin, AST, ALT, LDH, and alkaline phosphatase) and U/A with microscopic.

(e) Any other tests or procedures deemed appropriate by the examining physician.

(2) Each acute exposure examination shall include, as a minimum:

(a) A brief summary of the nature of the exposure and investigation of any symptoms or complaints.

(b) A total urinary phenol level (mg/L) or a urinary phenol adjusted for urinary creatinine (mg/g creatinine), plus a CBC and differential, with platelet count, and RBC indices (MCV, MCH, MCHC). Plasma folate and B12 levels to rule out megaloblastic anemia if the MCV is elevated.

(c) Any other test or procedure deemed appropriate by the examining physician may be performed, if available. CG medical providers are encouraged to contact Commandant (CG-113) for advise and consultation in selecting the most applicable test or procedure. Alternatively, medical providers may contact any certified Occupational Health clinic provider, available in the local community.

(d) If either the total urinary phenol level is below 50 mg phenol/L of urine, or the urinary phenol adjusted for urinary creatinine is less than 250 mg/g creatinine, and the CBC is normal, no further testing is required. Otherwise, contact Commandant (CG-113) for further requirements.

e. Specific written requirements. In addition to the general requirements specified in Section 12-B-4-b, the following must be addressed in writing by the examining Medical Officer:

(1) Any detected medical conditions, which would place the employee's health at greater than normal risk of material impairment from exposure to benzene.

(2) The Medical Officer's recommended limitations upon the employee's exposure to benzene or upon the employee's use of protective clothing or equipment and respirators.

(3) A statement that the employee has been informed by the Medical Officer of the results of the examination and any medical conditions resulting from benzene exposure which require further explanation or treatment.

4. Chromium Compounds, CG-6202.

a. Exposure effects. Hexavalent chromium compounds are known human carcinogens. They may also cause dermatitis, skin ulceration, occupational asthma, and nasal septum perforation. The primary routes of exposure are percutaneous absorption and inhalation. Chromates may be found in certain metal alloys, paints, and masonry cements. Within the CG, most chromate exposure is from the use of chromium containing paints.

b. Required surveillance. The CG MSALs are based on the ACGIH threshold limit values (TLVs). Medical surveillance is required for all personnel who are or may be exposed to chromium IV compounds at or above the current exposure action level 30 or more days per year.

c. <u>Information to Medical Officer</u>. The following information must be provided by the OMSEP coordinator to the examining physician prior to the examination taking place:

   (1) A description of the affected employee's duties as they relate to the employee's exposure.

   (2) The employee's representative exposure level or anticipated exposure level.

   (3) A description of any personal protective or respiratory equipment used or to be used.

d. <u>Examination protocols</u>. Each routine initial, annual (periodic), and exit examination must include:

   (1) A detailed history, which includes:

       (a) Past and current occupational exposures to chromate, asbestos, and/or any other pulmonary carcinogens at work and/or at home;

       (b) Smoking history and/or alcohol usage history;

       (c) Any past or current history of dry skin, skin ulcers—usually painless, nosebleeds, asthma, shortness of breath, wheezing, and/or cough;

   (2) A directed physical examination, with attention to the skin, mucous membranes, and respiratory tract, both upper and lower (ensure the patient is examined for erosion of the nasal mucosa and septum, respiratory rhonchi, dermatitis, and cutaneous ulcers).

   (3) A CBC, multichemistry panel (includes glucose, BUN, creatinine, total protein, total bilirubin, AST, ALT, LDH, and alkaline phosphatase), and a U/A with microscopic.

   (4) PFTs (including FVC & FEV1).

   (5) A PA CXR only for an initial/baseline or exit examination, unless there is a current clinical indication (cough, shortness of breath, wheezing, etc.).

   (6) Any other tests or procedures deemed appropriate by the examining physician.

COMDTINST M6000.1E

- e. <u>Specific written requirements</u>. Other than the general requirements specified in Section 12-B-4-b, the physician should address:

    (1) The periodicity of the next routine medical surveillance examination. Examinations will be provided annually unless the physician recommends a longer interval.

    (2) The employee's ability to use respiratory and other personal protective equipment (see Section 12-C-9), and any limitations thereof.

5. <u>Hazardous Waste, CG-6206</u>.

    a. <u>Exposure effects</u>. The OSHA medical surveillance protocol for hazardous waste operations and emergency response (HAZWOPER) [29 CFR 1910.120] involves medical surveillance for potential exposure to numerous metals and chemicals, usually in uncontrolled spill, fire, disposal situations. Therefore, there are no specific exposure effects to describe.

    b. <u>Required surveillance</u>.

        (1) Routine medical surveillance is required for employees involved in hazardous waste operations when any of the following conditions are met:

            (a) Exposure or potential exposure to hazardous substances or health hazards at or above the MSAL for that substance (as defined in Section 12-A-4), without regard to the use of respirators or personal protective equipment, for 30 or more days per year.

            (b) All hazardous waste operation employees who wear a respirator for 30 or more days per year or as required under Section 12-C-9 of this Manual.

            (c) All employees who are injured, become ill, or develop signs or symptoms due to possible overexposure involving hazardous substances or health hazards from an emergency response or hazardous waste operation.

            (d) Members of HAZMAT response teams, including all CG Strike Team members and firefighters.

        (2) In addition to routine surveillance requirements above, if an employee is exposed to a hazardous substance above the CG MSAL in an emergency (fire, spill) situation, a urine specimen will be collected as soon as possible thereafter, but not later than 24 hrs after the exposure, and an acute exposure examination will be performed within 72 hrs of the exposure.

c. Information to Medical Officer. The examining Medical Officer shall be provided, by the OMSEP coordinator, one copy of the OSHA HAZWOPER standard [29 CFR 1910.120] and its appendices, plus the following specific information:

  (1) A description of the employee's duties as they relate to the employee's exposures.

  (2) The employee's exposure levels or anticipated exposure levels.

  (3) A description of any personal protective equipment used or to be used, including any respirators.

d. Information from previous medical examinations of the employee which is not readily available to the examining physician.

e. Examination protocols.

  (1) Each routine (non-acute exposure) initial, periodic, and exit examination shall include, as a minimum:

    (a) A medical and occupational history which includes:

      (1) Past and current occupational exposure to hazardous chemicals, metals, dusts, fumes, and heat stress.

      (2) Any history of heat illness, allergies, sensitivities, or physical abnormalities.

      (3) Current medications, and immunization history.

      (4) Smoking history, and alcohol usage history.

      (5) A complete review of organ systems.

    (b) A complete physical examination with attention to the skin, eyes, nose, throat, and respiratory, cardiovascular, genitourinary, and neurologic systems.

    (c) A CBC and differential, with platelet count, and RBC indices (MCV, MCH, MCHC).

    (d) A multichemistry panel (includes glucose, BUN, creatinine, total protein, total bilirubin, AST, ALT, LDH, and alkaline phosphatase) and U/A with microscopic.

    (e) PFTs (including FVC & FEV1).

    (f) Vision screening.

(g) A PA CXR only for an initial/baseline or exit examination, unless there is a current clinical indication (cough, shortness of breath, wheezing, etc.).

(h) Any other tests or procedures deemed appropriate by the examining physician. (Consider a stool guaiac and/or electrocardiogram, if indicated by age or physical findings).

(2) Each acute exposure examination shall include, as a minimum:

(a) A brief summary of the nature of the exposure and investigation of any symptoms or complaints;

(b) A CBC and differential, with platelet count, and RBC indices (MCV, MCH, MCHC), a multichemistry panel (includes glucose, BUN, creatinine, total protein, total bilirubin, AST, ALT, LDH, and alkaline phosphatase) and a U/A with microscopic;

(c) PFTs (including FVC & FEV1);

(d) Appropriate biological monitoring tests (e.g., blood metal screen) depending on the exposure in question. Contact Commandant (CG-113) for further information and requirements.

f. <u>Specific written requirements</u>. Other than the general requirements specified in Section 12-B-4-b, the physician should address:

(1) Whether the employee has any detected medical conditions which would place the employee at increased risk of material impairment of the employee's health from work in hazardous waste operations or emergency response, or from respirator use.

(2) The employee's ability to use respiratory and other personal protective equipment (see Section 12-C-9), and any limitations thereof.

(3) The periodicity of the next routine medical surveillance examination. Examinations will be provided annually unless the physician recommends a longer interval.

6. <u>Lead, CG-6207</u>.

a. <u>Exposure effects</u>. In adults, excessive lead exposure can cause hypertension, anemia, peripheral neuropathy, encephalopathy, spontaneous abortions in women, and decreased fertility in men. The primary route of exposure in adults is inhalation of lead containing dust or fumes. Most exposure in the CG occurs during removal of previously applied lead-based paint coatings, or during environmental recovery of previously discarded lead-acid batteries. Some welders may be exposed to lead fumes.

b. Required surveillance. The CG MSAL is based on the OSHA PEL standard for shipyards [29 CFR 1915.1025]. Enrollment in the OMSEP is required for all personnel who are or may be exposed to lead at or above the current exposure action level for 30 or more days per year.

c. Information to Medical Officer. The OMSEP coordinator shall provide the Medical Officer with one copy of the OSHA lead standard [29 CFR 1915.1025] and its appendices, plus the following specific information:

   (1) A description of the employee's duties as they relate to the employee's exposure.

   (2) The employee's exposure level or anticipated exposure levels to lead and to any other toxic substance (if applicable).

   (3) A description of any personal protective equipment used or to be used, including any respirators (if known).

   (4) Prior blood lead determinations.

   (5) Information from previous medical examinations of the employee which is not readily available to the examining physician. This includes all available prior written medical opinions concerning the employee.

d. Examination protocols.

   (1) Biological monitoring or "blood lead only" examinations must be provided to each employee exposed at or above the OSHA action level (currently TWA of 30 mg/ m^3 air) every six months. Otherwise, only annual examinations must be performed, unless an employee's blood lead level is found to be elevated at or above 30 ug/100 ml of whole blood.

   (2) Each routine initial, periodic, exit, and acute exposure examination shall include, as a minimum:

      (a) A detailed work history and a medical history, with particular attention to:

         (1) Past lead exposure (occupational and non-occupational).

         (2) Personal habits (smoking, hand washing after work and before eating).

         (3) Past and current gastrointestinal, hematological, renal, cardiovascular, reproductive, and neurological problems.

(b) A complete physical examination with particular attention to:

(1) Occular fundi, teeth, gums, hematological, gastrointestinal, renal, cardiovascular, and neurological systems.

(2) Blood pressure (must be recorded).

(3) Pulmonary status should be evaluated if respiratory protection is to be used. (see Section 12-C-9).

(c) The following routine laboratory tests:

(1) A CBC and differential, with platelet count, and RBC indices (MCV, MCH, MCHC), plus examination of peripheral smear morphology.

(2) Blood lead level and zinc protoporphyrin (must be performed by a laboratory licensed by the CDC for proficiency in blood lead testing).

(3) A multi-chemistry panel (includes glucose, BUN, creatinine, total protein, total bilirubin, AST, ALT, LDH, and alkaline phosphatase).

(4) A U/A with microscopic examination.

(5) PFTs (including FVC & FEV 1).

(d) Any other tests or procedures deemed appropriate by the examining physician (pregnancy testing, laboratory examination of male fertility).

e. <u>Specific written requirements</u>. In addition to the general requirements specified in Section 12-B-4-b, the physician should address:

(1) Any detected medical conditions which would place the employee at increased risk of material impairment of the employee's health from exposure from lead, or from respirator use.

(2) The employee's ability to use respiratory and other personal protective equipment (see Section 12-C-9), and any limitations thereof.

(3) The results of the blood lead determinations.

7. <u>Noise, CG-6205</u>.

a. <u>Exposure effects</u>. The primary effect of excessive noise is to cause loss of hearing. This hearing loss may be described by three "p-words:" painless, progressive, and permanent. Cumulative overexposures to hazardous noise levels cause millions of people to lose hearing during their working lives.

b. <u>Required surveillance</u>. The CG MSAL is based on DoD Instruction 6055.12, DoD Hearing Conservation Program, as well as OSHA guidance [29 CFR 1910.95]. Enrollment in the OMSEP is required for all personnel who are exposed to hazardous noise at or above the current exposure action level. Surveillance can also be started regardless of the duration of noise exposure. Personnel who infrequently or incidentally enter designated "hazardous noise areas" need not be enrolled in the audiometric testing program.

(1) Enrollment is required in accordance with one of the following criteria:

(a) When the member is exposed to continuous and intermittent noise that has an 8-hour time-weighted average (TWA) noise level of 85 decibels A-weighted (dBA) or greater for 30 or more days per calendar year.

(b) When the member is exposed to impulse noise sound pressure levels (SPL's) of 140 decibels (dB) peak or greater for 30 or more days per calendar year.

(2) Reference (baseline) audiograms:

(a) All personnel shall receive a reference audiogram prior to any CG occupational noise exposure or before they are assigned to duties in "hazardous noise areas."

(b) Every effort should be made to schedule the reference audiogram on civilian workers in order to avoid conflicts with assigned duties; military personnel shall receive their reference audiogram at initial entry training.

(c) Testing to establish a reference audiogram shall be preceded by at least 14 hours without exposure to workplace noise. Hearing protectors that attenuate workplace noise below a TWA of 85 dBA, may be used to meet this requirement, in place of exclusion from the noisy workplace.

(3) Exit audiograms: shall be conducted on all employees, previously enrolled in the "hearing conservation program," if it is determined the employee no longer works in a designated "hazardous noise area," unless that employee is moving to another CG position that also involves work in such areas. However, if the employee's audiogram shows hearing losses (compared to the reference audiogram) equal to or greater than 25 dB in the speech frequencies (500 - 3000 Hz) the

employee must continue to receive annual audiograms until end of employment.

c. Information to Medical Officer. The OMSEP coordinator must provide the examining Medical Officer with a description of the employee's duties as they relate to the employee's exposure, the dB level of the hazardous work area and a description of any personal protective equipment used or to be used (e.g., earplugs or earmuffs).

d. Examination protocols.

(1) Each routine (non-acute exposure) initial, periodic, and exit examination shall include completion or updating of the indicated physical examination forms (i.e. History and Report of OMSEP Examination, CG 5447 or Periodic History and Report of OMSEP Examination, CG 5447A) and audiometric testing data (audiogram). All audiometric testing shall:

(a) Be performed by a licensed or certified audiologist, otolaryngologist, or other physician; or by a technician who is certified by the Council for Accreditation in Occupational Hearing Conservation. A technician who performs audiometric tests shall be responsible to an audiologist, otolaryngologist, or other physician. Standard instructions shall be given to individuals before testing.

(b) Be conducted in a testing environment with background octave band SPLs not greater than 21 dB at 500 Hz, 26 dB at 1000 Hz, 34 dB at 2000 Hz, 37 dB at 4000 Hz, and 37 dB at 8000 Hz. The test environment shall be surveyed annually to ensure these levels are not exceeded.

(c) Include pure tone, air conduction, and hearing threshold examinations of each ear at the test frequencies of 500, 1000, 2000, 3000, 4000, and 6000 Hz.

(d) Be performed on audiometers conforming to the most current calibration specifications of the American National Standards Institute (ANSI). Audiometers currently in operation must receive annual electroacoustic calibration to maintain certification.

(e) Occur on audiometers that have received a functional operations check before each day's use for specifications in the OSHA Occupational Noise Exposure standard [29 CFR 1910.95]

(f) Be recorded on the Reference Audiogram, DD-2215 or Hearing Conservation Data, DD-2216 or equivalent locally reproduced versions as appropriate.

(2) Significant Threshold Shift (STS). Transcribe the reference audiogram test results into the "Reference Audiogram" spaces on the DD Form 2216, Hearing Conservation Data (or equivalent). The reference levels are subtracted from the current levels at 2000, 3000, and 4000 Hz. The differences in hearing levels calculated at 2000, 3000, and 4000 Hz are added together and divided by three, for each ear. STS exists if the resulting average hearing loss in either ear is greater than or equal to ± 10 dB [29 CFR 1910.95]. Additionally, any change of ± 15dB at 2000, 3000, or 4000 Hz in either ear shall constitute an STS. Results shall be recorded on DD Form 2216 (or equivalent) as the "Reference Audiogram" results under the appropriate heading "Left" for left ear and "Right" for right ear. (Note: Occupational Safety and Health Administration (OSHA) age corrections shall <u>NOT</u> be applied when determining STS). (see How to Calculate a Significant Threshold Shift, CG-6215).

(3) A follow-up audiogram shall be conducted when an individual's audiogram shows an STS, in either ear, relative to the current reference audiogram. Medical evaluation is required to validate the existence of a permanent noise-induced threshold shift and/or to determine if further medical referral is required. An audiologist, otolaryngologist, or other knowledgeable physician shall perform the evaluation and determine if the noise-induced STS is/is not work-related or has/has not been aggravated by occupational noise exposure.

(4) When a negative STS (improvement in hearing threshold from the reference audiogram) is noted on the periodic audiogram, one 14-hour noise-free follow-up test is required. That may be administered on the same day as the periodic test. The results of the follow-up test may be used to create a re-established reference audiogram.

(5) When a positive STS (decrease in hearing threshold form the reference audiogram) is noted on the periodic audiogram, two consecutive 14-hour noise-free follow-up tests must be administered to confirm if the decrease in hearing is permanent. The follow-up exams may not be performed on the same day as the periodic audiogram The results of the second follow-up test may be used to reestablish a reference audiogram, if the required medical evaluation validates the existence of a permanent noise induced threshold shift (see Section 12-3-d.(3) above). If the results of the first follow-up test do not indicate an STS, a second follow-up test is not required.

(6) A new reference audiogram shall replace the original reference audiogram when the medical evaluation confirms that the STS noted during the annual and follow-up audiograms is permanent. The original reference audiogram shall be retained in the patient's medical record.

(7) Acute exposure examinations (formerly called the Detailed Surveillance Program). These examinations are designed to observe any dynamic hearing loss, to identify those who demonstrate unusual noise sensitivity, or to monitor personnel acutely exposed to unprotected high levels of noise (impulse >140dBA).

   (a) The initial acute exposure examination shall consist of all elements described in Sections 12-C-7.d. (1)-(6), above. Additional follow-up audiograms will be performed at 30 and 90 days, or at more frequent intervals at the discretion of the Medical Officer.

   (b) If any of the follow-up audiograms demonstrate an average loss of no more than 10 dB in 2000, 3000, and 4000 Hz in either ear, when compared to the revised reference audiogram, hearing may be considered stable. The reference audiogram (per Section 12-C-7-d (5) and (6)) remains the audiogram against which further testing is compared. The individual is returned to annual monitoring.

   (c) If these reevaluation audiograms exhibit a loss greater than an average threshold of 10 dB in 2000, 3000, and 4000 Hz in either ear when compared to the revised reference audiogram, the individual must be referred to an otolaryngologist for a consultation. Final disposition will depend on the consultant's diagnosis and recommendations.

   (d) Reporting requirements: In accordance with OSHA's Occupational Illness and Reporting Requirements effective January 1, 2003, the following rule applies: Any threshold shifts (+/- 10dB in either ear) that results in a total of 25dB level of hearing loss above audiometric zero, averaged over the 2000, 3000, and 4000 frequencies must be recorded and reported as a hearing loss case. Since most audiometers are designed to provide results referenced to audiometric zero no other calculations are required. NOTE: Any such event must be reported as a mishap in accordance with Chapter 3 of the Safety and Environmental health Manual, COMDTINST M5100.47 (series).

e. <u>Specific written requirements</u>. In addition to the general requirements specified in Section 12-B-4-b, the Medical Officer must do the following:

   (1) The employee shall be notified in writing within 21 days, when an audiologist or a physician confirms a threshold shift is permanent. Such determination must be entered in the employee's medical record.

(2) Supervisors shall be notified, in writing, that the worker has experienced a decrease in hearing. Release of medical information must conform to privacy act requirements.

(3) Document that the patient was counseled concerning the potential seriousness of repeated unprotected exposures to excessive noise and provided additional information on hearing protection and avoidance of hazardous noise exposures.

8. Pesticides, CG-6209.

   a. Exposure effects. There are over 1,200 chemical compounds currently classified as pesticides. However, this surveillance protocol is primarily concerned with only two classes of pesticides: organophosphate and carbamate insecticides, and chlorophenoxyacetic acid herbicides. Organophosphates and carbamates are inhibitors of the enzyme acetylcholinesterase and they cause parasympathetic nervous system hyperactivity (miosis, urination, diarrhea, defecation, lacrimation, salivation), neuromuscular paralysis, CNS dysfunction (irritability, anxiety, impaired cognition, seizures, coma), peripheral neuropathy, and depression of RBC cholinesterase activity. Chlorophenoxyacetic acid herbicides cause skin, eye, and respiratory tract irritation, cough, nausea, vomiting, diarrhea, abdominal pain, and peripheral neuropathy. In the past, some chlorophenoxyacetic herbicides were contaminated with dioxins during manufacture.

   b. Required surveillance. The CG MSALs for carbaryl, chlorpyrifos, malathion, parathion, 2,4, -D, and 2,4,5,-T are based on the ACGIH threshold limit values. Enrollment in the OMSEP is required for all personnel who are or may be exposed to any identified pesticide at or above the MSAL (as defined in Sect. 12-A-2) for 30 or more days per year.

   c. Information to Medical Officer. The OMSEP coordinator must provide the examining Medical Officer with:

      (1) A description of the employee's duties as they relate to the employee's exposure.

      (2) The employee's exposure level or potential exposure level to any pesticides.

      (3) A description of any personal protective equipment used or to be used, including any respirators.

   d. Examination protocols.

      (1) Biological monitoring or "RBC cholinesterase only" examinations must be provided at least every six months to each employee exposed

to organophosphate or carbamate pesticides at or above the MSAL. If an employee's RBC cholinesterase activity is found on any testing to be less than 80% of the pre-exposure baseline, the frequency of biological monitoring will be increased to at least every three months during the application season. Non-seasonal, acute exposures will be monitored at a frequency determined by the supervising Medical Officer based on exposure information data.

(2) Each routine (non-acute exposure) initial, periodic, and exit examination shall include, as a minimum:

   (a) A detailed work history and a medical history, with particular attention to:

   (1) Past and current exposure to pesticides or other chemicals (occupational and non-occupational).

   (2) Smoking and alcohol use history.

   (3) Any symptoms of eye, nose, or throat irritation; cough; nausea, vomiting, diarrhea, or abdominal pain; irritability, anxiety, difficulty concentrating, impaired short-term memory, fatigue, or seizures; numbness, tingling, or weakness in the extremities.

   (4) Allergic skin conditions or dermatitis.

   (b) A complete physical examination, with attention to the skin, respiratory, and nervous systems, including a mental status examination, should be performed. Pulmonary status must be evaluated if respiratory protection is used. (see Section 12-C-9).

   (c) The following routine laboratory tests:

   (1) A CBC, a multichemistry panel (includes glucose, BUN, creatinine, total protein, total bilirubin, AST, ALT, LDH, and alkaline phosphatase), and a dipstick U/A;

   (2) An erythrocyte (RBC) cholinesterase level.

   (3) Initial examination only-two RBC cholinesterase tests must be drawn at least 24 hrs. apart. The results of these two tests will be averaged to provide the pre-exposure baseline for future reference, unless they differ by more than 15% from each other, in which case, additional testing must be performed until successive tests do not differ by more than 15%. The pre-exposure baseline blood tests must be drawn after a period

of at least 60 days without known exposure to organophosphates.

- (d) Any other tests or procedures deemed appropriate by the examining physician (e.g., cognitive function testing). Pulmonary function testing should be performed at least once every 4 years if the employee wears a respirator.

(3) Each acute exposure examination shall include, as a minimum:

- (a) A medical and work history with emphasis on any evidence of eye, nose, or throat irritation; cough; nausea, vomiting, diarrhea, or abdominal pain; irritability, anxiety, difficulty concentrating, impaired short-term memory, fatigue, or seizures; numbness, tingling, or weakness in the extremities.

- (b) A complete physical examination with attention to any reported symptoms as well as the skin, respiratory, and nervous systems. A mental status examination must be performed.

- (c) An erythrocyte (RBC) cholinesterase level.

- (d) Any other tests or procedures deemed appropriate by the examining physician (e.g., CBC, CXR, cognitive function testing, urinary metabolites if less than 24 hrs. post acute exposure). Pulmonary function testing should be performed at least every 4 years if the employee wears a respirator.

e. Specific written requirements. In addition to the general requirements specified in Section 12-B-4, the physician should address:

(1) Any detected medical conditions, which would place the employee's health at increased risk from exposure to identified pesticides or from respiratory wear.

(2) Counseling on the possible increased risk of health impairment from working with certain pesticides, in the event that the employee was found to have skin disease, chronic lung disease, or abnormalities of the central or peripheral nervous system that could directly or indirectly be aggravated by such exposure.

9. Respirator Wear, CG-6208.

a. Exposure effects. The OSHA medical surveillance protocol for respirator wear is a means to assess the effectiveness of respiratory protection among exposed workers. Periodic examinations are required to assess continued fitness for duties and to assess whether the present respiratory protection program provides adequate protection against illness. Respirators are often extremely uncomfortable to wear for long periods. Workers with asthma, claustrophobia, angina, and other conditions may not be able to wear respirators effectively. The worker should be questioned for a history or symptoms of past and current exposures to hazardous chemicals; fumes and dusts; smoking and alcohol use histories; wheezing or abnormal breath sounds; clubbing; and cardiac arrhythmia.

b. <u>Required surveillance</u>.

(1) Medical Determination. An initial/baseline examination will be performed at the time of assignment to a job requiring respirator wear. Before an employee may be issued a respirator or assigned to a task that may require a respirator, that worker must complete a mandatory OSHA Respirator Medical Evaluation Questionnaire. This questionnaire will be provided, at the local unit by the cognizant SEHO, to all workers expected to require the use of a respirator. This questionnaire serves as the initial medical examination. A health care professional (nurse, nurse practitioner, physician assistant, and physician) must review this questionnaire to determine if a follow-up medical examination is required. Independent duty technicians (IDT'S) are authorized to review the questionnaire but must refer any positive Initial responses on questionnaire (or any other concerns) to the supervising Medical Officer for further review. Any employee who gives a positive response to any questions among questions 1-8 in section two of the questionnaire shall be subject to a follow-up medical examination. This examination will determine whether the worker is physically and mentally capable of performing the work and using a respirator [29 CFR 1910.134].

(2) Additional Medical Evaluation and Medical Examination.

(a) Additional medical examinations maybe required to assess continued fitness for duties involving respirator wear. The following conditions will dictate the need for a follow-up evaluation:

(1) The member reports signs and symptoms related to the ability to use a respirator;

(2) The health care provider, supervisor, or respirator program coordinator informs the command of the need for evaluation;

(3) Observations are made during fit testing, respirator use, or program evaluation that indicate the need for evaluation;

(4) When changes in workplace conditions such as physical work effort, protective clothing or climate conditions result in substantial increase in physiological burden;

(5) A member's scheduled quinqennial physical examination.

(b) Periodic physical examinations will be provided at least once every five years. The periodic physical examination requires a review and update of the respirator questionnaire. A health care provider must review the questionnaire to determine the need for a follow-up examination. A follow-up medical examination is required for anyone with positive responses to questions 1-8 in section two of the questionnaire.

c. Information to Medical Officer. The OMSEP coordinator must provide the examining Medical Officer with:

(1) A description of the employee's duties as they relate to the employee's respirator wear.

(2) The employee's exposures or potential exposures to any hazardous chemicals or physical agents.

(3) A description of the respirator(s) used or to be used.

d. Examination protocol. Each routine (non-acute exposure) initial and periodic examination shall include, as a minimum the completion of the mandatory OSHA Respirator Medical Evaluation Questionnaire.

e. Specific written requirements. In addition to the general requirements specified in Section 12-B-4, the physician should address:

(1) Any detected medical conditions that would place the employee at increased risk of material impairment of the employee's health from respirator use.

(2) Asthmatics with normal or mildly impaired lung function should be evaluated based on the job requirements, but disapproval should be strongly considered for asthmatics that require regular medications to maintain airflow, or who have a history of airway reactivity or sensitization to extrinsic materials (dusts, fumes, vapors, or cold).

(3) Note: As a general rule, anyone with documented respiratory impairment of moderate to severe degree (FEV_1 or FVC <70% of predicted) should not be routinely approved to wear a respirator.

10. Respiratory Sensitizers, CG-6210.

a. Exposure effects. Respiratory sensitizers include numerous compounds which cause both occupational asthma and/or hypersensitivity pneumonitis (extrinsic allergic alveolitis). Respiratory sensitizers include vegetable dusts and woods, molds and spores, animal danders, metals (platinum, chromium, nickel, cobalt, vanadium), and chemicals (isocyanates, formaldehyde, trimellitic anhydride).

b. Required surveillance. The CG MSALs for formaldehyde, toluene diisocyanate, and vanadium, are based on the ACGIH threshold limit values. Enrollment in the OMSEP is required for all personnel who are or may be exposed to any identified respiratory sensitizer at or above the MSAL (as defined in Section 12-A-2) for 30 or more days per year. In the CG, exposure to respiratory sensitizers is primarily associated with industrial operations, though some marine inspection activities may also lead to exposures.

c. Information to Medical Officer. The OMSEP coordinator must provide the examining Medical Officer with:

   (1) A description of the employee's duties as they relate to the employee's exposure.

   (2) The employee's exposure level or anticipated exposure level to any respiratory sensitizers.

   (3) A description of any personal protective equipment used or to be used, including any respirators.

d. Examination protocols.

   (1) Each routine (non-acute exposure) initial, periodic, and exit examination shall include, as a minimum:

      (a) A detailed work history and a medical history, with particular attention to:

         (1) Past and current exposure to respiratory sensitizers (occupational and non-occupational).

         (2) Smoking history.

         (3) Any symptoms of eye, nose, or throat irritation.

         (4) Chronic airway problems or hyperactive airway disease.

         (5) Allergic skin conditions or dermatitis.

      (b) In the event that the employee is not required to wear a respirator and the history and routine laboratory tests are unremarkable, the Medical Officer may determine that a complete physical examination is not required. Otherwise, at a minimum, a system specific physical examination with attention to the respiratory system must be completed. Pulmonary status must be evaluated if respiratory protection is used. (see Section 12-C-9).

   (c) The following routine laboratory tests:

      (1) a CBC, a multichemistry panel (includes glucose, BUN, creatinine, total protein, total bilirubin, AST, ALT, LDH, and alkaline phosphatase), and a dipstick U/A;

      (2) PFTs (including FVC & FEV_1).

   (d) Any other tests or procedures deemed appropriate by the examining physician (e.g., CXR, bronchial provocation tests).

(2) Each acute exposure examination shall include, as a minimum:

   (a) A medical and work history with emphasis on any evidence of upper or lower respiratory problems, allergic conditions, skin reaction or hypersensitivity, and any evidence of eye, nose, or throat irritation.

   (b) A directed physical examination with attention to the respiratory system.

   (c) PFTs (including FVC & FEV1).

   (d) Any other tests or procedures deemed appropriate by the examining physician (e.g., CBC, CXR, bronchial provocation tests).

e. <u>Specific written requirements</u>. In addition to the general requirements specified in Section 12-B-4-b, the physician should address:

   (1) Any detected medical conditions which would place the employee at increased risk of material impairment of the employee's health from exposure to identified respiratory sensitizers, or from respirator use.

   (2) The employee's ability to use respiratory and other personal protective equipment (see Section 12-C-9), and any limitations thereof.

11. <u>Solvents, CG-6213</u>.

   a. <u>Exposure effects</u>. There are over 30,000 industrial solvents. This protocol is designed to survey for the most frequent health effects of solvents when considered as an admittedly broad group. These effects are skin disorders (acute irritant dermatitis, chronic eczema), acute CNS effects (headache, nausea and vomiting, dizziness, light-headedness, vertigo, disequilibrium, fatigue, weakness, nervousness, irritability, depression, confusion, coma), and chronic CNS effects (chronic solvent intoxication, neurobehavioral abnormalities, cognitive dysfunction). Some other less frequent effects of solvents involve the hematopoietic, hepatic, peripheral nervous system, renal, reproductive, and respiratory systems. Most solvents are not carcinogenic to humans; benzene being a notable exception (see Section 12-C-3, above). In the CG, exposure to solvents is primarily associated with industrial and maintenance operations (e.g., painting).

b. Required surveillance. The CG MSALs for ethylene glycol, methyl ethyl ketone, VM & P naphtha, and xylene are based on the ACGIH threshold limit values. Enrollment in the OMSEP is required for all personnel who are or may be exposed to any identified hazardous solvent at or above the MSAL (as defined in Section 12-A-2) for 30 or more days per year. An acute exposure examination is required in the event of any documented overexposure (above the TLV or STEL) to a solvent or any presumed overexposure where symptoms are present. In the case of an acute overexposure, an appropriate urine or blood specimen should be collected as soon as possible after the overexposure incident.

c. Information to Medical Officer. The OMSEP coordinator must provide the examining Medical Officer with:

  (1) A description of the employee's duties as they relate to the employee's exposure.

  (2) The employee's exposure level or potential exposure level to any solvents.

  (3) A description of any personal protective equipment used or to be used, including any respirators.

d. Examination protocols.

  (1) Each routine (non-acute exposure) initial, periodic, and exit examination shall include, as a minimum:

    (a) A detailed work history and a medical history, with particular attention to:

      (1) Past and current exposure to solvents (occupational and non-occupational).

      (2) Smoking history and alcohol use history.

      (3) Any symptoms of dry skin, skin irritation, or dermatitis.

      (4) Any CNS symptoms, including headache, nausea and vomiting, dizziness, light-headedness, vertigo, disequilibrium,

fatigue, weakness, nervousness, irritability, depression, difficulty concentrating, mood changes, or confusion.

    (5) A review of symptoms with attention to the hematopoietic, hepatic, peripheral nervous system, renal, reproductive, and respiratory systems.

(b) A system specific physical examination, with attention to the skin and nervous systems, including a mental status examination, should be performed. Pulmonary status must be evaluated if respiratory protection is used. (See Section 12-C-9).

(c) The following routine laboratory tests:

    (1) A CBC and differential, with platelet count, and RBC indices (MCV, MCH, MCHC).

    (2) A multichemistry panel (includes glucose, BUN, creatinine, total protein, total bilirubin, AST, ALT, LDH, and alkaline phosphatase) and a U/A with microscopic.

(d) Consideration should be given to biological monitoring tests for ongoing overexposure to certain solvents, if specimens can be obtained in a timely manner during the exposure period. For non-acute exposures, a timely manner generally implies that the specimen be obtained at the end of a work shift or the end of a workweek.

    (1) For toluene, measure urinary hippuric acid, at the end of a full work shift.

    (2) For xylene, measure urinary methyl-hippuric acid, at the end of a full work shift.

    (3) For methylethylketone (MEK), measure urinary MEK, at the end of a full work shift.

    (4) For trichloroethylene, measure urinary trichloroacetic acid, at the end of a full workweek.

(e) Any other tests or procedures deemed appropriate by the examining physician (e.g., cognitive function tests. Note that skin (patch) testing is generally of little value in solvent-induced dermatitis, since the pathophysiology is generally not allergic. Pulmonary function testing should be performed at least once every 4 years if the employee wears a respirator.

(2) Each acute exposure examination shall include, as a minimum:

(a) A medical and work history with emphasis on any evidence of skin disorders or acute CNS effects (headache, nausea and vomiting, dizziness, light-headedness, vertigo, disequilibrium, fatigue, weakness, nervousness, irritability, depression, confusion, coma).

(b) A system specific physical examination with attention to the skin and nervous systems.

(c) If at all possible, a biological monitoring test for overexposure to the solvent in question should be performed, if such a test is available and a specimen can be obtained in a timely manner. For acute exposures, a timely manner implies within the first half-life of the chemical within the human body, generally a matter of a few hours after the overexposure.

(d) Any other tests or procedures deemed appropriate by the examining physician (e.g., CBC, CXR, and bronchial provocation tests).

e. Specific written requirements. In addition to the general requirements specified in Section 12-B-4-b, the physician should address:

(1) Any detected medical conditions, which would place the employee at increased risk of material impairment of the employee's health from any identified exposures to solvents, or from respirator use.

(2) The periodicity of the next routine medical surveillance examination. Examinations will be provided annually unless the physician recommends a longer interval.

12. Tuberculosis, CG-6212.

a. Exposure effects. Tuberculous droplet nuclei are coughed, spoken, or sneezed into the air by an individual with active pulmonary tuberculosis. Exposure to these airborne droplet nuclei may cause infection with the bacterium that causes tuberculosis.

b. Required surveillance. Employees who are occupationally exposed to active TB cases will be enrolled in the OMSEP.

c. Information to medical personnel. In order to assess whether the employee should remain under active surveillance for TB exposure, the OMSEP coordinator must provide the examining Medical Officer with the following information:

(1) A description of the employee's duties as they relate to the employee's exposure.

(2) The employee's exposure level or potential exposure level active TB cases.

(3) A description of any personal protective equipment used or to be used.

d. <u>Examination protocols</u>.

(1) For routine screening for exposed individuals follow the guidelines regarding testing, diagnosis, and treatment at www.cdc.gov/tb/.

(a) Personnel with a history of non-reactive tuberculin skin tests do not require annual skin testing unless directed by a Medical Officer.

(b) Personnel with a history of reactive skin test(s) will be monitored for development of symptoms of active TB (cough, hemoptysis, fatigue, weight loss, night sweats) annually. A health services technician or a Medical Officer may complete such monitoring.

(2) Guidelines for evaluation of personnel with newly reactive tuberculin skin tests or suspected active TB can be found at www.cdc.gov/tb/. A Medical Officer shall perform a physical examination and obtain a complete medical history in such personnel.

e. <u>Specific written requirements</u>. Medical personnel should make a written recommendation as to whether continued annual TB surveillance is required.

13. <u>Bloodborne Pathogens, CG-6211</u>.

a. <u>Exposure effects</u>. Bloodborne pathogens are defined as any pathogenic microorganism present in the blood of humans, which are able to cause human diseases. Prevention of Bloodborne Pathogens Transmission, COMDINST 6220.8 (series), includes definitions, prevention and control measures, and applicability, as well as discussing vaccination policy, and post exposure prophylaxis. Further instructions are found in Chapter 13 of this Manual which covers approved work practices and training requirements including discussions in Universal Precautions. The primary Bloodborne Pathogens (BBP's) include Human Immune Deficiency Virus (HIV), Hepatitis B (HBV), and Hepatitis C (HCV).

b. <u>Required surveillance</u>.

(1) Bloodborne Pathogen exposure surveillance is based on OSHA guidelines (29 CFR 1910.1030). Enrollment in OMSEP is required for all workers who reasonably anticipate contact with BBP's as a result of their duties. Determination of exposure must be based on the definition

of occupational exposure without regard to personal protective equipment. Exposures should be listed according to:

(a) Jobs in which all workers have occupational exposure (i.e. lab personnel, and EMTs) and,

(b) Jobs where only some of the workers may be exposed (i.e. alien migrant operations, and health care providers; sewage workers; health service technicians). In these circumstances all the specific tasks and/or procedures potentially causing the exposure must be clearly listed.

(2) All BBP enrollees will be entered into the OMSEP database for proper identification. Monitoring and post-exposure prophylaxis will be done in accordance with any reported or suspected acute exposure (see form CG-6211), and guidelines found in Chapter 13 of this Manual.

NOTE: Workers determined to be potentially exposed as part of their routine duties (section 12-C-13.b (1) a, will be followed in OMSEP for the duration of their careers and/or as medically indicated to rule out exposure, following termination of aforementioned duties. Workers potentially exposed as a result of casual non-routine related duties must be followed in OMSEP only until it is determined no exposure occurred.

c. Information to medical personnel. Since the potential for infectivity of patient's blood and body fluids is not routinely known, it is essential that all workers conform to blood and body fluid precautions, regardless of any lack of evidence of infectiousness. Acute viral hepatitis is a serious operational problem, which has significantly altered the course of many military operations. According to established classification acute hepatitis is a self-limited liver injury of <6 months duration and chronic hepatitis represents a hepatic inflammation >6 months. The usual course is six to 10 days of acute symptoms associated with a variable rise in ALT/AST and bilirubin. The common clinical presentation includes the symptom complex of anorexia, nausea, right upper quadrant pain and tenderness, hepatomegaly, and jaundice. Specific Bloodborne Pathogens are discussed in further detail:

(1) Hepatitis B (HBV), also known as "serum" hepatitis, is less of a risk for endemic outbreaks than other hepatitis viruses but is also less amenable to prophylactic measures. Serologic evidence precedes clinical symptoms by approximately 1 month. Hepatitis B is the leading cause of liver-related deaths from cirrhosis and hepatocellular carcinoma worldwide; is especially frequent in drug abusers, male homosexuals, and chronic dialysis patients; 5% to 10% of adults in the US have had the disease; and 10% develop a chronic carrier state and constitute an infectious pool. Important serological markers to follow include: HB_sAg, HB_eAg, HB_cAg, HB_sAb, HB_eAB and HB_cAb. The AST and

ALT should also be evaluated at monthly intervals following their initial rise and decline.

- (a) Hepatitis B surface antigen (HBsAg) is found in acute illness and becomes positive 1 to 7 weeks before clinical disease. It remains positive 1 to 6 weeks after clinical disease and in chronic carrier states. Blood-containing HBsAg is considered potentially infectious.

- (b) Hepatitis B antibody (Anti-HBs) is an antibody against the surface antigen of hepatitis B and appears weeks to months after clinical illness. The presence of this antibody confers immunity and indicates prior disease (if hepatitis B core antibody positive) or vaccination (if hepatitis B core antibody negative).

- (c) Anticore antibody (Anti-HBc) appears during the acute phase of the illness and its presence can be used to diagnose acute HBV infection especially in the "window period" when both HBsAg and HbsAb may be undetectable. Presence of HBcIgM denotes acute infection and IgG appears chronically. The latter may be protective against reinfection.

- (d) Hepatitis Be antigen (HBeAg) is a mark of infectivity both acutely and chronically.

- (e) Those who are hepatitis B carriers or have chronic active hepatitis will be HBsAg positive.

(2) Hepatitis C (HCV), formerly Non A- Non B hepatitis, is responsible for most cases of post-transfusion hepatitis and presents a significant risk for the development of hepatocellular carcinoma. It accounts for 20% to 40% of acute hepatitis in the United States. Hepatitis C also causes 90% of post transfusion hepatitis. The virus has an extremely high mutation rate and is thus not easily neutralized by the body's antibody response. Acute infection is usually asymptomatic; with 20% of patients developing jaundice, and 75% of those infected developing chronic disease. HCV hepatitis, to date, has no serological markers that have been exclusively associated with blood transfusions, making this a diagnosis of exclusion based on the appropriate clinical setting. Most patients with hepatitis C have a history of intravenous drug abuse. Other risk factors include history blood transfusion, tattoos, alcohol abuse and cocaine snorting. Epidemiological evidence suggests that it can be transmitted sexually with risk of transmission increasing with duration of a relationship but with a very low incidence (<5%).

(a) Diagnostic serologic tests that probe for antibodies produced in response to several viral antigens are now available for the diagnosis of hepatitis C. These tests are highly sensitive and specific. If testing low risk populations, RIBA (recombinant immunoblot assay) test should be obtained since the ELISA has a higher false-positive rate.

(b) Polymerase chain reaction (PCR) can detect minute quantities of HCV RNA present in blood as early as 1-2 weeks after infection. Qualitative PCR tests detect as few as 100 HCV RNA copies, and quantitative tests detect a lower limit of 500-2000 copies.

(c) Genetic heterogeneity of HCV identifies at least 6 distinct genotypes (with numerous subtypes). Different genotypes have geographic and epidemiological differences, and they are good predictors of response to interferon.

(3) Human Immunodeficiency Virus (HIV), is a retrovirus, which was recognized as an infectious cause of an unusual immunodeficiency syndrome, which is transmitted, in a similar mode to that of hepatitis B virus. Has been recognized as major public health problem for men and women, with between 5 and 10 million persons infected worldwide. It can be acquired through intimate homosexual or heterosexual contact, by receiving infected blood or blood products, or by inoculation via needles contaminated with infected blood (IV drug use, tattooing, etc). There is also good evidence that transmission via open skin wounds exposed to infected blood or saliva occurs, though such transmission is rare. The diagnosis is based on recognition of clinical symptoms in an at risk population and appropriate serological screening procedures:

(a) Clinical diagnosis. Some patients experience a flu-like illness when initially infected, but often there are no symptoms. A very variable, prolonged period may pass in which there are no signs or symptoms as immunosuppression proceeds. When the immune system is sufficiently impaired, infections with various organisms usually not pathogenic occur. The clinician should be attentive to signs of global dementia that occur in the absence of an opportunistic infection of the CNS. This appears to be a direct consequence of HIV viral infection and precedes any other clinical manifestation in between 10 and 25 percent of infected patients who develop AIDS. Initially, there are mild cognitive defects involving judgment and memory, which progress to a severe global dementia.

(b) Serological diagnosis. HIV ab test (western blot) serves as the screening tool during routine medical evaluations. This is a commercially available enzyme immunoassay (EIA) test. The median interval between infection and seropositivity is estimated at three months. Results are considered reactive only when a positive result is confirmed in a second test.

d. <u>Examination protocols</u>. Each examination should, as a minimum:

(1) Follow the post exposure guidelines found in Chapter 13 of this Manual.

(2) Ascertain source and exposed person's HCV exposure and immune status.

(3) Follow up any suspicious laboratory findings with a detailed work and medical history giving particular attention to:

(a) Past and present history of exposures to BBP's.

(b) Smoking and alcohol use history.

(c) Any symptoms of skin irritation, bleeding or recurrent dermatitis.

(d) Any CNS symptoms, including headaches, nausea, vomiting, dizziness, weakness, and disorientation.

(e) A review of the immunologic and hematopoietic systems.

(f) A system specific physical examination with attention to the skin, mucous membranes, respiratory, and nervous system including a mental status evaluation.

(g) The following laboratory tests are recommended (at the discretion of the attending medical provider): CBC, and WBC counts with differential, CD4 counts, immunoglobulins, platelet counts, liver enzymes and hepatitis profile and a multichemistry panel (including glucose, BUN, total protein and creatinine) and urinalysis.

(4) Provide a complete review of the medical record to confirm documentation of compliance with indicated immunizations and completion of baseline laboratory studies before assignment to specific tasks or procedures with potential risk of exposure.

e. <u>Specific written requirements</u>. In addition to the general requirements specified in Section 12-B-4-b, the physician should address:

(1) Any other medical conditions, which could place the worker at greater than normal risk.

(2) The periodicity of the next evaluation and/or referral to the appropriate specialty clinic.

(3) The recommended duty limitations, hygiene care and infectious disease precautions.

(4) The exposure risk (unprotected exposure) for HIV, HBV and HCV.

(5) "Universal Precautions"- defined as an approach to infection control where all human blood and body fluids are treated as if known to be infectious for blood borne pathogens. Specimens that entail "universal precautions" are all excretions, secretions, blood, body fluid, and any drainage. Personnel should protect themselves from contact with these specimens by using the appropriate barrier precautions to prevent cross-transmission and exposure of their skin and mucous membranes, especially the eyes, nose, and mouth. See Chapter 13 of this Manual for further guidance.

14. <u>Radiation (Ionizing/Non-ionizing) (Form CG-6214)</u>.

   a. <u>Exposure effects</u>. Humans are exposed routinely to radiation from both natural sources, such as cosmic rays from the sun and indoor radon, and from manufactured sources, such as televisions and medical x-rays and even the human body, which contains natural radioactive elements. There are many forms of radiation. For the purpose of Occupational Health Monitoring, only two major types of radiation will be addressed here: Ionizing and Non-ionizing radiation.

      (1) <u>Ionizing Radiation</u>. This type of radiation is defined as any electromagnetic or particulate radiation capable of producing ions. Ionizing radiation includes the following: gamma rays, X-rays, alpha particles, beta particles, neutrons, and protons. Biological effects are due to the ionization process that destroys the capacity for cell reproduction or division and causes cell mutation. Equipment or devices capable of generating ionizing radiation include: nuclear reactors, nuclear detonation devices, medical or dental radiological or fluoroscopic equipment, industrial radiographic equipment, and any contraband material capable of generating ionizing radiation.

      (2) <u>Non-Ionizing Radiation</u>. The term non-ionizing radiation refers to forms of radiation which do not have sufficient energy to cause the ionization of atoms or molecules. Sources of non-ionizing electromagnetic emissions include ultraviolet, visible or infrared light radiated by lasers, radars, radiofrequency (radio transmissions), and microwave sources. Broadband optical sources such as germicidal lamps, phototherapy, backlights, sunlamps, arc lights and projector

lamps used in many medical and industrial applications can also be sources of non-ionizing radiation exposure.

b. <u>Required surveillance</u>.

(1) Radiation surveillance is based on Federal regulations issued by the Nuclear Regulatory Commission (10 CFR 19, 20, and 71), Department of Health and Human Services, Department of Transportation (49 CFR), Department of Labor, Occupational Safety and Health Administration (OSHA), personnel exposures (29 CFR 1910.96, 1910.120), guidelines from the American Conference of Governmental Industrial Hygienists (ACGIH) and the Environmental Protection Agency (40 CFR). As an additional safeguard and in addition to these regulations, in order to decrease the risk of stochastic effects resulting from exposure, the nuclear industry follows the ALARA concept- <u>A</u>s <u>L</u>ow <u>A</u>s <u>R</u>easonably <u>A</u>chievable.

(2) Although the potential for radiation exposure in the CG is small, it is essential that all workers conform to established safety guidelines, regardless of any lack of suspected exposure. Procedures and guidance for the evaluation of suspected radiological exposures, during many operational activities, can be obtained from "Guidance for Actions when Encountering Radioactive Materials During Vessel Boarding, Cargo Inspections and Other Activities", COMDTINST 16600.2 (series),

(3) Enrollment in a medical surveillance program should be limited to those personnel who are clearly at risk of exposure to ionizing and/or non-ionizing radiation, above established exposure limits, as a result of their duties. Determination of exposure must be based on the definition of occupational exposure without regard to personal protective equipment. All personnel referred to the Radiation Exposure Protocol will be entered into the OMSEP database for proper identification. Monitoring will be based upon reported or suspected acute exposures. Enrollment should be considered for each of the following categories of workers:

(a) Field unit personnel exposed during daily operations, which may potentially lead to exposure to radiological materials. This would include: Marine Safety Inspectors; Port-Safety Control Boarding Teams; High Interest Vessel Boarding Teams; Recreational Boating Safety Inspectors; Container Inspection Inspectors (CIP); Spill Response Personnel and, Emergency Response personnel responding to incidents involving radiation.

(b) Medical and dental personnel, including dental and X-ray technicians as well as other dental paraprofessional staff, Research and Development (R&D) staff, and laboratory personnel.

(c) Aviation personnel exposed to cosmic radiation, radar emissions; shipment of radiation materials and radar, radio and video display terminal maintenance and repair personnel.

(d) NOTE: Exclusion from enrollment should apply to workers whose routine job activities have a low radiation exposure potential. For ionizing radiation this would include such activities as: the routine handling of radiation monitoring sources, electronic (radio) tubes, static eliminators, smoke detectors, weapon sights and certain gauging devices. For non-ionizing radiation this would include the routine handling of: microwave ovens, radio and radar equipment.

c. Information to medical personnel.

(1) Radiation effects fall into two broad categories: *deterministic and stochastic.* "Deterministic" effects usually manifest soon after exposure and have definite threshold doses. Examples include radiation skin burning, blood count effects, and cataracts. In contrast, "*stochastic*" effects are caused by more subtle radiation-induced cellular changes (including DNA mutations) that are random in nature and have no threshold dose. Cancer is a known clinical manifestation of radiation-induced stochastic effects.

(2) Radiation measures used in the United States include the following (the internationally used equivalent unit of measurement follows in parenthesis):

(a) Rad (radiation absorbed dose) measures the amount of energy actually absorbed by a material, such as human tissue (Gray=100 rads).

(b) Roentgen is a measure of exposure; it describes the amount of radiation energy, in the form of gamma or x-rays, in the air.

(c) REM (Roentgen Equivalent Man) accounts for the biological damage induced by radiation. It takes into account both the amount, or dose, of radiation and the biological effect of the type of radiation in question. A millirem is one one-thousandth of a rem (Sievert=100 rems).

(d) Curie is a unit of radioactivity. One curie refers to the amount of any radionuclide that undergoes 37 billion atomic transformations a second. A nanocurie is one one-billionth of a curie (37 Becquerel = 1 nanocurie).

(e) A conversion factor ("f" factor) is used to convert exposure (measured in air) into a more meaningful unit, the radiation absorbed dose (Rad), which is the energy deposited in a mass of tissue.

****Dose (in Rads)= 0.869 (f) (Roentgens)****

(3) OSHA's occupational limit for whole body exposure is 5 REM (50 mSv) per year. At this level the risk to individuals is considered to be very low. In the U.S., the average individual is exposed to a dose of approximately one REM (10 mSv) every 12 years, as a result of natural and medical procedures. The following table shows average radiation doses from several common sources of human exposure. (EPA's Rad facts)

Radiation Source	Dose (millirems)
Chest x-ray	10
Mammogram	30
Cosmic rays	31 (annually)
Human body	39 (annually)
Household radon	200 annually
Cross-country airplane flight	5

Table 12-C-1

(4) Most radiation exposure data should be made available to medical personnel at the time of the member's referral. The member or the member's Unit Safety Coordinator may provide this data based upon dose measurements from a personal radiation dosimeter. Information may also be obtained from the cognizant Safety and Environmental Health Officer (SEHO), who may have previously evaluated the worker or work task to obtain a representative dose. General principles that apply to the evaluation and monitoring of ionizing and nonionizing radiation induced health effects follow:

(5) Ionizing Radiation- The nature and extent of the radiation damage depend on the amount of exposure, the frequency of exposure, and the penetrating power of the radiation to which an individual is exposed as well as the sensitivity of the exposed cells. A given total dose will cause more damage if received in a shorter period of time (**dose rate**):

Acute Radiation Absorbed Dose (RAD)	Effect	Time
0-25	No observable effect	
25-50	Minor temporary blood changes	Hours
50-150	Possible nausea and vomiting; decreased WBC	2-3 weeks
150-300	Increased severity of above symptoms; diarrhea; malaise; decreased appetite; some death	3-4 weeks
0-500	Increased severity of above plus hemorrhaging; depilation; LD_{50} at 450-500 Rads	Within 2 months
> 500	Symptoms appear sooner; LD_{100} approx. 600 Rads	1-2 weeks

Table 12-C-2

(a) Acute Somatic Effects are the relatively immediate effects, which present in a person acutely exposed. Severity is dose dependent and death results from damage to bone marrow or intestinal wall. High doses of external irradiation can manifest as severe radiation sickness ("radiation poisoning). Skin effects (radiation dermatitis) are noted as an acute effect of radiotherapy and as a chronic effect of industrial exposure.

(b) Delayed Somatic Effects manifest as cancer, leukemia, cataracts, organ failure and abortion. The severity may be dose independent but the probability of the effect may be proportional to the dose received.

(c) Genetic Effects conveyed to offspring are usually irreversible and nearly always harmful. Radiation can cause changes in "DNA" leading to teratogenic or genetic mutations. The severity may be dose independent but the probability of the effect is likely to be proportional to the dose.

(d) Organs Effects are most significant in the hematopoietic and gastrointestinal systems (most susceptible are lymphocytes; bone marrow; gastrointestinal; gonads and other fast growing cells). The immune and cardiovascular systems can also be significantly affected, while the central nervous system is less susceptible.

(6) Non-Ionizing Radiation- the biological effects of non-ionizing radiation depend on the frequency and intensity of the electromagnetic emissions radiated by lasers, radiofrequency (RF), and microwave sources.

(a) Laser Radiation- lasers are designed to operate at various wavelengths in the ultraviolet, visible and infrared portions of the electromagnetic spectrum. Laser exposure can result in permanent and disabling eye injury. Laser exposure levels are set to protect the tissues from damage and are not the equivalent of comfortable viewing levels.

   (1) Lasers are grouped into four categories: Class I; II; III A and B and Class IV. Class I lasers are typically safe to view under all conditions, while Class IV can cause eye damage under most conditions. Laser exposures that are within the TLV produce no adverse biological effects.

   (2) Enrollment for laser surveillance should be limited to those personnel who are clearly at risk of exposure, typically associated with accidental injuries and not chronic exposures. Member's requiring surveillance include: Researched & Development (R&D) personnel and laboratory personnel who routinely work with Class III and IV lasers; Maintenance personnel who routinely repair Class III and IV lasers, and Engineering operators who routinely work with Class III and IV lasers.

(b) Radiofrequency (RF) Electromagnetic Radiation- RF exposure is primarily associated with operation of various radars, and communication systems.

   (1) Exposure limits are defined based upon whether the location can be characterized as a controlled or uncontrolled environment. Controlled areas are those where the personnel working in those areas are aware of and trained to protect themselves from the presence of RF radiation. Uncontrolled areas are public or berthing areas where exposures are not expected to be present.

   (2) Enrollment for RF surveillance should be limited to individuals who knowingly enter (work) areas where higher RF levels can reasonably be anticipated to exist, and those individuals exposed, in an uncontrolled area, where RF exposure levels have been determine to be over the TLV. The TLV's refer to time-averaged exposure values obtained by spatial averaging RF measurements over an area equivalent to the vertical cross section of the human body.

   (3) The farther away the individual is from the radiation source, the less the exposure. As a rule, if you double the distance, you reduce the exposure by a factor of four. Halving the

COMDTINST M6000.1E

        distance increases the exposure by a factor of four. This is promulgated by the fact that the area of the sphere depends on the distance from the source to the center of the sphere (radius). It is proportional to the square of the radius. As a result. If the radius doubles, the sphere surface area increases four times.

    (c) VDT/Microwave Radiation- no specific surveillance is required for VDT users. Precautions should be maintained for individuals with prosthetic heart valves working with or near microwave equipment.

d. <u>Examination protocols</u>. Each examination should, as a minimum:

  (1) Physical examination forms- Complete all clinical evaluation blocks of the physical examination forms: Report of Medical Examination, DD 2808 and Report of Medical History, DD 2807-1 and the Periodic History and Report of OMSEP Examination, CG 5447A and Acute Exposure Information Form, CG-6000-1, when applicable. The only exceptions are as follows: breast examinations are not required for females under the age of 36 years and digital rectal exams are not required for males under the age of 45 years. The Medical Officer should pay close attention to the preexisting medical and occupational work histories with particular attention to radiation exposures and malignancies, as well as accounting for the member's age and type of billet assignment.

  (2) Special Studies- the only required tests are a complete CBC and Urinalysis.

    (a) Any CBC (manual or automated) with a WBC count that falls outside the normal parameters of the laboratory reference values requires a differential white blood cell count. Any member with persistent abnormal blood counts, as per reference values, shall be removed from work pending a complete evaluation (consultation referral) with a Board Certified Hematologist. The evaluation and consultation referrals for an abnormal CBC should be directed toward the possible diagnosis of a malignant or premalignant condition.

    (b) The urinalysis will be tested for red blood cells using a standard clinical dipstick method or microscopic high power field (HPF). Any persistent hematuria (> 5 RBC's per HPF) on a repeat urinalysis will be considered disqualifying pending a definitive diagnosis. Other urine findings, such as WBC casts, albuminuria, glucosuria, low specific gravity, etc will require further evaluation by the Medical Officer but will not be considered disqualifying for the purposes of this protocol.

> (c) Additionally, any member who handles radioactive material that could reasonably be expected to exceed 10% of an annual limit on intake or in 1 year through inhalation should be evaluated for a partial body burden, by bioassay or external counting, at the initial assignment and at the time of termination. Periodic monitoring will be conducted on these individuals at the discretion of the Medical Officer. All personnel assigned to the handling of Radon should also have a Radon Breath Analysis or Radium Urine Bioassay at the initial and exit physicals.

e. <u>Physical Examinations</u>. Late or delayed effects of radiation may occur following a wide range of doses or dose rates. Although not anticipated, it is likely that if CG workers incur an exposure it would be the result of a single low-level accidental event. Low-level long-term exposure resulting in a Chronic Radiation Syndrome (CRS) is considered highly unlikely, providing safety practices are followed.

> (1) Initial/Baseline Examination - Any worker known to be potentially exposed or at risk (controlled environment), should have an Initial/Baseline examination performed. This includes all workers assigned to billets where radiation inspection duties are considered part of the employment criteria. Emergency Response personnel; dentists; dental technicians; other dental paraprofessionals; radiology technicians; nurses; laboratory and other medical personnel; as well as air crew members who may be sporadically exposed DO NOT require an initial / baseline examination.

> (2) Acute Exposure Examination- Any individual exceeding the radiation protection standards or who has ingested or inhaled radioactive material exceeding 50% of the TLV, or as deemed by the supervising Medical Officer, should be given an Acute Exposure examination with completion of CG 5447 A.

> (3) Personnel NOT required having a regular physical examination but who exceed 500 mrem (5mSv) exposure within a calendar year must have an Acute Exposure examination within 1 month of the time they exceeded the 500 mrem level.

> (4) Periodic Examination- Personnel routinely assigned to duties with potential radiation exposure must have a periodic examination not to exceed every 5 years until the age of 50. Thereafter, the examinations should be every 2 years until the age of 60 when the examinations should be performed yearly.

(5) Exit/ Separation Examination- Every reasonable effort should be made to ensure that workers who have had a history of radiation exposure complete an Exit physical examination upon separation or termination of employment or when permanently removed from the hazardous radiation exposure duties.

f. <u>Specific written requirements</u>. In addition to the general requirements specified in section 14-d (1&2) above the Medical Officer should address the following:

(1) Any preexisting condition or history of cancer; radiation therapy; polycythemia vera; cancerous or pre-cancerous lesions will be considerations for rejection or disqualification, unless adequately treated (e.g. Actinic keratosis, basal cell carcinomas, abnormal PAP smears)

(2) Any open lesions or wounds (including abrasions, lacerations, ulcerative, exfoliative or eruptive lesions) may be temporary or permanently disqualifying, depending on the condition, for any individual actively handling radioactive materials.

(3) Any history of gastrointestinal, pulmonary and ocular conditions, particularly vision impairment and cataracts, should be fully evaluated (Ophthalmology referral), to ensure that they are not related or aggravated by exposure to radiation. Any history of unconsciousness, e.g. epilepsy, vertigo, middle ear disease should also be investigated.

(4) Members under the age of 18 years and pregnant women need to be identified. Young workers should not be exposed to potential radiation and pregnancy is subject to special provisions in the exposure radiation regulations (reduced exposure limits). The main effects of ionizing radiation on the fetus are growth retardation, congenital malformations, fetal death and carcinogenesis.

(5) Preventive Practices/Basic Management. The spectrum of care will vary according to the level, intensity and nature of the radiological event. The medical provider should formulate a plan for the management of febrile, neutropenic patients, blast and thermal injuries, incidental wounds, ocular effects and psychological problems.

(a) Infections. Provide broad-spectrum antibiotics until patient is afebrile for 24 hours. Avoid aminoglycoside toxicity. Consider reverse isolation. Obtain blood cultures if possible.

(b) Thermal Injuries. Likely to be most common injury following nuclear detonation. Burns will be dictated by clothing pattern. Evaluate respiratory system for hot-gas effect. Intubate early. Provide IV hydration. High mortality expected.

(c) Ocular Injuries. Chorioretinal areas most affected following high-intensity visible and infrared radiation. Injury secondary to infrared energy along with photochemical reaction. Flashblindness is temporary, may last 30 minutes. Slit lamp exam should be considered.

(d) Skin Injuries. Radiation dermatitis results from high-level doses. Usually delayed and irreversible. Copious irrigation will help prevent beta skin damage. Clean and barrier all wounds to prevent absorption of radionuclides. If unable to remove contaminants, member must be referred for further assessment. Internal uptake of radionuclides should be considered on all contaminated open wounds. (See section d.2.c)

(e) Internal contamination. Results from absorbed, inhaled or ingested radioactive material. Treatment reduces the absorption dose and the risk of future biological effects. Use chelating or mobilizing agents as soon as possible. Gastric lavage and emetics may also be used. Purgatives, laxatives and enemas may help reduce retention time of radioactive substances in colon. Ion exchange resins may also be helpful. NOTE: If offending agent is identified contact DOD or REACTS for guidance. Blocking agents, such as iodine compounds, should be given as soon as possible (for radioiodine exposures)- radioiodine is blocked with a 300 mg dose of iodide.

(f) Acute High-Dose Radiation. The three principal situations for this exposure are a nuclear detonation; formation of a critical mass ("criticality") by high-grade nuclear material; and as a result of radiation dispersal from highly radioactive material (e.g. cobalt-60). In an Acute Radiation Syndrome situation the most highly radiosensitive organs that would be affected would be the gastrointestinal tract and hematopoietic systems. The severe radiation sickness resulting from these effects would be a primary medical concern. If appropriate medical care is not provided, the medial lethal dose, $LD_{50/60}$ (50% kill rate in 60 days) is estimated at 3.5 Gy.

  (1) Acute Radiation Syndrome. This represents a sequence of phased symptoms, which vary with individual radiation sensitivity, type of radiation, and the level of absorbed radiation.

  (2) Prodromal Syndrome. This is characterized by a rapid onset of nausea, vomiting and malaise. This is a non-specific clinical response, whose early onset, in the absence of trauma, represents a large radiation exposure. Radiogenic vomiting cannot be easily distinguished from psychogenic vomiting

resulting from stress or fear. Use of oral prophylactic antiemetics would be indicated for anticipated unavoidable high- dose radiation exposure

    (3) Latent Period. Manifest with an asymptomatic phase, which varies according to the dose absorbed. This phase may last from 2-6 weeks and is longest preceding the neurovascular syndrome and shortest prior to the gastrointestinal syndrome.

    (4) Manifest Illness. This phase presents with the clinical symptoms associated with the major organ systems affected. Earliest symptoms are found in the peripheral blood system occurring within 24 hours post radiation as a result of bone-marrow depression. Clinical evidence of anemia and decrease immunity (infections) will vary from 10 days to as long as 6-8 weeks following exposure. Erythrocytes are the least affected due to their short lifespan. The average time from clinical anemia to bleeding diathesis and decreased resistance to infection is from 2-3 weeks. The most useful laboratory procedure to evaluate bone marrow depression is the peripheral blood count. A 50% drop in lymphocytes within 24 hours indicates significant radiation injury.

g. NOTE: CG medical facilities are not equipped to handle large number of radiobiological injuries resulting from a nuclear detonation or a radiation dispersal device. Medical Providers should develop a referral, transportation, and consultation plan in coordination with local emergency services, medical specialty providers, and regional DoD MTF facilities. Participation is highly encouraged in USAMRIID's Chem-Bio training course and familiarization with guidelines provided in the "Medical Management of Radiological Casualties" handbook published by the Armed Forces Radiobiology Research Institute (AFRRI) http://www.afrri.usuhs.mil.

COMDTINST M6000.1E

CHAPTER 13
QUALITY IMPROVEMENT

Section A. Quality Improvement Program.

1. Mission 1
2. Background 1
3. Internal Quality Assurance Reviews 1
4. External Quality Improvement Reviews 1
5. Goals 2
6. Operational Health Readiness Program (OHRP) 2
7. Objectives 2
8. Definitions 3
9. Responsibilities 4
10. Confidentiality Statement 7
11. QIP Review and Evaluation 7

Section B. Credentials Maintenance and Review.

1. Background 1
2. Definitions 1
3. Pre-selection Credentials Review 2
4. Provider Credentials File (PCF) 3
5. Documentation 4
6. Verification 5
7. Contract Provider Credentials Review 6
8. Reverification 6
9. National Practitioner Data Bank (NPDB) 7
10. National Provider Identifiers Type 1 (NPI) 7

Section C. Clinical Privileges.

1. Purpose 1
2. Background 1
3. Definitions 1
4. Applicability and Scope 3
5. Clinical Privileges 4

Section D. Operational Health Readiness Program.

1. Background 1
2. Purpose 1
3. Overview 1
4. OHRP Compliance Process 2

Section E. Quality Improvement Implementation Guide (QIIG).

1. Background 1
2. Responsibilities 1

Section F. National Provider Identifiers.

1. National Provider Identifiers (NPI) Type 1 1
2. Clinic National Provider Identifiers (NPI) Type 2 1

Section G. Health Insurance Portability and Accountability Act (HIPAA).

1. Background 1
2. HIPAA Privacy/Security Officials (P/SO) 1
3. HIPAA Training Requirements 4
4. Handling HIPAA Complaints and Mitigation 7
5. Unintentional Disclosures of Protected Health Information 9
6. Protected Health Information and the Coast Guard Messaging System 10
7. Other CG Members Who Utilize Protected Health Information 10
8. Electronic Transmission of Protected Health Information 11

Section H. Quality Improvement Studies.

1. Background 1
2. Responsibilities 1
3. Definitions 1
4. General information 2
5. QIS Focus 2
6. QIS Process 2
7. QIS Report Form 2
8. Frequency of Quality Improvement Studies 2
9. Completing the QIS Report Form 2
10. Follow-up Reporting 5
11. Integration 5
12. Filing 5

Section I. Peer Review Program.

1. Background 1
2. Characteristics of a Peer Review Program 1
3. Responsibilities 1
4. Process 2
5. Definitions 2

Section J. Infection and Exposure Control Program.

1. Introduction 1
2. Policy 2
3. Standard Precautions 2
4. Precautions for Invasive Procedures 5
5. Precautions for Medical Laboratories 6
6. Handling Biopsy Specimens 6
7. Using and Caring for Sharp Instruments and Needles 7
8. Infection Control Procedures for Minor Surgery Areas and Dental Operatories 8
9. Sterilizing and Disinfecting 14
10. Clinic Attire 19
11. Storage and Laundering of Clinic Attire, PPE and Linen 19
12. Cleaning and Decontaminating Blood or Other Body Fluid Spills 20
13. Infectious Waste 20
14. Managing Exposures (Bloodborne Pathogen Exposure Control) 21
15. Training Personnel for Occupational Exposure 26

Section K. Patient Safety and Risk Management Program.

1. Purpose 1
2. Informed Consent 1
3. Adverse Event Monitoring and Reporting 4
4. Patient Safety Training 8

Section L. Training and Professional Development.

1. Definitions 1
2. Unit Health Services Training Plan (In-Service Training) 1
3. Emergency Medical Training Requirements 3
4. Health Services Technician "A" School 4
5. Health Services Technician "C" Schools 4
6. Continuing Education Programs 5
7. Long-Term Training Programs 6

Section M. Patient Affairs Program.

1. Patient Sensitivity 1
2. Patient Advisory Committee (PAC) 1
3. Patient Satisfaction Assessment 2
4. Patient Grievance Protocol 2
5. Congressional Inquiries 3
6. Patient Bill of Rights and Responsibilities 3

This page intentionally left blank

Chapter 13 Contents

Section A. Quality Improvement Program.

1. Mission. 1
2. Background. 1
3. Internal Quality Assurance Reviews. 1
4. External Quality Improvement Reviews. 1
5. Goals. 2
6. Operational Health Readiness Program (OHRP). 2
7. Objectives. 2
8. Definitions. 3
9. Responsibilities. 4
10. Confidentiality Statement. 7
11. QIP Review and Evaluation. 7

This page intentionally left blank.

Section A. Quality Improvement Program.

1. Mission. The Commandant and Director of Health, Safety, and Work-Life are committed to providing the highest quality health care to Coast Guard beneficiaries. The Health Services Quality Improvement Program (QIP) described here establishes policy, prescribes procedures, and assigns responsibility for Quality Improvement (QI) activities at CG health services facilities. It is intended to function as an integral component in a quality healthcare system aimed at improving patient outcomes while also achieving patient satisfaction. This is accomplished by using quantitative methods to continuously improve the health services program. It is essential that the QIP integrates into the CG's overall healthcare system in order to improve health care delivery at all organizational levels. The Health, Safety, and Work-Life Directorate, HSWL SC, unit COs, health care providers, and patients must cooperate to ensure successful implementation of the quality improvement concept in the health care arena.

2. Background. Healthcare quality, as defined by the Institute of Medicine (IOM), is "the degree to which health services for individuals and population increase the likelihood of desired health outcomes and are consistent with professional knowledge". For many years, CG health care facilities have conducted QI activities, usually as a normal outgrowth of complying with this Manual's directives and the consequence of CG practitioners' good medical and dental practices. Since Maintenance and Logistics Commands were established in 1987 and the Quality Assurance Division was reorganized in 1989 in the Office of Health and Safety, a concerted effort has been made to develop a CG-wide quality program designed to address quality-of-care issues at our facilities. This program has been tailored to CG medical and dental practices and incrementally phased it in over an extended time period. This program has been very successful in creating a quality foundation to the CG health care system. It is now time for us to expand this quality focus to broader views that reflect recommendations from health care quality studies in recent years.

3. Internal Quality Assurance Reviews. The CG first established an internal healthcare quality assurance (QA) program in the early 1990s to monitor the quality of healthcare delivered at its clinics. The MLCs (k) initially administered the program by conducting QA surveys at each clinic every three years by members of the MLC staff. Clinics passing the MLC survey were awarded a three-year certificate that verified the clinic met CG QA standards. In 2004 the internal QA review process changed to the current format which provides for an external accreditation organization to perform the Quality Improvement (QI) surveys of CG clinics and issue a one or three-year accreditation. The HSWL SC review process concentrates on CG-specific and Operational Health Readiness issues.

4. External Quality Improvement Reviews. The standard of healthcare in the U.S. is for QI program surveys to be conducted by external auditors. Additionally, external auditors help the CG meet DoD and TRICARE QA healthcare requirements. In 2004, the CG contracted an external accreditation organization to independently conduct CG clinic QI surveys. The external accreditation organization standards mirror many CG standards that were being implemented by clinics in accordance

with the Medical Manual, COMDTINST M6000.1 (series). The standard external survey cycle will be every three years. To receive a three-year accreditation, clinics must demonstrate compliance with the survey standards and Quality Improvement Studies (QIS) must be implemented on a continuous basis. The external accreditation organization is the sole accrediting body for CG clinics.

5. Goals. All CG health care facilities with medical or dental officers assigned shall have a QIP to organize efforts to achieve and document quality health care for eligible beneficiaries. The QIP described here contains the essential elements required at all CG facilities and assigns responsibilities for program initiatives. All active duty, reserve, and civilian health care providers treating patients at CG clinics must participate in on-going QIS designed to assess the quality and appropriateness of the services they provide.

6. Operational Health Readiness Program (OHRP). CG specific QI and operational health readiness issues will be managed and monitored by the HSWL SC under the Operational Health Readiness Program (OHRP) addressed in 13.D. The HSWL SC will no longer survey QA/QI issues that are addressed by the external accreditation surveyors nor provide a certification.

7. Objectives.

    a. Communicate information. Communicate important QI information to enable sound clinical and management decision-making at all organizational levels.

    b. Review credentials and approve privileges. Ensure a safe and professional health care team by reviewing credentials and approving privileges of health care providers that work in CG clinics.

    c. Standards. Establish criteria to assist and ensure that clinics meet external accreditation standards, by integrating quality improvement processes into daily health care delivery and to ensure clinics attain and sustain compliance with CG specific QI and operational health readiness issues.

    d. Monitor. Systematically monitor health services to identify opportunities to improve patient care, and use a systematic method of improvement changes to ensure effective improvements are made and sustained.

    e. Significant patterns. Integrate, track, and analyze patient care information to identify significant patterns that may require additional review or intervention.

    f. Resources. Identify and justify resources required to maintain high quality patient care standards.

    g. Risk assessment. Identify, assess, and decrease risk to patients and staff, thereby reducing liability exposure.

    h. Educational and training. Identify educational and training/professional development requirements and assure satisfactory education and training/professional development standards are established and maintained.

i. Patient satisfaction. Establish and maintain adequate systems to monitor and assess patient satisfaction; respond to patient and command concerns about access and quality of care.

8. Definitions.

    a. Quality. The desired level of performance as measured against generally accepted healthcare standards.

    b. Quality Health Care. According to the Institute of Medicine, quality health care is the degree to which health services for individuals and population increase the likelihood of desired health outcomes and are consistent with professional knowledge.

    c. Quality Assurance. Those functions that attempt to ensure the desired level of performance by systematically documenting, monitoring, evaluating, and, where necessary, adjusting healthcare to meet established standards. These functions must meet the minimum compliance with the Accreditation Association for Ambulatory Health Care (AAAHC) and the Coast Guard Medical Manual, COMDTINST M6000.1 (series) healthcare standards. QA functions do not necessarily contain QI functions.

    d. Quality Improvement. A system that attempts to proactively improve on the minimum healthcare standards established by the contracted external accreditation organization and the Medical Manual, COMDTINST M6000.1 (series). QI involves a continuous review of QA elements and operational procedures of healthcare delivery. QI always contains QA elements.

    e. Quality Improvement Studies (QIS). Those clinical processes that are identified as needing review for improvement. These initiatives demonstrate a commitment to making things better and always looking for and studying ways to improve. QIS help: evaluate the extent, severity and impact of a need or problem; assess and compare the effectiveness of various clinical or administrative approaches to resolution; identify areas for educational efforts; set performance goals, and track performance improvements. QIS replace the Monitoring and Evaluations.

    f. Professional Oversight. QIS provided by CG health care personnel and non-Federal providers, including among others, technical guidance and assistance, peer review, resource utilization review, external accreditation, and CG specific QI and operational health readiness issues managed and monitored by the HSWL SC to ensure compliance with the CG Health Care QIP and other CG directives.

    g. Governing Body. The agency that has ultimate authority and responsibility for establishing policy, maintaining quality patient care, and providing organizational management and planning. This is the Commandant (CG-11)

Executive Leadership Council. The Executive Leadership Council is comprised of Commandant (CG-112) (chair), Commandant (CG-11d), Commandant (CG-111), Commandant (CG-113), and the HSWL SC.

9. Responsibilities.

   a. Director of Health and Safety.

      (1) Establish at all CG health care facilities a comprehensive QIP which meets industry standards published by independent accrediting organizations. The HSWL SC implements the QIP as established by the Director of Health and Safety.

      (2) Govern CG health care facilities with delegated responsibilities to the Senior Health Services Officer (SHSO) at each facility.

      (3) Establish and promulgate health care policy including professional performance standards against which quality can be measured.

      (4) Establish and promulgate productivity and staffing standards for the health services program.

      (5) Conduct periodic Quality Improvement Meetings for Headquarters and HSWL SC QI staffs to coordinate and implement program policy at all organizational levels.

      (6) Review credentials and grant privileges for all CG medical and dental officers.

      (7) Develop and promulgate the Quality Improvement Implementation Guides.

      (8) Identify education and professional development training requirements and assure high quality standards are established and maintained. Coordinate and fund continuing professional education for all health services personnel.

   b. Health, Safety, and Work-Life Service Center (HSWL SC).

      (1) Ensure the Commandant's Health Care QI Program is executed at the field level.

      (2) Periodically conduct site assist visits to ensure compliance with external accreditation organization standards and Operational Health Readiness Program (OHRP) goals of all health services facilities in their area in accordance with Section 13.D.

      (3) Develop and maintain standard operating procedure manuals and/or health services support program guides necessary to provide operational guidance for clinic activities.

      (4) Develop and maintain Quality Improvement Self Assessment Checklists for assist visits.

(5) Perform utilization review of clinic expenditures, staffing, equipment, supplies, and facilities; review and process all requests for non-Federal medical care from units in its jurisdiction.

(6) Provide technical and professional advice regarding health services to units, as required.

(7) Conduct site visits on an appropriate schedule to verify standards compliance and to provide assistance in meeting the expectations of the Operational Health Readiness Program.

c. <u>Commanding Officers</u>.

(1) Ensure the unit actively pursues health services quality standards.

(2) Appoint in writing an individual to serve as Health Services Quality Improvement Coordinator in accordance with Paragraph 13.A.6.e.

d. <u>Senior Health Services Officer (SHSO)</u>. Represents the Governing Body locally for Quality Improvement and related activities.

e. <u>Health Services QI Coordinator</u>. The Health Services QI Coordinator should be a senior health services staff member with these characteristics:

(1) Demonstrates the ability and motivation to provide and ensure quality health care.

(2) Knows the requirements of the Medical Manual, COMDTINST M6000.1 (series).

(3) Communicates well in both writing and speaking.

(4) Well versed in delivering CG health care and supports the goals of health care quality improvement.

(5) Is an E-6 or above if military, or appropriate civilian employee.

f. <u>The Health Services QI Coordinator responsibilities</u>. The Health Services QI Coordinator responsibilities are as follows:

(1) Directs Health Services QI Focus Group activities.

(2) Implements the health care QI program locally by identifying and coordinating resolution of health care QI problems through design and implementation of QIS.

(3) Develops and promulgates an annual QI calendar which sets the agenda for all QI activities at the unit, including among other activities QI Focus Group meetings and all quality improvement studies.

(4) Other health care QI functions as necessary.

(5) Appoint health services staff members to serve on a Health Services Quality Improvement Focus Group in accordance with Paragraph 13.A.6.f.

(6) Forward copies of QI Focus Group meeting minutes to the HSWL SC.

g. <u>Alternate Health Services QI Coordinators</u>. The SHSO or Clinic Administrator may also be appointed as the Health Services QI Coordinator. However, this is not recommended in larger clinics since these two individuals are expected to provide necessary management expertise and clinical guidance in conducting the health care QI program and effecting any required program adjustments. The Health Services QI Coordinator's relationship to the SHSO is advisory.

h. <u>Accrediting Body</u>. An external accreditation organization will be used as the sole accrediting body for CG clinics. All facilities will be expected to be compliant with the current standards. The regular accreditation cycle is once every three years.

i. <u>Less than 3 year certification</u>. Facilities that do not receive a three-year accreditation will be resurveyed within 12 months of the initial survey.

j. <u>Health Services Quality Improvement Focus Group (QIFG)</u>.

(1) The Health Services QIFG shall consist of all clinic staff to a maximum of 15 members, depending on unit size, including both enlisted members and officers who broadly represent the health care services provided at that unit.

(2) Members will include at least a medical or dental officer, a clinic supervisor, and department representatives, e.g., pharmacy, physical therapy, x-ray, and laboratory. If desired, the QIFG at small units may operate as a "Committee of the Whole" of all staff members.

(3) The QIFG advises the SHSO about the quality of the facility's health care and performs these functions:

(a) Identifies and resolves problems which affect the quality of health care delivery at the facility. The SHSO may delegate investigating and resolving a particular QI problem to the staff member responsible for the clinical area where the problem has been identified (e.g., laboratory, patient reception).

(b) Ensures all required health services committee meetings are held according to the provisions of the CG Medical Manual, HSWL SC standard operating procedures and operational guides, and local instructions, including, among others, the Patient Advisory Committee.

(c) Uses existing CG standards, HSWL SC self assessment checklists, and QIS to review and evaluate the quality of services delivered both in-house and by contract providers.

(d) Performs systematic, documented reviews of health records for compliance and adherence to Medical Manual standards and HSWL SC standard operating procedures, health and safety support program guides, and self assessment checklists, and HIPAA privacy and security requirements.

(e) Solicits and monitors patient perceptions and satisfaction by surveys and questionnaires. Reports negative trends and potential solutions to the HSWL SC as a part of the QIFG meeting minutes.

(f) The QIFG shall meet at least quarterly and more often as local needs dictate. The clinic will maintain these meetings' original minutes for five years and will electronically forward copies of the minutes along with quality improvement studies through the chain of command to the HSWL SC for review on CG Central. The HSWL SC will provide electronic access to Commandant (CG-1122).

(g) Assists in obtaining and maintaining standards compliance necessary to achieve external accreditation.

10. <u>Confidentiality Statement</u>. All documents created under authority of this instruction are health services QI records and part of the CG's QIP. They are confidential and privileged under 14 USC 645 provisions. Releasing a health services QI document is expressly prohibited except in limited circumstances listed in 14 USC 645.

11. <u>QIP Review and Evaluation</u>. The Director of Health and Safety will annually review and evaluate the QIP. The review will reappraise the QI Plan and incorporate comments from the HSWL SC on implementation activities at field units during the preceding year.

    a. <u>QI Review and Evaluation Report</u>. By 30 November annually, HSWL SC shall provide to Commandant (CG-11) a written QI Review and Evaluation Report addressing these topics during the previous fiscal year:

    (1) Summary of clinic accreditations.

    (2) Summary of clinic Operational Health Readiness compliance.

    (3) Summary of significant clinical problems identified.

    (4) Summary of peer review activities.

    (5) Recommended QIP modifications.

    (6) HSWL SC QI Plan for upcoming calendar year.

COMDTINST M6000.1E

FIGURE 13-A-1

ORGANIZATIONAL CHART FOR QUALITY IMPROVEMENT PROGRAM

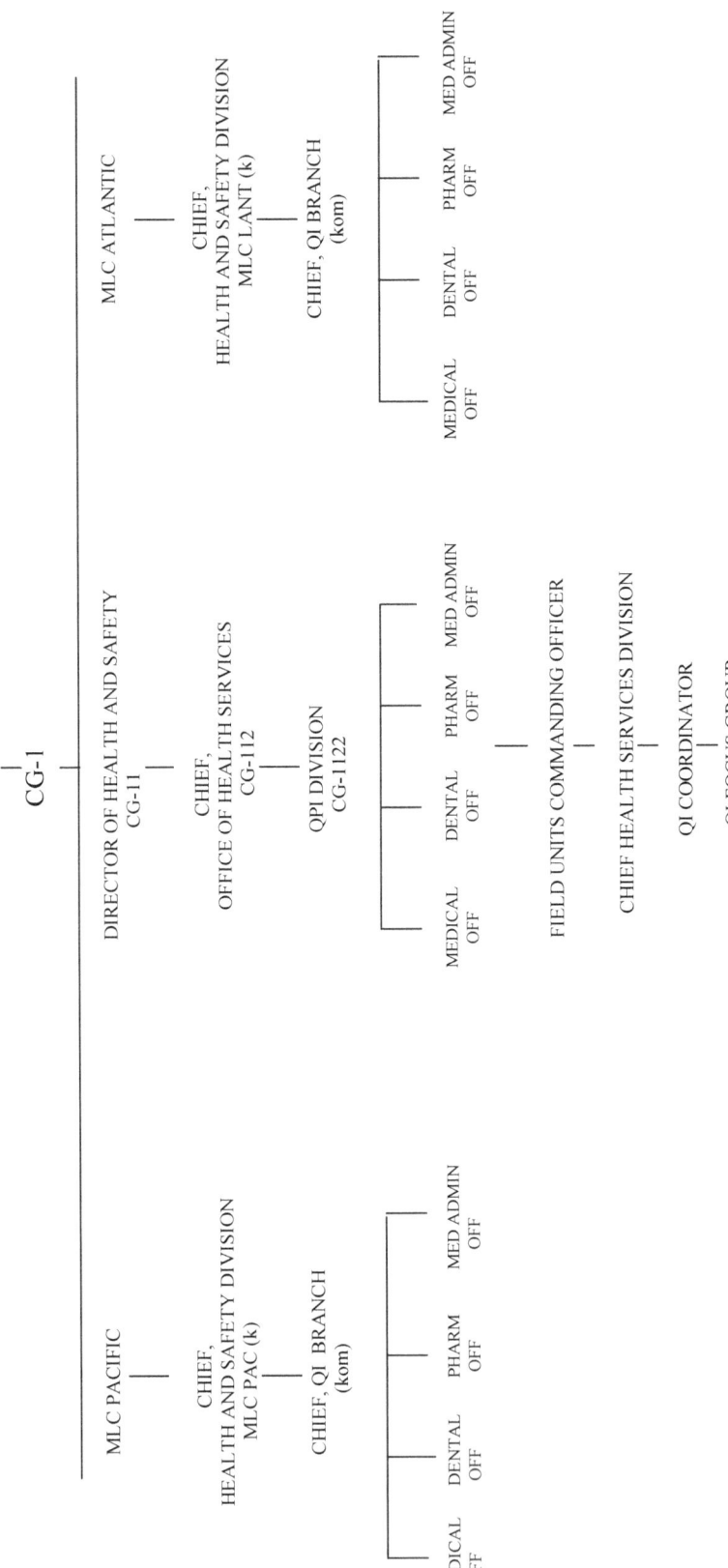

Chapter 13. A. Page 8

Section B. Credentials Maintenance and Review.

1. Background 1
2. Definitions 1
3. Pre-selection Credentials Review 2
4. Provider Credentials File (PCF) 3
5. Documentation 4
6. Verification 5
7. Contract Provider Credentials Review 6
8. Reverification 6
9. National Practitioner Data Bank (NPDB) 7
10. National Provider Identifiers Type 1 (NPI) 7

COMDTINST M6000.1E

This page intentionally left blank.

Section B. Credentials Maintenance and Review.

1. Background. Commandant (CG-11) is responsible for ensuring health care providers in CG facilities are competent and capable. Verifying licensed/certified healthcare providers qualifications are essential to assure providers are prepared for the scope of practice for which they are employed. Primary sources verification is needed. (Primary source verification is documented verification by an entity that issued a credential, such as a medical school or residency program, indicating that an individual's statement of possession of a credential is true). Primary sources must certify that certain valid credentials, including qualifying professional degree(s), license(s), graduate training, and references are met before a provider may practice independently in CG health care facilities. All candidates for CG employment, CG civil service employees, assigned PHS commissioned corps officers, CG Auxiliarist healthcare providers, and contract providers who provide direct patient care in CG health care facilities will comply with this chapter's provisions as applicable. The credentials shall be reviewed for each healthcare provider appointed to a position providing patient care. Privileges will be assigned based on this review.

2. Definitions.

    a. Contract Provider. An individual holding valid certification/licensure as a physician, dentist, dental hygienist, dental assistant, physician assistant, nurse practitioner, physical therapists or optometrists other than uniformed services personnel, who provide care in a CG health services facility under a contractual agreement with the CG. Contract providers will not be considered medical or dental officers as it relates to duties and responsibilities.

    b. Credentials. Documents constituting evidence of education, professional clinical training, licensure, experience, clinical competence and ethical behavior.

    c. Credentials Maintenance. Filing, updating, modifying or completing files, documents and databases about practitioner credentials.

    d. Credentials Review. The process of checking a practitioner's verified credentials and other supporting documents to evaluate potential assignments assign or rescind clinical privileges, or take administrative or personnel actions.

    e. Credentials Verification. The process of verifying a practitioner's license, education, training, and competence before initial assignment or employment.

    f. Dental Officer. A PHS commissioned officer assigned to the CG, who is a graduate of an accredited US school of dentistry and holds a valid, current state license to practice dentistry.

    g. License (Current, Unrestricted, Active). A certificate issued by one of the 50 states, District of Columbia or US Territories (Guam, Puerto Rico, Virgin Islands) that permits a person to practice medicine, dentistry, or other allied health profession.

h. **Medical Officer.** A commissioned CG or PHS officer assigned to the CG who has graduated from an accredited educational institution and is currently licensed as a physician, a nurse practitioner holding a valid certification by the American Academy of Nurse Practitioners or the American Nurses Credentialing Center or as a physician assistant holding valid certification from the National Association on Certification of Physician Assistants (exempt from licensing requirement).

i. **Pharmacy Officer.** A commissioned PHS officer assigned to the CG who graduated from an accredited US educational institution and is currently licensed as a pharmacist.

j. **Primary Source Verification.** Verification of a credential with an individual or institution possessing direct knowledge of the validity or authenticity of the particular credential.

k. **Privileges.** Type of practice activities authorized to be performed in the facility, within defined limits, based on the providers' education, professional license as appropriate, experience, current competence, ability, judgment, and health status.

l. **Provider.** A person granted individual clinical privileges to diagnose and treat diseases and conditions, including physicians, dentists, physician assistants, nurse practitioners, podiatrists, optometrists, and clinical psychologists.

3. **Pre-selection Credentials Review.**

    a. **PHS Liaison Officer.** The PHS liaison officer at Commandant (CG-112), in cooperation with the PHS Division of Commissioned Corps Assignments (DCCA) in the Office of Commissioned Corps Operations (OCCO) shall perform a pre-employment review and verify minimum standards before appointing Commissioned personnel. DCCA also screens individuals and certain credentials as part of the commissioning process. CG procedures are designed to complement DCCA's; the CG may alter its policies to reflect OCCO policy changes.

    b. **HSWL SC or local command.** The HSWL SC or local command by direction shall perform a pre-employment review of credentials of Civil Service employees and contractors providing care in CG health care facilities, and students.

    c. **Student credentials.** To review and verify student credentials, obtain a letter from the school stating the student is in good academic standing. Document malpractice coverage arrangements through an appropriate affiliation agreement. Student Externship Programs (SEP), COMDTINST 6400.1 (series).

4. **Provider Credentials File (PCF).** Through a Memorandum of Understanding between Commandant (CG-1122) and the Armed Forced Institute of Pathology

(AFIP) and the Department of Legal Medicine, the AFIP shall initiate and maintain PCFs for all Civil Service, Uniformed Service, Auxiliarist, and contracted licensed practitioners for the entire length of their employment or service. For contract providers (physician, dentist, PA/NP, physical therapists, optometrists or registered dental hygienist) the hiring entity (HSWL SC or HQ) will initiate the creation of the PCF upon offer or intent to hire the provider by sending the credentialing documents to AFIP as per 13. B. 5. a. Persons unable or unwilling to provide required information may be disqualified for employment or accession. These files must contain the following information:

a. Curriculum vitae. A curriculum vitae (CV) accounting for all time since the qualifying degree was received and prior to employment with the CG. For employed CG providers, their CV should remain current within three years.

b. Educational degrees. Copies of qualifying educational degrees (diploma, certificate) needed to perform clinical duties with the documents' primary source verification; see Section 13-B-6.

c. Postgraduate training certificates. Copies of required postgraduate training certificates for the area of work; for example, internship, residency, fellowship, nurse practitioner or physician assistant training, and primary source verification of these documents' authenticity.

d. State licenses. Copies of state licenses for all states in which the practitioner is licensed (active or inactive), current renewal certificates, and Educational Commission for Foreign Medical Graduates (ECFMG) certification if the practitioner graduated from a medical school not in the Continental US, Hawaii, Alaska, or from a medical school not accredited by the American Association Liaison Committee on Medical Education. The practitioner must attach a statement of explanation for lapsed state licenses or those subject to disciplinary action. The provider must maintain at least one unrestricted, current, and active license. The primary source must verify all licenses or renewal certificates.

e. Specialty board. Copies of specialty board and fellowship certificates with primary source verification of these documents.

f. Proof of competence and letters of reference. Proof of current (within one year) competence, i.e., two letters of reference for initial appointment/accession and a description of recent clinical privileges held (practitioner's supervisor(s) from last five years must note concurrence with applicant's position, scope of practice and approval of privilege performance).

   (1) The official, reviewing letters of reference, is authorized to contact the author of the letters to verify authorship and authenticity of letters. The official is also authorized to request a second letter of reference from an author when the first letter is deemed unclear. The official reviewing a letter of reference is authorized to contact the author via telephone in cases

in which the author declines to respond in writing. In such cases, the official will document in a telephone log the site, date, time, identity of call participants, and a detailed description of the conversation.

(2) Documents of reference submitted to DCCA for appointment in the USPHS may be used as letters of reference.

(3) In cases of a provider being acquired from other branches of the military, copies of officer fitness reports (OER) and/or performance assessment reviews (PARS) may be substituted for letters of reference.

g. Malpractice cases. A statement explaining any involvement in malpractice cases and claims, including a brief review of the facts about the practitioner's involvement.

h. Disciplinary action. A statement is needed explaining any disciplinary action from hospitals, licensing boards, or other agencies.

i. Basic Cardiac Life Support certification. A current Basic Cardiac Life Support (for Healthcare Providers), certification is required in accordance with Chapter 13 Section L of this Manual.

j. Advanced Cardiac Life Support. A current Advanced Cardiac Life Support certification is required for all active duty and reserve CG Medical Officers in accordance with Chapter 13 Section L of this Manual.

k. Drug Enforcement Agency (DEA). Copies of all current and prior Drug Enforcement Agency (DEA) registration, as appropriate.

l. National Practitioner Data Bank (NPDB). National Practitioner Data Bank (NPDB) query, current within two years.

m. Attestation Form.

n. Release of Information Letter.

o. National Provider Identifiers (NPI) Type 1. See Section F.

5. Documentation.

a. Credential Documents. Send the credential documents to AFIP and Commandant (CG-1122), via traceable means (e.g. DHS authorized Commercial Carriers FedEx or UPS); US Postal Service (USPS): 1) Express Mail or 2) Proof of Delivery using Extra Services which are either Certified, Delivery Confirmation, or Signature Confirmation. The technical review by the HSWL SC does not constitute official Coast Guard credentialing or privileging.

b. Confidentiality. AFIP will maintain files in a locked cabinet. PCFs and their contents are Class III (maximum security) records and protected from disclosure under the Privacy Act. Do not release documents in the PCF to any other individual or entity unless the provider has given express written permission.

c. Organization. Documents are placed in a six-section folder as follows:

(1) Section One. CG clinical privileging documents, Interagency Credentials Transfer Brief and Miscellaneous Supporting documents (i.e. support of supplemental privileges).

(2) Section Two. Letters/documents of reference, curriculum vitae (current within three years), National Provider Identification Number, and Release of Information/Attestation.

(3) Section Three. National Practitioner Data Bank queries, Health and Human Service Office of Inspector General List of Excluded Individuals/Entities, adverse actions, malpractice documents, proof of malpractice coverage, and statements about adverse information or malpractice claims.

(4) Section Four. Copies of license(s), diploma(s) or degree certificates, certificate (if applicable) from the Educational Commission for Foreign Medical Graduates (ECFMG), board certification, and Drug Enforcement Administration (DEA) number certificate.

(5) Section Five. Copies of post graduate training certificates, Accreditation Council for Graduate Medical Education letters, Basic Cardiac Life Support, (BCLS), Advanced Cardiac Life Support (ACLS), Pediatric Advanced Life Support (PALS), Basic Trauma Life Support (BTLS), Advanced Trauma Life Support (ATLS), and aviation/operational medicine courses.

(6) Section Six. Letter from the Joint Commission on Accreditation of Healthcare Organizations (JCAHO) Accredited Hospital regarding admitting privileges and privileges granted by other/previous institution(s).

6. Verification.

a. How to perform verification. To verify education, training, licensure or registration, certification, ECFMG and board certification, obtain either an original letter from the educational institution or certifying body attesting to successful completion of specialty training, print out of online internet verification, or verify by telephone call between the CG/AFIP representative and the educational institution or specialty board. Record telephone verification on the document itself and on official letterhead signed and dated by the person making the call. Place all verification documents with their source documents in PCF Section Six.

b. <u>AFIP verification</u>. AFIP will verify credentials of uniformed services providers before appointment/accession.

c. <u>MLC verification</u>. Before selection of Civil Service and contract providers, there will be a review of education, training, licensure, experience, certification or registration, and current competence completed by the HSWL SC as directed in section 3.b. All Civil Service and contract providers will require privileging to practice in CG facilities.

d. <u>Verify experience</u>. To verify experience and current competence requires at least two recommendation letters from appropriate sources as listed below. Commandant (CG-1122) or the HSWL SC shall receive direct letters from the person providing the reference. Verify descriptions of recent clinical privileges as above.

   (1) A letter either from the hospital chief of staff, clinic administrator, professional head, or department head if the individual has professional or clinical privileges or is associated with a hospital or clinic; or

   (2) A letter from the director or a faculty member of the individual's training program if he or she has been in a training program in the previous two years; or

   (3) A letter from a practitioner in the appointee's discipline who is in a position to evaluate the appointee's peer and a professional association or society association (mandatory if the appointee is self-employed).

7. <u>Contract Provider Credentials Review</u>.

   a. <u>Contracting agency</u>. The contracting agency has the responsibility for initial and ongoing primary source verification of credentials of all contract providers. Physician Assistants must be certified by the National Commission on Certification of Physician Assistants. Nurse Practitioners must be certified by the American Academy of Nurse Practitioners or the American Nurses Credentialing Center. Malpractice insurance must be provided and verified by the contracting agency.

   b. <u>Technical review</u>. At the contracting officer's request, HSWL SC will perform a technical review of the providers' credentials. This does not constitute a privileging authorization.

8. <u>Reverification</u>.

   a. <u>Renewable credentials</u>. These credentials are renewable and will be primary source verified on renewal: License, PA certification, Board certification, and contract providers' malpractice coverage. Reverify contract providers' updated credentials is at contract renewal.

b. Reverify these credentials by original letter or telephone contact. The person making the call will record telephone contact on the document or by a separate, signed memorandum.

9. National Practitioner Data Bank (NPDB).

    a. Commandant's role. Commandant (CG-11) possesses sole authority to report to the NPDB. Commandant (CG-1122) is designated as the appropriate entity for all NPDB queries. Coordinate all queries for patient care providers through this branch.

    b. NPDB requirements. A reply from the NPDB is not required before the practitioner begins providing services. However, any provider whose credential verification is not fully completed will be considered to have a conditional appointment until all credentials are verified as required.

10. National Provider Identifiers Type 1 (NPI).

    a. Requirement for NPI. All health care providers who furnish health care services or those who may initiate and/or receive referrals must obtain an NPI Type 1. NPI Type 1 is assigned at no fee by the Centers for Medicare and Medicaid Services (CMS) National Plan and Provider Enumeration System (NPPES). Providers shall apply for and will receive one and only one NPI Type 1. This NPI Type 1 will be a permanent identifier. CMS has an on-line NPI Type 1 application available at https://nppes.cms.hhs.gov.

    b. Filing the NPI. Once a provider obtains their NPI Type 1, they shall provide a copy to the CG credentialing office, Commandant (CG-1122). The information will be entered into the Centralized Credentials Quality Assurance System (CCQAS) database. A photocopy of the original hardcopy will be filed in the Practitioner Credentials File.

    c. Instructions. Instructions for obtaining and maintaining NPI Type 1 for health care providers are to be included in all privileging packages.

    d. HIPAA compliance. HIPAA compliance requires that NPPES be updated within 30 days of a change in the NPI Type 2 data.

    e. Privileging authority facility name. In order to ensure standardized addresses are being used in the mailing address and in the practice location fields on the NPI Type 1 application, providers (other than Reserve component providers) are to use the privileging authority facility name (USCG HQ, COMMANDANT (CG-1122)) as the address of record.

This page intentionally left blank.

Section C. Clinical Privileges.

1. Purpose 1
2. Background. 1
3. Definitions. 1
4. Applicability and Scope. 3
5. Clinical Privileges. 3

This page intentionally left blank.

Section C. Clinical Privileges.

1. Purpose. Granting individual clinical privileges to independent licensed providers who are providing services in health care organizations is an essential component of quality health care. Clinical privilege granting and rescinding activities define the provider's scope of care and services available to patients. The privileging process is directed solely and specifically at providing quality patient care; it is not a disciplinary or personnel management system. However, privileging actions may accompany administrative or judicial actions or engender them. Granting and rescinding clinical privileges is highly confidential, and must be conducted according to strict rules to prevent improper or prejudiced actions. This section establishes processes and procedures to grant and rescind clinical privileges. These provisions fall outside the scope of the Administrative Investigations Manual, COMDTINST M5830.1 (series).

2. Background. Commandant (CG-11) is responsible for planning, developing, and administering a comprehensive, high-quality health care program which must ensure the persons providing care have appropriate, verified licenses, education, and training. CG health care providers must adhere to commonly accepted standards for treatment and therapeutic modalities. In the CG, adherence to accepted standards is achieved by rigorous quality improvement (QI) and providers' peer reviews.

3. Definitions.

    a. Abeyance. The temporary removal of a health care provider from clinical duties while an inquiry into allegations of provider impairment or misconduct is conducted. Periods of abeyance provide privileging authorities the opportunity to review allegations while ensuring patient safety and protecting providers from unwarranted adverse privileging action. An abeyance terminates upon referral to a peer review hearing or at the end of 28 days, whichever occurs sooner. An abeyance is not an adverse action and is non-punitive.

    b. Adverse Privileging Action. Any action that denies, suspends, reduces, or revokes a provider's clinical privileges for greater than 30 days.

    c. Clinical Privileges. Type of practice activities authorized to be performed in the facility, within defined limits, based on the providers' education, professional license as appropriate, experience, current competence, ability, judgment, and health status.

    d. Convening Authority. Commandant (CG-11).

    e. Document Review. A review of medical record documentation and other pertinent data as defined by the Convening Authority.

f. Expiration of Credentials. It is ultimately the responsibility of the provider to ensure that all credentials required for clinical privileges are renewed prior to their expiration dates. If any credential required for clinical privileges is allowed to expire, the provider may have clinical privileges suspended or terminated. This will remove the provider from direct patient care and may render the provider ineligible to receive any special pay for clinical duties while the provider is in this status.

g. External Review. Administrative, non-judicial, or criminal investigations initiated by entities other than the CG health services program. This external review may be conducted by an outside agency.

h. Focused Review. An internal administrative mechanism to evaluate information about clinical care or practice. CG health services officers conduct focused reviews as part of the quality improvement program.

i. Full Staff Privileges. Unrestricted privileges as defined by "Clinical Privileges" above reevaluated and renewed every three years.

j. Impairment. Any personal characteristic or condition that may adversely affect the ability of a health care provider to render quality care. Impairments may be professional, behavioral, or medical. Professional impairments include deficits in medical knowledge, expertise, or judgment. Behavioral impairments include unprofessional, unethical, or criminal conduct. Medical impairments are conditions that impede or preclude a health care provider from safely executing his or her responsibilities as a health care provider.

k. National Practitioner Data Bank (NPDB). The agency established per regulations issued by the Department of Health and Human Services to collect and maintain data on substandard clinical performance and unprofessional conduct of health care providers. Requires reports of adverse privileging actions taken against providers and payments made to settle or satisfy claims or judgments resulting form medical malpractice of providers.

l. Peer Review. Review by an individual (or individuals) who possess relevant professional knowledge or experience, usually in the same discipline as the individual under review. This external review may be conducted by an outside agency.

m. Privileging. The process through which providers are given the authority and responsibility to make independent decisions to diagnose illnesses and/or initiate, alter, or terminate a regimen of medical or dental care.

n. Privileging Authority. Director, Health & Safety Commandant (CG-11) is the corporate privileging authority for all CG health care providers.

o. Professional Review Committee (PRC). A committee appointed by Commandant (CG-11). The committee shall be composed of the Deputy Director of Health and Safety, Commandant (CG-11d), the Chief of the Operational Medicine and Medical Readiness, Commandant (CG-1121), and the Chief of Quality Performance and Improvement Division, Commandant (CG-1122) or their designees. The committee shall have at least two Medical Officers (one of which shall be a physician and the other may be a PA or NP) and one Dental Officer. Other officers may participate as required (e.g. Auxiliarist Medical Officer).

p. Provider. For this chapter, an individual granted clinical privileges to independently diagnose and treat diseases and conditions. Physicians, dentists, physician assistants, and nurse practitioners and other professions so designated by the privileging authority are provider disciplines within the CG health services program.

q. Special Professional Review Committee. A Professional Review Committee designated by the Convening Authority to address allegation and/or complaints regarding a CG provider.

r. Summary of Suspension. The temporary removal of all or part of a provider's clinical privileges before the completion of due process procedures. A summary of suspension would be used during the period between an abeyance and the completion of due process procedures. Summary of suspension of privileges is not reportable to the NPDB unless the final action is reportable.

s. Suspension. The temporary removal of all or part of a provider's clinical privileges resulting from lack of current competence, negligence, or unprofessional conduct after due process procedures are completed. The suspension of privileges is reportable to the NPDB. Suspension of privileges would be used when in the privileging authority's judgment, additional training, education, or treatment may correct underlying deficiencies and allow reinstatement of full privileges. In such cases, the NPDB must be notified of the suspension, and then informed when privileges are reinstated, or if not reinstated, when privileges are reduced or revoked.

4. Applicability and Scope. All military, Civil Service, contract civilian, and auxiliarist CG health care providers shall have clinical privileges assigned. Health services personnel (other than providers) who function under a standard job or position description or standard protocol, policies, and procedures, or who must consult with another provider before or during medical or dental treatment will not receive clinical privileges.

5. Clinical Privileges.

a. General.

(1) Commandant (CG-11) will grant clinical privileges (to include initial appointment, reappointment and assignment or curtailment of clinical privileges) based on education, specific training, experience, license or certification status, current competence and needs of the service. He or she shall consider limitations (facility, support staff, equipment capability, etc.), which may prevent a provider from conducting certain activities. Commandant (CG-11) shall assign or require providers to perform professional duties only if their education, training, and experience qualify them to perform such duties. Commandant (CG-11) shall also consider the provider's health status and ability to treat coworkers and patients with dignity and respect when granting privileges.

(2) In order to request or renew privileges the provider shall use Request for Clinical Privileges, CG-5575. For core privileges, the provider shall sign, scan or route the request to the SME or SDE for signature. The SME or SDE shall sign, scan or route the request to the Professional Review Committee (PRC). The PRC will review the request and make recommendations to the Privileging Authority for a decision. If supplemental privileges are requested, supporting documentation verifying the training and experience for requested privileges should accompany the Request of Clinical Privileges, CG-5575. The requesting provider shall sign, scan or route the request to the SME or SDE for signature. The SME or SDE signs, scans or routes the request to HSWL SC Chief, Clinical Staff (HCCS) for signature with concurrence of the HSWL SC SME or SDE. HCCS reviews, signs, scans or routes the request to the PRC. The PRC will review the request and make recommendations to the Privileging Authority for a decision. A provider (AD, reserve, contract, auxiliary, and student) shall not be granted access authority in CHCS, PGUI, or ALHTA until their privileges have been approved by Commandant (CG-11).

(3) Absence of clinical privileges must not delay treatment in an emergency (a situation in which failure to provide treatment would result in undue suffering or endanger life or limb). In such cases the providers are expected to do everything in their power to save patients.

(4) On transfer, the provider shall submit a new Request of Clinical Privileges, CG-5575 as per 13.5.b.

(5) When providers in the CG are assigned TAD for greater than 90 days, the TAD orders issuing authority shall request that Commandant (CG-1122) transmit a copy of the provider's clinical privileges to the host SMO/SDO who will evaluate the privileges and advise the provider if any privileges will be restricted at that site.

(6) When providers from DoD are assigned TAD to CG clinics, their parent command shall transmit an Inter-agency Credentials Transfer Brief (ICTB) and a copy of their clinical privileges to the host command prior to their arrival. The SME/SDE will determine if any of the privileges should be restricted and shall contact Commandant (CG-1122) for clarification where needed.

b. <u>Procedures</u>.

(1) The CG PHS liaison in Commandant (CG-112) will inform new PHS providers assigned to the CG that they must request clinical privileges in writing before accession to active duty or formal employment, using the Request of Clinical Privileges, CG-5575. New PHS providers shall send written requests for clinical privileges to Commandant (CG-112) by mail at least 45 days before accession. The PHS provider must have a privileging authority approved the Request of Clinical Privileges, CG-5575 before finalizing assignment orders to the agency. For contract providers who require privileging the gaining SHSO/Supervisor shall verify that AFIP/Commandant (CG-1122) has received the required credentialing documents (per 13. B. 5.) and submit original, Request of Clinical Privileges, CG-5575 to Commandant (CG-1122) via traceable means (e.g. DHS authorized Commercial Carriers FedEx or UPS); US Postal Service (USPS): 1) Express Mail or 2) Proof of Delivery using Extra Services which are either Certified, Delivery Confirmation, or Signature Confirmation. Providers who have not received an approved Request of Clinical Privileges, CG-5575 from Commandant (CG-11) will not be authorized to perform any sort of health care tasks.

(2) Armed Forces Institute of Pathology, Department of Legal Medicine, (AFIP) is under contract to assist in the collection and review of appropriate credentialing information and presents this information at the PRC Meetings. AFIP shall maintain all original records of providers.

(3) AFIP shall maintain a paper Practitioner Credentials File in accordance with the CG Medical Manual that validates each MD/DO, DDS/DMD, PA, NP, Optometrist (OD), Physical Therapist (PT), and Dental Hygienist (RDH).

(4) AFIP shall complete the primary source verification and prepare each individual credentials portfolio within 30 days (45 days for foreign graduates) from the date all essential documents are received from the CG. These time frames may be extended when primary sources or references are slow or unresponsive. In such instances, partially-completed portfolios may be accepted by CG, with the understanding that the missing documents will be forwarded after receipt from the pertinent institution.

(5) AFIP shall monitor, maintain and keep the CG credentials files in Centralized Credentials Quality Assurance System (CCQAS) current, generate any letters and reports required, contact providers to request updated credentialing elements and otherwise update the files with new acquisitions and information on a regular basis.

(6) Primary source verification will be carried out in a timely and reasonable manner, and be fully documented. To the maximum extent possible, all appropriate documents will be verified at the primary source by telephone, fax, mail, electronically or otherwise.

(7) The CCQAS database will be used for all applicants. Data on new acquisitions will be entered into CCQAS as that information becomes available, including primary source verification information, and be maintained by the AFIP.

(8) Provisional clinical privileges are effective for one year, or until recommended for full privileges by PRC action. This status should be sought as an exception only. All efforts should made to request and obtain full privileges for clinical practice in a CG facility. When granting provisional privileges, the risks associated with the activities for which a new provider seeks privileges and the frequency with which he or she performs the procedures shall be considered. The SME, SDE, and SHSO shall evaluate the provider's provisional privileges after one year, or prior to that time if deemed appropriate. Providers may apply for full staff privileges after one year of successful performance or if recommended by the SME/SDE.

(9) Privilege request documents, PRC actions, and any other documents relating to the granting, maintaining, reviewing or rescinding clinical privileges will be maintained in the individual provider's credentials file.

(10) The PRC will evaluate full staff privileges every three years. Providers will submit written privilege requests to Commandant (CG-112) at least 90 days before privileges are due for renewal.

(11) Commandant (CG-1122) shall give notice to providers when privileges are due to expire, AFIP shall give notice when credentials are about to expire. Privileges and credentials expiration notification will be given 90 days prior so that the provider will have time to ensure currency.

(12) Although Commandant (CG-1122) will provide notice of renewal, it is ultimately the responsibility of the provider to ensure they maintain current credentials and privileges at all times. Current credentials and privileges are considered a condition of employment, therefore, expiration of credentials or privileges may result in an inability to provide patient care, which will affect the ability to renew special pay contracts.

(13) In the event that a new request for privileges has not arrived at Commandant (CG-1122) within 30 days of the current privileges expiration date, a letter/e-mail will be forwarded to the Commanding Officer and the provider, with a copy to the HSWL SC, notifying them that the provider's current privileges are due to expire in 30 days, and when expired the provider will no longer be allowed to provide patient care.

c. Routine Operations of the Professional Review Committee (PRC).

(1) The Quality Improvement (QI) Division, Commandant (CG-1122) is responsible for monitoring and administering the granting of clinical privileges for all providers in the Health and Safety Program that require clinical privileges to perform their duties.

(2) Commandant (CG-1122) will maintain a Practitioner Credentials File (PCF) for providers in the CG Health and Safety Program that will be used for granting clinical privileges.

(3) The local QI Coordinator at each field unit is responsible for maintaining a list of the expiration dates of all significant documents required to grant clinical privileges as stipulated in Section 13-B and will notify the provider when these documents are within 90 days of expiration.

(4) It is ultimately the responsibility of the provider to take appropriate actions to prevent these documents from expiring and to ensure that current documents are entered in the PCF.

(5) Commandant (CG-1122) and AFIP will also monitor the expiration dates on these documents and will notify provider of impending expiration dates.

(6) The PRC will make recommendations to Commandant (CG-11) on the granting of clinical privileges.

(7) The PRC will routinely review requests for clinical privileges for providers upon reporting to new CG duty stations and every 3 calendar years.

(8) The PRC can also be convened by Commandant (CG-11) to review PCFs for situations other than the routine review of clinical privileges. This is described further in Chapter 13. Section C.5.d.

(9) Commandant (CG-1122) will conduct a preliminary review of all requests for clinical privileges as well the entire PCF selected to be presented before the PRC.

(10) Commandant (CG-1122) will forward requests for clinical privileges as well as the PCFs, to the cognizant Program Manager who will evaluate the PCFs and decide if they should be presented before the PRC or if further information or action is required before submission to the PRC.

(11) After Commandant (CG-1122) and the cognizant Program Managers have decided which records will be presented to the PRC, Commandant (CG-1122) will prepare an agenda and will schedule a PRC meeting.

(12) The PRC will be comprised of Commandant (CG-11) staff to include:

    (a) Commandant (CG-11d) as Chair of the PRC.

    (b) At least 2 Medical Officers (at least 1 Physician and 1 PA or NP).

    (c) At least 1 Dentist.

    (d) Commandant (CG-1121)

    (e) Commandant (CG-1122)

    (f) One member acts as recorder.

    (g) Other members of Commandant (CG-11), including Auxiliarist assigned to Commandant (CG-1122) as necessary.

(13) The PRC will evaluate each PCF and recommend any of the following actions for each case:

    (a) Grant all requested privileges.

    (b) Revoke all current privileges or certain specific privileges.

    (c) Reduce all current privileges or certain specific privileges.

    (d) Suspend all current privileges or certain specific privileges.

    (e) Hold in abeyance all current privileges or certain specific privileges.

    (f) Monitored or supervised performance of clinical privileges.

    (g) Request any decision regarding privileges be deferred until additional supporting information is submitted to the PRC.

    (h) Maintain or modify current privileges while more information is forthcoming or an investigation is being conducted.

    (i) Request a document focused review or other type of internal investigation.

    (j) Request an external review or investigation.

    (k) Other actions as dictated by circumstances.

(14) The PRC will discuss each case but the decision to recommend approval or rejection of a privileging action will be made by Commandant (CG-11d).

(15) The PRC will forward its recommendations for privileging actions in the minutes of the meeting to Commandant (CG-11) via Commandant (CG-1122), Commandant (CG-112), and Commandant (CG-11d)

  (a) Commandant (CG-1122) will prepare the minutes for each meeting of the PRC.

  (b) The minutes will specify the recommended privileging action.

  (c) In the event of a recommendation by the PRC for any privileging action less than granting full privileges, the minutes shall specify the reasons or justification for that recommendation.

(16) After receiving the minutes, Commandant (CG-11) will make a decision on the recommendations of the PRC. In cases where the PRC has recommended the granting of full privileges, the Request for Clinical Privileges will be submitted to Commandant (CG-11) for final approval.

(17) In cases forwarded to Commandant (CG-0944) for a legal opinion, Commandant (CG-11) will have 3 working days after receiving the legal opinion from Commandant (CG-0944) to make a final decision on how to act. In all cases of granting less than full privileges, Commandant (CG-11) will attempt to contact the provider by telephone and inform him/her of the action;

  (a) Commandant (CG-11) will forward a letter to the provider by mail;

  (b) Commandant (CG-11) will inform the HSWL SC by letter; and

  (c) The HSWL SC will notify the provider's local command and the SHSO.

d. Adverse Privileging Actions.

  (1) All actions and processes on granting, reducing, suspending, and revoking clinical privileges are conducted in accordance with provisions of the CG health services Quality Improvement Program. The Privacy Act (5 USC§552a) and the medical quality assurance confidentiality statute (14 USC§645) protect all documentation related to these processes. These documents will be filed in the Practitioners' Credentials File, under the Privacy Act System of Record Notice (DHS/CG 052).

  (2) Actions to review, reduce, or withdraw clinical privileges will be taken promptly if reasonable cause exists to doubt a provider's competence to

practice or for any other cause affecting patient safety. Reasonable cause includes: a grossly negligent single incident; a pattern either of inappropriate prescribing or substandard of care; an incompetent or negligent act causing death or serious bodily injury; abuse of legal or illegal drugs or diagnosis of provider substance dependence; practitioner disability (physical and/or mental psychiatric conditions(s) impairing clinical duties); or a provider's significant unprofessional conduct.

(3) If a reasonable cause exists to doubt a provider's competence, or in the event of allegations of substandard or improper medical or dental treatment by a provider occurring in a CG health care facility, notification containing the allegations shall be forwarded by mail or facsimile to the Convening Authority. In cases where notification originates from military members or organizations, transmittal shall be via the chain of command to include the HSWL SC.

(4) Upon review of allegations, the Convening Authority shall, within 5 working days, designate appropriate follow-up action or disposition that may include the appointment of a Special Professional Review Committee (SPRC). The Convening Authority shall designate the composition of the SPRC when one is appointed.

(5) Once appointed, the SPRC shall convene and complete all review within a time not to exceed 15 working days. After reviewing the allegations, the SPRC shall make recommendations to the Convening Authority that may include: a focused review team, a documentation review, or other disposition as appropriate.

(6) Based on the nature of the allegation(s) and the recommendations of the SPRC, the Convening Authority may order a focused review team (on-site), a document review, or other disposition. In cases requiring further review, the Convening Authority will designate focused review team members or the document review officer through the HSWL SC within 10 working days from receipt of the SPRC's recommendation, and shall further define the particular review process based upon the nature of the allegations giving rise to the review.

(7) The focused review team or document reviewing officer shall initiate and complete the review action within 30 working days after the Convening Authority designates the review action.

(8) If the provider under review is a physician, the focused review team shall consist of at least three CG physicians. If the provider under review is a Flight Surgeon, Aviation Medical Officer (AMO), or Aeromedical Physician Assistant at least one of the reviewing physicians must be a Flight Surgeon. For a Dental Officer, the reviewing team shall consist of at least three CG Dental Officers. For a physician assistant or nurse

practitioner, the team shall consist of three Medical Officer reviewers, one of which must be a physician assistant or nurse practioner as applicable. The Convening Authority may assign additional team members (not to exceed 5 total team members) to assist in the review process.

(9) In cases requiring a document review officer, the HSWL SC, shall take measures to ensure the document review officer is impartial and will not represent any conflict of interest. The document review officer shall be of the same discipline as the provider under review, except when the provider being reviewed is a Physician Assistant or Nurse Practitioner; the document review officer may be a physician.

(10) The provider under review need not be present for records or other document review, but when possible should be available to answer questions for the focused review team or document review officer.

(11) The document review officer or focus review team shall brief the unit CO about significant findings at the end of the visit. Within 10 working days of concluding the review, the Convening Authority shall receive a written report for disposition containing findings, conclusions and specific recommendations, through the HSWL SC.

(12) Focused team or document review reports shall contain at least one of these recommendations:

   (a) No action.

   (b) Administrative action, such as verbal counseling.

   (c) Assignment to additional training.

   (d) Reassignment to another facility for observation, supervision, and/or additional training (may or may not involve reduction of privileges).

   (e) Privilege reappraisal.

   (f) Reduction of privileges (specify extent of reduction).

   (g) Privilege suspension (indefinite).

   (h) Permanent removal from clinical duties (privilege revocation).

   (i) Further review.

(13) If the document review officer or focused review team recommends immediate adverse privileging action, they shall contact the Convening Authority by the most expedient means possible.

(14) Upon review of the written report, the Convening Authority shall within three working days, determine further disposition that may include reconvening the SPRC for further review and recommendations. In the event that the written report recommends adverse privileging action, the Convening Authority shall reconvene the SPRC for further review and recommendations.

(15) If reconvened, the SPRC shall review all available records, may contact potential witnesses to assist in their deliberation, and shall provide recommendations to the Convening Authority within 30 working days.

(16) If the SPRC recommends adverse privileging action, the CG-112 Office Chief shall contact the provider under review the same duty day if possible, either by phone or in person. Written notification will be sent to the provider under review within five working days via traceable means (e.g. DHS authorized Commercial Carriers FedEx or UPS); US Postal Service (USPS): 1) Express Mail or 2) Proof of Delivery using Extra Services which are either Certified, Delivery Confirmation, or Signature Confirmation, which shall include notification that an adverse privileging action has been recommended against him or her and the reasons for the proposed action. The written notice shall further delineate that the provider has a right to request an appeal on the proposed action and the time limit (up to 30 working days) within which to request such an appeal in writing and specify the provider's rights in the appeal process.

(17) The provider's failure to request or appear at the appeal, absent good cause, constitutes a waiver of further appeal and appeal rights, and the proposed adverse privileging action shall be finalized by the Convening Authority.

(18) In the case where an adverse privileging action becomes final, all adverse privileging actions that restrict or suspend clinical privileges for longer than 30 days will be reported to the National Practitioner Data Bank (NPDB) according to the Memorandum of Understanding between the Department of Health and Human Services and Department of Homeland Security. Providers may dispute Data Bank information as provided in 45 CFR 60, "National Practitioner Data Bank for Adverse Information on Physicians and Other Health Care Practitioners."

e. <u>Appeal Process</u>.

(1) If a provider requests a hearing in writing within the time limit, CG-112 shall within 10 working days schedule the appeal hearing. Notification of the appeal hearing to the provider must state the hearing place, time, and date; which shall be convened not less than 30 days but not longer than 60

days after the date the written request for an appeal hearing was received by CG-112. The provider will also be given a written list of witnesses (if any) expected to testify at the hearing on behalf of the hearing committee.

(2) CG-112 will assign the hearing committee, consisting of three CG/PHS officers equivalent or higher in rank to the provider under review, not previously involved in the internal review process. The disciplines represented shall be the same as required for the focused review team. Each hearing committee member will have one vote.

(3) The provider under review has these rights:

(a) To consult with CG legal counsel or civilian legal counsel at his/her own expense. The provider shall request approval in writing to Commandant (CG-11) the services of CG legal counsel. While such counsel may attend the hearing and advise the provider during the proceedings, the counsel will not be allowed to participate directly in the hearing, (e.g., may not ask questions, respond to questions on behalf of the provider, or seek to enter material into the record).

(b) To obtain a transcript of the proceedings by paying any reasonable preparation charges.

(c) To call, examine, and cross-examine witnesses. The provider is responsible for arranging the presence of his or her witnesses and failure of the witnesses to appear will not constitute a procedural error or basis for delaying the proceedings.

(d) To present relevant verbal or written evidence regardless of its admissibility in a court of law.

(e) To submit a written statement at the close of the hearing.

(4) The hearing committee shall review all relevant records, hear all witnesses, and have the right to interview all witnesses. The hearing committee **should** request assistance from Commandant (CG-0944) throughout the hearing process.

(5) The hearing committee will base its recommendation on whether or not to sustain, reduce, suspend, or revoke a provider's clinical privileges on a preponderance of the evidence as judged by a majority vote. A report of the hearing committee's final recommendations will be reported to the Convening Authority within two working days after the hearing ends.

(6) The Convening Authority will review the hearing committee's recommendations within three working days of receiving their report; make a decision and notify the provider under review the day of the decision either by telephone or in person; and send written notice to the provider by DHS authorized commercial traceable means, within five working days after the hearing ends. The Convening Authority's decision shall be final.

Section D. Operational Health Readiness Program.

1. Background. 1
2. Purpose. 1
3. Overview. 1
4. OHRP Compliance Process. 2

This page intentionally left blank

D. Operational Health Readiness Program (OHRP).

1. Background. The CG established an internal healthcare quality assurance (QA) program in the early 1990s to monitor the quality of healthcare delivered at its clinics. The MLCs administered the program by conducting QA surveys at each clinic every three years by members of the MLC staff utilizing Quality Assurance Checklists. Clinics passing the MLC survey were awarded a three year certificate that verified the clinic met CG QA standards. QA survey items were retroactively reviewed. The internal QA certification program was augmented by an external accreditation program in 2004. However, the need for a program that ensures clinic compliance with CG specific healthcare issues and health readiness still exists. CG specific QA and operational health readiness issues are monitored by the HSWL SC under the Operational Health Readiness Program.

2. Purpose. The intent of the OHRP is to assist and ensure all clinics monitor and comply with CG specific healthcare-related requirements not reviewed by the external accreditation organization surveyors.

3. Overview.

    a. Definitions.

        (1) Operational Readiness. Standards established by the CG that determine whether individual members and units are prepared to meet their assigned missions.

        (2) Quality Assurance, Quality Improvement – See Chapter 13. Section A.5.a-d

    b. Program Elements. The OHRP is designed for clinics to monitor those healthcare-related QA issues not reviewed by external surveyors and to ensure units within their area-of-responsibility (AOR) are operationally ready in accordance with CG standards. There are three issues that require oversight. One, QA items historically reviewed by HSWL SC during their triennial surveys, but not reviewed by the external accreditation organization. Two, policies and procedures that apply to operational health readiness. Three, areas of interest that are not directly related to operational health readiness, but involve a supportive role. These three issues will be overseen by the HSWL SC on a continuous basis.

    c. Collaborative Program. The primary mission of the CG clinics is to maintain the operational health readiness of active duty and reserve personnel by assuring their availability to physically and mentally meet worldwide deployment standards in accordance with the Medical Manual COMDTINST M6000.1 (series). Maintaining a high level of health readiness involves collaboration between providers, commands, clinics and the HSWL SC.

    d. Monitoring the OHRP. Clinics must review the operational health readiness of active duty/reserve members within their AORs on a regular basis. It is the Command's responsibility to ensure medical and dental readiness of the active duty/reserve members in their AOR. It is the responsibility of the SHSO to develop and maintain a plan that ensures optimal health readiness for all active duty/reserve members within the designated AOR in accordance with guidance provided in this instruction. The HSWL SC will review CG-specific QA and operational health readiness issues on a continual basis and provide needed assistance to clinics to ensure a high level of health readiness. Operational health readiness compliance will be accomplished through reviews of each individual clinic's information posted in OHRP databases, QA public folders on CG Central and the MLC assist visits. A post-visit OHRP evaluation report will be provided to the clinics through the CO.

   e. Assistance Program. The OHRP is designed to provide an environment in which QI and operational health readiness of clinics are monitored on a continuous, versus retroactive, basis. The OHRP is an assistance program designed to ensure a high level of care is provided at CG clinics and that a high level of operational health readiness is maintained. The program assists clinics in meeting both AAAHC and CG readiness and QI standards.

   f. Accreditation. The OHRP assessment does not confer accreditation or certification status. Operational readiness is a command-directed process. The MLCs provide assistance in meeting OHRP goals, QA/I standards and preparation for the AAAHC survey. The AAAHC is the sole healthcare quality assurance/improvement accrediting body recognized by the CG.

4. OHRP Compliance Process.

   a. Responsibility.

      (1) Unit. The unit CO is responsible for ensuring the command's health care facility complies with standards set forth in the Coast Guard Medical Manual and the HSWL SC OHRP.

      (2) Clinics. The SHSO is responsible for routinely monitoring the progress of medical, dental, pharmacy readiness within their AOR and the implementation of the OHRP.

      (3) HSWL SC. Responsible for developing and coordinating process checklists, self-assessment tools, assist visits to the clinics, and process reviews

      (4) Headquarters. Chief, Directorate of Health and Safety coordinates and directs the program, adjudicates appeals, and promulgates appropriate standards governing CG providers' delivery of health care and policies on managing and operating CG health care facilities.

   b. Process Checklist. The process checklists show QA and/or operational readiness tasks that clinics must address on a regular basis. The checklists are not all-inclusive because they do not list tasks that do not directly apply to QA or operational readiness (e.g. "take out trash"). Clinics must determine what tasks they do on a regular basis and have mechanisms in place to ensure these tasks get completed. The HSWL SC will assist in this effort. To view the most current OHRP compliance checklist go to the HSWL SC microsite on CG Central.

   c. Self-Assessment. Health readiness and policy adherence is a continuous process and must be routinely reviewed by the clinic and HSWL SC. Self-assessment tools serve as a guide to assess how well the intent of the OHRP is being met through the daily operations of the clinic. Clinics that are diligent in addressing the issues listed on the self-assessment sheets should meet AAAHC QI and CG OHRP standards. The self assessments mirror the previous MLC QA checklist items formerly used for certification surveys.

d. Quality Improvement Studies (QISs). Clinics must demonstrate that they have a system in place to monitor healthcare delivery. Previously this was done through retroactive data reviews of given topics (i.e. monitoring and evaluation reports). With external accreditation, clinics must review areas of concern or interest and implement quality improvement studies. QISs may be adapted for operational readiness or other issues not reviewed by the external accreditation organization.

e. CG Central. CG Central serves as the primary repository for OHRP QA/QI documents such as QIFG meeting minutes, SOPs, and Letters of Designation, and other items listed on Quality Improvement Calendar, CG-6000-5.

f. Public QA/I Folders. Public folders may be used for depositing QA/QI documents (e.g. CBRN antidote inventories) but do not take the place of using CG Central.

This page intentionally left blank.

Section E. Quality Improvement Implementation Guide (QIIG).

   1. Background. 1
   2. Responsibilities. 1

This page intentionally left blank.

E. Quality Improvement Implementation Guide (QIIG).

1. Background. The QIIG is a series of exercises designed to assist commands in meeting Health Services QI Program requirements and to augment policy that is outlined in the Medical Manual. Serving as a guideline, the QIIG minimizes the QI program administrative requirements by providing direction and, in many cases, templates for addressing critical quality issues. The exercises often eliminate the need for each clinic to develop its own policies and procedures by providing generic frameworks clinics can adapt to local conditions. In some cases, clinics may be required to submit evidence of completing an exercise to the HSWL SC for data evaluation purposes.

2. Responsibilities.

    a. Commandant (CG-112). Commandant (CG-112) develops exercises as needed on critical quality issues for inclusion in the QIIG and posts them on **http://www.uscg.mil/hq/cg1/cg112/cg1122/QIIG.asp**.

    b. HSWL SC. HSWL SC ensures exercises are available to Commands for clinic personnel to complete and also reviews clinic's use of the QIIGs as part of the Operational Health Readiness Program.

    c. Unit QI Coordinator. Unit QI Coordinators ensure staff promptly complete all QIIG exercises and maintain a complete, updated QIIG folder.

This page intentionally left blank.

Section F. National Provider Identifiers.

   1. National Provider Identifiers (NPI) Type 1 (NPI). 1
   2. Clinic National Provider Identifiers (NPI) Type 2. 1

This page intentionally left blank.

F. National Provider Identifiers.

1. National Provider Identifiers (NPI) Type 1 (NPI).

    a. Who must have a Type 1 NPI. All health care providers who provide health care services or those who may initiate and/or receive referrals must obtain an NPI Type 1. A NPI Type 1 is assigned at no fee by the Centers for Medicare and Medicaid Services (CMS) National Plan and Provider Enumeration System (NPPES). Providers shall apply for and will receive one and only one NPI Type 1. This NPI Type 1 will be a permanent identifier unique to that provider. CMS has an online NPI Type 1 application available at https://nppes.cms.hhs.gov.

    b. Copies of the NPI. Once a provider obtains their NPI Type 1 they shall provide a copy to Commandant (CG-1122). The information will be entered into the Centralized Credentials Quality Assurance System (CCQAS) database. A photocopy of the original hardcopy will be filed in the Practitioner Credentials File.

    c. Obtaining and maintaining a NPI. Instructions for obtaining and maintaining NPI Type 1 for health care providers are to be included in all privileging packages.

    d. Updates. HIPAA compliance requires that NPPES be updated within 30 days of a change in the NPI Type 1 data. (Example: provider changes their name or provider changes their duty station).

    e. Privileging authority address. In order to ensure standardized addresses are being used in the mailing address and in the practice location fields on the NPI Type 1 application, providers (other than Reserve component providers) are to use the privileging authority facility name (USCG HQ, COMDT (CG-1122)) as the address of record.

2. Clinic National Provider Identifiers (NPI) Type 2.

    a. Who must have a NPI Type 2. Per the HIPAA NPI Final Rule, 45 CFR, Part 162, all health care facilities that provide health care services must have an NPI Type 2. The NPI Type 2s are assigned at no fee by the Centers for Medicare and Medicaid Services (CMS), National Plan and Provider Enumeration System (NPPES). CMS has an online NPI Type 2 application available at https://nppes.cms.hhs.gov.

    b. SHSO. Each SHSO is responsible for submitting the initial NPI application and updates. Once a clinic obtains their NPI Type 2 they shall provide a copy to Commandant (CG-1122). The clinic shall maintain the NPI Type 2 in a permanent record.

    c. Updates. HIPAA compliance requires that NPPES be updated within 30 days of a change in the NPI Type 2 data. (Example: Address change).

This page intentionally left blank.

COMDTINST M6000.1E

Section G. Health Insurance Portability and Accountability Act (HIPAA).

1. Background 1
2. HIPAA Privacy/Security Officials (P/SO) 1
3. HIPAA Training Requirements 4
4. Handling HIPAA Complaints and Mitigation 7
5. Unintentional Disclosures of Protected Health Information 9
6. Protected Health Information and the Coast Guard Messaging System 10
7. Other CG Members Who Utilize Protected Health Information 10
8. Electronic Transmission of Protected Health Information 11

This page intentionally left blank.

COMDTINST M6000.1E

G. Health Insurance Portability and Accountability Act (HIPAA).

1. Background.

   a. Health Insurance Portability and Accountability Act, (HIPAA). On 21 August 1996, the Health Insurance Portability and Accountability Act, (HIPAA), was signed into law as Public Law 104-191. The Act included provisions for health insurance portability and renewability, preventing fraud and abuse, medical liability reform, tax-related health provisions, group health plan requirements, revenue offset provisions and administrative simplification requirements. Title II, Subtitle F on Administrative Simplification required the Secretary of Health & Human Service to publish standards for electronic exchange, privacy and security of health information.

   b. Federal Regulations. The promulgated regulations, known as the Privacy Rule are found at 45 Code of Federal Regulations (CFR) Part 160 and Part 164, Subparts A and E. The Security Standard is found at 45 CFR Part 164, Subpart C. These regulations became effective as of April 21, 2003, and must be complied with as of April 21, 2006. These regulations are available at the following web sites:

      (1) http://www.hhs.gov/ocr/privacy/hipaa/understanding/summary/ or

      (2) Parallel Department of Defense implementing regulations are found at http://www.dtic.mil/whs/directives/corres/html/602518r.htm

2. HIPAA Privacy/Security Officials (P/SO). 45 CFR Part 164.530 (a) requires (1) the designation of a privacy official responsible for the development and implementation of policies and procedures and (2) the designation of a contact person who is responsible for receiving complaints and providing further information about matters covered under the Notice of Privacy Practices. 45 CFR Part 164.308 (a) (2) requires that the CG "identify the security official who is responsible for the development and implementation of the policies and procedures required by this subpart for the entity."

   a. The CG Privacy and Security Official.

      (1) The Chief, Office of Health Services Commandant (CG-112) shall designate an officer as the CG Privacy and Security Official, residing within Commandant (CG-1122). This official shall serve as the Privacy and Security Official (P/S O) for the CG Health Care System and as the CG Service Representative to the TRICARE Management Activity (TMA) Privacy Office.

      (2) Responsibilities of the CG Privacy and Security Official are:

         (a) Provide coordination between the CG and Tricare Management Activity (TMA) Privacy Office on all HIPAA related issues.

         (b) Maintain current knowledge of applicable Federal and State privacy laws, accreditation standards and CG regulations. Monitor advancements in emerging privacy and health information security technologies to ensure that the Coast Guard is positioned to adapt and comply with these advancements.

- (c) Establish, modify and disseminate CG HIPAA policy.
- (d) Serve as the CG HIPAA liaison to receive complaints and provide further information about matters covered by the notice required by the HIPAA Privacy Rule, 45 CFR Parts 160 and 164, from Health and Human Services (HHS), Tricare Management Activity (TMA), and Congress.
- (e) Serve as the local P/SO for the Health, Safety, & Work-Life Directorate and Commandant (CG-11).

b. <u>HSWL SC Privacy and Security Official</u>.

(1) The Commanding Officer, HSWL SC, shall designate a junior officer as Privacy and Security Official for the CG Health Care System who will provide reports to the CG-1122 Privacy and Security Official.

(2) Responsibilities of the HSWL SC Privacy and Security Official are:

- (a) Serve as the CG HIPAA liaison to receive complaints and provide further information about matters covered by the notice required by the HIPAA Privacy Rule, 45 CFR Parts 160 and 164, from all Coast Guard commands and all Regional Practice Privacy and Security Officials.
- (b) Maintain a log of all Regional Practice Privacy and Security Officials and a file of all letters of designation.
- (c) Develop Standard Operating Procedures (SOPs) for Regional Practice implementation of the HIPAA Privacy and Security Regulation requirements.
- (d) Establish and recognize best practices relative to the management of the privacy and security of health information.
- (e) Serve as a liaison to other P/SOs.
- (f) Review all system-related information security plans throughout the local health care network to ensure alignment between security and privacy practices, and act as liaison to the information systems department.
- (g) Serve as the point of contact for HIPAA Privacy and Security compliance, monitoring and assuring staff compliance with HIPAA training requirements. The officer will administrate the databases that track data disclosures and complaints; conduct Privacy and Security risk assessments; participate in the HIPAA compliance quality assurance and improvement process; and report findings to the CG P/SO.

c. <u>Regional Practice Privacy and Security Officials</u>.

   (1) The Regional Practice Privacy and Security Official serve as the point of contact for CG treatment facilities within the AOR/Regional Practice. The P/SO oversees activities related to the implementation and maintenance of Regional Practice HIPAA SOPs covering the access to and privacy of patient health information.

   (2) The Regional Manager is responsible for designating in writing the HIPAA Privacy and Security Official for their respective Regional Practice. The designee must be of the rank of E-7 or above. A copy of this letter of designation shall be forwarded to the HSWL SC Privacy and Security Official. Whenever there is a change in the Regional Practices's P/SO the Regional Manager must designate another member as P/SO, notify HSWL SC of the change by email, and fax or email a copy of the letter of within 10 working days of the effective date of such letter.

   (3) Responsibilities of the Regional Practice Privacy and Security Official are:

   (a) Oversee, direct, monitor and ensure delivery of initial HIPAA privacy and security training and orientation to all clinical staff. Ensure annual refresher training is conducted in order to maintain workforce awareness and to introduce any changes to HIPAA privacy or security policies to the health care workforce. The P/SO may share or delegate responsibilities for monitoring compliance with HIPAA training requirements to another appropriately trained health care workforce individual as a HIPAA Training Administrator at the unit.

   (b) Perform initial and periodic information privacy and security risk assessments and conduct related ongoing compliance monitoring activities in coordination with applicable CG directives. Report findings as required.

   (c) Ensure a mechanism is in place within all respective treatment facilities for receiving, documenting, tracking, investigating all complaints concerning the organization's privacy and security policies and procedures in coordination and collaboration with other similar functions, and, when necessary, legal counsel.

   (d) Document disclosures of Protected Health Information (PHI) using the Protected Health Information Management Tool (PHIMT) to allow patients and other qualified individuals to review or receive reports on such activity as required by law.

   (e) Understand the content of health information in its clinical, research and business context.

   (f) Understand the decision-making processes that rely on health information. Identify and monitor the flow of information within the clinic and throughout the local health care network.

(g) Serve as privacy/security liaison for users of clinical and administrative systems.

(h) Collaborate with other health care professionals to ensure appropriate security measures are in place to safeguard protected health information and to facilitate exchange of information between entities.

(i) Initiate, facilitate and promote activities to foster information privacy awareness within the organization and related entities.

(j) Serve as the advocate for the patient relative to the confidentiality and privacy of health information.

3. <u>HIPAA Training Requirements</u>.

   a. <u>45 Code of Federal Regulations (CFR)</u>. 45 CFR 164.530 (b) specifies the training requirement standards under HIPAA. All CG health care workforce members are required to complete designated training within 30 working days of reporting on duty to the CG or being assigned to a specific CG unit. Meeting with the Regional Practice Privacy and Security Official should be included as a required element of all in-processing for health care workforce members.

      (1) The Regional Practice P/SO will provide the individual with the domain identification number for their respective unit to complete web-based training requirements. When a health care workforce member leaves the treatment facility, the local P/SO should direct the member to change the domain identifier to that of the receiving treatment facility where the member will be assigned.

      (2) Required training includes at least (1) those courses corresponding to the appropriate HIPAA Job Position provided through the TRICARE Management Activity (TMA) Privacy Office on the Military Health System's Training Portal; (2) training on the Regional Practice policies and procedures; (3) any other HIPAA privacy and security training as determined by the Regional Practice Privacy and Security Official.

      (3) Training shall be completed by utilizing the web-based training courses available through the Military Health System's Training Portal, MHS Learn, at https://mhslearn.satx.disa.mil/. Each individual should choose the "HIPAA Job Position" which is most closely aligned with their functional responsibilities.

         (a) These requirements apply to all active duty and reserve members, contract staff and Auxiliarists within the CG health care workforce.

         (b) Completion of the HIPAA core and refresher training courses is required prior to obtaining access and for continued access to the electronic health record system such as CHCS and PGUI. Individuals who are greater than ninety (90) days overdue for their annual refresher training will have their access deactivated.

         (c) CG health care workforce members are required to complete annual HIPAA refresher training during their birth month.

(d) Health Service technicians shall choose the "Nursing" job position for their training requirements.

(e) P/SOs shall choose the "Senior Management" job position for their training requirement.

(f) Clinic Administrators who are not P/SOs shall choose the "Medical Records" job position for their training requirement.

(g) The following table provides narrative descriptions of each of the HIPAA Job Positions found at the MHS Learn website.

HIPAA Job Positions and Descriptions

HIPAA Job Position	Description
Ancillary Clinical	Ancillary clinical staff including technicians: *Behavioral Health personnel, Work-Life staff, Optometrist, Pharmacist, Physical Therapist, Podiatrist, Social Worker, Medical Laboratory Technician, Medical Technologist, X-ray Technician, Clinical support volunteers. Audiologist Chiropractor, Clinical Psychologist, Dietician, Occupational Therapist Optician Speech Pathologist Dental Laboratory Technician, Dermatology Technician, Histopathology Technician, Respiratory Therapy Technician*
Patient Services	Patient Assistance staff or Administrative Support Staff: *Administrative Support Staff, Administrative Assistants, Executive Assistants, Receptionists, and File Clerks.*
Operations and Finance	Resource Management, Personnel staff, Medical Operations *(Readiness, Education, Training, Security)*, Business & Finance personnel
Support Services	All non-clinical support personnel: *(Biomedical Repair, Chaplain/Religious Services, Environmental Health Services, Facilities Management- Janitorial, Housekeeping, Maintenance, Food Service, Industrial Hygiene/Safety, Logistics, Occupational Health, Transportation, Supply)*
Information Systems	Information Management/Information Technology staff, Telecommunication; Mailroom, Biomedical Illustrator; Photographer
Medical Records	Clinic Administrators, Health Benefits Advisors, Medical Records staff, Patient Admin staff, Coders, Transcriptionists, Clinical/Ward Admin staff, Administrative volunteers
Nursing	Staff Nurse- RN/LPN/LVN, Nurse Mid-wife, Nurse Anesthetist, Medical Assistants, Dental Hygienist, Dental Assistants, Health Service Technicians, Corpsmen, Medics, Emergency Medical Technicians
Providers	Physicians- all specialties, Physician Assistants, Dentists- all specialties, Nurse Practitioners, Research Clinicians, Dental Science and Research
Senior Management	Commanders, Executive staff/leadership, general administration staff, hospital legal staff, Public Affairs /Marketing staff, Medical Administration Officers

Table 13-G-1

COMDTINST M6000.1E

4. Handling HIPAA Complaints and Mitigation.

   a. Requirements. The CG Health Care Program must be prepared to address beneficiary inquiries, concerns and complaints related to the protection of the individual's health information. The Privacy Rule of the Health Insurance Portability and Accountability Act (HIPAA) of 1996 and the Notice of Privacy Practices describe how the MHS/CG Health Care Program may use and disclose an individual's protected health information (PHI) and outlines patient rights regarding the use and disclosure of PHI.

   b. Inquiries or complaints. Beneficiaries may file complaints regarding perceived misuse or disclosure of their PHI. This information includes demographics such as age, address, or e-mail address and others, and relates to past, present or future health information and related health care services. Inquiries or complaints may be received at any level of the organization, or TRICARE Management Activity (TMA) by mail. Individuals also have the right to make inquiries or address complaints directly to the Department of Health and Human Services (HHS). The HHS Office for Civil Rights (OCR) Web site gives instructions to individuals who wish to make a HIPAA complaint about a covered entity when they perceive that their protected health information has been used or disclosed in a manner not compliant with the covered entity's privacy policies. The CG Health Care Program, the covered entity, should try to resolve patient and individual complaints before they become complaints to OCR. Privacy incidents do happen, and may be inadvertent disclosures (technical/practical errors that are not generally deliberate, planned, or malicious disclosures). It is realistic to expect that complaints will occur.

   c. HIPAA Complaints Received at the Local Treatment Facility.

      (1) A Privacy/Security Official (P/SO) will generally be the initial contact for response to privacy incident. If an individual arrives in person to complain, talk with him or her about his or her complaint. The P/SO will inform the individual about the complaint form on the TRICARE HIPAA site. There are advantages of asking the individual to fill out the form, including getting the complaint in his or her own words, obtaining the individual's signature, and making sure all the information is completed.

      (2) Beneficiary complaints should be directed in writing to the respective Regional Practice P/SO. The beneficiary also has the right to submit complaints to the TMA Privacy Officer or HHS if he/she feels the issue has not been appropriately addressed at the local level. The address and complaint form for submission to TMA can be found on the website http://tricare.osd.mil/tmaprivacy/hipaa/hipaacompliance/beneficiaries/index.htm. The address and form for HHS is on their website http://www.hhs.gov/ocr/privacy/hipaa/complaints/index.html. The complaint must include:

         (a) Beneficiary's name, address, phone number, social security number and clinic accessed for care

Chapter 13. G. Page 7

(b) Date complaint taken/submitted

(c) Description of complaint and approximate date incident occurred

(d) Facility and location where incident occurred

(3) The Regional Practice P/SO is responsible for ensuring the investigation into the complaint is conducted and if necessary any further actions taken. The P/SO determines whether a complaint is a HIPAA complaint, a grievance under another privacy law, or not a HIPAA complaint. In investigating an incident, the CG Administrative Investigation process shall be used. As necessary, witnesses, managers and staff can be interviewed, the scene of the incident can be visited, action can be taken to limit scope of incident, and copies of relevant files should be retrieved. Disclosures may be identified as incidental to routine business, accidental or due to malicious intent.

(4) The Regional Practice P/SO shall notify the HSWL SC and CG P/SOs of all complaints received at the treatment facility so that CG P/SO can provide assistance, guidance and review of the response and facilitate any coordination necessary with the TMA Privacy Office or legal counsel.

(5) A summary and corrective action plan can include: a summary of the incident, the cause of the incident, any procedural changes required, any training changes required, the staff involved and sanctions applied, and any specific corrective actions to implement.

(6) Once this process is complete, the Regional Practice P/SO will provide a written response to the beneficiary and a copy will be sent to the HSWL SC and CG P/SOs. In the case of complaints made by beneficiaries directly to the HHS and forwarded to TMA for resolution, responses are required to be provided to the TMA Privacy Office for review and endorsement to HHS. Direct communication to the complaining beneficiary will be at the discretion of HHS.

(7) The complaining party must receive a written response in a timely manner. The designated review authority (P/SO) shall reply within 30 days of the date of receipt of the complaint. If additional review is necessary, the reviewer can request an extension for an additional 30 days. When this occurs, the individual must be notified in writing that the issue is under investigation and the extension is being put into effect.

(8) Written documentation of the complaint and its disposition must be maintained by the activity receiving the inquiry or complaint. Each Regional Practice is required to ensure appropriate documentation. The complaint and any accounting of a disclosure must be recorded in the Protected Health Information Management Tool (PHIMT). If the issue required action at the TMA level, the TMA Privacy Officer will keep the file as well as all correspondence related to a complaint processed by TMA. Documentation must be maintained for a minimum of six years from the submission of the complaint.

d. Complaints Received at Commands Other Than Treatment Facilities.

   (1) Whenever possible, complaints received at Commands other than CG treatment facilities, should be redirected to the appropriate Regional Practice P/SO for investigation and response.

   (2) Commands shall notify immediately the HSWL SC P/SO and CG P/SO Commandant (CG-1122) by email of all other complaints. The HSWL SC P/SO will assist and advise the Command's investigating officer; coordinate the response with legal counsel, where necessary; and review the written response of the investigating officer. The CG P/SO will coordinate the response with the TMA Privacy Office, where necessary. The Command's investigating officer should comply with the guidance provided in Chapter 13.Section G.4.c.(2).

5. Unintentional Disclosures of Protected Health Information.

   a. Breach of security. If anyone within the CG discovers evidence or circumstances which would suggest that a breach of security of a system containing protected health information (PHI) or of an unintentional disclosure of PHI may have occurred, this information shall be immediately brought to the attention of the Commanding Officer and Regional Practice Privacy/Security Official (P/SO).

   b. Procedures of Commanding Officer. The CO shall follow the guidance set forth in Commandant Instruction 5260.5, "Privacy Incident Response, Notification, and Reporting Procedures for Personally Identifiable Information (PII)".

   c. Procedures of Regional Practice P/SO. The Regional Practice P/SO shall receive, document, and initiate an investigation of the incident, including conducting interviews of all individuals knowledgeable of the circumstances of the incident, or of the technical systems or administrative procedures which may have lead created the vulnerability.

   d. Notification of the CG P/SO. The Regional Practice P/SO shall notify the HSWL SC and CG P/SOs of the incident via email or telephonically. The Regional Practice P/SO may confer with the HSWL SC or CG P/SO on any issue related to investigation or mitigation of the incident.

   e. Time line. The Regional Practice P/SO through the local command authority shall provide notification of all individuals who's PHI may have been compromised within 10 business days of the conclusion of the investigation of the incident. This notification shall:

      (1) Identify the nature and scope of the incident and the circumstances surrounding the loss, theft, compromise or disclosure of the PHI.

      (2) What specific data was involved?

      (3) The actions taken by the local facility to remedy the vulnerability.

      (4) The potential risks incurred by the affected individuals as a result of the disclosure, compromise, loss or theft of PHI.

(5) Actions which the individuals can take to protect against potential harm.

(6) A resource for obtaining further information and/or a point of contact to address any further questions the individual may have related to the potential compromise of PHI.

f. <u>Final report</u>. A final report containing a description of the findings of the investigation, efforts made to mitigate any harm resulting from the disclosure, and corrective actions take to remedy weakness of technical systems, or administrative policies or procedures which lead to the vulnerability shall be made in writing, either electronically or by paper to the HSWL SC P/SO and CG P/SO within Commandant (CG-1122).

g. <u>Lessons learned</u>. The HSWL SC P/SO will disseminate lessons learned from the incident to all Regional Practice P/SOs and appropriate command authorities so that local systems, policies and procedures can be review and appropriate corrective action and/or training can be completed.

6. <u>Other CG Members Who Utilize Protected Health Information</u>. Other members of the CG may routinely or occasionally have access to or utilize protected health information in the course of their duties. Although these members are not considered part of the "health care workforce," and therefore, are not required by law and implementing regulations (see 45 CFR 164.530 (b)) to complete HIPAA training, it is critical that these members are aware of the intent of HIPAA and maintain the privacy and confidentiality of protected health information with which they are entrusted. To accomplish this objective, members assigned to the following organizations or performing duties in the following roles should complete appropriate HIPAA training:

(1) National Maritime Center

(2) CG Personnel Command/Physical Disabilities Evaluation Board

(3) Special Needs Program staff

(4) Command Drug and Alcohol Representatives/ Drug and Alcohol Program staff

(5) Others as deemed necessary by COs

Members may complete HIPAA training through the Military Health System's Training Portal, MHS Learn, at https://mhslearn.satx.disa.mil/ by self-registering using the "Senior Management" HIPAA Job Position. Each member must select "MTF\Location\Unit" and "HIPAA Job Domain" identifiers. Select the domain established specifically for your organization such as "(CGPSC) USCG Personnel Support Center" or "(CGNMC) USCG National Maritime Center." These HIPAA Job Domains may be located using the search function to the right of the block by clicking on the "flashlight," expanding the "plus box" to the left of CG, selecting the appropriate choice and then clicking on "OK" at the bottom of the window. Contact your local HIPAA P/S O for all registration questions. After completing the core courses, registrants will be automatically reminded by email to complete Annual HIPAA Refresher Course during their birth month of each year.

7. Electronic Transmission of Protected Health Information.

   a. Coast Guard Messaging System. Messages should not contain personally identifiable health information. This includes listing the name of the individual and any disease code (i.e., International Classification of Disease (ICD-9 or ICD-10) or Common Procedural Terminology (CPT)) which be used to identify the disease or condition of the individual. Messages requiring transmission of personally identifiable health information shall use the Inpatient Hospitalization Message format (see paragraph 7.b below).

   b. Inpatient Hospitalization Messages. Protected Health Information (PHI) will be sent utilizing the procedure described in Chapter 7.B.(3)(b) for the Disease Alert Report or Chapter 2.A.(2)(b) utilizing the Inpatient Hospitalization system. Send only the minimum necessary information to accomplish the intended purpose of the use, disclosure or request via e-mail to HQS-DG-HSWL Inpatient Hospitalization, as appropriate. This e-mail will only be viewed by limited command designated individuals at HQ and HSWL SC with a need to know. No other individuals shall be included or copied on this e-mail, nor shall the e-mail containing PHI be forwarded after the fact.

   c. Faxing Protected Health Information. Any individual who has access to protected health information (PHI) in the course of their duties is obligated to maintain the security of that information. Best practices to maintain the security of PHI include only faxing PHI to secure faxes, in other words, faxes in secured spaces where only those who utilize PHI have access to the secure fax. If information is sent to any other non-secure fax, it is required that the sender alert the receiver to stand by and receive the fax so that the fax containing PHI cannot be inadvertently intercepted by someone without authorization to receive and use PHI. The receiver should then contact the sender to acknowledge safe receipt of the fax containing PHI.

   d. Recommended Disclaimer on Protected Health Information Sent Electronically. The following disclaimer statement is recommended by the TMA Privacy Office. It may be placed in the footer of a Fax Cover Sheet for the transmission of PHI or may be used at the end of an email containing PHI. The word "Confidential" in bold should be placed at the beginning of the footer above this disclaimer as depicted below:

CONFIDENTIAL

This document may contain information covered under the Privacy Act, 5 USC552(a), and/or the Health Insurance Portability and Accountability Act (PL 104-191) and its various implementing regulations and must be protected in accordance with those provisions. Healthcare information is personal and sensitive and must be treated accordingly. If this correspondence contains healthcare information it is being provided to you after appropriate authorization from the patient or under circumstances that don't require patient authorization. You, the recipient, are obligated to maintain it in a safe, secure and confidential manner. Redisclosure without additional patient consent or as permitted by law is prohibited. Unauthorized redisclosure or failure to maintain confidentiality subjects you to application of appropriate sanction. If you have received this correspondence in error, please notify the sender at once and destroy any copies you have made.

COMDTINST M6000.1E

Section H. Quality Improvement Studies.

1. Background 1
2. Responsibilities 1
3. Definitions 1
4. General information 2
5. QIS Focus 2
6. QIS Process 2
7. QIS Report Form 2
8. Frequency of Quality Improvement Studies 2
9. Completing the QIS Report Form 2
10. Follow-up Reporting 5
11. Integration 5
12. Filing 5

This page intentionally left blank.

H. Quality Improvement Studies.

1. Background. In the early 1990s the CG established a Monitoring and Evaluation (M&E) program to examine areas of clinical care the CG deemed important in order to assess how well clinics provided this care. The M&E program centered on the review of historical data and, thus, was a retroactive program. Further, the program was strictly a QA program in that it was designed to ensure a set standard of care was met in specific areas. M&Es did not necessarily seek to improve care beyond a set standard. Quality Improvement Studies (QISs) will replace M&Es as the primary tool for evaluating healthcare delivery in clinics. M&Es will no longer be used as a QA tool. QISs provide a framework so that current QA clinic standards of care themselves are reviewed for improvement. Further, QISs are proactive versus retroactive in nature because data from QISs are reviewed as they become available.

2. Responsibilities.

    a. HSWL SC. Monitors the QIS Program activities. The HSWL SC provides guidance to the program.

    b. Quality Improvement Coordinator. The QI Coordinator ensures that at least four QISs are completed annually, in a timely manner, and in the proper format and are documented in the QI Focus Group (QIFG) meeting minutes. The QI Coordinator ensures that delegated tasks are completed by the appropriate clinic personnel.

    c. Quality Improvement Focus Group. The QIFG meets at least quarterly and is responsible for approving and monitoring the QISs conducted in the clinic. The QIFG provides guidance to QIS investigators and other members of the staff involved in implementing QISs. On-going QISs are discussed in QIFG meetings and documented in its minutes. The QIFG, which includes providers and administrators, participates in the resolution of the problem or issue identified.

    d. Clinic personnel. Ensure important problems that address clinical, administrative or cost issues, and patient outcomes are brought before the QIFG to initiate as QISs. All personnel participate in the identification and resolution of problems.

3. Definitions.

    a. Problem. Any question to be considered, resolved, or answered in order to meet or improve upon Accreditation Association if Ambulatory Health Care (AAAHC) or Chapter 13 of the Medical Manual quality of care standards.

    b. Quality Improvement Study. In a healthcare setting, a tool used to systematically review a single problem of healthcare delivery or operations within a clinic in order to determine if there is an improved and sustainable solution to the problem.

    c. Quality Assurance, Quality Improvement. See Chapter 13 Section A 8 for the definitions of Quality Assurance and Quality Improvement.

4. General information. The QIS Program must be active (implements at least 4 studies per year), organized (utilizes a systematic, "closed loop" process), peer-based (results reviewed by the QIFG, documented in the QIFG minutes, posted in clinic public folder for HSWL SC review), and integrated (includes issues from all clinical and administrative departments within the clinic, incorporates results into the clinic standard operating procedures, and provides staff training when necessary).

5. QIS Focus. QISs address or identify issues including standards of care, quality of care delivered, effectiveness of healthcare delivery, efficiency of operations, and additional issues or concerns unique to individual clinics. The QIS process must focus on one problem or issue per study although the clinic may conduct more than one QIS concurrently.

6. QIS Process. The QIS process is a sequential process that roughly parallels the scientific method. The process is outlined in a flow-sheet (See Figure 13-H-1).

    a. Step 1: Identify problem.

    b. Step 2: Gather information on problem.

    c. Step 3: Develop solution to problem.

    d. Step 4: Conduct training on solution.

    e. Step 5: Implement solution to problem.

    f. Step 6: Report results of implemented solution.

    g. Step 7: Evaluate solution to problem.

7. QIS Report Form. Clinic QI activities are reported on the Quality Improvement Study Report Template, CG-6000-6 which follows the stepwise QIS process.

8. Frequency of Quality Improvement Studies. Quality improvement is a continuous process therefore clinics must initiate a minimum of four QISs per calendar year. QISs should be spread throughout the year when possible and involve different clinical areas when possible (e.g. lab, pharmacy, medical, administration).

9. Completing the QIS Report Form.

    a. Overview. The QIS Report form is a major component of implementing a successful QI program. It serves as the building block for QI interventions and a record of QI activities. This section describes the major components of the form and how to complete it.

    b. Name of study. Concise yet descriptive such as "health record tracking," "lab results monitoring," or "prescription error rate."

    c. Investigator. The person responsible for completing the QIS and presenting its findings to the QIFG.

    d. Study. Select if the QIS is an initial study or a follow-up study.

    e. Date completed. The date on which the current QIS Report form was completed.

f. Problem Statement. The specific problem is described in one or two sentences. The name of the study should reflect what the problem is. Each QIS addresses a single problem. Each QIS must only address one problem. If there are multiple problems, a QIS must be done for each one.

g. Background to problem/Known facts of problem. The background to the problem is described and the known facts of the problem are listed (who, what, when, where, how). Information on the problem is evaluated for reliability.

h. Parameters of problem. The parameters that define the problem are determined. Problems with greater negative consequences that occur frequently should take precedence over those with lesser consequences that occur less frequently.

i. Area of Care. Select the area of care that best describes the nature of the problem:

   (1) Administrative. Examples include health record completeness, record tracking system, referral tracking, staffing utilization, staff satisfaction, medical/legal issues, cost issues, patient flow, health readiness, quality controls in clinic departments, monitoring of care, assessing patient satisfaction, wasteful practices, access to care.

   (2) Ancillary. Examples include monitoring abnormal results, radiograph retakes.

   (3) Clinical. Examples include tracking management of contagious disease cases, assessing for appropriateness of care according to standard guidelines, assessing changes in outcomes based on changes in practice, medications or ancillary treatments.

   (4) Dental. Examples include annual Type 2 exam process, ensuring proper sterilization of instruments, and endodontic and periodontal treatment follow-up.

   (5) Medical. Examples include physical exam process, diagnostic testing procedures, practice patterns of providers, and comparisons to national standards of care.

   (6) Patient outcome. Examples include adverse events, medication errors, deviation from standard of care, clinical procedure processes, and peer review findings.

   (7) Pharmaceutical. Examples include Non-Formulary Medication Utilization, Appropriate Use of Antibiotics to treat URIs, and Improving Patient Medication Outcomes.

j. Parameters of problem Consequence. Determine what happens if solution to problem is not found. This step may assist clinics to determine on which issues to focus their efforts.

   (1) Devastating. Problem results in intolerable outcome, loss of life, injury, economic penalty or legal issues.

(2) <u>Serious</u>. Problem could result in injury, hazard or economic penalty.

(3) <u>Moderate</u>. Problem will probably not cause hazard or economic penalty.

(4) <u>Low</u>. Problem does not have much implication to health or economics.

k. <u>Standards used to evaluate problem</u>. This element usually applies to clinical QISs that involve the comparison of clinic standards of care against national treatment or practice guidelines. Complete if applicable.

l. <u>Proposed solution to problem</u>. Describe how and what information was gathered to determine course of action. Describe specifically what steps the clinic will take to address the problem. This will take a paragraph to describe.

m. <u>Desired outcome of solution</u>. Discuss specifically what the clinic hopes to attain by implementation of the solution.

n. <u>Training Date</u>. Give date on which the staff was trained on the proposed solution to the problem. Must ensure staff is trained so they know how to implement the solution and what is expected of them.

o. <u>Training Aids</u>. Check applicable boxes. Generally, solutions that involve tasks with higher levels of consequence if an error occurs or those that involve tasks that occur less frequently require greater training intervention than those that have less consequences or occur more frequently. The QIFG must determine what training strategies to use in order to successfully implement the corrective solution. Training must involve at least two strategies that include memory tools, lectures, checklists, flow charts and practice/rehearsal.

p. <u>Implement solution to problem</u>. Each task must have a person assigned to it who is responsible for its completion by a specified date. These tasks include those that originate from the statements listed under "proposed solution to problem." Tasks are implemented concurrently or sequentially depending on the problem. As each task is completed the date is noted in the "completion date" column. The responsible party does not have to be the investigator. Progress is reported in the meeting minutes of the QIFG. The QIFG determines if the results achieved by the intervention provide sustainable improvements. If the solution involves a long-term project (i.e. one over six months to implement or review) such as an area renovation, check the appropriate box noting this fact. Interpret the QIS Flowchart in light of the time adjustments required for long-term projects.

q. <u>Report results of the implemented solution</u>. Complete the "Initial QIS" section for the first study, the "Follow-up QIS" section for the second study and the "Additional QIS" section if a third study is warranted. For long term projects note the appropriate follow-up dates in the text.

r. <u>Evaluate solution to problem: Initial QIS</u>. Check whether the solution was sustained or not sustained and fill-in the appropriate boxes. Note when the findings were documented in the QIFG meeting minutes.

s. <u>Evaluate solution to problem: Follow-up QIS</u>. Check whether the solution was sustained or not sustained after the follow-up study was concluded. If sustained, check the appropriate boxes for what actions were taken to integrate the solution into clinic operations. Check what training tools were used to educate staff on new proposed solution. Note when the findings were documented in the QIFG meeting minutes.

t. <u>Evaluate solution to problem: Additional QIS (if needed)</u>. For QISs that involve areas of high risk to patients or could result in devastating consequences if not resolved, an additional evaluation may be desired. Check whether the solution was sustained or not sustained after the additional study was initiated. Check what training tools were used to educate staff on new proposed solution. A new QIS Report Form must be started if the implemented solution is not sustained after a third study. Note when the findings were documented in the QIFG meeting minutes.

u. <u>Evaluate solution to problem: HSWL SC assistance</u>.

10. <u>Follow-up Reporting</u>. The QIS Report Form is designed to be used for the initial and follow-up study (or studies) for a particular problem. For follow-up or additional QISs add the findings to the "Report Results of Implemented Solution" section. Results are recorded in the QIFG minutes.

11. <u>Integration</u>. Once a follow-up or additional QIS results in a sustainable solution, the corrective solution must be incorporated into the SOP and results reported in the QIFG minutes.

12. <u>Filing</u>. The HSWL SC will establish a filing process for the clinics such as public folders or microsite on CG Central to ensure sharing of information.

COMDTINST M6000.1D   Figure 13-H-1

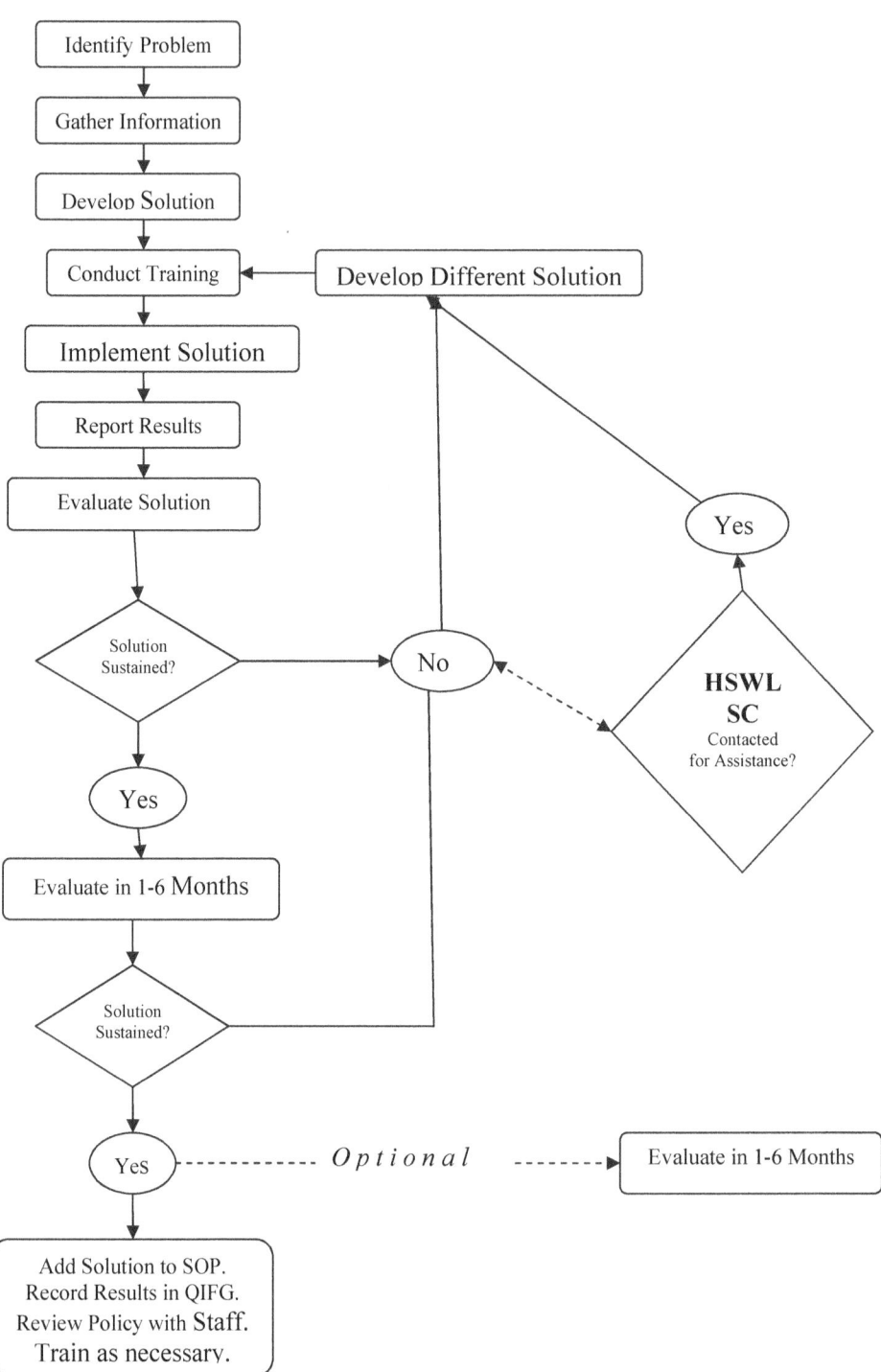

Chapter 13. H. Page 6

Section I. Peer Review Program.

1. Background. 1
2. Characteristics of a Peer Review Program. 1
3. Responsibilities. 1
4. Process. 2
5. Definitions. 2

This page intentionally left blank.

I. Peer Review Program.

1. Background. In striving to improve the quality of care and promote more effective and efficient utilization of facilities and services, an accredited organization maintains an active, integrated, organized, peer-based program of quality management and improvement that links peer review, quality improvement activities, and risk management in an organized, systematic way.

2. Characteristics of a Peer Review Program. The CG peer review program maintains an active and organized process for peer review that is integrated into the quality management and improvement program, evidenced by the following characteristics.

   a. Health care providers. Health care providers understand, support and participate in a peer review program through organized mechanisms and are responsible to the governing body. The peer review activities are evidenced in the quality improvement program. Health care providers participate in the development and application of the criteria used to evaluate the care they provide.

   b. Commandant (CG-1122). Commandant (CG-1122) provides ongoing monitoring of important aspects of the care provided by physicians, dentists, mid-level providers, and other health care professionals. Monitoring important aspects of care by individual practitioners is necessary for monitoring individual performance and establishing internal benchmarks.

   c. Data criteria. Data related to established criteria are collected in an on-going manner and periodically evaluated to identify acceptable or unacceptable trends or occurrences that affect patient outcome.

   d. Clinical privileges. Results of peer review activities are used as part of the process for granting continuation of clinical privileges.

   e. Peer review activities are not designed to be punitive in nature, but can be used to identify trends requiring improvements, to enhance or improve professional competence, skill, and quality of performance of health care providers, and to guide educational programs and activities consistent with the CG mission, goals, and objectives.

3. Responsibilities.

   a. Commandant (CG-112). Establish and maintain contract with an external peer review organization. Collaborate with the HSWL SC to agree on specific ICD-9/CPT and CDT codes/medical and dental clinical guidelines to be used for each annual review. Coordinate with external peer review organization and clinics to schedule on-site peer reviews.

   b. HSWL SC. Collaborate with Commandant (CG-1122) to identify specific ICD-9/CPT and CDT codes/medical and dental guidelines for each annual review. Conduct second level review, if necessary, based on report from the peer review organization.

   c. Clinic Administrator. Select up to ten (10) patient records per provider based on the selected clinical guidelines as determined by Commandant (CG-1122) and HSWL SC.

d. <u>External Peer Review Organization</u>. Conduct reviews utilizing the CG developed peer review instruments and clinical guidelines available on the Commandant (CG-112) website at http://www.uscg.mil/hq/cg1/cg112/default.asp. Reviewers are required to be experienced, clinically practicing physicians and dentists.

4. <u>Process</u>.

   a. <u>Review of Providers</u>. Annually, Commandant (CG-1122) and the external peer review organization will establish a schedule for reviewing all active duty and contract privileged providers (dentists, physicians, physician assistants, and nurse practitioners). Commandant (CG-1122), with input from the HSWL SC, will provide the specific medical and dental clinical guideline for each annual review. The schedule and information, including the peer review instrument and the appropriate medical/dental clinical guideline will be provided to the clinics by the HSWL SC.

   b. <u>8 Weeks Prior to Review</u>. Eight weeks before a scheduled peer review, Commandant (CG-1122) will contact the Clinic Administrator to verify the date. Once confirmed, the external peer review organization and HSWL SC will be notified of the confirmed date.

   c. <u>2 Weeks Prior to Review</u>. Two weeks before the scheduled visit, the clinic will be contacted by the peer review organization to arrange for access to the clinic and an in-brief with the Command.

   d. <u>During the review</u>. During the review, reviewers will engage the health care provider under review for any clarifications and input. At the conclusion of the review, reviewers will provide an out-brief to the Clinic Administrator, Quality Improvement Coordinator, and/or SHSO. Health care providers will be given their individual peer reviews – this will serve as a teaching tool to improve performance and/or identify needed training. Individual reviews are not sent to Commandant (CG-1122).

   e. <u>Commandant CG-1122</u>. Commandant (CG-1122) will use data provided from the reports to track enterprise-wide trends and establish benchmarks for improvement.

   f. <u>Findings</u>. Findings determined to warrant a second review will be conducted by HSWL SC per guidance from Commandant (CG-1122).

5. <u>Definitions</u>.

   a. <u>Current Procedural Terminology (CPT)</u>. The CPT is an acronym for Current Procedural Terminology. CPT codes are published by the American Medical Association, and the fourth edition, the most current, is used. The purpose of the coding system is to provide uniform language that accurately describes medical, surgical, and diagnostic services.

b. <u>International Classification of Diseases, 9th Revision, Clinical Modification (ICD-9-CM)</u>. The ICD-9-CM coding system is used to code signs, symptoms, injuries, diseases, and conditions.

c. <u>Code on Dental Procedures and Nomenclature (CDT)</u>. CDT is an acronym for Code on Dental Procedures and Nomenclature. The American Dental Association's (ADA) Code on Dental Procedures and Nomenclature (CDT) is used to record and report dental procedures. It is the dental equivalent of Current Procedure Terminology (CPT) codes for other-than-dental procedures. Hence the ADA's choice of the official abbreviation CDT rather than CDPN.

d. <u>Benchmarking</u>. A systematic comparison of products, services, or work processes of similar organizations, departments or practitioners to identify best practices known to date for the purpose of continuous quality improvement.

This page intentionally left blank.

Section J. Infection and Exposure Control Program.

1. Introduction 1
2. Policy 2
3. Standard Precautions 2
4. Precautions for Invasive Procedures 5
5. Precautions for Medical Laboratories 6
6. Handling Biopsy Specimens 6
7. Using and Caring for Sharp Instruments and Needles 7
8. Infection Control Procedures for Minor Surgery Areas and Dental Operatories 8
9. Sterilizing and Disinfecting 14
10. Clinic Attire 19
11. Storage and Laundering of Clinic Attire, PPE and Linen 19
12. Cleaning and Decontaminating Blood or Other Body Fluid Spills 20
13. Infectious Waste 20
14. Managing Exposures (Bloodborne Pathogen Exposure Control) 21
15. Training Personnel for Occupational Exposure 26

This page intentionally left blank.

Section J. Infection Control Program (Exposure Control Plan).

1. Introduction.

    a. Standard Precautions. Identifying potentially infectious patients by medical history, physical examination, or readily available laboratory tests is not always possible. Extended periods often exist between the time a person becomes infected with a microbial agent and the time when laboratory tests can detect the associated antigens or antibodies. Consequently, even if a patient tests negative, he or she may still be infectious. Health care personnel must assume that all blood/body fluids and contaminated instruments and materials are infectious and routinely use Standard Precautions to protect themselves and patients.

    b. Safety Procedures. All procedures should be available to minimize the sources and transmission of infections, including adequate surveillance techniques.

    c. Protection. All CG systems must provide for the protection of patients, staff and the environment.

    d. Exposure. While CG health services personnel and emergency medical technicians must be seriously concerned with the risk of exposure to human immunodeficiency virus (HIV), the risk of contracting other infectious diseases, such as hepatitis B virus (HBV), is much greater. HBV infection can result in serious physical debilitation and adversely affect a practitioner's ability to provide health care. Once infected, a person also poses a potential risk to future patients as an HBV infection "carrier." Infection control practices that prevent HBV transmission also prevent HIV transmission. Since 1982 a safe, effective vaccine to prevent Hepatitis B has been available; it stimulates active immunity against HBV infection and provides over 90% protection against the virus for 7 or more years after vaccination.

    e. Occupational Safety and Health Administration (OSHA). The OSHA Blood borne Pathogens (BBP) Standard requires the use of Standard Precautions to protect the healthcare worker from exposure to bloodborne pathogens. The basic principle of Standard Precautions is the assumption that all patients are potentially infectious. Therefore, the risk of exposure to blood or other potentially infectious materials (OPIM) posed by a procedure dictates the level of precautions, rather than the perceived infectivity of the patient. In 1996, the Hospital Infection Control Practices Advisory Committee (HICPAC) issued guidelines for transmission-based precautions in hospitals. In addition to precautions for BBP, airborne, droplet and contact isolation procedures were also included. Under this regime, procedures to protect health services personnel from BBP are referred to as Standard Precautions, previously identified as Universal Precautions. All CG Health Services will adopt the use of standard blood and body fluid precautions as recommended by the CDC and OSHA.

2. Policy.

   a. Health services personnel. Health services personnel will adhere to infection-control principles, general hygiene measures, and the Center for Disease Control and Prevention's (CDC's) "standard precautions" to prevent transmitting infectious disease between themselves and their patients.

   b. Mandatory vaccination. Hepatitis B vaccination is mandatory for all CG active duty and reserve members and all civilian health care providers. The civilian administrative staff is exempt; however, these personnel are encouraged to receive Hepatitis B vaccination. Civilian clinic administrative personnel declining to receive Hepatitis B vaccination must sign this statement on an SF-600, and it shall be retained in the individual's health record:

   > I understand due to my occupational exposure to blood or other potentially infectious materials I may be at risk of acquiring Hepatitis B virus (HBV) infection. I have been given the opportunity to be vaccinated with the hepatitis B vaccine, at no charge to myself. However, I decline Hepatitis B vaccination at this time. I understand that by declining this vaccine, I continue to be at risk of acquiring hepatitis B, a serious disease. If, in the future, I continue to have occupational exposure to blood or other potentially infectious materials and I want to be vaccinated with hepatitis B vaccine, I can receive the vaccination series at no charge to me.

   c. Emergency Medical Technicians. Emergency Medical Technicians will adhere to the "standard precautions" described in Chapter 13-J-3.

   d. OSHA Blood-Borne Pathogen (BBP) Standard. Under the OSHA Blood-Borne Pathogen (BBP) Standard, all health services administrative and clinical personnel are potentially occupationally exposed. All clinics shall provide the health care professional responsible for vaccinating employees with Hepatitis B vaccine a copy of the OSHA BBP Standard.

3. Standard Precautions.

   a. Background. Since medical history and examination cannot reliably identify all patients infected with HIV or other blood-borne pathogens, health services personnel must consistently use blood and body-fluid precautions with all patients, including those in emergency care settings in which the risk of blood exposure is greater and the patient's infectious status usually is unknown. CDC currently recommends the "standard blood and body-fluid precautions" approach or "standard precautions."

   (1) All health care workers will routinely use appropriate barrier precautions to prevent skin and mucous membrane exposure when anticipating contact with any patient's blood or other body fluids. Personnel will wear gloves to touch patients' blood and body fluids, mucous membranes, or broken skin; to handle

items or surfaces soiled with blood or body fluids; and to perform venipuncture and other vascular access procedures. Personnel will change gloves after contact with each patient. Personnel will wear masks and protective eyewear or face shields during procedures likely to generate blood droplets or other body fluids to prevent exposure to oral, nasal, or optic mucous membranes. Personnel will wear gowns or aprons otherwise identified under Personal Protective Equipment (PPE) during procedures likely to generate blood splashes or other body fluids. All protective clothing must be removed before leaving the work area.

(2) Hand Hygiene

(a) During the delivery of healthcare, avoid unnecessary touching of surfaces in close proximity to the patient to prevent both contamination of clean hands from environmental surfaces and transmission of pathogens from contaminated hands to surfaces.

(b) When hands are visibly dirty, contaminated with proteinaceous material, or visibly soiled with blood or body fluids, wash hands with either a nonantimicrobial soap and water or an antimicrobial soap and water.

(c) If hands are not visibly soiled, or after removing visible material with nonantimicrobial soap and water, decontaminate hands in the clinical situations described in 2.c.1-6. The preferred method of hand decontamination is with an alcohol-based hand rub. Alternatively, hands may be washed with an antimicrobial soap and water. Frequent use of alcohol-based hand rub immediately following handwashing with nonantimicrobial soap may increase the frequency of dermatitis. Perform hand hygiene:

(1) Before having direct contact with patients.

(2) After contact with blood, body fluids or excretions, mucous membranes, nonintact skin, or wound dressings.

(3) After contact with a patient's intact skin (e.g., when taking a pulse or blood pressure or lifting a patient).

(4) If hands will be moving from a contaminated-body site to a clean-body site during patient care.

(5) After contact with inanimate objects (including medical equipment) in the immediate vicinity of the patient.

(6) After removing gloves.

(3) All health services personnel will take precautions to prevent injuries caused by needles, scalpels, and other sharp instruments or devices during procedures or when cleaning used instruments, disposing of used needles, and handling sharp instruments after procedures. To prevent needle stick injuries, personnel will not by hand directly recap needles, purposely bend or break them, remove them from disposable syringes, or otherwise manipulate them. After using disposable syringes and needles, scalpel blades, and other sharp items, personnel will dispose of them by placing them in puncture-resistant containers located as close to the use area as practical. The CG prohibits the use of reusable needles.

(4) Per CFR 1910.1030 Subpart Z (2001), OSHA requires: a) the use of sharps protection devices with engineered sharps injury protection, b) evaluation by employers with input from non-managerial employees involved in the use of the devices, and c) documentation of efforts to implement requirements. Employers must consider, and where appropriate, use effective engineering controls. Effective being defined as a device, that based on reasonable judgment, will make an exposure incident less likely to occur in the application in which it is used. The evaluation and documentation shall include the following:

   (a) Methods of evaluation.

   (b) Results of evaluation.

   (c) Justification for selection decision.

(5) Although research has not definitively implicated saliva in HIV transmission, it is prudent to use appropriate protective barriers such as mouthpieces, resuscitation bags, or other ventilation devices instead of direct mouth-to-mouth resuscitation. These devices must be available for use in areas where the need for resuscitation is predictable.

(6) Health care workers who have exuding lesions or weeping dermatitis will not provide any direct patient care or handle patient care equipment until the condition resolves.

(7) Eating, drinking, smoking, applying cosmetics or lip balm, and handling contact lenses are prohibited in work areas with a reasonable likelihood of occupational exposure to BBP.

(8) Personnel shall not keep food and drink in refrigerators, freezers, shelves, drug storage areas, or cabinets or on counter tops or bench tops where blood or other potentially infectious materials are present.

(9) Personnel shall perform all procedures involving blood or other potentially infectious materials in a manner that prevents droplets of these substances from splashing, spraying, and splattering.

(10) Pregnant health care workers apparently do not face greater risk of contracting HIV infection than non-pregnant health care workers; however, if a health care worker develops HIV infection during pregnancy, the infant risks infection due to prenatal or perinatal transmission. Therefore, pregnant health care workers will thoroughly learn and strictly adhere to standard precautions to minimize the risk of HIV transmission.

b. Implementation. Implementing standard blood and body fluid precautions for all patients eliminates the need for the "Blood and Body Fluid Precautions" isolation category CDC previously recommended for patients known or suspected to be infected with blood-borne pathogens. Personnel will use isolation precautions as necessary if they diagnose or suspect associated conditions, such as infectious diarrhea or tuberculosis.

4. Precautions for Invasive Procedures.

   a. Aseptic techniques. Acceptable aseptic techniques are to be used by all persons in the surgical area. Environmental controls are implemented to ensure a safe and sanitary environment.

   b. When to use standard precautions. The standard blood and body fluid precautions listed above and those listed below shall be the minimum precautions for all invasive procedures, defined as surgical entry into tissues, cavities, or organs; repair of major traumatic injuries in an operating or delivery room, emergency department, or out-patient setting, including both physicians' and dentists' offices; a vaginal delivery; manipulating, cutting, or removing any oral or perioral tissues, including tooth structure, during which bleeding occurs or the potential for bleeding exists.

   c. Types of precautions. All health care workers who routinely participate in invasive procedures shall take appropriate barrier precautions to prevent skin and mucous membrane contact with all patients' blood and other body fluids. Personnel shall wear gloves and surgical masks for procedures that commonly generate droplets, splash blood or other body fluids, or generate bone chips, such as those using rotary dental instrumentation. Personnel shall wear gowns or aprons made of materials that provide an effective barrier during invasive procedures likely to splash blood or other body fluids.

   d. Accidents. If a glove is torn, cut, or punctured, the wearer will remove it, re-scrub, and put on a new glove as promptly as patient safety permits. The needle or instrument involved in the incident shall also be removed from the sterile field.

5. Precautions for Medical Laboratories. Blood and other body fluids from all patients will be considered infectious. To supplement the standard precautions listed above; the following precautions are recommended for health care workers in clinical laboratories.

    a. Blood and body fluid specimens. All blood and body fluid specimens shall be placed in a well-constructed, labeled container with a secure lid to prevent leaking during transport, taking care when collecting each specimen to avoid contaminating the container's exterior or the laboratory form accompanying the specimen.

    b. Equipment. All persons obtaining or processing blood and body fluid specimens (e.g., removing tops from vacuum tubes) shall wear gloves. Personnel shall wear masks and protective eyewear if they anticipate contact with mucous membrane with blood or body fluids, change gloves, and wash hands after completing specimen processing.

    c. Routine procedures. For routine procedures such as histological and pathologic studies or microbiologic culturing, a biological safety cabinet is not necessary. However, personnel shall use biological safety cabinets (Class I or II) whenever performing procedures with a high potential for generating droplets, including activities such as blending, sonicating, and vigorous mixing.

    d. Pipetting. Use mechanical pipetting devices to manipulate all liquids in the laboratory. Never pipette by mouth.

    e. Needles. When using needles and syringes, personnel will follow the recommended standard precautions to prevent needle injuries.

    f. Decontamination. Decontaminate laboratory work surfaces with an appropriate chemical germicide after spilling blood or other body fluids and completing work activities. Decontaminate contaminated materials used in laboratory tests before reprocessing or place such materials in bags and dispose of them according to institutional policies for disposing of infectious waste. Decontaminate scientific equipment contaminated with blood or other body fluids with an appropriate chemical germicide and clean such equipment before repairing it in the laboratory or transporting it to the manufacturer.

    g. Hand washing. All persons shall wash their hands after completing laboratory activities and remove protective clothing before leaving the laboratory.

6. Handling Biopsy Specimens. Generally, personnel must put each specimen in a sturdy container with a secure lid to prevent leaking during transport and take care when collecting specimens to avoid contaminating the container's exterior. If the outside of the container is visibly contaminated, clean and disinfect it or place it in an impermeable bag before delivery to the appropriate destination for examination.

7. Using and Caring for Sharp Instruments and Needles.

a. <u>Sharps</u>. Personnel will consider sharp items (needles, scalpel blades, dental burs, and other sharp instruments) potentially infectious and handle them with extreme care to prevent unintentional injuries.

b. <u>Disposal items</u>. All generating personnel must place disposable syringes, tube holders, needles, scalpel blades, anesthetic carpules and other sharp items in closable, leak-proof, puncture-resistant containers. Cardboard containers are not appropriate for this purpose. To prevent unintentional needle stick injuries, personnel will not directly recap disposable needles by hand, purposefully bend or break needles, remove them from disposable syringes or tube holders, or otherwise manipulate them after use.

   (1) At the discretion of the Clinic Administrator, a clinic may elect to receive sharps from patients for proper disposal. If so, then the following criteria must be met.

   (a) The sharps container must be:

   (1) Installed in a non-sensitive area to allow for disposal by patients.

   (2) Accessible by wheelchair bound patients.

   (3) Out of the reach of children.

   (4) Maintained regularly and replaced when ¾ full.

   (b) Patients must dispose of their own sharps into an appropriate sharps container.

   (c) Patients will be instructed to maintain lancets, needles, and other sharps in a leak-proof, puncture-resistant container such as a bleach container or 2-liter soda bottle.

   (2) The Clinic Administrator must maintain policies and procedures for the handling of sharps brought into the clinic.

c. <u>Recapping needles</u>. If multiple injections of anesthetic or other medications from a single syringe are required, personnel may use these techniques in lieu of directly recapping by hand:

   (1) Use an approved shielding device specifically designed to recap safely (e.g., "On-Guard").

   (2) Use the "scoop" recapping technique. Affix the empty needle sheath to a flat surface and "scoop" it onto the exposed needle. A hand does not touch the sheath until the needle is securely inside.

(3) Use a hemostat to recap by securing the empty sheath well away from the health care worker's hand.

d. <u>Needle sticks protocol</u>. All CG Health Care Units shall establish a needle stick protocol; see Section 13-J-14. If a needle stick occurs, the affected person shall report the accident to his or her immediate supervisor, who will document the incident in a memorandum to the SHSO or health services department head, with a copy to the affected person. The memorandum will detail the needle stick's time, date, and circumstances and any medical treatment received. The SHSO or health services department head shall ensure the established needle stick protocol is observed in all cases.

8. <u>Infection Control Procedures for Minor Surgery Areas and Dental Operatories</u>.

   a. <u>Medical History</u>. Always obtain a thorough medical history. For dental procedures, have the patient complete a Dental Health Questionnaire, CG-5605. Amplify this information by asking the patient specific questions about medications, current illnesses, hepatitis, recurrent illness, unintentional weight loss, lymphadenopathy, oral soft tissue lesions, results of last HIV test, or other infections. Completely review the individual's health record or consult with a physician if the history reveals active infection or systemic disease.

   b. <u>Using Personal Protective Equipment and Barrier Techniques</u>.

      (1) Health services personnel (HCW) in CG medical/dental treatment facilities must comply fully with 29 CFR, Part 1910, OSHA Occupational Exposure to Blood Borne Pathogens. OSHA has determined that health care workers face a significant health risk as a result of occupational exposure to blood and "other potentially infectious materials" (OPIM) that may contain potentially harmful blood borne pathogens. This risk can be minimized or eliminated by the practice of standard precautions including the use of PPE.

      (2) PPE is defined in CFR 1910.1030 as specialized clothing worn by an employee for protection against a blood borne hazard. PPE must be removed daily, when visibly soiled, or when leaving the work area and must be commercially laundered at the unit's expense. Under no circumstances shall employees take PPE or contaminated clinic attire from the workplace for self-laundering.

      (3) Health services personnel will consider all patients' blood, saliva, and other body fluids infectious. To protect themselves and patients, personnel must always wear gloves when touching:

         (a) Blood.

         (b) Saliva.

         (c) Body fluids or secretions.

         (d) Items or surfaces contaminated by the above.

(e) Mucous membranes.

(4) Further, personnel must completely treat one patient, if possible, and wash and re-glove hands before performing procedures on another patient. Repeatedly using a single pair of gloves is not allowed; such use can produce defects in the glove material, which reduce its effectiveness as a barrier to microorganisms. Additionally, when gloves are torn, cut, or punctured, the wearer immediately must remove them, thoroughly wash his or her hands, and put on new gloves before completing minor surgical or dental procedures.

(5) Personnel shall wear surgical masks and protective eyewear or a chin-length plastic face shield. Personnel shall change masks after lengthy examinations or procedures, most especially after any, which produce spatter. Patient protective eyewear shall be provided during all treatment procedures likely to splash or spatter blood, saliva, gingival fluids, or foreign objects. Personnel will use rubber dams, pre-procedural mouth rinsing, high-speed evacuation, and proper patient positioning, when appropriate, to minimize droplet generation and spatter in the dental operatory.

(6) Clinic attire is defined in section 10.

c. Hand Hygiene.

(1) Hand hygiene includes hand washing, alcohol-based hand rubs, and surgical/aseptic hand washing. Wearing gloves does not replace the need for hand hygiene.

(2) Indications for hand hygiene are: before and after treating patients (e.g. before glove placement and after glove removal), after barehanded touching of inanimate objects likely to be contaminated by blood or saliva, before regloving after removing gloves that are torn, cut, or punctured, and before leaving the dental operatory.

(3) At the beginning of the day, hand washing with plain soap is adequate, since soap and water will remove transient microorganisms. Wet hands with water, apply product, rub hands together for at least 15 seconds, rinse and dry with a disposable towel. Whenever possible wash hands at sinks that provide hot and cold water through a single mixing valve.

(4) During the rest of the day, for routine dental procedures, alcohol-based hand rubs are recommended. Apply product to palm of one hand, rub hands together covering all surfaces until dry. The appropriate volume of product is based on manufacturer. Alcohol based hand rubs should NOT be used if hands are visibly soiled or contaminated.

(5) For surgical procedures, personnel must use an antimicrobial surgical hand scrub. Scrub hands and forearms for the length of time recommended by manufacturer (2-6 minutes). Clinics may need to stock non-allergenic soap and sterile gloves for allergic individuals.

(6) Health services personnel who have exuding lesions or weeping dermatitis must refrain from all direct patient care and handling patient-care equipment until the condition resolves.

(7) Health services personnel should avoid wearing artificial nails and keep natural nails short as to minimize harboring bacterial growth.

d. Dental equipment. Sterilizing and Disinfecting Dental Hand Pieces, Ultrasonic Scalers, Dental Units, and Dental Laboratory equipment by the following procedures:

(1) After each use with each patient, personnel will sterilize dental hand pieces (including high-speed, low-speed components used intra-orally and ultrasonic scalers) because the device may aspirate a patient's blood, saliva, or gingival fluid into the hand piece or waterline. Clinics should purchase sufficient numbers of autoclavable hand pieces to meet this requirement. Dry heat is the recommended method of sterilizing dental burs.

(2) Disinfect all dental unit surfaces with a suitable chemical germicide between patients or cover such surfaces during use. Use impervious backed paper, aluminum foil, or clear plastic wrap to cover surfaces difficult or impossible to disinfect (e.g., light handles or x-ray tube heads). Remove the covering while gloved, discard the covering, remove used and don fresh gloves, and then recover with clean material after each patient.

(3) Dental laboratory personnel will observe infection control protocols. They will thoroughly, carefully clean blood and saliva from material used in the mouth (e.g., impression materials, occlusal registrations), especially before polishing and grinding intra-oral devices. They will clean and disinfect contaminated materials, impressions, and intra-oral devices before handling them in the dental laboratory and before putting them in a patient's mouth. They will disinfect laboratory instruments (e.g. spatulas, knives, and wax carvers), plastic benches, chucks, handles, switches, tubing, air hoses, and lab hand pieces every day. Rubber mixing bowls require overnight immersion to disinfect. Workstations, including exposed equipment, drawers, work surfaces, and sinks, require weekly surface disinfecting. Because of the increasing variety of dental materials used intra-orally, dental providers should consult with manufacturers about specific materials' stability in disinfecting procedures.

e. Dental Unit Waterlines.

(1) Background: Studies have demonstrated that dental unit waterlines are colonized with a wide variety of microorganisms including bacteria, fungi, and protozoa. Microorganisms colonize and multiply on the interior surfaces of the waterlines resulting in the formation of biofilms. Although oral flora may enter and colonize dental water systems, the public water system is the primary source of the microorganisms found in waterline biofilms.

(2) Discussion: Current dental water systems cannot deliver water of optimal microbiologic quality without some form of intervention by the user. The literature supports the need for improvement in dental unit water quality. Improving the microbiologic quality of water used in dental treatment shows commitment to high-quality patient care. All CG dental clinics should take prudent measures to provide quality water for dental treatment and to ensure a safe and healthy environment for their patients and employees.

(3) All CG dental clinics shall follow the Centers for Disease Control and Prevention (CDC) recommendation that only sterile solutions be used for surgical procedures that involve the cutting of bone.

(4) The number of colony forming units (CFU) in water used as a coolant or irrigant for non-surgical dental treatment should be as low as reasonably achievable. The ceiling limit for acceptable dental water quality is </=500 CFU/mL of heterotrophic plate count bacteria, the regulatory standard for safe drinking water. Non-surgical procedures include most subgingival scaling or restorative procedures and for initial access into the dental pulp.

(5) Water Quality Improvement: There are several options for improving dental unit water quality. They are:

(a) Flushing: Flush waterlines for 2-3 minutes at the beginning of the day, 20-30 seconds between patients to eliminate any retracted oral fluids, and 3 minutes at the end of the day. Mechanical flushing is an interim measure and has no effect on biofilms. However, flushing between patients will remove patient material potentially retracted during treatment, and should be continued even when other methods to control biofilms are used.

(b) All water lines should be completely drained and air purged at the end of the day. This procedure will remove all existing water, dry the lines and discourage the re-growth of microorganisms.

(c) An independent water reservoir will eliminate the inflow of municipal water into the dental unit and provides better control over the quality of source water for patient care. Independent water reservoirs are available as optional equipment on most new dental units and can be retrofitted to existing equipment. Use of independent reservoirs when used with a routine disinfection protocol, can virtually eliminate bacterial and fungal contamination.

(d) Periodic monitoring should be preformed to assess compliance with recommended protocols and to identify technique errors or non compliance. Dental staff should be trained regarding water quality, biofilm formation, water treatment methods, and appropriate maintenance protocols for water delivery systems. Clinical monitoring of water quality can ensure that procedures are correctly performed and that devices are working in accordance with the manufacturer's previously validated protocol. Dentists should consult with the manufacturer of their dental unit or water delivery system to determine the best method for maintaining acceptable water quality (i.e., </= 500 CFU/mL) and the recommended frequency of monitoring.

(e) If the dental unit manufacturer does not provide a recommendation for frequency of monitoring then monthly testing on a semi-random basis is recommended, (e.g. daily, weekly, monthly so it is easy to remember to perform the testing). Water should be tested at each exit point of the unit. If a unit fails to test </=500 CFU/mL, the unit shall be re-treated (under supervision if need be). This does not preclude the continued use of the dental unit.

(f) Monitoring of dental water quality can be performed by using commercial self-contained test kits or commercial water-testing laboratories. Because methods used to treat dental water systems target the entire biofilm, no rationale exists for routine testing for such specific organisms as *Legionella* or *Pseudomonas*, except when investigating a suspected waterborne disease outbreak.

f. Dental Radiology Sterilization and Disinfecting Procedures.

(1) Film-Holding and Aiming Devices. Film-holding and aiming devices will be heat-sterilized.

(2) Panoramic Unit Bite Blocks. Use disposable bite block covers between patients. If disposable covers are not available, treat bite blocks similarly to film-holding devices.

(3) The use of film with barriers is highly recommended. The following outlines the protocol of film handling with barriers:

(a) Place paper towel on work surface in darkroom.

(b) Place container with contaminated films next to paper towel.

(c) Put on gloves.

(d) Take one contaminated film out of container.

(e) Tear open barrier.

(f) Allow film to drop onto paper towel.

(g) Do not touch film with gloved hands.

(h) Dispose of barrier.

(i) After removing all barriers, dispose of container.

(j) Remove gloves, wash hands or use alcohol-based hand rub.

(k) Secure door, turn out darkroom lights.

(l) Unwrap/process films.

(4) The following outlines the protocol of film handling without barriers:

(a) Place paper towel on work surface in darkroom.

(b) Place container with contaminated films next to paper towel.

(c) Secure door, turn out darkroom lights.

(d) Put on gloves.

(e) Take one contaminated film out of container.

(f) Open film packet tab and slide out lead foil backing and black paper.

(g) Discard film packet wrapping.

(h) Rotate foil away from black paper and discard.

(i) Open black paper wrapping without touching film.

(j) Allow film to drop onto paper towel.

(k) Do not touch film with gloved hands.

(l) Discard black paper wrapping.

(m) After all film packets have been opened, dispose container.

(n) Remove gloves, wash hands or use alcohol-based hand rub.

(o) Process films – handle by edges.

(5) X-ray Chair. Between patients wipe arm- and headrests with a chemical surface disinfecting solution. If using paper or plastic headrest covers, replace them after each patient.

(6) Intra-oral X-ray Tubehead and Exposure Buttons. Wipe these items with a surface disinfectant or cover them after each patient visit. Do not allow disinfectant liquid to leak into the tubehead seams or the exposure button switch.

(7) Digital Sensors. Digital sensors will be covered with a disposable plastic sleeve.

9. Sterilizing and Disinfecting.

   a. Background. The rationale for sterilization is to kill all microbes remaining on the instruments and help assure patient safety.

   b. Instrument Categories (Spaulding Classification). The Spaulding Classification defines as critical instruments that normally penetrate soft tissue, teeth, or bone (e.g., forceps, scalpels, bone chisels, scalers, surgical burs, etc.). They must be heat-sterilized after each use. Instruments not intended to penetrate soft or hard tissues (e.g., amalgam carvers, plastic instruments, etc.) but which may come into contact with tissues are semi-critical and also should be heat-sterilized after each use. If heat sterilization is not possible, semi-critical instruments must receive chemical sterilization. Non-critical instruments never contact tissue. Sterilization is recommended for non-critical instruments, but high-level disinfection is acceptable.

   c. Instrument Processing.

      (1) Designate a central processing area and divide into:

         (a) Receiving, cleaning, and decontamination.

         (b) Preparation and packaging.

         (c) Sterilization.

         (d) Storage.

      (2) Cleansing Instruments. Instruments must be cleansed for sterilization to be effective. Use automated cleaning equipment (ultrasonic cleaner, instrument washer). Use a container or wrapping material compatible with then type of sterilization process. Hand-scrubbing instruments is prohibited. Persons who cleanse instruments must wear heavy-duty ("Nitrile") rubber utility gloves to reduce the risk of injury. Inspect instruments for cleanliness before preparing them for packaging. Use only FDA-cleared medical devices for sterilization.

      (3) Packaging and Wrapping Instruments. Depending on intended use, wrap or package most instruments individually or in sets. Packaging in metal or plastic trays reduces set-up time; instruments and other materials arranged systematically are more convenient. Package size and sterilization method generally determine the best wrapping material, most commonly paper/plastic peel pouches, nylon plastic tubing, cloth, sterilization wrap, or wrapped cassettes. Seal packages by heat, tape, and self-sealing methods. Wrap instruments loosely to allow the sterilizing agent to circulate freely throughout the pack. Pack scissors, hemostats, and hinged instruments in the open position so the sterilizing agent can reach all parts. When

wrapping in an easily punctured material, cover the tips of sharp instruments with 2 x 2 gauze or cotton roll. If using plastic or nylon sterilization tubing, the pack should be approximately 20% larger than the longest instrument to allow the inside air to expand when heated. Clear tubing is relatively puncture-resistant and enables rapid identification of contents. When using cloth to wrap critical items, use a double thickness. Package instruments/cassettes with microbial barriers. Allow packages to dry in the sterilizer before they are handled to avoid contamination. Do not use liquid chemical sterilants for surface disinfection or as holding solutions.

   d. Heat Sterilization. The best way to minimize cross-contamination is to sterilize all instruments that can withstand sterilizing conditions. The most practical, dependable sterilization method, heat, when appropriate, is preferable to chemical means. These are the most common heat sterilization techniques:

   (1) Steam Vapor under Pressure Sterilizer (Autoclave). Steam vapor under pressure is an excellent sterilization method. Moist heat kills the bacteria by causing their proteins to denature and coagulate within the microbial cell. The steam's high temperature, not the pressure, kills the microorganisms. Steam can rust cutting edges made of carbon steel; however, antirust agents reduce this process.

   (2) Chemical Vapor under Pressure Sterilizer (Chemiclave). This sterilizer uses chemical vapor under pressure and kills bacteria in much the same manner as the steam sterilizer. It is an excellent sterilization method. Because chemical vapors are less corrosive than steam, they do not dull sharpened instruments. Chemical vapor sterilizers use a specific mixture of formaldehyde, alcohols, ketone, acetone, and water. If the manufacturer's recommended chemical solution is not available, distilled water may be used for a short time. Chemical solutions shall be used only once. A disadvantage of the chemical vapor sterilizer is the residual chemical vapor that escapes into the air when the chamber door is opened. While non-toxic and non-mutagenic, its odor can be objectionable. Allowing the sterilizer to cool for at least 20 minutes before opening will significantly reduce the residual vapor level. A commercial purging system that reduces residual vapor levels is available.

   (3) Dry Heat Sterilizer. Dry heat kills bacteria by an oxidation process. Dry heat sterilization will not corrode instruments, but dry heat sterilizers can destroy metal instruments' temper and melt solder joints if not monitored properly. Some dry heat units are not able to sterilize large trays and require special wrapping and bagging materials. For these reasons, dry heat sterilization is not recommended for critical instruments, and should be monitored carefully and used judiciously with semi-critical and non-critical instruments. Because sterility is destroyed as soon as items are touched or

left open to the environment, do not place loose instruments in dry heat sterilizers. Wrap and bag all instruments; they must remain wrapped or bagged until used.

e. Sterilization Monitoring.

(1) All sterilization procedures must be monitored and recorded in a log book for compliance.

(2) Mechanical Monitoring. Correct time, temperature and pressure is monitored to demonstrate that the physical parameters of the sterilization process have been achieved with every load. Use mechanical monitoring with each load.

(3) Chemical Monitoring. Chemical indicators show that every package has been exposed to sterilizing conditions in a heat sterilizer. They do not guarantee the instruments are sterile. External chemical indicators (autoclave tape or sterilizing bags with heat-sensitive printing) identify at a glance which instruments have been processed but show that only the outside of the pack was exposed to an elevated temperature. An external chemical indicator must be on every pack processed. If using see-through packages, a chemical indicator placed inside the pouch is acceptable. Internal chemical indicators, available in strips, cards, or labels, react to time/temperature/ sterilizing agent combinations – use an internal chemical indicator inside each package. Do not use instrument packages if mechanical or chemical indicators suggest inadequate processing.

(4) Biological Monitoring (Spore testing). Bacterial spores are used to demonstrate that the sterilization procedure kills highly resistant microbes (bacterial spores). Place them in the most challenging area of the load being tested and wrap the pack in the usual fashion. Monitor all chemical vapor, water vapor, and dry heat sterilizers with a spore test either weekly or each cycle, whichever is less frequent.

(a) These systems require either a medical laboratory service or an in-house incubator to incubate the test spore. Dry heat sterilizers require an alternate system using a glassine envelope with enclosed spore strips. Regardless of the system used, document spore monitoring, including identification test date, test results, and operator, and maintain the records for two years.

(b) In the case of a positive spore test, take the sterilizer out of service and review procedures to determine if operator error could be responsible. Re-test the sterilizer using biological, chemical, and mechanical indicators after correcting any procedural problems. If repeat test is negative and the chemical and mechanical tests are normal, put the sterilizer back in service. If the repeat spore test is positive do not use the sterilizer until it has been inspected or repaired or the problem identified. Recall and reprocess items from the suspect loads. Re-test the sterilizer with spore tests in three consecutive empty chamber sterilization cycles after the cause of the failure has been determined and corrected before putting it back into service.

(5) <u>Storage and Shelf Life</u>. Implement practices based on date- or event-related shelf life for the storage of wrapped, sterilized items. Materials are considered indefinitely sterile unless packaging is torn, ripped, punctured or exposed to water. At a minimum, place the date of sterilization and which sterilizer was used on the package. Examine wrapped sterilized packages before opening them to ensure the barrier wrap is in tact. Re-clean, re-pack and re-sterilize packages that are compromised. Store sterile packages in dry closed cabinets.

f. <u>Chemical Sterilization and High-Level Disinfection</u>.

(1) Although heat is the preferred sterilization method, certain instruments and plastics will not tolerate heat sterilization and require chemical sterilization or high-level disinfection. These disinfectants destroy microorganisms by damaging their proteins and nucleic acids. Most formulae contain 2% glutaraldehyde and come in two containers. Mixing the proper amounts from each container activates the solution. Sterilization monitors cannot verify glutaraldehyde sterilization. The solution is caustic to the skin, so use forceps or rubber gloves to handle instruments immersed in glutaraldehyde and *always* follow manufacturer's directions *carefully*. Label each container of fresh solution with an expiration date.

(2) Uninterrupted immersion for 7 to 10 hours in a fresh glutaraldehyde solution usually will achieve sterilization; uninterrupted immersion for 10 minutes will kill most pathogenic organisms, but not spores. Heavily soiled or contaminated instruments render glutaraldehydes ineffective. Debride instruments thoroughly to disinfect effectively. <u>Glutaraldehydes are not recommended for surface disinfection.</u>

g. <u>Surface Disinfection</u>.

(1) Extraordinary efforts to disinfect or sterilize environmental surfaces such as walls, floors, and ceilings generally are not required because these surfaces generally do not transmit infections to patients or health care workers. However, routinely clean and remove soil from them.

(2) After contamination, wipe all other treatment room surfaces such as countertops, dental chairs, light units, exam tables, and non-sterile objects in the operating field with absorbent toweling to remove any extraneous organic material, and then disinfect them with a suitable chemical germicide. Personnel shall wear heavy-duty ("Nitrile") rubber utility gloves when applying surface disinfectants. Many different chemical disinfectants possessing varying degrees of effectiveness are available. The following three surface disinfectants are recommended.

(a) <u>Iodophor</u>. Iodophor compounds contain 0.05 to 1.6% iodine and surface-active agents, usually detergents, which carry and release free iodine. Iodophor's antimicrobial activity is greater than that of iodine alone: 10 to 30 minutes of contact produces intermediate levels of disinfection. Iodophors are EPA-approved as effective when diluted 1:213 with water. Because iodine's vapor pressure is reduced in iodophor, its odor is not as offensive. In addition, iodophors do not stain as readily as iodine.

(b) <u>Phenolics</u>. In high concentrations, phenolic compounds are protoplasmic poisons. In low concentrations, they deactivate essential enzyme systems. As disinfectants, phenolics are usually combined with a detergent; 10 to 20 minutes of contact produces disinfection. Phenolics are less corrosive to treated surfaces.

(c) <u>Sodium Hypochlorite</u>. Sodium hypochlorite is thought to oxidize microbial enzymes and cell wall components. A 1:10 dilution of 5.25% sodium hypochlorite in water produces a solution which disinfects at an intermediate level in 10 minutes. Sodium hypochlorite solution tends to be unstable, so prepare a fresh solution daily. It possesses a strong odor and can harm eyes, skin, clothing, upholstery, and metals (especially aluminum).

(3) Chemical Disinfectants Not Recommended For Use.

(a) <u>Alcohol</u>. Alcohol is bactericidal against bacterial vegetative forms by denaturing cellular proteins. Diluted in water, a 70 to 90% solution is more effective than a more concentrated solution. Alcohol's disadvantages are: (1) rapid evaporation, (2) lack of sporicidal or viricidal activity, and (3) rapid inactivation by organic material. Since alcohol interferes with proper surface cleansing, it has no place in the disinfection protocol.

(b) <u>Quaternary Ammonium Compounds</u>. In the past, benzalkonium chlorides and other "quats" were used as disinfectants because they were thought to be safe and inexpensive and have low surface tension. Their biocidal activity breaks down the bacterial cell membrane, producing an altered cellular permeability. As a group, these compounds have serious deficiencies. Being positively charged, they are attracted to not only bacteria but also to glass, cotton, and proteins, which decrease their biocidal activity. Common cleaners, soaps, and other compounds negatively charged ions neutralize "quats." Research has shown some "quats" support the growth of gram-negative organisms. Quats are ineffective against most spore formers, the Hepatitis B virus, and the tubercle bacillus.

10. <u>Clinic Attire</u>.

a. <u>Definition</u>. Clothing ensembles worn during routine direct patient encounters when not anticipating exposure to blood or OPIM is considered clinic attire.

b. <u>Approved clinic attire</u>. Approved clinic attire is defined as military uniforms or surgical scrubs only. Clinical attire is NOT intended to be PPE and must be supplemented by PPE whenever exposure to blood or OPIM is reasonably anticipated. Surgical scrubs worn as clinic attire shall be worn in designated direct patient care work areas of the clinic, only when engaged in direct patient care activities and shall not be worn outside the clinic. Undergarments worn under scrubs will be the same as those required to be worn under military uniforms. Under no circumstances should long-sleeve undergarments be worn. When arms need to be covered when performing procedures, long sleeve PPE should be worn. The work area is defined in OSHA BBP plan as the area where potential blood borne exposure exists, including corridors or passageways in direct patient care areas.

c. <u>Soiled Clinic attire</u>. Clinic attire that is visibly soiled with blood, OPIM or that had been exposed to contaminated spray or splatter is considered contaminated. PPE is always considered contaminated even if no visible evidence of contamination is present. At no time shall PPE or contaminated clinic attire be worn in administrative areas, break areas, or areas where food or potable drink are stored, prepared or consumed.

d. <u>PPE or contaminated clinic attire</u>. Except for commercial laundering, PPE or contaminated clinic attire shall not be removed from the clinic's direct patient care area, nor shall it be stored in personal clothing lockers nor removed from the clinic.

e. <u>Name tags</u>. When wearing surgical scrubs, military uniforms and civilian clothing as clinical attire, HCWs must also wear a name tag that includes name, rank and occupation (i.e. Physician, Dentist, Physician Assistant, Nurse Practitioner, and Health Service Technician) clearly visible to all patients.

11. <u>Storage and Laundering of Clinic Attire, PPE and Linen</u>.

a. <u>Laundering clinic attire and PPE</u>. Military uniforms and civilian clothing worn as clinic attire that is visibly soiled with blood or OPIM or have been exposed to contaminating spray and spatter is considered contaminated laundry and shall be commercially laundered only at the expense of the unit. PPE is considered contaminated even if no visibly evidence of contamination is present and shall be commercially laundered at the expense of the unit. All linen shall be commercially laundered at the expense of the unit. All surgical scrubs, even if not contaminated will not be taken home for self-laundering and shall be commercially laundered only at the expense of the unit.

b. Handling contaminated laundry. Contaminated laundry, including scrubs, shall be placed and transported in bags labeled or color-coded in accordance with OSHA Regulation, Bloodborne Pathogens Standards, 1910.1030(g)(1)(i). (If contaminated laundry is wet, bags or containers must prevent leakage or soak-through). Gloves and other appropriate PPE will be worn when handling contaminated laundry.

c. Linen. Although research has identified soiled linens as a source of large numbers of certain pathogenic microorganisms, the risk of linens actually transmitting disease is negligible. When handling soiled linen, it is recommended to always wear gloves. Handle it as little as possible and with minimum agitation to prevent gross microbial contamination of the air and persons handling the linen. Carefully check linen for sharps objects and remove them before washing. Bag all soiled linen where used; do not sort or rinse it in patient care areas.

12. Cleaning and Decontaminating Blood or Other Body Fluid Spills. Use an EPA-approved germicide or recommended surface disinfectant agent to promptly clean all blood and blood-contaminated fluid spills. Health care workers must wear gloves. First remove visible material with disposable towels or other appropriate means that prevent direct contact with blood. If anticipating splashing, wear protective eyewear and an impervious gown or apron that provides an effective barrier to splashes. Next decontaminate the area with disinfectant solution or an appropriate EPA-approved germicide. Clean and decontaminate soiled cleaning equipment or put it in an appropriate container and dispose of it according to clinic policy. Use plastic bags clearly labeled as containing infectious waste to remove contaminated items from the spill site. Remove gloves; then wash hands.

13. Infectious Waste.

a. Medical waste. Epidemiological evidence does not suggest most clinic waste is any more infectious than residential waste. However, public concern about the risk of medical wastes must not be ignored. Identifying wastes for which special precautions are necessary include those wastes which potentially cause infection during handling and disposal and for which special precautions appear prudent, including sharps, microbiology laboratory waste, pathology waste, and blood specimens or products. While any item that has touched blood, exudates, or secretions potentially may be infectious, it is usually not considered practical or necessary to treat all such waste as infectious. Materials containing small amounts of blood, saliva, or other secretions such as tainted gauze pads, sanitary napkins, or facial tissues are not considered infectious waste. Generally, autoclave or incinerate infectious waste before disposing of it in a sanitary landfill. Infectious waste autoclaving standards are different from normal sterilization standards. Carefully pour bulk blood, suctioned fluids, excretions, and secretions down a drain connected to a sanitary sewer. Or for materials capable of it, grind and flush such items into sanitary sewers (some states prohibit this practice).

b. Environmental Protection Agency classification. The Environmental Protection Agency classifies health care facilities as generators of infectious waste based on the weight of waste generated. CG classification is based on facility type. All CG clinics are considered generators. Each CG health care facility must have a written infectious waste management protocol consistent with state and local regulations in the unit's area.

c. Biohazard. Biohazard warning labels shall be affixed to regulated waste containers; refrigerators, and freezers containing blood or other potentially infectious material; and other containers used to store, transport, or ship blood or other potentially infectious materials with these exceptions:

   (1) Substitute red bags for labels on regulated waste bags or containers. OSHA believes red bags protect personnel because they must comply with OSHA BBP Standard Paragraph (g)(2)(iv)(M), which requires training personnel to understand the meaning of all color-coding.

   (2) Individual containers of blood or other potentially infectious materials placed in a labeled container during storage, transport, shipment or disposal.

14. Managing Exposures (Bloodborne Pathogen Exposure Control).

   a. Exposure.

      (1) An exposure occurs if a health care worker comes in contact with blood or other body fluids in one of these ways:

         (a) Parenteral—through a needle stick or cut;

         (b) Mucous membrane—from a splash to the eye or mouth;

         (c) Cutaneous—contact with large amounts of blood or prolonged contact with blood when the health care worker's exposed skin is chapped, abraded, or afflicted with dermatitis.

      (2) After an exposure, if the source of the exposure is known, obtain the source person's consent (if applicable), making sure to follow local laws governing consent for testing non-active duty source persons and incompetent or unconscious persons.

      (3) The treating healthcare provider will perform an initial screening of the exposure incident to determine if the "source" is known to be HIV positive. This should be done within 15 minutes of the exposure. If the "source" is known to be HIV positive, the treating physician will contact the nearest

hospital with infectious disease services, notify them of the exposure and arrange a time for the exposed worker to be seen ASAP.

(4) Post-exposure prophylaxis (PEP) should be initiated as soon as possible, preferably within hours rather than days of exposure. If a question exists concerning which antiretroviral drugs to use, or whether to use a basic or expanded regimen, the basic regimen should be started immediately rather than delay PEP administration. The optimal duration of PEP is unknown, however the CDC recommends a 4 week period for PEP. The nearest local hospital with infectious disease services should be consulted for additional guidance.

(5) If the HIV status of the source is not known, a rapid HIV antibody test should be performed on the source at the nearest local hospital or USMTF (protocol for clinic use of rapid HIV antibody testing will be developed soon). Each clinic should have a local hospital point of contact who can assist with obtaining stat HIV results. Viromed should not be utilized for stat testing because the results will not be available until 48 hours post-exposure. If the test is positive, the treating physician should prescribe HIV PEP based on CDC guidelines.

(6) In addition to determining the HIV status of the source, a blood sample should be drawn and tested for, Hepatitis B Surface Antigen, Hepatitis C Antibody, and for the ALT status of the source person. Provide the source person post-test counseling and treatment referrals. Inform the exposed person of the source person's test results and applicable laws and regulations on disclosing the source person's identity and infectious status. It is extremely important all persons who seek consultation for any HIV-related concerns receive appropriate counseling from a USMTF or other medical facility capable of providing this service.

(7) After an exposure, any worker (active duty, civilian, or contractor) incurring an exposure to blood/body fluids will wash or flush the area for at least 5 minutes, and then report the exposure immediately to their supervisor. The exposed individual is to then to seek medical attention immediately. Workers reporting to an outside facility initially should follow-up at a CG clinic on the next day (during regular business hours).

(8) Recommendations for Hepatitis B PEP and HIV PEP are located in paragraphs (b) and (c). Currently, there is no recommendation for Hepatitis C PEP. Both active duty and civilian workers will be followed by the local CG clinic. Contract workers will be contacted by a healthcare provider to educate them on their need to follow-up with their private physician and to provide them the results on the "source'.

(9) All clinics shall ensure the health care professional evaluating a worker after an exposure incident has this information:

(a) A copy of the OSHA BBP Standard;

(b) A description of the exposed employee's duties as they relate to the exposure incident;

(c) Documentation of the route(s) of exposure and circumstances under which exposure occurred; and

(d) Results of the source individual's blood tests, if available; and all records on the employee's appropriate treatment, including vaccination.

(10) The SME shall obtain and give the exposed person a copy of the evaluating health care professional's written opinion within 15 days after the evaluation is complete. The healthcare professional's written opinion for post-exposure evaluation and follow-up shall be limited to the following:

(a) Written opinion for Hepatitis B vaccination shall be limited to whether Hepatitis B vaccination is indicated for an employee, and if the employee has received such vaccination.

(b) The employee has been informed of the results of the evaluation.

(c) The employee has been told about any medical conditions resulting from exposure to blood or other potentially infectious materials which require further evaluation or treatment.

(11) A copy of the SME's written opinion will also be provided to the SHSO or health services department head. The QI coordinator or his or her designee also will retain a copy and ensure all required follow-up treatment and testing is documented. The SHSO or health services department head shall ensure that the following this management protocol is adhered.

(12) Utilize CG-6201, Bloodborne Pathogen Exposure Guidelines.

b. <u>Hepatitis B Virus Post-exposure Management</u>.

(1) For a worker exposed to a source individual found to be positive for HbsAg:

(a) The exposed worker who has not previously received Hepatitis B vaccine will receive the vaccine series. A single dose of Hepatitis B immune globulin (HBIG) if it can be given within 7 days of exposure is also recommended.

(b) Test the exposed worker who has previously received Hepatitis B vaccine for antibody to Hepatitis B surface antigen (anti-HBs). If the antibody level in the worker's blood sample is inadequate (i.e., less than 10 SRU by RIA, negative by EIA) give the exposed employee one dose of vaccine and one dose of HBIG.

(2) If the source individual is negative for HbsAg and the worker has not been vaccinated, the worker shall receive Hepatitis B vaccination.

(3) If the source individual refuses testing or cannot be identified, the unvaccinated worker should receive the Hepatitis B vaccine series. Consider administering HBIG on an individual basis if the source individual is known or suspected to be at high risk of HBV infection. At his or her discretion the responsible Medical Officer will manage and treat as needed previously vaccinated workers who are exposed to a source who refuses testing or is not identifiable.

(4) Additional guidance on Hepatitis B PEP be found at the CDC Updated USPHS Guidelines for the Management of Occupational Exposures to HBV, HCV, and HIV and Recommendations for Postexposure Prophylaxis, MMWR, June 29, 2001 / 50(RR11):1-42 – http://www.cdc.gov/mmwr/preview/mmwrhtml/rr5011a1.htm

c. <u>Human Immunodeficiency Virus Post-exposure Management</u>.

(1) Workers who have an occupational exposure to HIV should receive follow-up counseling, post-exposure testing, and medical evaluation regardless of whether they receive PEP. In view of the evolving nature of HIV post-exposure management, the health care provider must be well informed of current CDC guidelines on this subject. The basic regimen includes:

(a) Zidovudine (Retrovir, ZDV, AZT) plus lamivudine (Epivir, 3TC) which is available as Combivir. The preferred dosing is - ZDV: 300 mg twice daily or 200 mg three times daily, with food; total: 600 mg daily plus 3TC: 300 mg once daily or 150 mg twice daily or as Combivir: one tablet twice daily (300 mg ZDV + 150 mg 3TC); OR

(b) Zidovudine (Retrovir, ZDV, AZT) plus emtricitabine (Emtriva, FTC). The preferred dosing is - ZDV: 300 mg twice daily or 200 mg three times daily, with food; total: 600 mg/day, in 2-3 divided doses plus FTC: 200 mg (one capsule) once daily; OR

(c) Tenofovir (Viread, TDF) plus lamivudine (Epivir, 3TC). The preferred dosing is - TDF: 300 mg once daily plus 3TC: 300 mg once daily or 150 mg twice daily; OR

(d) Tenofovir (Viread, TDF) plus emtricitabine (Emtriva, FTC) which is available as Truvada. The preferred dosing is - TDF: 300 mg once daily plus FTC: 200 mg once daily or as Truvada: one tablet daily.

(2) For alternate basic regimens, consult an infectious disease physician or refer to the CDC Updated USPHS Guidelines for the Management of Occupational Exposures to HIV and Recommendations for Postexposure Prophylaxis, MMWR, September 30, 2005 / 54(RR09):1-17 - http://www.cdc.gov/mmwr/preview/mmwrhtml/rr5409a1.htm. If a provider prescribes Lopinavir/ritonavir (Kaletra) – the preferred dosing listed in the CDC reference is erroneous. The correct dosing is LPV/RTV: 400/100 mg.

(3) The Bloodborne Pathogen Exposure Control Plan Instruction, COMDINST M6220.8 (series), offers additional guidance on HIV PEP. If PEP is used, workers should be monitored for drug toxicity by testing at baseline and again 2 weeks after starting PEP. The scope of testing should be based on medical conditions in the exposed person and the toxicity of drugs included in the PEP regimen. Minimally, laboratory monitoring for toxicity should include a complete blood count and renal and hepatic function tests. If toxicity is noted, modification of the regimen should be considered after expert consultation; further diagnostic studies might be indicated.

(4) Exposed workers who choose to take PEP should be advised of the importance of completing the prescribed regimen. Information should be provided about potential drug interactions and drugs that should not be taken with PEP, side effects of prescribed drugs, measures to minimize side effects, and methods of clinical monitoring for toxicity during the follow-up period. Evaluation of certain symptoms (e.g., rash, fever, back or abdominal pain, pain on urination or blood in the urine, or symptoms of hyperglycemia (e.g., increased thirst or frequent urination) should not be delayed.

(5) After the initial test at the time of exposure, retest seronegative workers 6 weeks, 12 weeks, and 6 months after exposure to determine whether HIV transmission has occurred. Extended HIV follow-up (e.g., for 12 months) is recommended for workers who become infected with the HCV after exposure to a source coinfected with HIV and HCV. During this follow-up period (especially the first 6 to 12 weeks after exposure, when most infected persons seroconvert), exposed workers must follow CDC recommendations to prevent transmitting HIV, including refraining from blood donation, informing health care workers rendering treatment of his or her status, and using appropriate protection during sexual intercourse. During all phases of follow-up, it is vital to protect worker confidentiality.

(6) Advise the exposed worker to report and seek medical evaluation for any acute febrile illness occurring within 12 weeks after exposure. Such an illness, particularly one characterized by fever, rash, or lymphadenopathy, may indicate recent HIV infection. HIV testing should be performed on any exposed worker who has an illness compatible with an acute retroviral syndrome, regardless of the interval since exposure. A person in whom

HIV infection is identified should be referred for medical management to a specialist with expertise in HIV treatment and counseling.

(7) If the source individual's tests are seronegative, perform a baseline testing of the exposed worker with optional follow-up testing 12 weeks later if the worker desires or the health care provider recommends it. After the initial test at the time of exposure, at the responsible Medical Officer's discretion, retest consenting seronegative source individuals at 12 weeks and 6 months afterward.

(8) If the source individual cannot be identified, decide appropriate follow-up on an individual basis. All workers concerned they have been infected with HIV through an occupational exposure should undergo serologic testing.

(9) Follow CDC recommendations for preventing HIV and HBV transmission to patients during exposure-prone procedures, defined as those invasive procedures with a recognized risk of percutaneous injury to health care workers.

(10) All health care workers shall adhere to standard precautions. Health care workers with exuding lesions or weeping dermatitis shall refrain from all direct patient care. Health care workers shall comply with current CDC guidelines for disinfecting and sterilizing equipment and supplies.

(11) All health care workers performing exposure-prone procedures shall know their HIV and HBV status.

(12) All health care workers who are HIV or HBV positive shall refrain from performing exposure-prone procedures.

15. <u>Training Personnel for Occupational Exposure</u>. All Health Services Divisions or Branches will inform and train personnel in occupational exposure initially on assignment and annually thereafter. Personnel who have taken appropriate training within the past year need to receive additional training only on subjects not previously covered. The training program shall contain at least these elements:

   a. An accessible copy and explanation of the regulatory text of this standard (Federal Register 56 (235): 64175, December 6, 1991 [29 USC 1910.1030]).

   b. A general explanation of the epidemiology and symptoms of bloodborne diseases.

   c. An explanation of bloodborne pathogen transmission modes.

   d. An explanation of the exposure control plan outlined in Section 13-J.

e. An explanation of the appropriate methods to recognize tasks and other activities that may involve exposure to blood and other potentially infectious materials.

f. An explanation of methods to reduce or prevent exposure, such as barrier techniques, and their limitations.

g. Information on the types and properly using, locating, removing, handling, decontaminating, and disposing of personal protective equipment.

h. An explanation of the basis for selecting personal protective equipment.

i. Hepatitis B vaccine. Information on the Hepatitis B vaccine, including efficacy, safety, administration, and benefits. This vaccination is mandatory for active duty and reserve personnel.

j. Information on appropriate actions to take and persons to contact in an emergency involving blood or other potentially infectious materials.

k. Explanation of the procedures. An explanation of the procedure to follow if an exposure incident occurs, including the method of reporting the incident and available medical follow-up described in Section 13-J-13.

l. Information on the post-exposure evaluation and follow-up the Senior Medical Officer (SMO) or designee is required to provide for the employee after an exposure incident.

m. An explanation of the signs, labels, and/or color coding required for sharps and biohazardous materials.

n. A question-and-answer period with the person conducting the training session.

This page intentionally left blank.

Section K. Patient Safety and Risk Management Program.

1. Purpose... 1
2. Informed Consent... 1
3. Adverse Event Monitoring and Reporting.. 4
4. Patient Safety Training 8

This page intentionally left blank.

K. Patient Safety and Risk Management Program.

1. Purpose.

    a. Background. The patient safety and risk management program supports quality medical care by identifying, analyzing, and preventing actual and potential risks to patients and staff. The program provides mechanisms to detect and prevent medical errors, accidents and injuries and reduces the cost of claims and loss of other resources. Patient safety involves a variety of clinical and administrative activities that identify, evaluate and reduce the potential for harm to beneficiaries and to improve the quality of health care.

    b. Responsibilities. Patient safety and risk management programs are most effective if they are prospective, preventive, and comprehensive. All staff members, beneficiaries, contract providers, and volunteers shall be aware of risks in the clinical environment and act safely and responsibly to implement program requirements. Patient safety and risk management activities are not limited to claims activities but examine all instances of actual and potential risk or loss. Successful patient safety programs facilitate a non-punitive, interdisciplinary approach to decrease unanticipated adverse health care outcomes. The organizational focus is on continued learning about risks and risk management strategies and reengineering systems/processes to reduce the chance of human error.

2. Informed Consent.

    a. Background. Every person, with a few exceptions, has the right to be examined and treated only in the manner they authorize. This individual prerogative is based on the concept a competent patient has the right to make informed decisions about health care. Consent for health care must be informed, voluntary, competent, and specific, and is clearly an important issue in quality patient care. The objective of informed consent is improved patient-provider communication in non-emergent situations, which should result in patients' realistic expectations about the nature of treatment and the expected outcome, and reduced liability for the government. Clear documentation demonstrating the patient was properly informed is necessary to protect the patient, the provider, and the government. Although patients must be informed of treatment options, military members who refuse treatment necessary to render them fit for duty (including immunization) are subject to separation and/or disciplinary action (see Chapter 2-Section A. 4. b.).

    b. Responsibilities.

        (1) SHSO: The SHSO must publish facility-specific implementing instructions that ensure providers carry out the spirit and intent of this Section. The SHSO and HSWL SC should monitor compliance with consent policies and procedures as a regular part of medical and dental records review.

(2) Health Care Providers: Responsible health care providers must counsel patients before treatment and document receiving the patient's informed consent.

c. Types of Consent.

(1) Expressed Consent: This type of consent is obtained by open discussion between the provider and patient and must include a statement the patient consents to the proposed procedure. Expressed consent may be oral or written.

(2) Oral Consent. Except where this regulation specifically requires written consent, oral consent is sufficient authorization for treatment. However, oral consent is difficult to prove. If a health care provider receives oral consent to treatment, he or she must document it by an entry in the treatment record. Consent received from competent authority by telephone is a form of oral expressed consent; a person not directly involved in the patient's care should witness such consent; and it must be documented by an entry in the treatment record.

(3) Conditions Requiring Written Consent. Document written consent by having the patient sign forms authorizing treatment and including an entry in the treatment record that discusses the requirements outlined in Paragraph 13-K-4. Except in emergencies, written consent is required for these situations:

(a) All surgical procedures (including, among others, placing sutures, incision and drainage, removing a foreign body(s), cauterizing, removing wart(s), injecting medications into a joint(s), etc.)

(b) Invasive tests and procedures to diagnose and treat disease or remove tissue specimens (e.g., biopsies), except routine phlebotomy.

(c) Anesthesia, including local dental anesthesia.

(d) All dental procedures.

(e) Genitourinary procedures including vasectomies, IUD insertion or removal, etc.

d. Implied Consent. Implied consent is derived from the patient's conduct even if he or she does not communicate specific words of consent. Assume implied consent only if one can reasonably presume the patient knows the risks, benefits, and alternatives to treatment. For example, a patient's presence at dental sick call is implied consent for a dental exam. Never accept implied consent to treatment involving surgical therapy or invasive diagnostic procedures except in emergencies.

e. Emergencies. Consent before treatment is not necessary when immediate. treatment is required to preserve the patient's life or limb. The provider will document the existence and scope of the emergency and describe the events precluding obtaining consent.

f. Who May Consent. Generally, competent adult patients who have the capacity to manage their own affairs who present themselves for treatment have the authority to consent. If a patient is incompetent due either to statutory incompetence (e.g., a minor) or mental impairment, then it must determined who the individual with legal capacity to consent and obtain his or her consent before examining or treating the patient. Laws defining minors and to what they may legally consent differ by state. The law of the state where the facility is located governs legal capacity to consent. Each clinic will develop a policy for treating minors.

g. Information to Provide. The provider must advise the patient of the nature of his or her condition; describe the proposed treatment in terms the patient can understand; and explain the material risks and expected benefits of the proposed treatment course, available alternative health care options, and the option of non-treatment. A material risk is one a reasonable person likely would consider significant in deciding whether to undertake therapy and is a function of the likelihood of occurrence, the severity of the injury it threatens to cause, and existing reasonable alternatives. A provider is not required to explain risk that are considered extremely remote unless the patient requests an explanation or the potential adverse consequences are so grave a reasonable person in the patient's particular circumstances would consider the risk important.

h. Informing the Patient. Health care providers will provide information in a manner that allows a patient of ordinary understanding to intelligently weigh the risks and benefits when faced with the choice of selecting among the alternatives or refusing treatment altogether. Health care providers must communicate in language one can reasonably expect the patient to understand. Although open discussions between the responsible health care provider and the patient should be the standard, each department may develop internal methods to acquaint patients with the benefits, risks, and alternatives to procedures requiring consent. In some departments, prepared pamphlets or information sheets may be desirable.

i. Documentation. Regardless of the method used to inform the patient or the form of consent (oral or written), the provider must document the disclosure and the patient's reactions in the medical or dental record. It is highly recommended to document this in progress notes even if the patient has signed a preprinted "consent" form. Progress notes written to document disclosing information to the patient will be specific about the information provided. The notes must specifically enumerate risks, alternative forms of treatment, and expected benefits the provider discussed with the patient. Use the Request for Administration of Anesthesia and for Performance of Operations and Other

Procedures, SF-522 to document consent in all surgical, anesthetic and reproductive procedures.

j. <u>Witness to Consent</u>. All consent forms require a witness's signature. The witness may be a health care facility member who is not participating in the procedure or treatment. Patients' relatives are not acceptable as witnesses. The witness confirms the patient signed the form, not that he or she received all relevant information.

k. <u>Duration of Consent</u>. Consent is valid as long as no material change in circumstances occurs between the date the patient consented and the procedure or treatment date. Obtain new consent if a material change in circumstances occurs, for example the provisional diagnosis changes. If more than seven (7) days elapse between the date the patient signed the consent and the date treatment begins, provider and patient must re-sign, re-initial, and re-date the consent form. A new consent is not required for each stage in a series of treatments for a specific medical condition (e.g., repeated application of liquid nitrogen to warts).

3. <u>Adverse Event Monitoring and Reporting</u>.

    a. <u>Definitions</u>.

        (1) Action Plan: The end product of a Root Cause Analysis that identifies the risk reduction strategies to prevent the recurrence of similar adverse events.

        (2) Adverse Event: An occurrence or condition associated with the provision of health care or services that may result in harm or permanent effect. Adverse events may be due to acts of omission or commission. Incidents such as falls or erroneous administration of medications are also considered adverse events even if there is no harm or permanent effect.

        (3) Contributing Factors: Additional reasons for an event or series of events that may result in harm, which could apply to individuals, systems operations or the organization.

        (4) Near Miss: An event or situation that could have resulted in harm but did not either by chance or timely intervention.

        (5) Root Cause: The most basic reason that a situation or treatment did not turn out as planned or as expected.

        (6) Root Cause Analysis: A process for identifying the basic or contributing causal factor(s) associated with a sentinel event, an adverse event or close call. The review is interdisciplinary and includes those who are closest to the process, and focuses on systems and processes, not individual performance. An ad hoc Root Cause Analysis Team, with membership as

necessary depending on the event, is identified by the patient safety official to develop the Root Cause Analysis and Action Plan.

(7) Safety Assessment Code: A risk assessment tool that considers the severity of an adverse or near miss event together with the probability of the event's recurrence. The score, or Safety Assessment Code, assigned to the event determines the type of action that should be taken, e.g., Root Cause Analysis (score 3), intense analysis (score 2 or 1) or no action. Severity is divided into four categories – catastrophic, major, moderate, and minor. Probability is divided into three categories – high, medium, and low. This provides a standardized process for prioritizing actions and applying resources where there is the greatest opportunity to improve safety.

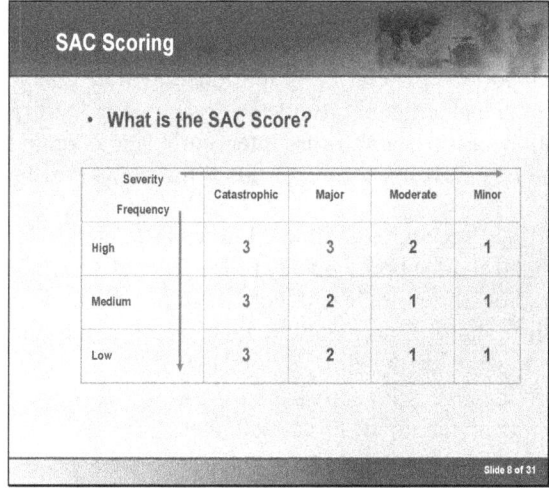

Table 13-K-1

(8) Sentinel Event: An unexpected occurrence involving death or serious physical or psychological injury, or the risk thereof that is not related to the natural course of an individual's illnesses or underlying condition. Such events signal the need for immediate investigation and proactive response on the part of the organization.

b. <u>Significant Events</u>. Events are not reviewed to place blame or discipline those involved, but rather to assess the health care process (es) and systems involved and identify potential areas for improvements in patient safety. The CG Health Care Program uses the resulting recommendations to determine health care policy, personnel, equipment and training needs to prevent future adverse health care outcomes or patient injuries. A significant event may result in initiating a Mishap Board as the Safety and Environmental Health Manual, COMDTINST M5100.47 (series), requires and a legal investigation conducted concurrently with a medical incident review of the same event (e.g., a vessel collision with injuries). In most cases however, an adverse event review will occur solely within a CG health care facility or the CG Health Care Program.

c. <u>Responsibilities</u>.

   (1) SHSO: The SHSO must publish facility-specific implementing instructions that ensure providers carry out the spirit and intent of this Section.

   (2) Health Care Providers: Identification and reporting of near misses and adverse events must be encouraged as an expectation of everyday practice by CG health care. Prevention of harm to patients and reporting all potential and/or adverse events is a performance expectation for all CG health care program staff.

d. <u>Immediate Actions</u>. Upon identification of a patient safety event, the staff member will immediately perform necessary health care interventions to protect and support the patient(s). Practitioners will be contacted as soon as possible to report the incident and provide an update. The staff member/practitioner will take all necessary health care interventions to contain risk and to present event-related materials that may be needed for analysis or investigation.

e. <u>Reporting Procedure</u>. Within 24 hours after an adverse event occurs, the command shall submit copy(s) of Emergency Care and Treatment Report, SF-558 and/or Chronological Record of Care, SF-600 for events occurring within the clinic and/or Emergency Medical Treatment Report, CG-5214 for events occurring outside the clinic to the HSWL SC. Clearly mark "Patient Safety Report" in large print across the top of these forms. Stamp or print this statement on the top of each document: "This is a medical quality assurance document. It is protected by Federal law." HSWL SC shall send copies of the documents to Commandant (CG-112) within three days of receipt.

f. <u>Review Procedure</u>. On receiving one of the three forms, HSWL SC conferring with Commandant (CG-112), shall review the document(s); verify the event meets the Paragraph 13-K-3 criteria for an adverse event or near miss; determine whether an on-site medical review or Root Cause Analysis shall be conducted; and designate a single point of contact at Commandant (CG-112). A Root Cause Analysis must be conducted and an Action Plan completed for all adverse events with Severity Assessment Code 3.

   (1) If HSWL SC after conferring with Commandant (CG-112), determines a medical incident review is unnecessary, they shall notify the command by letter within 10 working days of the event and send a copy of the letter to Commandant (CG-112).

   (2) If an on-site medical incident review or Root Cause Analysis is indicated, HSWL SC shall notify the involved command as soon as possible and designate a clinic professional staff member to conduct a review or convene a panel of qualified professional staff members from the involved facility,

to review all aspects of the incident. To ensure confidentiality, the panel shall consist of only the designated facility point of contact and the persons HSWL SC appoint.

(3) If a patient safety event is an intentional unsafe act that results from gross negligence or possible criminal activity, the event shall be reported to the appropriate authorities for investigation.

g. <u>Incident review officer or Root Cause Analysis Team</u>. The incident review officer or Root Cause Analysis Team shall request and review all relevant documents and reports, interview personnel as required, and when the review is complete, submit a written letter report with this information on the incident to Commandant (CG-112) through the HSWL SC:

(1) Synopsis. A brief summary of the incident and injuries and/or fatalities involved.

(2) Factual Information. Factual information and data about the incident and personnel involved shall consist of at least these topics:

(a) History. The chronological order of any significant event preceding, during, and after the incident, including any written logs or transcripts of radio logs substantiating this chronology, such as the Emergency Care and Treatment, SF-558, the Emergency Medical Treatment Report, CG-5214, or the Chronological Record of Care, SF-600.

(b) Injuries. Describe each injury, or in the case of fatalities, the cause of death. Include autopsy findings when available.

(c) Professional qualifications of all persons who delivered health care, if relevant, including all recent applicable training and certificates (e.g., ACLS, BLS, EMT, HS, etc.).

(d) Equipment Performance. List all pertinent medical equipment used during the incident and any failures due to mechanical malfunction, operator error, inadequate training, or other factors. Describe whether equipment involved was maintained or serviced according to manufacturers' specifications.

(e) Applicable Medical and/or Dental Guidelines.

(3) Analysis and Conclusions. The analysis and conclusion should contain the individual's or panel's hypothesis of the circumstances surrounding the event, emphasizing the health care aspect, including a brief conclusion about the health care rendered and how it contributed to the event's outcome.

(4) Action Plan. The action plan comprises recommended modifications and risk reduction strategies in policy, staffing, equipment, training, or other health care delivery system aspects that need improvement to avoid similar incidents in the future. The action plan should address responsibility for implementation, oversight, pilot testing (if appropriate), timelines and the metrics to be used in evaluating the effectiveness of the actions taken.

h. Routing Patient Safety Review Reports.

(1) The completed root cause analysis report will be sent from the clinic to Commandant (CG-112) thru HSWL SC for review and appropriate action.

(2) Staff members who submit patient safety event reports shall receive timely feedback on the actions being taken as a result of their report. Management efforts and activities shall focus on improving the systems and processes that may have contributed to the patient safety event.

(3) In cases involving an unanticipated outcome of care, a qualified health care provider shall inform the patient. QI-protected information shall not be released or provided to the patient. During the communication, at least one other health care program staff member should be present. The provider shall document in the patient's record what was communicated.

4. Patient Safety Training.

a. All health care program staff shall receive patient safety, risk management and teamwork education during their initial orientation and on an as-needed basis.

b. Patient safety topics shall include an overview of the patient safety and risk management program, roles and responsibilities in reporting patient safety events, patient education in safety and effective communication strategies.

Section L. Training and Professional Development.

1. Definitions.. 1
2. Unit Health Services Training Plan (In-Service Training). 1
3. Emergency Medical Training Requirements. 3
4. Health Services Technician "A" School. 4
5. Health Services Technician "C" Schools. 4
6. Continuing Education Programs. 5
7. Long-Term Training Programs. 6

This page intentionally left blank.

Section L. Training and Professional Development.

1. Definitions.

    a. ACLS (Advanced Cardiac Life Support). Sponsored by the American Heart Association (AHA) and American Safety and Health Institute (ASHI), this 16-hour program (8 hours for recertification) emphasizes cardiac-related diagnostic and therapeutic techniques and grants a completion certificate valid for two years on completion. An ACLS certificate of completion recognizes a person completed the course and does not in any way authorize him or her to perform skills taught there. ACLS also sometimes refers to the cardiac component of Advanced Life Support. Online ACLS courses without hands-on skills proficiency testing are not accepted substitutes for the ACLS courses noted above.

    b. Advanced Life Support (ALS). A general term applied to pre-hospital skills beyond the basic life support level including, among others, EKG interpretation, medication administration, and advanced airway techniques.

    c. Basic Life Support (BLS) for the Health Care Provider. Health care providers must successfully complete and maintain proficiency in a program sponsored by any of the following: The Military Training Network, American Heart Association (AHA), American Red Cross (ARC), American Safety & Health Institute (ASHI) or the American College of Emergency Physicians (ACEP). (The Military Training Network is the preferred choice). Successful completion grants certification for 2 years. The course curriculum of all programs includes basic skills (e.g. airway maintenance, cardiac compression and use of the automatic external defibrillator) necessary to sustain heart and brain function until advanced skills can be administered.

    d. Emergency Medical Technician (EMT). A general term referring to the certification of pre-hospital care providers. Three skill levels (EMT-Basic, EMT-Intermediate, EMT-Paramedic) are recognized, but functions performed at each level vary significantly by jurisdiction. When the term EMT is used alone, it refers to EMT-Basic, which performs BLS skills. The term EMT applies to all CG personnel with EMT training and certification regardless of rating.

    e. Paramedic. An individual certified by the National Registry of Emergency Medical Technicians as an Emergency Medical Technician-Paramedic (NREMTP) or certified by a local governing body to perform ALS procedures under a physician's license.

2. Unit Health Services Training Plan (In-Service Training).

    a. Health Services Units. These personnel must have an on-going in-service training program aimed at all providers with emphasis on the Health Services Technicians' professional development. It is expected of clinic staff members attending outside training to share new information with other staff members.

In-service training sessions allow clinics to ensure issues of clinical significance are presented to their staff.

b. <u>Clinic Training Program must include these topics, among others</u>.

(1) Quality Improvement Implementation Guide Exercises.

(2) Annual review of clinic protocols on suicide, sexual assault, and family violence.

(3) Patient satisfaction issues.

(4) Patient sensitivity.

(5) Patient confidentiality to include HIPAA guidelines.

(6) Emergency I.V. therapy.

(7) Emergency airway management.

(8) Cardiac monitor and defibrillator familiarization.

(9) Cervical spine immobilization and patient transport equipment.

(10) Emergency vehicle operator's training (where operated).

(11) Section 13-J: Infection and Exposure Control Program.

c. <u>Health Services Training Coordinator (HSTC)</u>. The SHSO must designate in writing a Health Services Training Coordinator (HSTC) who coordinates clinic in-service training, distributes a quarterly training schedule, and maintains the unit's health services training record. The HSTC's responsibilities include these:

(1) Establishes and maintains a Health Services Training Record to document all training conducted within the clinic. Records should include presentation outline, title, program date, name of presenter, and list of attendees. Maintain training records for 3 years from the date on which training occurred.

(2) Ensures all emergency medical training is documented in the individual's CG Training Record, CG-5285 for credit toward the 48-hour National Registry EMT continuing education requirement.

(3) Maintains a Training Record section that records personnel certifications including CPR, ACLS, EMT, and flight qualifications, including expiration dates and copies of the current certificate. The HSTC should ensure assigned personnel obtain recertification before current certificates expire.

3. Emergency Medical Training Requirements.

    a. BLS Certification. All active duty, civilian, and contract civilian personnel working in CG clinics and sick bays shall maintain current BLS certification at the health care provider level (AHA "C" Course or equivalent).

    b. SAR or MEDEVAC. Every Health Services Technician, or other CG EMT (eg Rescue Swimmer), who participates in SAR or MEDEVAC operations must be a currently certified EMT by NREMT or equivalent state organization. The Flight Surgeon may authorize, in writing, EMTs to perform BLS and ALS skills in the course of their assigned SAR/MEDEVAC duties.

    c. Emergency Vehicles. At least one currently certified EMT will staff CG Emergency Vehicles. CG Emergency Vehicles will, at a minimum, meet standards established under Federal Specification KKK-A-1822E and as defined under CFR 42 Part 410 Section 41. Unit CO shall ensure HS's are trained in sufficient numbers under Section 13-L-3.h to meet this requirement. This staffing requirement does not apply to general-purpose vehicles used by the medical department. However, general-purpose vehicles shall not be equipped with emergency warning lights and/or sirens nor shall they display a "star of life" insignia or other emblem implying emergency medical capabilities. Emergency vehicles shall be equipped to provide basic life support (BLS) only. The clinic shall maintain equipment (monitor-defibrillator, advanced airway kit etc.) and medications to provide ALS services in a reserve status and add them when necessary if authorized ALS providers are available.

    d. ACLS Certification. All Medical Officers serving in clinical assignments will maintain current ACLS certification. Only licensed or certified physicians, nurse practitioners, physician assistants, or nationally registered advanced life support providers (EMT-P and EMT-I) will perform ALS procedures, except as Section 13-L-3.e stipulates. Paramedics may perform functions authorized by their certifying jurisdiction's protocols with written Medical Officer authority. Other than those described this section, persons who have completed an ACLS course should note certification means only they have completed the course and does not convey a license to perform any skill. Individuals completing ACLS courses shall serve as a clinic resource on current standards for pre-hospital care in training and equipment areas. ACLS classes that are electronic only (e-ACLS) do not satisfy this certification requirement. Individuals with documented training and demonstrated proficiency may request and obtain written authorization by a local CG Medical Officer to perform emergency medical procedures not normally associated with EMT-B skill sets (e.g. use of Combitube).

    e. EMT training (basic course or recertification). Commands shall use local military sources if available. Usually most public service training agencies or community colleges offering training can accept CG personnel. If the required training is not available from a civilian or military source within a 50-mile radius, commands may use other cost-effective training sources. Submit requests through the chain of command to Commandant (CG-112) with these items:

(1) Short-Term Resident Training Request, CG-5223;

(2) Request, Authorization, Agreement and Certification of Training, SF-182;

(3) Requests for training outside a 50-mile radius which incur per diem expense require the unit CO's or officer-in-charge's statement local training sources are unavailable.

4. Health Services Technician "A" School.

   a. The Office of Personnel and Training operates the 14-week introductory course for Health Services Technicians, including the Emergency Medical Technician (EMT) course, at TRACEN Petaluma. As program manager, Commandant (CG-1121) provides professional comments to the TRACEN on curriculum and qualifying requirements. Commandant (CG-132) controls HS "A" School personnel quotas. The Training and Education Manual, COMDTINST M1500.1(series), outlines selection requirements and procedures.

   b. All HS "A" School students must successfully pass the NREMT-B examination in order to advance to HS3 upon graduation.

5. Health Services Technician "C" Schools.

   a. Training. Due to the specialized nature of health care, the CG requires some Health Services Technicians to complete training in medical specialty fields such as aviation medicine, preventive medicine, medical and dental equipment repair, physical therapy, laboratory, radiology, pharmacy, and independent-duty specialties. The usual sources are Department of Defense training programs and through IDHS training which is conducted at CG Training Center Petaluma.

   b. Selection for HS "C" Schools. Selection for HS "C" Schools is based on qualification code requirements for HS billets at clinics and independent duty sites as specified in personnel allowance lists. Secondary selection criteria include command requests, personnel requests, and deficiencies noted on HSWL SC Quality Improvement Site Surveys.

   c. Training Request. HS personnel should submit a Short-Term Resident Training Request CG-5223, with Command endorsement to Commandant (CG-1121) through the appropriate chain of command. Commandant (CG-1121) must receive this request at least 45 days before the training convening date. HS personnel wishing to pursue "C" school training in courses of 20 weeks or longer require a permanent change of duty station coordinated by Commander, Personnel Service Center (PSC-epm-2).

6. Continuing Education Programs.

    a. Licensing. All PHS and CG Physician Assistants must maintain active professional licenses and/or certification to practice their professional specialty while assigned to the CG. Licensing and/or recertification requirements often demand continuing professional education, which enhances the practitioner's skills and professional credentials.

    b. Funding. The Director of Health and Safety encourages one continuing education course annually for all licensed health services professionals. The funding command using HSC 30 funds will approve the Short Term Training Requests. This program is in addition to the operational medicine (AFC 56) training program (see Medical Manual Chapter 1. Section C). Generally training should provide at least six documented continuing education credits per day pertinent to the applicant's CG billet. Personnel should obtain training at the nearest possible geographic location.

    c. Licensing and Certification Exams. Medical and Dental Officers' licensing and certification exams will not be funded as continuing education. CG-sponsored Physician Assistant (PA) programs' graduates may request funding for examination fees (primary care only), travel to the testing site nearest their current duty station, and per diem associated with obtaining initial certification from the National Commission on Certification of Physician Assistants. The CG funds this one-time exception because it sponsors the PA training program and requires certification for employment. PA's may take the recertification examination in conjunction with the annual physician assistant conference. Travel and per diem will be authorized as annual CME. The member pays recertification examination fees.

    d. Healthcare Provider Training. There are several required medical, dental, leadership, CBRNE, and Disaster training courses. These are listed at http://www.uscg.mil/hq/cg1/cg112/cg1121/medtraining.asp.

    e. Procedures. Except for Health Service Technician "C" School applicants, Health and Safety Program personnel requesting continuing education must follow these procedures:

        (1) Each person requesting training must complete Short-Term Resident Training Request, CG-5223 with proper endorsements.

        (2) Accompany each training request with course literature (e.g., a descriptive brochure) or a brief written description.

        (3) Submit Request, Authorization, Agreement and Certification of Training, SF 182 (10 parts) with proper endorsements if using a government purchase order to pay tuition or fees.

        (4) Send all completed forms to Commandant (CG-112) for processing. Send one information copy of the Short Term Training Request, CG-5223 to the

appropriate Maintenance and Logistics Command, Quality Assurance Branch.

(5) Training requests must arrive at Commandant (CG-112) 8 weeks before the anticipated training convening date. Coast Guard Training Quota Management Center (TQC), Portsmouth, VA, processes approved requests and issues orders.

7. Long-Term Training Programs.

   a. Long-Term Post-graduate Training. Long-Term Post-graduate Training for Medical Officers (Physicians, Physician Assistants, and Nurse Practitioners). This 1- to 2-year program for Medical Officers principally emphasizes primary care (family practice, general internal medicine). Consideration may be given for non-primary care specialties such as sports medicine, occupational health, public health, and preventive medicine. Training in orthopedics is a potential option for mid-level practitioners only. The Health Services Program Manager will consider non-primary care post-graduate medical training only when needed. Applicants also must have applied to their chosen training program and meet its requirements before requesting training. Applicants should have served with the CG Health Services Program for at least 2 years for each year of training received. For physician applicants, highest consideration will be given first to those who have not completed an initial medical residency. Commandant (CG-112) has more information.

   b. Comprehensive Dental Residency. This 2-year program provides Dental Officers advanced training in general dentistry, enabling them to give more effective, comprehensive dental care to CG beneficiaries. The Naval Postgraduate Dental School, National Naval Medical Center, Bethesda, MD, conducts the training, designed to qualify Dental Officers to meet the American Dental Association and the American Board of General Dentistry requirements for specialty board examination. Dental Officers chosen for this program are expected to pursue board certification. For program prerequisites and applications procedures, see the Training and Education Manual, COMDTINST M1500.1 (series).

   c. Health Services Administration. This program provides instruction in facility and personnel management, program planning, cost containment, quality assurance, third-party payment and liability, and medical-legal issues. The program provides training at the undergraduate (bachelor's degree) level for Chief Warrant Officers and senior enlisted HS personnel (Medical Administrators) and post-graduate (master's degree) level for officers in grades O-2, O-3, and O-4. See the Training and Education Manual, COMDTINST M1500.1 (series) for eligibility requirements, prerequisites, and application procedures.

   d. Physician Assistant Program. Conducted at the U.S. Inter-service Physician Assistant Program, Fort Sam Houston TX, this program trains CG personnel interested in becoming Physician Assistants. Program graduates receive a baccalaureate degree from the University of Nebraska. If they meet eligibility requirements, graduates are offered a direct commission as ensigns as described in the Personnel Manual, COMDTINST M1000.6 (series), Article 1.A.7. Each year, up to three Coast Guard students are selected for training based on Service needs. Training at other institutions is not authorized. See the Training and Education Manual, COMDTINST M1500.1 (series) for eligibility requirements, prerequisites, and application procedures.

This page intentionally left blank.

COMDTINST M6000.1E

Section M. Patient Affairs Program.

1. Patient Sensitivity 1
2. Patient Advisory Committee (PAC) 1
3. Patient Satisfaction Assessment 2
4. Patient Grievance Protocol 2
5. Congressional Inquiries 3
6. Patient Bill of Rights and Responsibilities 3

This page intentionally left blank.

COMDTINST M6000.1E

M. Patient Affairs Program.

1. Patient Sensitivity.

    a. The importance of patient sensitivity. The CG considers patient sensitivity issues of paramount importance in delivering health care. Important issues in this area include medical record confidentiality, appropriate privacy during medical examination and treatment, respect for patient concerns and cultural backgrounds, and enhancing the patient's perception of the quality of services delivered. Patients are always treated with respect, consideration and dignity.

    b. Training. All clinics shall conduct continuing patient sensitivity training.

2. Patient Advisory Committee (PAC).

    a. Purpose of the PAC. The CG's health services program provides primary health care to a wide array of beneficiaries authorized by law and regulation. Medical Treatment Facilities (MTFs) often are unaware of their population's health problems until patients voice complaints or criticisms to the command. To enable beneficiaries to express their concerns, a PAC must be available to open lines of communication between health care providers and care recipients.

    b. Each CG MTF shall establish a PAC and specify criteria for committee functions. PACs shall include one officer and one enlisted member not assigned to the clinic; an active duty representative from each CG command in the clinic's service area; an active duty representative from each of the other uniformed services using the MTF; a retired representative; and an active duty dependent representative from both officer and enlisted communities.

    c. Meeting Frequency. MTF shall conduct PAC meetings at least quarterly.

    d. The SHSO or his or her designee shall chair the meeting. Meeting minutes shall include recommended actions and an attendance list; and will be forwarded to the CO with a copy to each PAC member. Specific PAC objectives include:

        (1) Advise the SHSO on the range of services the beneficiary population requires.

        (2) Serve as a communications link between the MTF and the beneficiaries the members represent.

        (3) Serve as patient advocacy groups to assure all patients are accorded their rights as described in the Commandant's Patient Bill of Rights and Responsibilities.

        (4) Patients are provided, to the degree known, complete information concerning their diagnosis, evaluation, treatment and prognosis. When it is medically inadvisable to give such information to a patient, the information

ids provided to a person designated by the patient or to a legally authorized person.

(5) Patients are given the opportunity to participate in decisions involving their healthcare, except when such participation is contraindicated for medical reasons.

(6) Assist the SHSO in advising patients of their responsibilities as described in the Commandant's Patient Bill of Rights and Responsibilities. Patients are informed about procedures for expressing suggestions to the organization and policies regarding grievance procedures and appeals.

(7) Assist the SHSO in establishing patient education programs.

(8) Advise the SHSO on the acceptability and convenience of the services provided.

3. Patient Satisfaction Assessment.

   a. Patient satisfaction. Assessing patient satisfaction through patient satisfaction surveys has become an effective, efficient method to investigate and measure the quality of the CG health care delivery system from the patient's perspective.

   b. Satisfaction Form Availability. A patient satisfaction survey form shall be available to every patient who receives care at a CG facility. Locally prepared patient satisfaction surveys are authorized for use.

   c. Survey Frequency. Satisfaction surveys will be conducted at least annually for all patient visits during a randomly selected one-week period.

   d. Patient satisfaction survey results. Patient satisfaction survey results shall be provided to the quality improvement focus group for discussion and action and will be documented in meeting minutes. Survey results shall be reported and actions for improvement recommended to the unit CO, HSWL SC, and Commandant (CG-1122).

   e. Care received from civilian providers. Persons distant from a CG clinic can comment about care received from civilian providers by sending a mail-in HSWL SC survey form available from unit Health Services Technicians.

4. Patient Grievance Protocol.

   a. Overview. The CG expects health services personnel to maintain a professional attitude at all times. Our goal to provide the highest quality health care within allotted resources to all beneficiaries with the least personal inconvenience. Despite our best efforts, occasionally a patient will be dissatisfied with the care received.

b. Individuals with grievances. Whenever possible individuals with grievances should seek out or be referred to the clinic supervisor, health benefits advisor (HBA), or Clinic Administrator (CA) for complaint resolution before leaving the clinic. Refer written or telephone complaints to the appropriate clinic staff member. At a minimum, the complainant shall be given the name of his or her unit Patient Advisory Committee representative, and advise the complainant of the time and place of the next PAC meeting.

c. Chain of command. If the clinic supervisor, HBA, or CA cannot resolve the complaint, he or she shall refer the complainant to the senior medical or dental officer as appropriate.

d. Unresolved complaint. Refer the complainant to the CO or higher authority only if the patient believes the clinic or PAC has not resolved the complaint.

e. Review of complaint. HSWL SC shall review concerns reported on forms mailed to the HSWL SC for quality improvement purposes, action, or referral to an appropriate level for resolution and follow up.

5. Congressional Inquiries.

   a. Congressional liaison staff. Occasionally, circumstances arise in which beneficiaries exercise their right to solicit assistance from their elected Congressional Representative to resolve their complaint with the CG health care system. The CG maintains a Congressional liaison staff to direct inquiries to the appropriate Headquarters office that can best address the issue and respond satisfactorily. Normally Commandant (CG-11) replies to health care problems.

   b. Investigation. Congressional inquiries require a complete investigation of the circumstances surrounding the issues the beneficiary addresses. To this end, the command, health care facility, and individuals involved must supply supporting documentation and/or statements to assist in the investigation.

6. Patient Bill of Rights and Responsibilities.

   a. Posting the Bill of Rights. Each CG health care facility shall conspicuously display the Commandant's "Patient Bill of Rights and Responsibilities."

   b. Clinic administrator's responsibility. The "Patient Bill of Rights and Responsibilities" is periodically reviewed and updated by Commandant (CG-1122). The clinic administrator shall assure that the most recent edition of the "Patient Bill of Rights and Responsibilities" is displayed in the clinic.

This page intentionally left blank

COMDTINST M6000.1E

CHAPTER 14

MEDICAL INFORMATION SYSTEM (MIS) PROGRAM

Section A. Medical Information Systems (MIS) Plan.

1. Purpose 1
2. Background 1
3. Privacy rights 2
4. Applicability and Scope 4
5. Objectives 5
6. Definitions 5
7. Organizational Responsibilities 6

Section B. Medical Information System.

1. Background 1
2. Systems 1

Section C. Medical Readiness Reporting System (MRRS).

1. Description 1
2. Recorded tests 1
3. Questions Related to MRRS 1
4. Access Instructions 1

Section D. Medical Information Implementation Guide (MIIG).

1. Background 1
2. Responsibilities 1

COMDTINST M6000.1E

This page intentionally left blank

Chapter 14 Contents

Section A. Medical Information Systems (MIS) Plan.

1. Purpose..1
2. Background..1
3. Privacy rights 2
4. Applicability and Scope..4
5. Objectives. 5
6. Definitions...5
7. Organizational Responsibilities. 6

This page intentionally left blank.

A. <u>Medical Information Systems (MIS) Plan</u>.

1. <u>Purpose</u>. The Medical Information System (MIS) program described here follows the policy established by the Office of Health Services Commandant (CG-112), outlines systems and assigns responsibility for the administration of the MIS. The MIS is a key component for the overall management of CG clinics and sickbays. MIS is a dynamic tool, which will provide a comprehensive electronic solution for tracking operational medical readiness, health systems management, and patient access to care. The Health and Safety Directorate, HSWL SC, unit COs, and health care providers are responsible for ensuring successful implementation of the CG MIS.

2. <u>Background</u>.

    a. There is an ongoing need for Commandant, Area Commanders, and field level COs to assess medical and dental operational readiness. As one of the offshoots of this need, along with assurance of medical safety, the President and Congress have mandated the use of the Electronic Health Record (EHR) in military services. Additionally, the CG Health Services program needs to accurately capture workload, performance, and productivity through standardized methodology. Proper analysis of health care data provides the ability to realign assets where they are most needed to deliver timely, quality health care. The full implementation of the Composite Health Care System (CHCS), the military EHR, Armed Forces Health Longitudinal Technology Application (AHLTA), Medical Readiness Reporting System (MRRS), Dental Common Access System (DENCAS), and future enhancements to AHLTA will significantly enhance our ability to provide this information as needed.

    b. Federal statutes impose strict requirements for managing government information. The most pertinent Federal statutes that govern information include:

        (1) Federal Records Act (Public Law 81-754): Sets policy for and mandates establishment of agency programs for the management of Federal records.

        (2) Freedom of Information Act (Public Law 90-23): Provides policy to ensure public access to Federal government information.

        (3) Paperwork Reduction Act (Public Law 96-511): Recognizes information as a Federal resource and directs agencies to establish specific programs for management of the resource and associated elements.

        (4) Paperwork Reduction Reauthorization Act (Public Law 99-500): Defines information resources management and directs further program management requirements.

(5) A suspected or confirmed breach/compromise shall be reported in accordance with the Privacy Incident Response, Notification, and Reporting Procedures for Personally Identifiable Information (PII), COMDTINST 5260.5 (series).

(6) Privacy Act (Public Law 93-579): Provides policy and safeguards to protect privacy of individuals.

(7) Health Insurance Portability and Accountability Act (HIPAA), (Public Law 104-191): Requires health plans to assure the security and privacy of individually identifiable health information, and to use specified standards and code sets for electronic transactions involving medical information.

3. Privacy rights. CG policy concerning the privacy rights of individuals and the CG's responsibilities for compliance with operational requirements established by The Coast Guard Freedom of Information (FOIA) and Privacy Acts Manual, COMDTINST 5260.3 (series), Privacy Act and HIPAA are as follows:

   a. Privacy.

   (1) Protect, as required by the Privacy Act of 1974, as amended, and HIPAA, the privacy of individuals from unwarranted intrusion. Individuals covered by this protection are living citizens of the US and aliens lawfully admitted for permanent residence.

   (2) Collect only the personal information about an individual that is legally authorized and necessary to support CG operations. Disclose this information only as authorized by the Privacy Act and HIPAA, and described in Chapter 4 of this Manual.

   (3) Keep only personal information that is timely, accurate, complete, and relevant to the purpose for which it was collected.

   (4) Safeguard personal information to prevent unauthorized use, access, disclosure, alteration, or destruction.

   (5) Let individuals know what records the CG keeps on them and let them review or get copies of these records, subject to exemptions authorized by law.

   (6) Permit individuals to amend records about themselves contained in CG systems of records, as authorized by HIPAA, which they can prove are factually in error, not up-to-date, not complete, or not relevant.

   (7) Allow individuals to ask for an administrative review of decisions that deny them access to or the right to amend their records.

(8) Maintain only information about an individual that is relevant and necessary for CG purposes, as required to be accomplished by statute or Executive Order.

(9) Act on all requests promptly, accurately, and fairly.

b. Security.

(1) Facility Access Controls:

(a) The CG will continually access potential risks and vulnerabilities to individual protected health information in its possession, and develop, implement and maintain appropriate administrative, physical and technical security measures in accordance with HIPAA.

(b) Clearly define the security perimeter of the premises and building. Ensure that the perimeter is physically sound. Ensure all external doors are adequately secured against unauthorized access by installing locks, alarms or other access control devices.

(c) Define the instances in which visitors are allowed, including the areas they may visit and any escort requirements.

(d) Ensure all doors to interior areas requiring compartmentalization or added security are adequately protected against unauthorized access by installing locks, alarms, or other access control devices.

(2) Workstation Use and Security

(a) Comply with all applicable CG information system security policies.

(b) Log off every time prior to leaving the terminal

(c) Inspect the last logon information for consistency with actual last logon; report any discrepancies.

(d) Comply with all applicable password policies and procedures, including not storing written passwords.

(e) Close files and systems not in immediate use.

(f) Perform memory-clearing functions to comply with security policies.

(3) Workforce Security

(a) Identify the extent of authorization each class of workforce members will require when accessing electronic protected health information, considering the criticality and sensitivity of the information to be handled.

(b) Workforce member, contractors and others shall access only those areas and the applicable health information to which they are authorized.

(c) Ensure appropriate training is completed before access to MIS components is granted or reinstated.

(4) Information Systems Activity Review

(a) Assign personnel to conduct a regular review of electronic protected health information systems' activities.

(b) Reviewers should have appropriate technical skills to access and interpret audit logs correctly.

(5) Contingency Plan

(a) Identify the hardware, software, applications and information sets that receive, manipulate, store and/or transmit electronic protected health information. Define information sets for the purpose of criticality rating.

(b) Identify backup methods and materials to be used, and the frequency of performing backups

(c) Monitor storage and removal of backups and ensure all applicable access controls are enforced.

4. <u>Applicability and Scope</u>. All health care facilities (clinics, satellite clinics, and sickbays) shall comply with the MIS operating guidelines as set forth. The MIS program described here contains the essential elements required at all CG facilities with medical personnel assigned and assigns responsibilities for the program's initiatives. The SHSO shall ensure all healthcare providers and support staff; which include Medical Officers, Dental Officers, Pharmacy Officers, Clinic Administrators, HS's; HSD's and Medical and Dental contractors; shall participate. Information technology is not static in nature but rapidly changing and dynamic, and requires the diligence of all concerned to create and maintain a sound program.

5. Objectives.

   a. The Director of Health and Safety Commandant (CG-11) has established a MIS that provides necessary tools and capabilities to assist in making sound business decisions for those Commands having healthcare facilities.

   b. Identify and justify resources required to maintain a quality MIS.

   c. Establish access and connectivity for CG-wide comprehensive utilization of AHLTA, ensuring local DoD host site affiliation for electronic referrals and consultations and access to the Central Data Repository for all military health system beneficiary medical records.

   d. Establish and maintain clinic and sickbay Microcomputer Allowance Lists (MAL) that provide appropriate access to medical information systems for managing clinical and administrative operations.

   e. Establish a standardized equipment list for peripherals. (e.g. pharmacy printers, Lab barcode readers, thin terminal clients devices, etc.).

   f. Identify systems training requirements and ensure required education and training standards are established and maintained.

   g. Provide direction as new adjuncts to existing programs are developed and deployed.

   h. Participate in DoD sponsored software and product development for use in the medical arena.

6. Definitions.

   a. The short list of acronyms and definitions below is provided for clarification of Chapter 14 terms:

      (1) Intranet. A privately owned network based on the Transmission Control Protocol/Internet Protocol (TCP/IP) suite.

      (2) Internet. A voluntary interconnected global network of computers based upon the TCP/IP protocol suite, originally developed by the U.S. Department of Defense Advanced Research Projects Agency.

      (3) NIPERNET. Non-Classified Internet Protocol Routing Network. The Defense Information Systems network (DISN) Internet line for unclassified DoD and federal agency Internet traffic.

      (4) CGDN+. CG Data Network Plus. The secure CG-wide area network (WAN).

(5) <u>Firewall</u>. Security measure which blocks unwanted/unauthorized entry to computer systems from outside the internal system.

(6) <u>Host (site)</u>. Medical facility where a CHCS server platform resides.

(7) <u>TelNet</u>. Telecommunications Network. A protocol that facilitates remote logins to host site server and functions via the Internet. Restricted by CG IT authorities.

(8) <u>IP address</u>. Internet Provider address. An assignable 32 bit numeric identifier, which designates a device's location on an intranet network or on the Internet.

(9) <u>LIU</u>. Local Area Network Interface Unit. Device designed to provide external access and interface with the local area network (LAN).

7. <u>Organizational Responsibilities</u>. A detailed list of Organizational responsibilities and actions for each will be published in the Medical Information Implementation Guide (MIIG).

Section B. Medical Information System.

1. Background. 1
2. Systems. 1

This page intentionally left blank.

B. **Medical Information System.**

1. **Background.** Information technology is dynamic in nature and rapidly changing. Commandant (CG-112) is responsible for ensuring that the Health, Safety, and Work-Life Directorate's MIS continues to evolve. The MIS has evolved from manual data collection systems to automated systems such as CLAMS to the DoD's hospital-based Composite Health Care System (CHCS). The advent of TRICARE in the mid 1990's necessitated integration of the CG's health care information with that of DoD's infrastructure.

2. **Systems.** The following outlines current automated information systems, applications and program components that come under the CG MIS program.

    a. **Provider Graphic User Interface (PGUI) and AHLTA.** A graphical user interface is software that makes CHCS easier to understand and use. The PGUI currently used in the CG will transition to AHLTA as DOD resolves the connectivity, efficiency, security, and other issues.

    b. **Medical Readiness Reporting System (MRRS).** Section C of this Chapter provides further details.

    c. **Dental Common Access System (DENCAS).** The Dental Common Access System is an enterprise-wide, world class e-business system that functions seamlessly between ship and shore to provide a complete picture of Navy and CG personnel dental readiness. DENCAS also provides an accurate, real-time, comprehensive administrative reporting system.

    d. **Protected Health Information Management Tool (PHIMT).**

        (1) The Privacy Rule of the Health Information Portability and Accountability Act (HIPAA) requires a covered entity (i.e., the CG Health Care Program) to maintain a history of when and to whom disclosures of Protected Health Information (PHI) are made for purposes other than for treatment, payment and health care operations. The covered entity must be able to provide an accounting of these disclosures to an individual upon their request. Authorizations and Restrictions to disclosures from an individual to a covered entity are included in the information that is required for accounting purposes. Disclosures that are permitted but also must be must be accounted for are those made within six years of the date of request, in the following 12 categories:

            (a) As required by law, statute, regulation or court orders.

            (b) For public health reports, communicable disease control, FDA reports, and OSHA reports.

            (c) To government authorities regarding victims of abuse or domestic violence.

(d) To health oversight agencies.

(e) To judicial or administrative proceedings through an order from a court or administrative tribunal (or a subpoena if notice to the individual is provided).

(f) As required by law or court order, to identify a suspect, or to alert law enforcement of a crime.

(g) To funeral directors, coroners or medical examiners as authorized by law.

(h) To facilitate organ, eye or tissue donation.

(i) For research, as approved by a Review Board.

(j) To prevent a serious threat to health or safety.

(k) For execution of the military mission and other essential government functions.

(l) To comply with workers' compensation laws.

(2) To comply with the requirements for accounting for disclosures, the TMA has developed and provided and electronic disclosure tracking tool. The Protected Health Information Management Tool (PHIMT) stores information about disclosures, Authorizations and Restrictions that are made for a particular patient. The PHIMT also has a functionality that can provide an accounting of disclosures by individual patient, upon request.

(3) Use of the PHIMT is password protected, and several user roles are defined:

(a) A regular user can create disclosures and Authorization/Restriction requests.

(b) A user administrator can add/modify users within their Service.

(c) A Privacy/Security Officer can approve/deny disclosures, Authorizations and Restrictions, and generate the associated letters.

(4) A User Guide and an Administrator Guide for the PHIMT can be accessed through the HIPAA Learning Management Tool at www.HIPAAtraining.tricare.osd.mil using the student ID and password used for the HIPAA Privacy training module.

COMDTINST M6000.1E

Section C. Medical Readiness Reporting System (MRRS).

1. Description. 1
2. Recorded tests…………..…… 1
3. Questions related to MRRS 1
4. Access Instructions: 1

This page intentionally left blank.

C. Medical Readiness Reporting System (MRRS).

1. Description. The Medical Readiness Reporting System (MRRS) is the CG's medical readiness reporting system adopted from the Navy. It is designed for use by clinics, independent duty health services technicians and CG Personnel Command. MRRS contains the following functional elements:

   a. Immunization data.

   b. Primary Physical Exam data.

   c. Periodic Health Assessment data.

   d. Medical Readiness data.

   e. Blood type/ tests data.

   f. Visual Acuity/ insert requirements.

   g. Dental Exam and classification.

   h. Pre/Post Deployment History.

   i. Forms

   j. Health record tracking.

2. Recorded tests. MRRS is designed to track medical readiness parameters (e.g. HIV test, TST, DNA specimen submission, G6PD, sickle test, blood type, primary physical exam currency, periodic health assessment currency, and immunizations. The system is tailored to meet all Department of Defense (DoD) and CG medical readiness reporting requirements.

3. Questions related to MRRS. Questions on policy related to MRRS may be directed to COMDT (CG-1121).

4. Access Instructions. Members requiring access to MRRS need to request permissions from their local (clinic) MRRS Security Officer. Upon completion of mandatory MRRS training, members will receive access to MRRS after faxing or sending via electronic mail a completed DD-2875, System Access Request Form to the appropriate Security Officer. This form is available on the MRRS website at https://mrrs.sscno.nmci.navy.mil.

This page intentionally left blank.

Section D. Medical Information Implementation Guide (MIIG).

1. Background 1
2. Responsibilities 1

COMDTINST M6000.1E

This page intentionally left blank.

D. Medical Information Implementation Guide (MIIG).

1. Background. The MIIG is a series of guides designed to assist commands in meeting the requirements of the Health Services MIS Program requirements and to augment policy that is outlined in the Medical Manual. Serving as both policy and guidelines, the MIIG utilizes the same principal used in the QI program (as contained in chapter 13), by outlining administrative requirements and by providing direction and policy for addressing critical MIS issues. The exercises provide generic frameworks adaptable to local conditions. In some cases, clinics may be required to submit evidence of completing an exercise to the HSWL SC for data evaluation purposes.

2. Responsibilities.

   a. Commandant (CG-112). Commandant (CG-112) develops exercises as needed on critical MIS issues for inclusion in the MIIG and posts them on http://www.uscg.mil/hq/cg1/cg112/cg1123/default.asp.

   b. HSWL SC. The HSWL SC ensures guides are available to Commands for all clinic personnel to complete and also reviews clinic's use of the MIIGs as part of the Operational Health Readiness Program.

   c. Unit Clinic Administrators (CA) & System Administrators (SA). Unit CA & SA shall ensure all clinic staff promptly comply with all MIIG guides and maintain a complete, updated MIIG folder.

www.ingramcontent.com/pod-product-compliance
Lightning Source LLC
Chambersburg PA
CBHW082016300426
44117CB00015B/2256